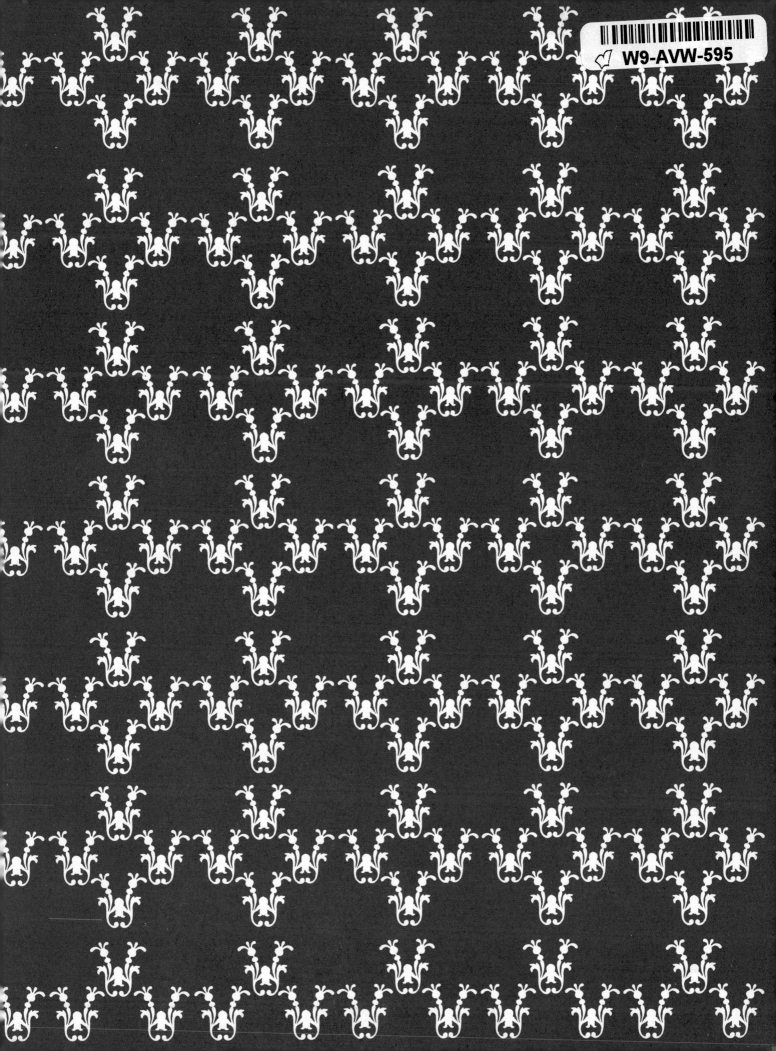

GYNECOLOGIC SURGERY AND UROLOGY

GYNECOLOGIC SURGERY
AND
UROLOGY

THOMAS L. BALL, M.D.

Associate Clinical Professor of Obstetrics and Gynecology, University of California School of Medicine at Los Angeles;
Consulting Obstetrician and Gynecologist, Queen of Angels Hospital, Los Angeles, Calif.; formerly Associate Professor
of Clinical Obstetrics and Gynecology, Cornell University Medical College,
and Associate Attending Obstetrician and Gynecologist,
The New York Hospital, New York, N. Y.

with Foreword by
R. GORDON DOUGLAS, M.D.

Professor of Obstetrics and Gynecology, Cornell University Medical College;
Obstetrician and Gynecologist-in-Chief, The New York
Hospital, New York, N. Y.

Illustrated with 198 full-page plates by
DAISY STILWELL

SECOND EDITION

THE C. V. MOSBY COMPANY · ST. LOUIS · 1963

FOREWORD TO SECOND EDITION

Gynecologic surgery, a substantial part of the total number of operations performed in any general hospital, has become increasingly complex in recent years. More extensive and radical surgery in the management of cancer of the female genitalia has established itself as a very important part of our therapeutic armamentarium in the management of cancer. A better understanding of the function of the female bladder and the process of micturition has led to increasingly complicated procedures for the management of recurrent urinary incontinence. The close relationship between the urinary and the genital systems and, to a somewhat lesser extent, the lower bowel, has made it imperative that pelvic surgeons be trained who are competent to deal with many problems encountered in the process of gynecologic surgery. This second edition of *Gynecologic Surgery and Urology* further emphasizes the concept of regional pelvic surgery that was stressed in the first edition.

All of Dr. Ball's practical experience in gynecologic and urologic surgery has been obtained at The New York Hospital-Cornell Medical Center. It is quite natural then that all the operations included in this book have been performed in this Center. All patients with carcinoma of the cervix, incontinence, urinary tract infections, and many other conditions are investigated preoperatively in our own departmental cystoscopic clinic.

An increasing number of residents trained in this discipline are doing a larger percentage of the gynecology in this country each year. The number of trained gynecologists is such at this time that smaller communities present attractive openings for these newly trained residents. This book should prove very helpful to the residents in training and to the practicing gynecologist. Unlike many other texts in this discipline, this book is not designed for the average medical student because it contains a considerable amount of technical detail that is not a part of the educational program of the medical student. However, this detailed knowledge is of great help to the practicing gynecologist.

The management of urinary incontinence and the reconstruction of the decompensated pelvic floor were emphasized in the first edition and have been enlarged upon extensively in this edition. These chapters alone will add substantially to this book's usefulness as a teaching guide in the educational program of future pelvic surgeons.

In the long history of organ transplantation, many investigators have been fascinated with the possibility of ovarian transplantation. Up to the present time, successful transplantation of any part of the genital tract has not been successful. With the rapid advances in immunology, it would seem reasonable to prognosticate that, in the not too distant future, the problem of host resistance will be solved and an era of organ replacement will be at hand. The opportunities for such transplantation are immediately apparent to any gynecologic surgeon.

When the problem of immunization is solved, the gynecologist must then be prepared to use his special skills not only to diagnose accurately the lesion or defect, but also to plan and carry out the technical procedures indicated. The technical aspects of this problem should not be too difficult for any well-trained gynecologic surgeon.

I have had Dr. Ball as a medical student, a resident, and on my attending staff since the completion of his resident educational program. He has been an able and efficient teacher during these years, and I hope that his teaching will reach a larger number of gynecologists in practice and residents undergoing their educational experience and that they may profit from his teaching, as have the residents at The New York Hospital-Cornell Medical Center.

T. Gordon Douglas

FOREWORD TO FIRST EDITION

Both the theory and the practice of gynecology have made many significant advances over the past two decades. One of the results of these developments has been the accumulation of a volume of periodical and textbook literature so vast that it is well-nigh impossible for the student of gynecology, let alone the busy practicing specialist, to become thoroughly conversant with it. Furthermore, the different schools of thought and conflicting opinions in some phases of this field may make it difficult for the gynecologic surgeon to locate information on the best modern practices.

The staff of the Department of Obstetrics and Gynecology of The New York Hospital-Cornell Medical Center has been constantly testing and evaluating both the theories and the practices of modern gynecology. Dr. Thomas Ball has been an active participant in this endeavor as teacher, investigator, and clinician since his resident training in this Department. In some respects, this book represents not only his own opinions and practices, but also the consensus of the accumulated studies and experiences of his colleagues in the Department. *Gynecologic Surgery and Urology* may be considered, then, a compendium of standard accepted procedures in the field as they have been evaluated, modified, and developed by Dr. Ball and his colleagues at this Center.

This volume is not, however, merely another textbook of pelvic surgery. Adopting, as it does, the concepts held by those who adhere to the regional surgery school of thought, it correlates and integrates all of the significant theoretical and practical information essential to the gynecologist who wishes to prepare himself to treat the varied conditions which arise in the female pelvis. Unlike the surgeon of the specialty school, who confines himself to the treatment of disorders of one organ system, or the cancer surgeon, who treats malignancies wherever they may occur in the human body, the regional surgeon deals with all contingencies in the region of his specialty—in this case, the pelvis. This book will be valuable in teaching the regional approach to gynecology and gynecologic surgery both to the resident surgeon and to the practicing specialist who wishes to keep abreast of the most acceptable modern developments in this field.

Dr. Ball has made a contribution to gynecologic knowledge, to medical education, and to the welfare of the gynecologic patient.

R. Gordon Douglas

5

PREFACE TO SECOND EDITION

Many things encouraged me to write the second edition of *Gynecologic Surgery and Urology*. First and most gratifying was the widespread use of this textbook in the teaching of resident physicians in obstetrics and gynecology. For this reason alone, an up-to-date and available edition was in order. Second, several surgical advances in gynecology over a five-year period had to be included. Third, sections of the text and illustrations that required elaboration and expansion were pointed out in numerous helpful and informative letters from many fine surgeons. And, fourth, I felt that this edition would provide a forum where some of my own ideas could be expressed concerning the aims of gynecologic surgery.

The competency and self-assurance that I have observed among the residents oriented to the regional approach to pelvic surgery has more than justified my insistence that they extend their training to include surgery of the gastrointestinal tract and lower urinary tract. Training many men and constantly urging them to expand their surgical skills rather than to compartmentalize their endeavors to the female genital system is gratifying. More so, to observe how confidently they learn to recognize and manage the many complications of the bladder and the bowel that are attendant upon gynecologic surgery. This second edition expands and amplifies the concept of the regional pelvic surgeon.

A surgical text such as this cannot illustrate and describe every known, acceptable, and proved method of performing an operation. It could not include all the variations in technique of a basic operation designed to correct the condition. Certainly this is true in the plastic operations on the pelvic floor. However, it can concisely explain and illustrate what the author considers one or more sound and logical operations for a specific disease based on the surgical anatomy of the part to be removed, the supports to be reconstructed, or, in the event of malignant disease, an adequate operation that ensures the patient the best possible chance of cure or maximum palliation. Within these limitations of space, I have attempted to present all the basic operations in gynecologic surgery and female urology by one or more techniques that have been found almost universally successful among my associates, residents in training, and myself.

Which operative techniques should be included and which should be omitted is certain to stimulate controversy among my many respected colleagues. Since we have not all been trained by the same teachers and since we have subsequently developed ideas of our own, many differences will exist. But all this is stimulating and has educational value in itself. Moreover, the residents in training always have the unique privilege of selecting the best of what they see (just as we did) and then utilizing the sum total of all the knowledge of their various teachers to develop their surgical skills and gain wisdom in the management of their patients. They, in turn, advance the specialty of gynecology as they become the practitioners and teachers for the next generation.

Should a textbook of surgery usurp just a little of the function of the medical journals in presenting some new procedures used successfully by the author? I think so. There is such a discouraging time lag from the death of an outmoded procedure and its burial by the profession that many patients do not receive the best accepted and current therapy as evaluated in the major centers of teaching and research. For example, how long is it going to take for the operation of a primary uterine suspension of the uterus to die? By contrast, in one decade after World War II, a dedicated group of gynecologists and urologists extensively studied the physiology of micturition in the female and produced an imposing amount of useful, informative medical literature on the subject that is being successfully applied by clinicians here and abroad. Many factors in the diagnosis of the defects rendering women incontinent were discovered. Several new operations were devised that substantially increased the percentage of cures among patients operated upon for urinary stress incontinence. But we must not stop with these achievements. Thus, in this second edition are included some new operations that meet all the requirements of sound surgical practice to correct the anatomic defects or pathologic physiology of the condition for which they were designed.

One is of my own device. The second is an extensive revision of a procedure used many years ago for the hypertonic, low-capacity bladder whether due to intrinsic disease, or, as is more common today, the result of surgery that failed. The third, recognizing the necessity of correcting rectal prolapse coincident with and of the same etiology as vaginal prolapse, is designed to simultaneously repair both conditions. Advances in any field of surgery to correct conditions heretofore considered hopeless create a certain share of complications. The sling and periosteal suspension operations for urinary incontinence, when they fail, create a frozen bladder syndrome in the space of Retzius. The scar tissue created requires a resection of this useless bladder wall. The technique of this operation is included in this edition. Not infrequently, a hypertonic, secondarily contracted, irritable bladder is a component in the symptom complex presented by the patient seeking aid from the gynecologist. These patients require an operation that will render the bladder less irritable by appropriate nerve resection. This operation, in selected patients, could replace the sounds, silver, and sympathy that urologists have thrust upon these unfortunate women for generations. The third operation is a composite procedure for the correction of complete decompensation of the pelvic floor involving the vagina, urethra, bladder neck, bladder, and rectum. It represents the ultimate in technical detail in the plastic surgery of the female genital tract and the understanding of the statics of the female pelvic viscera. I felt the usefulness of these new procedures warranted their being presented to surgeons for consideration now rather than await formal reports in the journals.

I trust this revision will aid in the teaching of the future specialists in obstetrics and gynecology as well as contribute to the sum total of our knowledge of gynecologic surgery and urology.

Thomas L. Ball, M.D.

PREFACE TO FIRST EDITION

The traditional subdivision of the female pelvic organs into the specialties of urology, gynecology, and proctology must be modified to conform to modern surgical concepts and progress. Surgeons who specialize in one organ system should be capable of performing operations on adjacent structures when complications arise during the primary procedure. Nevertheless, proponents of the specialty concept that limits a surgeon's endeavors by sex and organ system are still in the great majority. This is not in the best interest of the gynecologic patient. Regional pelvic surgeons should be trained in their specialty and receive additional experience in other procedures relevant to the primary surgical condition. If gynecologists will embrace the regional surgery concept, the inclusiveness of gynecologic surgery will expand to include all of the complications arising in the lower urinary and intestinal tracts rather than contract to the mere suturing of the sagging sex canal.

Many departures from the traditional chapter arrangement of textbooks of gynecologic surgery are made to emphasize the regional concept and to extend the scope of pelvic surgery. The surgical anatomy of an organ or region is described immediately before the operative technique to which it applies. A Study Plan for Review of the Surgical Anatomy of the Female Genitalia and Lower Urinary Tract and the Regional Anatomy of the Large and Small Bowel Pertinent to Gynecology is provided for those who wish to use the book to study the female pelvic anatomy. The psychosomatic aspects of gynecologic surgery are emphasized, particularly in the management of patients with pelvic cancer. Urologic and proctologic conditions encountered by the gynecologist, together with the common operations within these areas, are thoroughly covered. Chapters are introduced on experimental gynecologic cancer, hormonal control of pelvic cancer, radiation and isotope methodology, and chemotherapy of malignant disease. A section on gynecologic and obstetric emergencies contains chapters on cardiac arrest and traumatic injuries of the female genitalia. Pediatric gynecologic surgery is separately treated to emphasize the special problems of the surgery of infants and children.

Gynecologic Surgery and Urology is written to incorporate the best features of atlas-type books and encyclopedic reference works. The essential information is given in as condensed a form as possible and is neither too scant on the one hand nor buried in an endless word mass on the other. The bizarre "useful adjuncts to our armamentarium" are eliminated. Newer concepts and techniques not only accepted at The New York Hospital-Cornell Medical Center but also proved elsewhere are presented.

For their help in this task, I want to thank Professor R. Gordon Douglas, M.D., the head nurses and their associates in the operating rooms, and my friends and associates of the attending staff, as well as the fine group of residents who come to us for training.

Thomas L. Ball

CONTENTS

STUDY PLAN

for review of the surgical anatomy of the female genitalia and lower urinary tract and the regional anatomy of the large and small bowel pertinent to gynecologic surgery

Organ, region, or related anatomic structure	Principal description and plates of surgical anatomy	Supplemental description and plates of operative dissections and surgical pathology
Developmental anatomy	51-53, 613, 614	56-61, 613-616
Surgical anatomy of the common genital anomalies	51-53, 63, 64	56-61, 63-72
Vulva	298, 299, 300, 301-303	404, 405, 406, 407, 408
Perineum	298, 299, 300, 302, 303	116, 117, 119
Surgical anatomy of the sensory nerves supplying the vulva, perineum, and perianal skin	95, 96, 97	300, 301
Lymphatics and structures in radical groin dissection	404, 405, 406, 407, 408	300, 301, 410, 411-413
Vagina	312, 313	119, 310, 311
Cervix of the uterus	317-320	321, 324, 623, 624, 625, 626, 627
Internal cervical os	623, 624, 625, 626, 627	317-320
Fundus of the uterus	317-320	330-336, 340-342
Fallopian tubes	347, 348, 349-351	37, 353, 632, 635
Ovaries	347, 348, 349-351	353, 632
Anus	271-274, 278, 281	285
Rectum	271-274, 278, 281, 287, 288	292-294, 295
Bladder	180-183	188-192, 252, 255
Urethra	181, 182	112, 113, 230, 248
Pelvic arteries and veins	521, 522, 528, 529, 532-536	446-450
Sympathetic and parasympathetic nerves of the pelvis	209, 210, 211, 212-214	216-222
Muscles of the buttocks, deep branches of the hypogastric artery and veins, and the lumbosacral plexus	531, 532, 534	533-536
Pelvic ureter	539, 540	254, 255, 257, 258, 261, 262, 264, 444-454
Levator ani and pelvic floor	103, 104, 105, 106-108	300, 302, 303
Pelvic parietal and visceral connective tissue	103, 104, 105	300, 301-303
Pelvic floor aperture	103, 104, 105	300, 301-303

Numbers in boldface type indicate pages on which plates appear.

Organ, region, or related anatomic structure	Principal description and plates of surgical anatomy	Supplemental description and plates of operative dissections and surgical pathology
Pudendal hernia	105, 106-108	145, 146, 147, 148, 149-159, 160-163
Surgical anatomy of the decompensated pelvic floor	287, 288, 289	147, 148, 149-159, 160-163
Gracilis muscle	236-239	240, 241
Obturator fascia and membrane	440, 441	449, 450, 473, 483
Adjacent muscle groups of the pelvic floor	465, 466	473, 488
Vessels, nerves, and lymphatics of the pelvic floor	406, 408	414, 472, 473
Prelumbar (presacral) plexus	359-361, 362	209, 210, 217, 218
Prepubertal female genitalia	603, 604	607, 610
Abdominal wall	558-560, 561-563	567, 568
Inguinal canal	571, 572	576, 578
Femoral canal	571, 573	576, 580
Small bowel	583, 584	585
Cecum	591-593	588, 589
Appendix	591, 592	588, 589
Large bowel	591-593	595, 596
Omentum	498, 500	499
Surgical anatomy of the larynx and trachea	556	555

GYNECOLOGIC SURGERY AND UROLOGY

Section I · MINOR SURGERY AND OFFICE PROCEDURES

1 · Dilatation and Curettage, Minor Surgery, and Infertility Studies

DILATATION AND CURETTAGE
Indications

Few diagnostic procedures in medicine are as fruitful of information as dilatation and curettage performed by an astute pelvic surgeon. While the operation is usually considered a minor procedure, it should not be performed by anyone who is incapable of handling any of the complications of the operation, whether they involve pelvic organs, bowel, or lower urinary tract.

The operation is done either for diagnostic purposes or as a form of therapy for a variety of pelvic conditions. The most common indication is the presence of abnormal uterine bleeding. In the older age group it is done when there is a suspicion of a carcinoma of the endometrium. Common pathologic diagnoses that can be made by performing the procedure include submucous myomas, hyperplasia of the endometrium, uterine polyps, and a variety of congenital abnormalities of the uterus. In the study of infertility the phase of the menstrual cycle is determined and the operation is performed in the latter half of the cycle to determine the existence of ovulation. This is confirmed by finding a secretory endometrium. With few exceptions the operation should precede all gynecologic surgery, especially when the diagnosis and any complications are not clear. As a therapeutic measure, it is commonly performed in primary dysmenorrhea when the pain is in the midline and particularly when it radiates posteriorly toward the hollow of the sacrum. A slow dilatation of the cervix results in improvement for a variable length of time up to six months. Dilatation and curettage are done as a preliminary measure before performing an amputation of the cervix, a Fothergill-Hunter operation, and many other procedures upon the cervix. The cervix is dilated prior to the insertion of radium, and the extent to which the cervix is dilated is governed by the size and distribution of the radium sources that are employed. This operation is of such importance to the gynecologist that a list of surgical principles and some indications are given below even though they are repeated in many instances in the discussion of individual diseases.

Dilatation and curettage can be performed on an out-patient basis if the patients are properly screened. Patients with probable ectopic pregnancy, suspected uterine malignancy with a large soft uterus, severe uterine bleeding with secondary anemia, and similar disorders should be admitted to the hospital. Simple diagnostic curettage for menometrorrhagia, infertility, or postmenopausal bleeding can be done safely on an out-patient basis with Pentothal induction and gas-oxygen inhalation anesthesia. The patient may return home the same afternoon the surgery is performed.

However, the gynecologist should take into account the common practice in his community and certainly have every facility available for any complications before adopting this practice.

Thirty-Two Surgical Principles

1. The cervix is almost routinely biopsied prior to dilatation and curettage. In this way not only can a rare early carcinoma of the cervix be diagnosed, but also a histologic record of the cervical cellular strata of the patient can be obtained. This biopsy should be done before dilating the cervix so the appearance of suspicious areas in and about the mucocutaneous junction is not altered.

2. A blunt tenaculum of the Jacobs type is used to grasp the anterior lip of the cervix. A bullet tenaculum is more likely to result in tearing. The type of tenaculum employed will, of course, vary with the different situations and anatomic differences in the cervix.

3. In performing a dilatation and curettage after a Fothergill-Hunter operation or previous surgical amputation, multiple bullet tenaculi can be used around the scar tissue of the new external os. These divide the traction over several areas, thus avoiding tearing and possible injury to the bladder.

4. In the presence of a large cervical myoma the cervix may be completely effaced, and the operator will have to devise some means of making traction upon the myoma or adjacent structures to determine the position and course of the cervical canal.

5. Sounding of the uterus requires gentleness on the part of the operator. The sounds are molded so as to follow the probable contour of the uterine cavity determined on bimanual examination. Situations where sounding of the uterus is inadvisable will be enumerated later.

6. When the external os has been almost completely obliterated, a small malleable probe is useful in locating it.

7. Should the patient have a congenitally small external os (pinhole os), the surgeon should consider plastic enlargement of the external os rather than simple dilatation; otherwise a pinhole os may return to its original size.

8. The surgeon should be alert to the possibility of a stenosis of the cervical canal. A false canal may be created by forceful insertion of a probe or of dilators.

9. Each operator should develop some method of breaking the force of the dilating hand, such as pressing the extended small finger against the patient's buttocks. This provides a method of controlling the dilating instrument should it suddenly pass through the internal os and into the uterine cavity under considerable pressure.

10. A senile uterus is easily perforated because of its thin and atrophic walls. In sounding, dilating, and curetting such a uterus, the small depth of the uterine cavity must be appreciated.

11. A larger uterus that harbors a malignancy or a degenerated myoma is easily perforated. The depth and any distortion of the canal are gently determined before vigorously curetting or removing tissue from the cavity with an ovum forceps.

12. The usefulness of mechanical dilators of the Goodell or Wylie type has been questioned by many surgeons. These instruments exert a tremendous force and, even if used correctly (with the regulators constantly adjusted), they are capable of rupturing the cervical canal of a normal uterus. Except for unusual situations, it is better not to have these instruments on the operating table, since they may tempt the operator to perform a rapid dilatation in an operation in which a patient, slow performance is desirable.

13. In performing a dilatation of the cervix for dysmenorrhea, it is even more important that the dilatation be done gradually. It can be continued to a No. 12 Hegar dilator without tearing tissue.

14. If the dilatation proceeds with unusual difficulty, the surgeon should be aware that an artificial canal may have been created and he should stop and explore the cervix further.

15. During the course of a dilatation, and in the absence of a pregnancy or a recently pregnant uterus, the dilators may pass with unusual ease. The possibility of an incompetent cervical os may be raised by this observation. This is particularly true if the patient has given a history of repeated miscarriages or premature termination of pregnancies.

16. As with the passage of the sounds, the dilators should be passed in a direction that conforms to

any variation in flexion of the uterus from that of its normal anteflexion.

17. This operation may be performed after previous intracavitary radium. The cervix is atrophic or flush with the vaginal vault. It is important during the dilatation and sounding of such a cervical canal to recognize the proximity of the bladder and rectum due to the retraction of tissues.

18. Damage to the cervix during the course of a dilatation is suggested by brisk arterial bleeding from the os. Usually the lesion consists of a lateral laceration on one side or other of the cervix with the rupture of some small cervical branches of the uterine artery. The bleeding is usually controlled by the cervix contracting about the vessel.

19. The rupture of a larger artery or of the uterine artery itself in the course of this procedure is followed by profuse bleeding from the external os. This should be recognized and dealt with immediately by performing an anterior hysterotomy and ligating the uterine vessels by this means. If not accessible by this approach, the uterine artery should be exposed in the same manner as it is approached during the course of a vaginal hysterectomy and specifically ligated. It is folly to depend on the use of an intrauterine or intracervical pack, and, in fact, dangerous to do so. Rupture of the artery commonly results in a dissecting hematoma into the broad ligament and retroperitoneally into the flank up to the perinephric space. The insertion of a cervical pack only encourages the dispersion of the blood in this manner and masks the seriousness of the bleeding, and the patient may be found in shock as the first indication that a serious internal hemorrhage is in process. Once again, in obstetrics and gynecology, the use of a pack to control serious bleeding has dubious usefulness.

20. The perforation of the anterior wall of a retroverted uterus by the introduction of a sound or dilator in the direction usually assumed for normal anteversion should not occur. In almost every instance it represents the cardinal gynecologic sin of failing to perform an examination under anesthesia prior to any pelvic procedure. The position of the uterus and its state of retroversion and retroflexion must be accurately ascertained prior to this operation.

21. The depths of penetration of any sound or dilator should be correlated with the length of the cervix and the size of the fundus as determined on bimanual examination.

22. An unanticipated pyometra may be encountered by the gynecologist as the dilatation of the cervix or exploration of the uterus is done. The most conservative therapy includes the insertion of a small rubber tube for drainage and discontinuance of the operation at this time. Perforation of the uterus under these circumstances has serious complications.

23. During the dilatation or exploration of the uterus, an unanticipated hematometra may be recognized. The possibility of congenital anomalies or other acquired causes will have to be investigated further. The hematometra is drained, with subsequent exploration of the uterus after the retained blood has been evacuated.

24. Much of the information to be obtained in this procedure is frequently obviated by the failure of the surgeon to use a variety of ovum forceps or common duct exploration forceps to search for polyps and pedunculated submucous myomas within the cavity of the uterus.

25. The use of a forceps, however, is a double-edged sword, since the serious bowel and omental complications that result from perforation of the uterus usually result from the use of a crushing instrument and traction upon the structures.

26. If malignancy is suspected from the vaginal smear studies or from the patient's symptoms, a fractional curettage is done. This consists of curetting the cervical canal and placing the curettings in a separate fixative. Then the lower uterine segment and finally the fundus of the uterus are curetted and each of the specimens fixed and identified separately.

27. The operator should develop a systematic way of curetting the uterus even though a fractional curettage is not indicated. This can usually be divided into five stages: (1) the curetting of the anterior wall; (2) the curetting of the posterior wall; (3) the curetting of the right cornu; (4) the curetting of the fundus of the uterus; and (5) the curetting of the left cornu. In this way all areas of the uterine cavity are covered in the diagnostic procedure.

28. The operator should be on the alert for a septum in the uterus which may simulate a submucous myoma or a large pedunculated polyp. Such a septum frequently appears on a hysterogram as a persistent defect in the cavity of the uterus, regardless of the position or the degree of distention of the uterus by radiopaque substance.

29. In performing the operation on a duplex uterus with a double cervix, the dilatation of each

PLATE 1

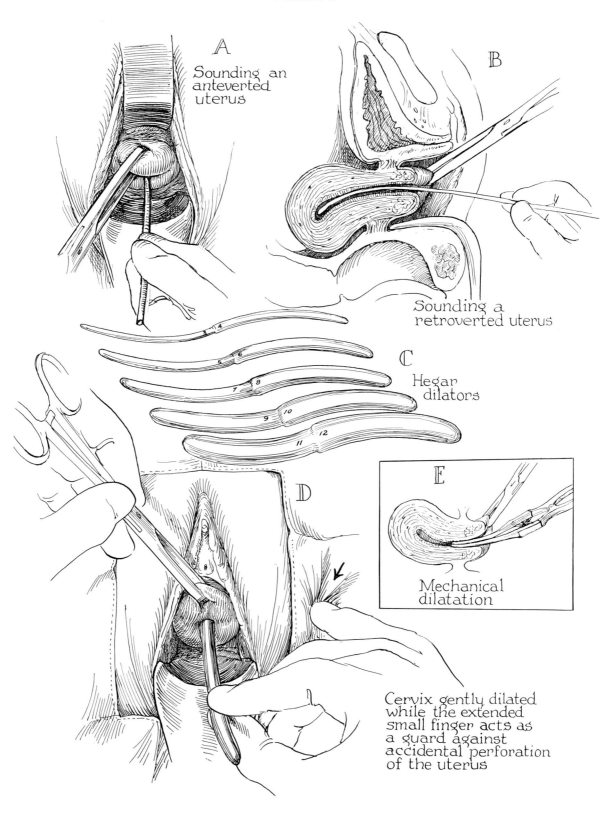

A

Sounding an
anteverted
uterus

B

Sounding a
retroverted uterus

C

Hegar
dilators

D

E

Mechanical
dilatation

Cervix gently dilated
while the extended
small finger acts as
a guard against
accidental perforation
of the uterus

PLATE 1 (Concluded)

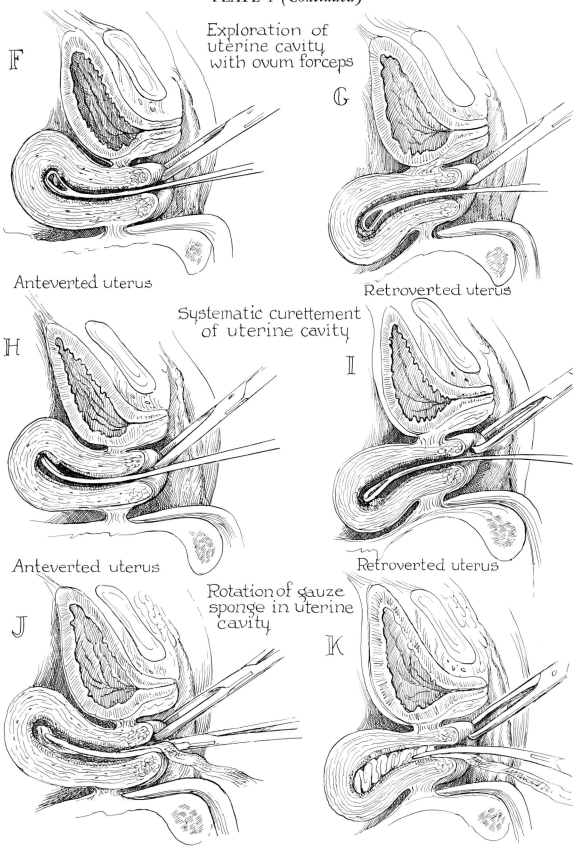

Exploration of
uterine cavity
with ovum forceps

F

G

Anteverted uterus

Retroverted uterus

Systematic curettement
of uterine cavity

H

I

Anteverted uterus

Retroverted uterus

Rotation of gauze
sponge in uterine
cavity

J

K

cervix is done with considerable gentleness. The possibility of one cervix originating from a blind horn should be kept in mind. The sounding of the uterus is done in anticipation of the possibility of such a congenital anomaly.

30. The presence of multiple submucous myomas with a large distorted cavity impresses the operator with the shortcomings of the procedure. Under such circumstances it is sometimes impossible to get a complete picture of the entire endometrial cavity since it cannot be reached either by the sound or the curette. In these patients further surgery is usually indicated, and either the uterine cavity can be explored from above or, if a hysterectomy is indicated, the specimen opened to reveal the character of those portions of the endometrial surface that have not been curetted.

31. In the event of perforation of the uterus the patient should be observed for signs of bleeding and shock, and if these appear, abdominal exploration is indicated. If there is any suspicion that the bowel has been perforated or that a pyosalpinx or other pelvic abscess has been opened into the pelvic and abdominal cavities, a laparotomy is likewise indicated.

32. All curettings should be diligently saved and sent to the laboratory. They should be separated from any biopsies taken of the cervix. In a fractional curettage the areas from which suspicious tissue is curetted are noted. The curettings are placed in as many bottles of fixative as are necessary to identify the intrauterine site of the tissue.

Steps of the Operation

1. A weighted retractor is placed in the vagina and a small Sims or Deaver retractor is placed anteriorly to expose the cervix. The cervix is grasped with a Jacobs tenaculum placed on the anterior lip. The direction of the cervical canal is determined by sounding with a blunt probe (Plate 1, A), and with the uterus in an anteverted position (determined by the examination under anesthesia) and no contraindication to sounding the interior of the uterus, the depth of the uterine cavity is determined. A note is made of any obstruction or distortion in the uterine cavity.

2. If it has been determined on bimanual examination that the uterus is retroverted, the sound is molded to conform to the presumed direction of the uterine cavity and cervical canal with the uterus in this position (Plate 1, B).

3. Plate 1, C, shows the common type of Hegar dilators, No. 3 to No. 12. This set of graduated dilators is recommended by most surgeons since

each dilator is of the same diameter throughout its entire length except for the tip. Dilators that are graduated from the tip to the shank permit the tip of the instrument to pass the internal os, while the full thickness of the dilator is still in the cervical canal. This gives the operator a false impression as to the degree he has dilated the internal os.

4. The cervix is gradually dilated and the operator proceeds to the next higher caliber after he is able to withdraw the dilator with ease. Plate 1, D, shows a technique of extending the little finger in "teacup" fashion and pressing it against the patient's thigh to break or cushion the force used by the operator in performing the dilatation and so prevent an accidental perforation of the uterus.

5. Except where the use of ordinary graduated dilators fails to effect a dilatation of the cervix, the use of mechanical dilators has been abandoned by many pelvic surgeons. The mechanical dilator (Plate 1, E) exerts its force in a lateral direction, with only a small amount of the force of the dilatation being exerted against the anterior and posterior aspects of the cervical canal. The force, then, is directed toward the margin of the large vessels supplying the internal os and cervix. Further laterally the uterine arteries may be avulsed.

6. A curved or straight ovum forceps is introduced into the uterine cavity to explore for pedunculated polyps or myomas (Plate 1, F). The use of common duct exploration forceps permits exploration through a cervix dilated to a No. 8 Hegar. This exploration is done with great gentleness, since it is a crushing instrument perforating the uterine wall that can cause serious damage to bowel or omentum if either of these structures is grasped and drawn into the uterine cavity.

7. Plate 1, G, shows the introduction of an ovum forceps into a retroverted uterus. The operator should not presume that a uterus reposed in the anesthesia room during a preoperative bimanual examination has remained in place while the patient has been moved to the operating room. The direction of the cavity is carefully ascertained before the instrument is opened and closed. The cavity of the retroverted and retroflexed uterus is systematically explored and polypoid structures within the cavity are removed.

8. The uterine cavity is systematically curetted with a sharp curette (Plate 1, H). The largest size that can be admitted through the os after the dilatation is used. The anterior wall, the posterior wall, the right fornix, the right cornu, the left

cornu, the fundus of the uterus, and then the left fornix are systematically curetted. A blunt curette will slide over most of the structures within the uterine cavity and, except as an accessory means of exploring the uterine cavity, is of little value. A serrated curette is also of dubious value and may cause some harm in that its inefficiency may be compensated for by the operator's more vigorous movements and an increase in the possibility of rupture and perforation.

9. Plate 1, *I,* shows the same procedure in a retroverted and retroflexed uterus. The operator starts with the posterior wall in the curettement of the uterine cavity.

10. Fragments of endometrium or other tissues dislodged in the course of the curettement are removed by the rotation of a hot, wet, gauze sponge within the uterine cavity (Plate 1, *J* and *K*). Experience shows that with present-day antisepsis this does not increase the risk of infection.

11. The cervix is observed for several minutes to determine whether there is any active bleeding either from the cervical canal or uterine cavity. The exocervix is observed for any active bleeding from the biopsy sites or the tenaculum.

12. If there is no active bleeding, the retractors are withdrawn and the operation is concluded. If there is some slight ooze from the cervix that does not warrant suture ligature or cauterization, a 4 by 4 leaded gauze sponge is left in the vagina until the afternoon or following morning. In place of this some operators prefer to place a packing of iodoform or plain gauze.

TECHNIQUE OF ENDOMETRIAL BIOPSY AND MINOR SURGICAL PROCEDURES ON THE CERVIX

1. Plate 2, *A,* shows the technique of endometrial biopsy for determination of the menstrual phase and histologic study of the endometrium. A serrated curette is used, and strong suction is made by means of a Luer-Lok syringe. Representative fragments from the anterior and posterior walls and from both cornua of the uterus are obtained. The precautions observed during dilatation and curettage are observed during this diagnostic procedure to prevent perforation of the uterus.

2. The method of management of a chronic cystic cervicitis is shown in Plate 2, *B* and *C*. Nabothian cysts are first punctured with a needle to remove their contents and destroy the cyst wall. The needle electrode is replaced by a ball-point and the cervix is coagulated in a linear fashion throughout its circumference. This allows small islands of epithelium to remain to cover the cervix during the healing process.

3. The method of a cautery conization of the cervix is illustrated in Plate 2, *D, E,* and *F*. A cervical malignancy is excluded by vaginal smears and multiple biopsies prior to this operation. The heating of the tissue that occurs during this method causes cellular changes in the specimen submitted for histologic examination, and therefore cautery conization is frowned upon by most pathologists as a diagnostic method. The loop electrode is introduced into the cervical canal, and with the apparatus set for a cutting current, the loop is rotated through 360 degrees. The entire mucocutaneous junction and a considerable portion of the endocervical canal are removed (Plate 2, *D* and *E*). The cutting loop is removed and a ball-point needle inserted. The current is changed to coagulation and any bleeding points not controlled by the cutting current are coagulated (Plate 2, *F*). Because of the danger of postoperative hemorrhage, this method has been largely replaced by the cold knife technique and the procedure performed in the hospital under anesthesia.

4. Several methods are used in the excision of endocervical polyps. Endocervical polyps are removed as an office procedure when the base of the polyp can be positively identified and a complete excision done. Large polyps with sessile pedicles that extend high in the canal are removed under anesthesia. The base of such polyps may contain blood vessels of considerable size. Many polyps can be grasped with an Allis forceps and, by rotating the tumor, torsion is placed on the pedicle (Plate 2, *G*) and the polyp removed with a minimum of bleeding. The polyp may be grasped with an Allis clamp and excised with knife or scissors. Plate 2, *H* and *I,* shows such an excision. The base of the polyp is fulgurated to ensure completeness of removal and prevent recurrence. Regardless of the method, the base of such a polyp is fulgurated to ensure its complete removal and to prevent bleeding (Plate 2, *I*). The surgeon may elect to remove the polyp by means of a cautery with a strong coagulation or cutting current. Coagulation of the exocervix (Plate 2, *J*) is carried out at the same time. A tonsil snare is useful in removing some polyps (Plate 2, *K*), particularly if the pedicle extends some distance in the cervical canal. The snare not only amputates the polyp, but also crushes the pedicle near its base and removes the polyp with a minimum of bleeding. The base of the pedicle is treated by further coagulation to ensure its complete removal.

25

PLATE 2

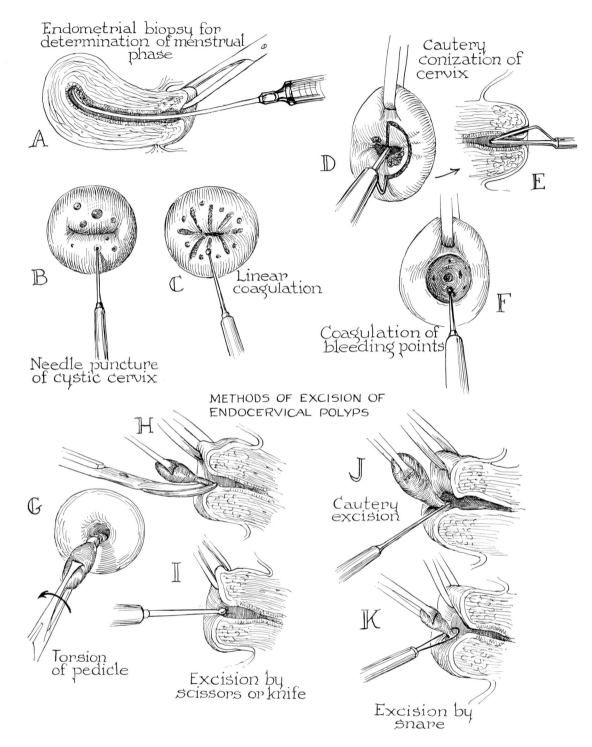

Endometrial biopsy for
determination of menstrual
phase

A

Cautery
conization of
cervix

D

E

B

Needle puncture
of cystic cervix

C

Linear
coagulation

F

Coagulation of
bleeding points

METHODS OF EXCISION OF
ENDOCERVICAL POLYPS

H

G

Torsion
of pedicle

I

Excision by
scissors or knife

J

Cautery
excision

K

Excision by
snare

ENDOMETRIAL BIOPSY
and
TECHNIQUE OF MINOR SURGICAL PROCEDURES OF THE CERVIX

PLATE 3

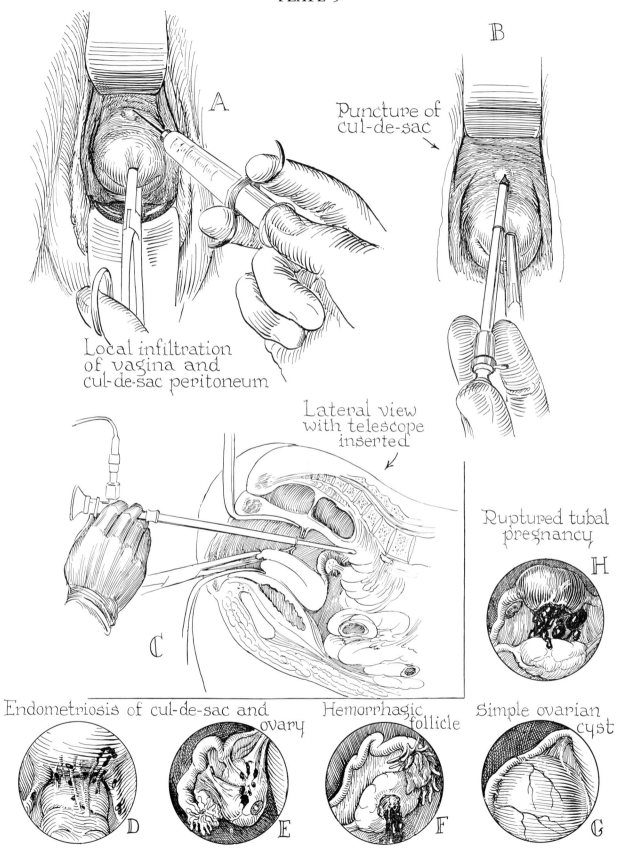

A

Local infiltration
of vagina and
cul-de-sac peritoneum

B

Puncture of
cul-de-sac

Lateral view
with telescope
inserted

C

Ruptured tubal
pregnancy

H

Endometriosis of cul-de-sac and
ovary

D

E

Hemorrhagic
follicle

F

Simple ovarian
cyst

G

Postoperative Care

Sexual relations and douching are interdicted until the cervix has healed. The use of local antibiotics after this minor surgery is of dubious value, particularly if the base of the preparation acts as a foreign body in the healing wound.

POSTERIOR COLPOTOMY AND CULDOSCOPY
Steps of the Operation

1. A posterior colpotomy is performed, for most purposes, in the lithotomy position. The operation is done in the knee-chest position as a part of a culdoscopy prior to inserting the observation telescope. With the patient awake, the most dependent portion of the cul-de-sac is infiltrated with local anesthesia (Plate 3, *A*). This extends deep enough to infiltrate the peritoneum.

2. The sheath and trocar of the culdoscope are introduced into the pelvic cavity at the site of local infiltration while strong traction is made anteriorly on the cervix by means of a Jacobs tenaculum (Plate 3, *B*).

3. The observation telescope is introduced and the posterior aspect of the cul-de-sac and uterus inspected. The tubes and ovaries are systematically observed while the uterus is manipulated by the tenaculum. As shown in Plate 3, *C,* the position of the patient is of the utmost importance. Introduction of the trocar permits air to enter the peritoneal cavity, and with the back properly arched and the abdomen above the level of the table, the small bowel and sigmoid colon will fall away from the field of observation unless they are adherent because of some disease.

4. Plate 3, *D,* shows moderately advanced endometriosis of the cul-de-sac. It is possible to visualize the characteristic nodules of endometriosis along the uterosacral ligaments and rectum. Disease of this extent may necessitate a laparotomy, so that the procedure may be terminated at this time.

5. Endometrial implants on the tube or ovary are readily identified (Plate 3, *E*) provided the disease is not extensive and the adnexa are not obscured by adherent bowel or omentum.

6. A hemorrhagic follicle (Plate 3, *F*) can be observed by this method and the cause of lower abdominal pain determined without resorting to a useless laparotomy. Operative procedures upon the adnexa for minor conditions are better per-formed through an exploratory colpotomy rather than by instruments inserted through any type of endoscope.

7. The clear wall of a simple ovarian cyst (Plate 3, *G*) is noted by this method and the need for removal determined. Frequently removal can be done through a colpotomy incision when the surgeon has been reassured by culdoscopy that the cyst is not adherent to vital structures that would make vaginal removal hazardous.

8. A tubal pregnancy, ruptured (Plate 3, *H*) or unruptured, as well as a tubal abortion with minimal bleeding, is observed by this method. Removal of an ectopic pregnancy by the vaginal route depends on the ability of the operator to obtain adequate exposure and to perform a salpingectomy with complete control of any bleeding.

Postoperative Care

The puncture site need not be sutured unless bleeding is profuse. Antibiotic therapy is administered if an inflammatory process is found or may be activated by the manipulation of the pelvic organs.

EXPLORATORY COLPOTOMY
Indications and Surgical Principles

The use of the culdoscope, vaginoscope, and peritoneoscope for endoscopic procedures requires that the operator be familiar with the appearance of structures through a lens system. Not infrequently the technical difficulties of introducing the instrument and obscuring of the field by bleeding invalidate the procedure, and the operator is left uninformed about the condition of the pelvic structures.

Recently there has been a revival of the use of an exploratory colpotomy in order to visualize the uterus, tubes, ovaries, pelvic peritoneum, rectum, and even the appendix. This is a different procedure from the colpotomy used in the treatment of pelvic abscesses. It is also a different procedure from simple aspiration of the cul-de-sac for the presence of blood in diagnosing an ectopic pregnancy. For a simple posterior colpotomy, a long scissors or knife is used to incise the posterior fornix. The opening is enlarged with a long Kelly clamp to drain the contents of the cul-de-sac, and a

PLATE 4

EXPLORATORY COLPOTOMY

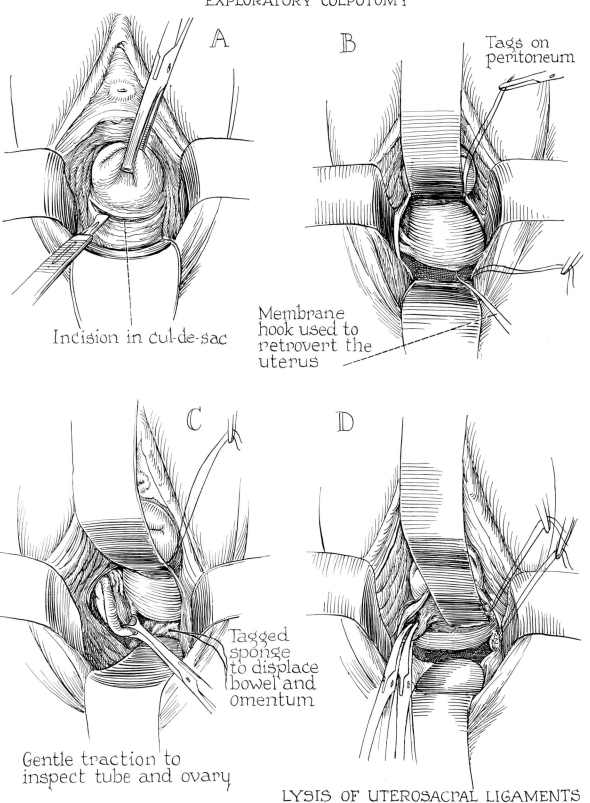

A

Incision in cul-de-sac

B

Tags on peritoneum

Membrane hook used to retrovert the uterus

C

Tagged sponge to displace bowel and omentum

Gentle traction to inspect tube and ovary

D

LYSIS OF UTEROSACRAL LIGAMENTS

finger is introduced to break up loculations. In an exploratory colpotomy, however, the cul-de-sac is opened the full distance between the uterosacral thickenings. This procedure is used to visualize directly the tubes, ovaries, and other pelvic structures and to determine the presence of endometriosis, tuberculosis, ectopic pregnancy, or simple cysts of the ovary. It permits a biopsy under direct vision. By this technique and with the proper instruments, ectopic pregnancies have been removed without resorting to laparotomy. Bleeding from a ruptured follicular cyst can be controlled by this simple expedient, and many small benign lesions of the tubes and ovaries can be corrected surgically without subjecting the patient to a major abdominal procedure. It is not used when exploration of the upper abdomen, in addition to the pelvis, is indicated.

Steps of the Operation

1. The longest instruments available to the surgeon are used in this operation. Long Deaver retractors, long straight and right-angle retractors, large Sims retractors, long Kelly clamps, right-angle clamps, long Babcock clamps, and long needle holders all facilitate the procedure.

2. A Jacobs tenaculum is placed on the posterior lip of the cervix and is drawn sharply anteriorly. An incision is made in the cul-de-sac (Plate 4, *A*) through the full thickness of the posterior vaginal wall until the peritoneum of the cul-de-sac is visualized. Bleeding vessels in the incision are ligated so as not to obscure the operative field.

3. The peritoneum is incised and the incision carried laterally until it reaches the uterosacral ligaments. This gives ample space to insert long retractors. A digital exploration is made of the pelvis, and in some instances the tubes and ovaries can be brought into the field of vision by the operator's finger. The mobility of the uterus and the presence of adhesions of the tubes and ovaries to the surrounding structures are noted. A thorough palpation of the pelvic sidewalls is carried out. If the uterus is already retroverted, it is a rather simple matter to bring the tubes and ovaries into view, provided they are not adherent to structures at a higher level. It is sometimes possible to retrovert the uterus gently by means of a membrane hook or bullet tenaculum (Plate 4, *B*) and to bring the adnexa into the field by this means.

4. A tagged sponge or baby lap pad is used to displace the bowel and omentum out of the field of operation while the retractors are moved to one side or the other to inspect the tube and ovary (Plate 4, *C*). A long Babcock clamp is used to grasp the ovarian ligament if this can be readily recognized. By gentle traction on this structure, the tube and ovary are brought into view unless they are firmly adherent to surrounding structures. If the tube must be grasped in order to inspect it thoroughly, this must be done very gently or bleeding may be induced in the mesosalpinx. A similar procedure is carried out to inspect the other tube and ovary.

5. Any diagnostic or operative procedures that seem feasible are carried out by this approach. It is frequently possible to resect an early, unruptured, ectopic pregnancy or to remove the products of a tubal abortion without resorting to laparotomy. Endometrial implants, either on the tube and ovary or on the cul-de-sac peritoneum, may be biopsied for histologic confirmation of the disease. This approach may also be used in patients who are suspected of having pelvic tuberculosis rather than simple pelvic inflammatory disease.

6. The field is inspected for hemostasis and the peritoneum closed with a running suture. If the patient has had severe, midline dysmenorrhea as part of her gynecologic complaint, the uterosacral ligaments may be lysed in the closure of the exploratory colpotomy incision. This will be described separately. After the closure of the peritoneum, the vaginal vault is closed by interrupted sutures of 00 chromic catgut, a pack is placed in the upper vagina to prevent a hematoma behind the posterior vaginal wall, and a catheter is placed in the bladder until the pack is removed the following morning.

Postoperative Care

If active inflammatory disease is discovered at the time of operation, the patient should be placed on antibiotic therapy. There are usually no postoperative complications, and the patient may be discharged on or about the third postoperative day.

LYSIS OF UTEROSACRAL LIGAMENTS
Indications and Surgical Principles

Lysis of the uterosacral ligaments is indicated in patients who have severe dysmenorrhea of a midline character and particularly pain that radiates toward the sacrum. It is a simple procedure compared with a presacral neurectomy. The latter requires a laparotomy and subsequent dissection about the great vessels with displacement of the ureters. A presacral neurectomy interrupts only the sympathetic fibers found in the presacral plexus, whereas a section of the uterosacral ligaments will interrupt a considerable number of both the sympathetic and parasympathetic fibers of the uterus.

The operation is preceded by a slow dilatation of the cervix and curettage. The dilatation itself helps to relieve this type of menstrual pain. After resection of the ligaments the peritoneum is placed between the resected ends. This, on theoretical grounds, should prevent the re-establishment of continuity in those nerves that have been resected. After the interposition of peritoneum between the ligaments, the latter can be resutured together to contribute whatever they can to the support of the uterus and to the maintenance of its normal anteversion. This, however, is based on theoretical grounds. It is quite probable that even though the ligaments are not specifically sutured together, firm union takes place during the process of healing. This serves the same purpose as suturing them together.

Steps of the Operation

1. An exploratory colpotomy is performed. The operator determines that no organic lesion that needs correction has been overlooked. In closing the peritoneum of the colpotomy wound, the angles of the peritoneum are left open, and only the central portion is closed to keep the bowel and omentum out of the field of operation. Long Kelly clamps are then placed on the uterosacral ligaments which are resected and ligated with 00 chromic catgut (Plate 4, *D*).

2. The edges of the peritoneum at each angle are then interposed between the resected ends of the uterosacral ligaments by interrupted sutures. At the operator's discretion, one or more sutures may be used to reapproximate the uterosacral ligaments with the peritoneum interposed.

3. The vaginal wall is then closed with interrupted sutures of 00 chromic catgut, a pack placed in the vagina, and a catheter left in the bladder until the following morning.

Postoperative Care

No special postoperative treatment is necessary unless some inflammatory disease was found in the pelvis, in which case antibiotic therapy is begun. The patient should be told that she may experience a feeling of pressure in the rectum for several weeks following this procedure, and mild catharsis should be advised so that a hard, dry mass is not passed at the time of defecation. The patient can usually be discharged on the third postoperative day.

INFERTILITY STUDIES
General Considerations

Infertile women may be divided into two main groups: (1) those with organic or congenital disease that precludes conception, for whom we can do little, and (2) those emotionally disturbed, sensual, aggressive, resentful, anxious, and obsessive women who crowd our sterility clinics and offices, proclaiming with a wry smile that they want to become pregnant, for whom we can do little. Here, too, as in other branches of medicine, it is seldom that a patient can be exclusively classified. Several factors contribute to the infertility of a mating, and the husband's deficiencies, organic and psychic, are equally important in any study.

The second group may be further divided into two types: (1) those who are subjected to a complete infertility study, some of whom become pregnant, and (2) those for whom nothing is done, some of whom become pregnant. Recent, well-controlled, statistical studies suggest that, without psychosomatic or psychoanalytic therapy, the patient can take her choice as to treatment. It is not difficult to single out those patients whose sensuality and aggressiveness find them lacking in motherliness and femininity despite their insistence to the contrary. If their tubes are open and their husbands have some motile sperm, there is little doubt as to the direction any therapy should take. It is probable that the psychotherapy of infertile couples will show more concrete progress in the problem as a whole than any of the other minor procedures that really have not changed much since Cary washed out the tubes with normal saline.

Routine Diagnostic Procedures

An orderly investigation of an infertile couple is done to exclude the patients for whom there is no treatment available and to minimize the time and expense for those for whom something can be done. The woman is given a test or tests for tubal patency by air insufflation or hysterosalpingography. The husband has a sperm count. After having established the fact that the wife's tubes are open and the husband has some motile sperm, it is best to stop and evaluate the woman psychologically before proceeding with the many paracentric tests which, although advocated in the study of these patients, actually have little to do with attaining a favorable outcome.

Psychiatric Evaluation of an Infertile Female—General Considerations

The simple adaptive devices that women use to handle the stresses concerned with menstruation, conception, pregnancy, and parturition provide the line of questioning and prompting which the gynecologist pursues in deciding whether he or an analyst should be treating the patient. I do not wish to infer that the many tests in the infertility ritual do not help in repressing psychogenic factors responsible for a sterile union. I do wish to place them in their proper perspective. The authority of the gynecologist, whether he understands the emotional substructure of an infertile female or not, will have some success even if his therapy consists only of explaining to the patient that her cervical mucus is hostile to the sperm, the sperm are not particularly motile or aggressive, or some such other fantasy. Strength and reassurance will be given to a woman's harassed ego by simply telling her that husbands are at fault 50 per cent of the time (plus or minus a 10 per cent standard deviation of the mean). Neither the gynecologist nor the patient need have any insight at this point. Nor is it to be inferred that the

occupational therapy provided by basal body temperatures or the spinnbarkeit of the cervical mucus does not divert the patient from her conflicts and provide much needed rest, during which she may become pregnant. The analytically oriented gynecologist soon diagnoses those patients requiring formal psychotherapy and decides whether it is within his capabilities or not. I will state now and repeat again that many symptoms serve an important purpose to many patients and they should not be removed indiscriminately or prematurely by a physician before the patient has a better solution to her conflicts. The symptoms associated with rejection of conception may be protecting her from more serious psychopathologic developments into which she would regress. The useless repetition of minor sterility examinations by the organically minded gynecologist in a patient with deeply ingrained emotional conflicts inhibiting conception is not without danger. This deception and mishandling confuses many patients and fixes their symptoms so that future psychotherapy is difficult, hazardous, or impossible. Realizing that emotional disorders tend to be phasic, with periods of intermission and relapse, the gynecologist pursues his psychosomatic evaluation of the patient with due regard to this fact and the menstrual cycle. Statistical analysis might prove the contrary, but it is impressive to note the number of women who present themselves with a chief complaint of sterility during the emotionally laden premenstrual phase of the cycle and not just after a period, when they should be suffering regret for not having conceived. Reduced to the most simple terms, the interview should answer the following basic question, and the answer should be evaluated by determining the patient's attitude toward some well-known female desires.

Can this patient depart from her daily way of life and adjust herself to the psychologic and biologic experience she must face in pregnancy, childbirth, and motherhood?

1. Has she shown interest in the care of the helpless and weak? Does she impress you as

one who is sincerely aware of this simple quality of motherliness?

2. Has she ever shown aggressiveness in the defense of other children that would suggest that she will make sacrifices for the well-being of her own child? Does this suggest that she will suffer pain and deprivation in pregnancy, delivery, and the care of her infant?

3. Discuss with the patient her mother's motherliness. What was her mother's attitude toward labor and child raising? Has her mother's influence affected the patient's femininity and desire to be a mother?

4. How strongly is, or was, she attached to her father or his memory? Did he regard her as a girl and later as a woman and potential mother? Has the Oedipus complex persisted into maturity and her marriage?

5. What birth and pregnancy theories have persisted to plague her as a mother? Were her mother's subsequent pregnancies, if any, presented to her as a child in a frightful and undesirable manner?

6. In the normal pubertal activities of baby sitting, baby care, and homemaking, has she shown active interest without maternal encouragement, with maternal encouragement, or in spite of a mother who cannot accept her own femininity?

These simple questions serve to guide the gynecologist in permitting the patient to ventilate. They obviously represent only a small part of the emotional content that may be brought to light. More important, however, is the information that will determine whether this patient wants to or is equipped to be a mother at all. Certainly it would be an empty therapeutic triumph to achieve a conception between two treatment-resistant psychoneurotics, support the woman so she does not abort, stand by both of them during parturition, and deliver one more individual almost sure to join the battalions of neurotics. Before proceeding with the various infertility tests on both husband and wife over and beyond the basic determinations of patent tubes and motile sperm, the gynecologist should now decide whether they will do more harm than good. As the patient is put through the gamut of tests and therapeutic measures, she should receive psychosomatic guidance. Subjecting her to the various manipulations and quasi-scientific procedures may have some success even if the emotional substructure is ignored or not understood by the physician. It does not, however, represent modern thinking in this field and certainly results in statistical studies with a mass of misinformation.

Miscellaneous Diagnostic Tests in the Female

The timing of ovulation may be determined by a basal body temperature record, endometrial biopsy, and vaginal smears. Observation of the cervical mucus, grossly and microscopically, shows characteristic thinning and clearing at or about the time of ovulation. Study of the pattern of crystallization of the mucus (spinnbarkeit) shows this to be related to hormonal activity. Further studies of cervical mucus arborization and its chemical structure promise to be informative and may provide a means of regulating hormonal therapy.

Intracervical and intrauterine postcoital examinations are used to study the survival of the sperm and compatibility of the cervical mucus. Urethral and cervical smears and cultures are obtained to diagnose specific and nonspecific infections that might be significant. The length of the cervix and total length of the uterus (uterine index) may be determined, the vaginal glycogen studied, and the pH of the cervical mucus and the combined secretions found in the posterior fornix ascertained. All of these are interesting. Many other endocrinologic tests are being studied that may prove useful. Patients in whom a general case history has not been obtained and who have not had a physical examination and a basal metabolism test or other tests of thyroid function by the referring physician should have these completed. The psychosomatic evaluation of the patient relative to pregnancy is the responsibility of the gynecologist who usually will care for the patient should conception, perchance, occur.

TECHNIQUE OF THE COMMON INFERTILITY TESTS
Uterotubal Insufflation (Cary-Rubin Test)

Innumerable devices and adjunct apparatuses are available for uterotubal insufflation, which requires, basically, a cannula and a well-controlled source of carbon dioxide or air. Plate 5, *A*, diagrammatically illustrates some of the surgical principles involved in the test. The cervix is grasped with a tenaculum, and the external os and canal are swabbed with alcohol. A sound is gently passed into the uterine cavity and the depth measured. A note can be made of the length of the cervical canal and the depth of the uterine cavity above the internal os (uterine index). An acorn tip or other similar cannula is introduced and held firmly in the cervical canal. Traction is made in the opposite direction with the tenaculum. The nurse can hold the instruments at this time unless the operator uses one of the many types of automatic devices available. A gradually increasing volume and pressure of carbon dioxide is introduced by a controlled device while the physician auscultates the lower abdomen, first over the one tube and then over the other. The pressure should never exceed 180 mm. Hg, and as little carbon dioxide is introduced as possible. Patency is evidenced by hearing the gas enter the peritoneal cavity and observing the fall in pressure within the closed system of the apparatus employed. Further evidence of patency of one or both tubes may be obtained by fluoroscopy or x-ray in the erect position to note subdiaphragmatic pneumoperitoneum. Shoulder pain, usually on the right side, reported by the patient is the more simple and common method of confirming the existence of air in the peritoneal cavity.

This test can be done after the administration of sedatives and antispasmodic drugs to study the effects of tubal spasm. Studies of tubal peristalsis by kymography and a variety of other common tools of the physiologist are in progress.

Hysterosalpingography

Hysterosalpingography is one of the most useful tests in the evaluation of an infertile couple. The test shows the patency of the tubes or the site of obstruction. It gives information not obtainable with the insufflation technique about each tube. Iodine in an oil base is used if tubal patency is the basic information desired. A twenty-four-hour plate can be taken with this medium. Iodine in a water-soluble base is used to demonstrate intrauterine lesions or anomalies that distort the normal contour of the cavity (Plate 5, *B*).

A hysterogram with a water-soluble medium is performed as follows. A cannula is inserted and connected to a syringe containing the radiopaque material. One milliliter of material is injected and a picture taken. Depending on the size of the uterus, pictures are taken after the injection of material in 1 or 2 ml. increments until the cavity is full and the material enters the tubes. The patient will complain of pain in the lower abdomen if much pressure is exerted. Lateral pain suggests that the fluid is entering the tubes. The uterus is best outlined under fluoroscopic control if the equipment is available. Instruments and patient are rotated to the right for a right oblique or lateral picture and then to the left for additional plates (Plate 5, *B*). The operator should make traction on the cervix to retrocess the uterus (Plate 5, *B*). This gives a full view of the cavity without areas being superimposed on each other. If the radiopaque material is suspended in oil, a twenty-four-hour plate is taken to observe dye in the peritoneal cavity and between the loops of bowel. A plate at this time is also valuable to note collections of dye in a diseased tube and some of the finer details of the cornu.

The accuracy of hysterosalpingography has been challenged by Sweeney at the New York Hospital–Cornell Medical Center. His study was based on one thousand x-rays. Five hundred seventy-eight patients had abnormalities in reading their hysterograms. Two hundred eighteen patients were admitted with 232 preoperative diagnoses. Of the total preoperative diagnoses, 55.2 per cent were not confirmed at operation, 35.6 per cent were confirmed by the operator, and 10.5 per cent were equivocal.

PLATE 5

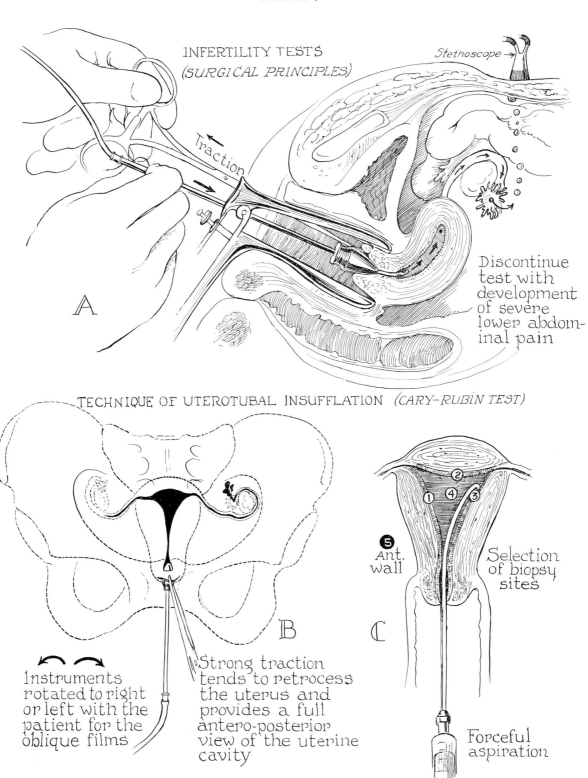

INFERTILITY TESTS
(SURGICAL PRINCIPLES)

Stethoscope →

Traction

A

Discontinue
test with
development
of severe
lower abdom-
inal pain

TECHNIQUE OF UTEROTUBAL INSUFFLATION *(CARY-RUBIN TEST)*

B

Instruments
rotated to right
or left with the
patient for the
oblique films

Strong traction
tends to retrocess
the uterus and
provides a full
antero-posterior
view of the uterine
cavity

HYSTEROSALPINGOGRAM

C

⑤
Ant.
wall

Selection
of biopsy
sites

Forceful
aspiration

ENDOMETRIAL BIOPSY

35

The conclusion is that this method is only an ancillary procedure with a limited degree of accuracy.

Endometrial Biopsy

An endometrial biopsy gives indirect evidence that ovulation has taken place. The presence of a secretory endometrium does not ensure that a normal, mature ovum capable of being fertilized was produced. Other diseases of the endometrium such as hyperplasia and a rare cancer have been diagnosed fortuitously. The test is done in the luteal phase of the cycle, preferably during the premenstrual period before the first day of menstruation. The study of the tissue is correlated with the basal temperature chart. One of the several types of endometrial curettes is introduced into the uterine cavity (Plate 5, C). Multiple fragments of tissue are obtained by forceful aspiration as the curette is moved over the endometrial surface. In the following order, samples are taken from the endometrium: right lateral wall, fundus, left lateral wall, posterior wall, and finally the anterior wall. The surgeon should be alert for any intrauterine pathology such as polyps, septa, submucous myomas, and malignant disease.

SURGICAL MANAGEMENT OF OCCLUDED FALLOPIAN TUBES
Indications and Surgical Principles

The number of term pregnancies resulting from surgery on diseased and occluded tubes would contraindicate these operations were it not that we cannot stand still in our effort to solve the problem. Perhaps, with the advent of new drugs to prevent subsequent closure and constriction, the many operations and their bizarre variations will produce a procedure that is more productive. At the present time the patient should be promised nothing should she wish to submit to a salpingostomy or implantation. Statistics that include the reimplantation of normal tubes into the uterus after a previous ligation should never be included in a report of the results of these operations. That would be comparable to including in the same quasi-scientific statistical study the results

of a nasal reconstruction after cancer or destructive radiation and a simple insertion of a piece of cartilage in the nose to make it bigger, smaller, or Grecian.

The tragic loss of children or the remarriage of a patient who has had her tubes ligated after several cesarean sections is indication for operation. I always ligate the tubes in young patients close to the uterus and bury the end in the broad ligament. Women react much better to an operation that they feel can be temporary or permanent and that permits reimplantation with a reasonable assurance of success. Operations on diseased tubes are a different matter. Two standard procedures are illustrated.

Steps of the Operation—Tubal Implantation

1. The occluded or previously ligated proximal end of the tube is resected and the remainder of the tube tested for patency by passing air through it with a syringe and adapter (Plate 6, A).

2. The cornu of the uterus is resected and the endometrial cavity entered and explored with a curette (Plate 6, B). An adequate amount of the myometrium is removed so the tube can be placed in the wall of the uterus without constriction.

3. The end of the tube is split and traction sutures are placed on the everted ends. The needle is passed into the uterine cavity and back out through the uterine wall to draw the end of the tube well within the uterus (Plate 6, C).

4. Several sutures of fine catgut are used to close the resected cornu of the uterus without constriction of the new intramural tube (Plate 6, D).

Steps of the Operation—Salpingostomy

1. The occluded end of the tube is opened with the least possible instrumentation. Traction sutures of fine 0000 catgut on atraumatic needles are used to hold the tube during the procedure (Plate 6, E).

2. The patency of the rest of the tube is determined by the insufflation of air (Plate 6, F). The air can be observed to pass through the tube into the uterine cavity.

3. The patency of the tube is assured by passing a piece of fine polyethylene tubing into the uterine cavity. The end is brought out of the abdominal incision. An alternate method is to extract it from

PLATE 6

IMPLANTATION OR REIMPLANTATION OF THE PROXIMAL SEGMENT OF THE TUBE

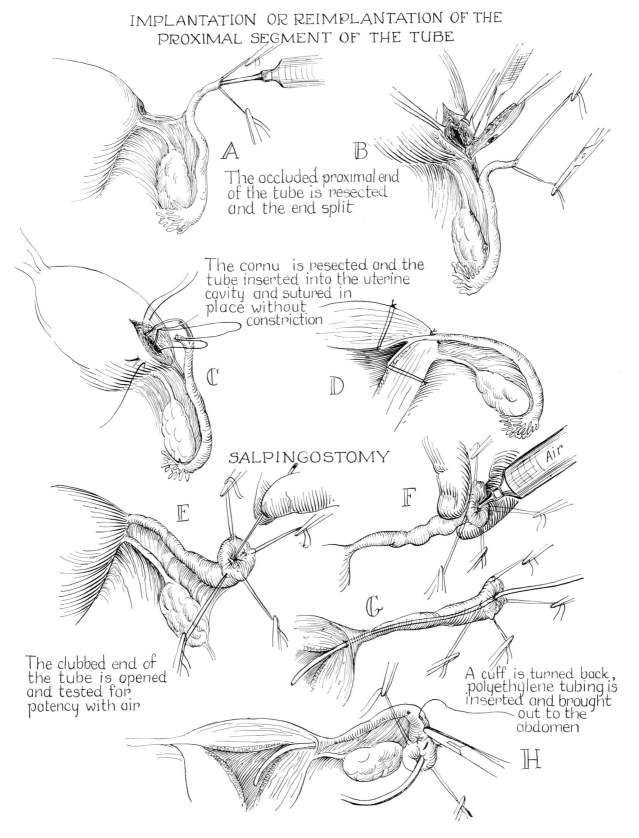

A

B

The occluded proximal end of the tube is resected and the end split

The cornu is resected and the tube inserted into the uterine cavity and sutured in place without constriction

C

D

SALPINGOSTOMY

E

F
Air

G

The clubbed end of the tube is opened and tested for patency with air

A cuff is turned back, polyethylene tubing is inserted and brought out to the abdomen

H

the uterine cavity. In Plate 6, *G,* the tube has been passed into the uterine cavity.

4. Several sutures of 0000 catgut on atraumatic needles suture the fimbriated end of the tube in a manner to evert the mucosa (Plate 6, *H*).

Postoperative Care

Patients in whom reimplantation of normal tubes is done require no special medication. A tubal insufflation on the sixth postoperative day will usually reveal that the air passes without difficulty. With the abnormal tubes the problem is different. The patients are placed on antibiotic therapy for an extended period of time, and this may involve medication for several weeks. The polyethylene tubing, whether it is doing good or damage, is extracted from the abdominal wound or through the uterus on or about the sixth day. Air or saline can be passed through the tubes at intervals after this to prove that air or saline will pass. What it has to do with the ultimate patency of the diseased tube is a matter of conjecture. What any operation to restore the patency of diseased tubes has to do with the production of term pregnancies needs a painful and creditable appraisal.

References

Abrams, B. S., and Hughes, A.: Pneumocography as an Aid in the Diagnosis of Gynecologic Disease, Am. J. Obst. & Gynec. 70: 1115, 1955.

Andrews, M. C., and Andrews, W. C.: Plastic Reconstruction of the Fallopian Tubes Using Polyethylene Catheters, Am. J. Obst. & Gynec. 70: 1232, 1955.

Asherman, J. G.: The Myth of Tubal and Endometrial Transplantation, J. Obst. & Gynaec. Brit. Emp. 67: 228, 1960.

Bailey, K. V.: Ovarian Changes Concerned With Gonadotrophic Dysfunction and Associated With Amenorrhea and Infertility; Treatment by Ovarian Wedge Resection and Eversion With Gilliam Suspension, J. Obst. & Gynaec. Brit. Emp. 65: 556, 1959.

Ball, T. L., and Javert, C. T.: Fertility and Dysgerminoma Ovarii, J. Clin. Endocrinol. 8: 694, 1948.

Barr, D. P.: Hazards of Modern Diagnosis and Therapy— the Price We Pay, J. A. M. A. 159: 1452, 1955.

Beaton, J. H., Nanzig, R. P., and Aldridge, C. W.: Transvaginal Operation in Gynecologic Problem Cases, Am. J. Obst. & Gynec. 79: 965, 1960.

Becker, S.: The Value of Hysterosalpingography in the Diagnosis and Therapy of Infertility, J. Am. M. Women's A. 12: 332, 1957.

Benson, R. C., and Miller, J. N.: Surgical Curettage; Its Value in Abnormal Uterine Bleeding, Obst. & Gynec. 8: 523, 1956.

Berezin, D., and others: Treatment of Amenorrhoea With Small Doses of Methyloestrenolone (Orgasteron), Acta obst. et gynec. scandinav. (Suppl. 1) 40: 1, 1961.

Berkow, S.: A Replacement for the Vaginal Douche, Obst. & Gynec. 15: 773, 1960.

Berman, R., and Sonnenblick, B. P.: Intravaginal Measurement of Radiation Dose Incident to X-ray Pelvimetry and Hysterosalpingography, Am. J. Obst. & Gynec. 74: 1, 1957.

Birnberg, C. H., Wexler, D., and Eisen, I.: Ethiodol in Hysterosalpingography, Obst. & Gynec. 11: 196, 1958.

Brown, A. B., and Crocker, K. M.: Culdoscopy, Am. J. Obst. & Gynec. 80: 25, 1960.

Buxton, L., and Southam, A.: A Critical Survey of Present Methods of Diagnosis and Therapy in Human Infertility, Am. J. Obst. & Gynec. 70: 741, 1955.

Buxton, C. L., and Southam, A.: Ovarian Dysfunction as an Infertility Problem, Obst. & Gynec. 8: 135, 1956.

Caldwell, J.: The Routine Colpotomy, Am. J. Obst. & Gynec. 72: 1227, 1956.

Carey, L. C., Cian, L. C., Davis, H. J., Boving, B., and Jones, H. W.: Experimental Substitution of an Isolated Segment of Ileum for the Uterine Tube, Obst. & Gynec. 11: 156, 1958.

Cary, W. H.: Note on Determination of Patency of Fallopian Tubes by the Use of Collargol and X-ray Shadow, Am. J. Obst. 69: 462, 1914.

Castallo, M. A., and Wainer, A. S.: Polyethylene Intubated Salpingoplasty; a Newer Approach to Closed Tube Sterility, Am. J. Obst. & Gynec. 66: 385, 1953.

Cauwet, R. W.: Surgical Management of the Tubal Factor in Infertility, J. A. M. A. 168: 991, 1958.

Charny, C. W.: Treatment of Male Infertility With Large Doses of Testosterone, J. A. M. A. 160: 98, 1956.

Crews, R., Holford, F., and Ferguson, J.: Culdocentesis at the Jackson Memorial Hospital—400 Cases, Am. J. Obst. & Gynec. 75: 914, 1958.

Cronquist, M., and Kullander, S.: The Effect of Enovid, a Synthetic 19-nor-Steroid (Norethynodrel) on Postmenopausal Vaginal and Uterine Mucosa, Acta obst. et gynec. scandinav. 40: 43, 1961.

Dahl, E. V., and Herrick, J. F.: A Vascular Mechanism for Maintaining Testicular Temperature by Counter-Current Exchange, Surg., Gynec. & Obst. 108: 697, 1959.

Davids, A. M.: X-ray Diagnosis of Uterine Pathology, Am. J. Obst. & Gynec. 65: 1167, 1953.

Decker, A.: Culdoscopy; A New Technic in Gynecologic and Obstetric Diagnosis, Philadelphia, 1952, W. B. Saunders Co.

Decker, A., and Decker, W. H.: Tubal Function Test, Obst. & Gynec. 4: 35, 1954.

Doyle, J. B.: Cervical Tampon and Spoon, Obst. & Gynec. 12: 433, 1958.

Doyle, J. B.: Cervical Tampon—Synchronous Test for Ovulation; Simultaneous Assay of Glucose From Cervix and Follicular Fluid From Cul-de-sac and Ovary by Culdotomy, J. A. M. A. 167: 1464, 1958.

Doyle, J. B., and Ewers, F. J.: The Fertility Testor, J. A. M. A. 170: 45, 1959.

Doyle, J. B., Ewers, F. J., and Sapit, D.: The New Fertility Testing Tape, J. A. M. A. 172: 1744, 1960.

Duboff, G. S., Behrman, S. J., and Hawver, D.: Halochromogens in Human Urine Associated With Pregnancy and Ovulation, Am. J. Obst. & Gynec. 81: 630, 1961.

Ehrmann, R. L., McKelvey, H. A., and Hertib, A. T.: Secretory Behavior of Endometrium in Tissue Culture, Obst. & Gynec. 17: 416, 1961.

Englund, S., Ingelman-Sundberg, A., and Westin, B.: Hysteroscopy in Diagnosis and Treatment of Uterine Bleeding, Gynaecologia 143: 217, 1957.

Friedman, E. A., Little, W. A., and Sachtleben, M. R.: Enzymatic Debridement of Cervical Erosions, Am. J. Obst. & Gynec. 79: 474, 1960.

Furuhjelm, M.: Transplantation of Foetal Membranes in Cases of Secondary Amenorrhea, Caused by a Non-Reacting Endometrium, Acta obst. et gynec. scandinav. 38: 453, 1959.

Furuhjelm, M.: Classification and Treatment of Oligomenorrhea and Amenorrhea, Acta obst. et gynec. scandinav. **39**: 593, 1960.

Furuhjelm, M., and others: The Quality of the Human Semen in Relation to Perinatal Mortality, Acta obst. et gynec. scandinav. **39**: 499, 1960

Garcia, C., Pincus, G., and Rock, J.: Effects of Three 19-Nor Steroids on Human Ovulation and Menstruation, Am. J. Obst. & Gynec. **75**: 82, 1958.

Geijerstam, G. A.: The Importance of Psychological Factors in Female Infertility, Acta obst. et gynec. scandinav. **38**: 457, 1959.

Hodgson, J. E.: Pregnancy Testing in Tranquilized Patients, J. A. M. A. **170**: 1890, 1959.

Horne, H. W.: Therapeutic Results in Infertility, Obst. & Gynec. **10**: 202, 1957.

Hunter, C. A., Howard, W. F., and McCormick, C. O.: Amelioration of the Hypertension of Toxemia by Postpartum Curettage, Am. J. Obst. & Gynec. **81**: 884, 1961.

Ingelman-Sundberg, A.: Testicles and Reproduction in Vitamin E–Deficient Guinea Pigs, Acta endocrinol. **17**: 165, 1954.

Jailer, J. W.: Therapy of Common Endocrine Disorders, Bull. New York Acad. Med. **34**: 650, 1958.

Javert, C.: Fertility After Cervical Dilatation, Am. J. Obst. & Gynec. **78**: 974, 1959.

Johnson, T. H.: Cyclical Changes of Electrolytes in Endometrial Tissue, Am. J. Obst. & Gynec. **75**: 240, 1958.

Jones, G., and Woodruff, J.: Effect of a Radiation Opaque, Water-Soluble Medium on the Histopathology of the Endometrium, Am. J. Obst. & Gynec. **80**: 337, 1960.

Karlson, S.: The Influence of the Seminal Fluid on the Motility of the Non-Pregnant Human Uterus, Acta obst. et gynec. scandinav. **38**: 503, 1959.

Kay, F. M.: Spontaneous Uterine Rupture Through Perforation Scar of Previous Curettement, Obst. & Gynec. **6**: 228, 1955.

Keettel, W. C., and others: Report of Pregnancies in Infertile Couples, J. A. M. A. **160**: 102, 1956.

Kistner, R. W.: Observations on the Use of a Nonsteroidal Estrogen Antagonist; I. Cystic Disease of the Breast, Am. J. Obst. & Gynec. **81**: 233, 1961.

Kobak, A. J., and Sadove, M. S.: Combined Paracervical and Pudendal Nerve Blocks—a Simple Form of Transvaginal Regional Anesthesia, Am. J. Obst. & Gynec. **81**: 72, 1961.

Kovar, W., Giblin, H., and Roddy, J.: Vaginal Tampons and Their Relationship to the Cervix Uteri as Determined by Roentgenography, Obst. & Gynec. **13**: 269, 1959.

Kucharczuk, J. B., and Greene, J. W.: Preliminary Report on the Use of Ileum as Oviduct in the Dog, Am. J. Obst. & Gynec. **72**: 528, 1956.

Kupperman, H. S., and others: Induction of Ovulation in the Human: Therapeutic and Diagnostic Importance, Am. J. Obst. & Gynec. **75**: 301, 1958.

Kurland, I. I., and Loughran, C. H.: Corticosteroids in the Treatment of Nonpatent Fallopian Tubes, Am. J. Obst. & Gynec. **81**: 243, 1961.

Lang, W. R.: Benign Cervical Erosion in Nonpregnant Women of Childbearing Age; a Colposcopic Study, Am. J. Obst. & Gynec. **74**: 993, 1957.

Lang, W. R., Rakoff, A. E., and Tartarian, G.: Cytologic and Histologic Correlation of Colposcopic Findings, Surg., Gynec. & Obst. **108**: 717, 1957.

Lindahl, P. E., and others: The Sperm Anti-agglutinic Factor in Women, J. Obst. & Gynaec. Brit. Emp. **63**: 363, 1956.

Luraschi, C.: Miscroscopical Examination of the Capillaries by Reflected Light During the Menstrual Cycle and the Puerperium (Microscopia capillare a luce riflessa in rapporto al cicle mestruale e allo stato puerperale), An. ostet. y ginec. **78**: 441, 1957.

MacLeod, J.: The Present Status of Human Male Infertility, Am. J. Obst. & Gynec. **69**: 1256, 1955.

Mastroianni, L.: Causes and Treatment of Infertility, Connecticut M. I. **21**: 332, 1957.

Müller, H. J.: Damage to Posterity Caused by Irradiation of the Gonads, Am. J. Obst. & Gynec. **67**: 467, 1954.

Norment, W. B.: The Hysteroscope, Am. J. Obst. & Gynec. **71**: 426, 1956.

Olson, A. W., and Nichols, E. E.: Colposcopic Examination in a Combined Approach for Early Diagnosis and Prevention of Carcinoma of the Cervix, Obst. & Gynec. **15**: 372, 1960.

Parks, R. D., Scheerer, P. P., and Greene, R. R.: The Endometria of Normal Postmenopausal Women, Surg., Gynec. & Obst. **106**: 413, 1958.

Peel, J. H.: The Role of Major Surgery in Infertility, Am. J. Obst. & Gynec. **71**: 706, 1956.

Perloff, W. H., and Channick, B. J.: Effect of Prednisone on Abnormal Menstrual Function, Am. J. Obst. & Gynec. **77**: 138, 1959.

Pfaltz, H., and Severinghaus, E. L.: Effects of Vitamin Deficiencies on Fertility, Course of Pregnancy, and Embryonic Development in Rats, Am. J. Obst. & Gynec. **72**: 265, 1956.

Pratt, J. H., Banner, E. A., and Huang, M.: Reconstructive Operations for Obstruction of the Fallopian Tubes, Am. J. Obst. & Gynec. **71**: 1097, 1956.

Riva, H. L., Hatch, R. P., and Breen, J. L.: Culdoscopy, Obst. & Gynec. **12**: 610, 1958.

Rubin, I. C.: Röntgendiagnostik der Uterustumoren mit Hilfe von intrauterinen Collargolinjektionen, Zentralbl. Gynäk. **38**: 658, 1914.

Sandberg, F., and others: In Vitro Studies of the Motility of the Human Uterus, J. Obst. & Gynaec. Brit. Emp. **64**: 334, 1957.

Sandberg, F., and others: In Vitro Studies of the Motility of the Human Fallopian Tube; Part 1. The Effects of Acetylcholine, Adrenaline, Noradrenaline, and Oxytocin on the Spontaneous Motility, Acta obst. et gynec. scandinav. **39**: 506, 1960.

Salzer, R. B.: Colposcopy—an Aid in the Detection of Early Cancer and Precancerous Conditions of the Cervix, Obst. & Gynec. **13**: 451, 1959.

Schwartz, M., and Soule, S.: Estradiol 17-Beta-Cyclopentyl-propionate, a Long-acting Estrogen, Am. J. Obst. & Gynec. **70**: 44, 1955.

Seiger, H. W.: New Inflatable Uterotubal Cannula for Gas Insufflation or Liquid Injection, Obst. & Gynec. **17**: 364, 1961.

Shettles, L. B.: Cervical Factors in Reproduction, Obst. & Gynec. **14**: 635, 1959.

Siegler, A. M.: The Cervical Glucose as an Indicator of Ovulation, Am. J. Obst. & Gynec. **79**: 1169, 1960.

Smith, J., and Morris, J.: Posterior Colpotomy: An Avenue for Definitive Pelvic Operations, Am. J. Obst. & Gynec. **79**: 52, 1960.

Smith, O., Smith, G., and Gavian, N.: Urinary Estrogens in Women, Am. J. Obst. & Gynec. **78**: 1028, 1959.

Solomon, C., Panagotopoulos, P., and Oppenheim, A.: The Use of Urinary Sediment as an Aid in Endocrinological Disorders in the Female, Am. J. Obst. & Gynec. **76**: 56, 1958.

Southam, A. L.: Clinical Application of Enovid and Other Progestational Agents in Control of Dysfunctional Uterine Bleeding and Correction of Amenorrhea, Proc. Symposium on Enovid, Searle Research Laboratories, 1958.

Stavorski, J., and Hartman, C. G.: Uterotubal Insufflation; a Study to Determine the Origin of Fluctuations in Pressure, Obst. & Gynec. **11**: 622, 1958.

Stein, I. F., and Leventhal, M. L.: Amenorrhea Associated With Bilateral Polycystic Ovaries, Am. J. Obst. & Gynec. **29**: 181, 1935.

Steinberg, W.: Hysterosalpingography With Ethiodol, Am. J. Obst. & Gynec. **75**: 144, 1958.

Sundelin, G.: Intrasellar Tumour Treated With Surgery and X-ray Followed by Complete Restoration of Gonadotrophic Function, Acta obst. et gynec. scandinav. **38**: 699, 1959.

Sweeney, W. J.: Hysterosalpingography: I. Accuracy of Preoperative Hysterosalpingograms, Obst. & Gynec. **11**: 640, 1958.

Sweeney, W. J.: Hysterosalpingography: II. Postoperative Hysterograms, Obst. & Gynec. **12**: 83, 1958.

Sweeney, W. J.: Hysterosalpingography With a New Water

Soluble Medium, Diatrizoate Iodipamide Methylglucamine, Obst. & Gynec. 14: 677, 1959.

Taylor, E. S., and McCallin, P. F.: A Correlation of the Cytology of the Urinary Sediment With Endometrial Histology, Am. J. Obst. & Gynec. 63: 1009, 1952.

Taylor, E. S., and others: Urinary Estriol Determinations in Normal Pregnancy, Am. J. Obst. & Gynec. 81: 625, 1961.

Taymor, M. L., and others: Menorrhagia due to Chronic Iron Deficiency, Obst. & Gynec. 16: 571, 1960.

Tyler, E. T., and Singher, H. O.: Male Infertility—Status of Treatment, Prevention and Current Research, J. A. M. A. 160: 91, 1956.

Vermeeren, J., Chamberlain, R. R., and Te Linde, R. W.: 10,000 Minor Gynecologic Operations on an Outpatient Basis, Obst. & Gynec. 9: 139, 1957.

Wade, R., and Jones, H.: Inhibition of Human Endometrial Adenosine Triphosphatase by Progesterone, Obst. & Gynec. 3: 608, 1954.

Werner, P., and Sederl, J.: Abdominal Operations by the Vaginal Route, London, 1958, Pitman Medical Publishing Co.

Wolfe, L. A.: Colpomicroscopy: Its Value in the Microscopic Examination of the Uterine Cervical Epithelium in Vivo, Am. J. Obst. & Gynec. 76: 1163, 1958.

Woltz, J. H., and others: Complications of Hysterosalpingography, Am. J. Obst. & Gynec. 76: 736, 1958.

Word, B., Gravlee, R. C., and Wideman, G. L.: The Fallacy of Simple Uterine Curettage, Obst. & Gynec. 12: 642, 1958.

Zondek, B., and Rozin, S.: Cervical Mucus Arborization, Obst. & Gynec. 3: 463, 1954.

2 · Gynecology and the Sprained or Decompensated Back

BACKACHE

Backache is an almost universal complaint in the practice of gynecology. The ability of most women to associate their wombs with any pain from the costal margin to the coccyx is a projection the most erudite Freudian might study for a lifetime. To explain the symptoms of a sprained or decompensated back by the presence of a retroverted uterus was fashionable (but dishonest) several decades ago. Today it would represent the worst medical chicanery. It might be reasonable to believe that a chronically infected cervix could contribute to some pelvic discomfort and, combined with an orthopedic cause for backache, result in the patient's symptom complex. It might also be reasonable to believe that a herniation of the pelvic floor (prolapse) and a backache of mechanical origin may combine to form the sum total of the patient's pelvic complaints. However, when the symptom of backache is honestly appraised, it is almost always found to rest on an orthopedic basis. That, seemingly, should end this chapter were it not that some element of comprehensive care should exist in all specialities.

One qualification for certification of a gynecologist should be a basic knowledge of psychosomatic techniques and psychopathology. He should recognize abnormal dynamisms and not associate the uterus with every female complaint. With this release of some puzzling and disturbing things in the psychosexual sphere, most of us will be capable of an exacting diag-

nosis. After we have desensitized the sagging multipara to her husband's criticism, she can then be taught how to adjust to her life situation without using her backache as a subterfuge.

Organic causes, the result of parturition and strictly gynecologic disease, contribute to abnormal body mechanics and to nerve and joint injuries. We are responsible for the recognition of these lesions and should consult the orthopedist in their management. This chapter is written for our orthopedic friends—that they may enjoy a well-earned rest from women with a simple backache complicated by some pelvic disease and turn their talents to more stirring problems.

Normal Body Mechanics

Body mechanics was defined by the Subcommittee on Body Mechanics of the 1931 White House Conference on Child Welfare as "the mechanical correlation of the various systems of the body with reference to the skeletal, muscular, and visceral systems and their neurological association." What constitutes normal body mechanics of all types of habitus has not been completely determined. The standards will also vary with age and occupation, so that the effect of an individual's body mechanics on the function of the various organ systems must be interpreted with these and many other factors in mind. It represents a step in the right direction for the gynecologist to think in terms of the entire body and skeleton, for the pelvic floor—his special region of endeavor—receives the brunt of many derangements of the body mechanics.

The Subcommittee on Body Mechanics listed some requirements for good posture and appearance of the head, thorax, abdomen, and extremities.

1. The head is drawn somewhat back so that a line let fall from the tip of the chin passes through the sternal notch and perpendicular to the ground. This starts to line up the head so that it is balanced above the shoulders, hips, and ankles.

2. The costal angle of the thorax is made wide by drawing in the abdomen and makes the sternum the farthest forward part of the body.

3. The lower abdomen is held in and flat.

4. The lower extremities are so aligned with the trunk and head that the lower ends of the femurs and the upper ends of the tibias oppose each other in such a manner as to support the body weight with a minimum amount of muscular exertion or tonus. The maintenance of the weight-bearing lines of the lower extremities that will best protect the joint mechanism of the feet requires a little effort at pronation as the supinator muscles of the lower legs and feet are slightly stronger than the opposing pronator group of muscles.

The Subcommittee was primarily interested in children and not parous women, so these ideals must be projected into an older generation who may have been subjected to a distortion of the pelvic floor and abdominal musculature by multiple pregnancies. These criteria are not without practical application to the adult parous female if the observer will allow for the inevitable consequences of age and pregnancy.

Abnormal Body Mechanics

No clear line of demarcation exists between a normal and abnormal patient in the study of body mechanics. An abnormal posture may be the result of organic disease rather than the latter being caused by faulty body mechanics. An obviously obese patient (short and stocky with bulging jowls and a massive, sagging, and hanging panniculus) requires little study to determine the existence of abnormal body mechanics. Certain simple observations in the normal and underweight group will shed light on their back pain and the part faulty body mechanics may play in the syndrome. The pathomechanics of posture is an exceedingly complex orthopedic problem, but certain simple observations by the gynecologist are of practical application in the management of simple backache aggravated by gynecologic disease.

Steindler states that:

"The characteristic difference between normal and abnormal posture lies in the fact that in the former compensation takes place in the spine itself and not in the hip or knee joint, so that the relations of the line of gravity to the spine or the points of intersection remain the same; whereas in the abnormal posture the deflection of the line of gravity persists and results in abnormal relations to sacro-iliac, hip, and knee joints, balance being ultimately recovered by the position of the feet. In geometrical terms, normal posture means compensation of the spinal deflections within the spine itself. Malposture means that a deflection of the spinal column in relation to the line of gravity is compensated by the body as a whole by abnormal positions of the pelvis, hips, and knees."*

With this simple rule to follow, it is seen that in pregnancy or paralysis of the back extensors the line of gravity is posterior to the sacroiliac joint. The patient compensates by increasing the lumbar curve and in turn tries to balance this by increasing the dorsal curve (kyphosis). This accounts for some of the back trouble in pregnancy. Other patients with the same backward displacement may compensate by hyperextending the hips, decreasing the pelvic inclination, and causing the abdomen to protrude. By estimating where the center of gravity passes in relation to the sacroiliac and hip joints, Steindler distinguishes four types of posture.

In the first type the weight-bearing line falls between the hip joint and the sacroiliac articulation. There is more or less normal inclina-

---

*From Steindler, A.: Mechanics of Normal and Pathological Locomotion in Man, Springfield, Ill., 1935, Charles C Thomas, Publisher.

tion of the pelvis and a straight or round back with a good lumbar curve. This is a securely balanced frame and is to be considered normal and physiologic. In a second type the weight line is moved forward in relation to the spine owing to a flexion deformity or flexion contracture of the hip joint. Compensation for this is accomplished by bending the knees, which carries the supporting surfaces far enough backward to receive the line of gravity. The third type is very frequent. It is seen with the common postural anomaly associated with weakness and lack of tone of the abdominal muscles. Here the center of gravity moves backward, which causes hyperextension of the hip joint and a throwing backward of the entire trunk to compensate. In the fourth type, osteoarthritis of the spine or senile kyphosis causes forward flexion of the trunk and a moving forward of the center of gravity. Compensation takes place here by a compensatory flexion of the hip and flexion of the knee joint.

An understanding of several fundamentals in the statics of the abdominal viscera and pelvic articulations during pregnancy will clarify the diagnosis of many back problems in women. All three articulations (lumbosacral, sacroiliac, and the symphyseal) undergo relaxation during pregnancy. It is most marked in the symphysis and less in the other joints. The degree of relaxation is more frequent and more marked in the multipara than in the primipara. In addition, the multipara has lost some tone in her abdominal muscles and carries slightly larger babies. The sacroiliac pain in pregnancy suggests the same etiology as the night backache, where relaxation develops with a deep sleep in the recumbent position or where the articulation is relaxed during operation and deep anesthesia.

The mechanics of sprain in the pelvic articulations involve three common motions. Forces acting in the anteroposterior plane most frequently derange the lumbosacral articulation. Lateral strains pass through the lumbosacral joint to involve the sacroiliac joints secondarily. Rotatory movements are the most important, for, if the force is not spent in motion, it ultimately is transmitted to the sacroiliac joint, although not strictly confined to one joint.

A systematic outline for the study of backache by the gynecologist is presented in Chart I. It will guide him in deciding the necessity for orthopedic consultation and x-ray studies of the lumbosacral spine and pelvis.

Pouching of the lower abdomen (visceroptosis) reflects the position of the abdominal viscera (enteroptosis) in a patient with poor posture, poor muscular development, and poor muscular tone. A longitudinal section of the abdomen in a patient with good body mechanics reveals the abdominal viscera to occupy a space resembling an inverted pear, the bulk of the contents being in the upper abdomen. With poor posture, development, and tone, the opposite obtains and the large and small bowel are crowded into the lower abdomen and pelvis, with the thick end of the pear toward the extremities. Between the diaphragm and the levator ani are enclosed the abdominal and pelvic contents, all of which have insufficient ligamentary supports to keep them in position were not other factors operating that are much more important. The suction of the diaphragm, the tone and development of the abdominal musculature, the statics of the female pelvic floor, and the statics of the lumbosacral spine all contribute to the shape of the abdominal cavity which, in turn, reflects the patient's body mechanics (Chart I).

The lumbar curve is a readily observed landmark that provides much information about the support of the abdominal and pelvic viscera (Chart I). A deep curve can be recognized by palpating the fourth and fifth lumbar vertebrae through the abdomen as well as by measuring the depth of the curve in relation to the rest of the back. In good body mechanics the anterior surfaces of the fourth and fifth lumbar vertebrae are nearer the abdominal wall than the back. This causes a shelf on which the viscera, as well as the kidneys and their fatty envelope, even though they are retroperitoneal, may partially impinge. The lumbar curve also indicates whether there is a favorable pelvic tilt with rotation of the sacrum

CHART I

EVALUATION OF LOW BACK PAIN BY THE GYNECOLOGIST

1. Gynecologic history
   A. Relationship of back pain to menstruation

   _____

   B. Relationship of onset of back pain to childbirth

   _____

   C. Onset subsequent to surgery in the lithotomy position

   _____

   D. Associated lower abdominal and bladder symptoms

   _____

   E. Psychosomatic considerations

   _____

2. Orthopedic history

   _____

3. History of back injury

   _____

4. Gynecologic examination

   _____

5. Palpation of nerves and ligaments on rectovaginal examination
   A. Sacrotuberous and sacrosciatic ligaments

   _____

   B. Lumbosacral plexus

   _____

   C. Pelvic sidewalls and obturator fossae

   _____

   D. Coccyx

   _____

6. Examination of posture and body mechanics
   A. Posture type (thin, intermediate, stocky, remarks)

   _____

Thin type   Intermediate type   Stocky type

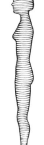 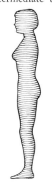 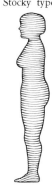

CHART I (Concluded)

EVALUATION OF LOW BACK PAIN BY THE GYNECOLOGIST

B. Weight _____ (actual) _____ (accepted normal)

_____

C. Muscular tone (good, fair, poor, remarks)

_____

D. Muscular development (good, fair, poor, remarks)

_____

E. Enteroptosis (none, slight, marked, remarks)

_____

7. Examination of the back
   A. Lumbar curve and pelvic tilt (normal, moderate, marked, remarks)

   _____

Good curve   Bad curve

65°   LESS THAN 65%

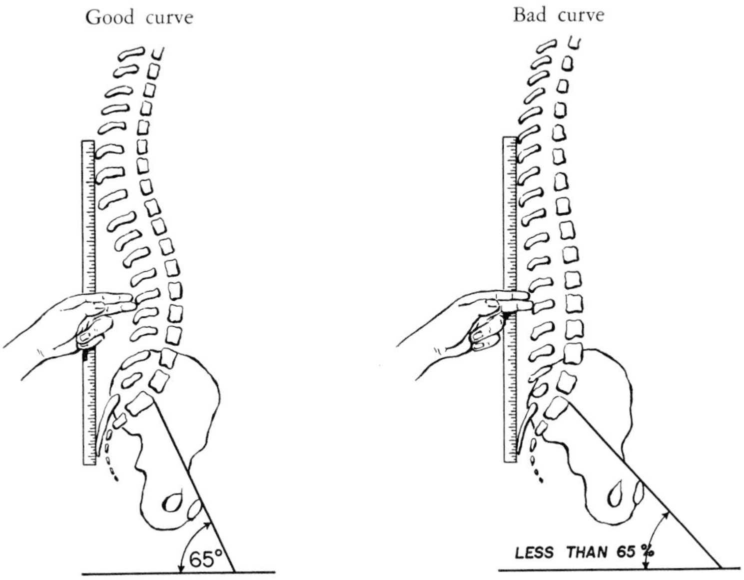

B. Generalized spasm and rigidity (none, moderate, marked, remarks)

_____

C. Degree of pain (minimal, moderate, marked, remarks)

_____

D. Location of trigger areas

_____

8. Plan of treatment
   A. Necessity for orthopedic consultation

   _____

   B. Correction of aggravating gynecologic conditions

   _____

   C. Medical management and exercises

   _____

downward and backward. The angle the true conjugate forms with the horizontal is increased and the pelvic floor receives the stress of the abdominal contents less directly than when the pelvic inlet is more horizontal.

The pelvic congestion syndrome is probably aggravated, if not caused, by faulty body mechanics and the erect posture. The pelvic organs are drained by a group of venous plexuses named from the organ of origin, but all of them anastomose freely with each other. These veins have thin walls and no valves. In the multipara, large varicosities of the pelvic veins are common, especially in the broad ligament, the infundibulopelvic pedicle, and about the rectum and cul-de-sac. It is quite understandable that these engorged vessels, aggravated by the additional pressure created by poor posture and muscular tone, can give rise to a "bearing-down" or "dragging-down" sensation in the lower abdomen and back.

The urologic origins of backache are more diverse than the gynecologic when the nerve pathways above the pelvic brim and extending to the kidneys are added to the picture. Stimuli of sympathetic visceral terminals along the course of the renal pelvis and ureter are transmitted to the cord and, by some unknown mechanism, incite adjacent sensory cells to react and transmit the feeling of pain to somatic segments. The renal parenchyma is insensitive, but the renal capsule, renal pelvis, and ureter are exquisitely sensitive to distention and refer pain to many areas. The tenth, eleventh, and twelfth dorsal and the first lumbar segments of the cord supply sympathetic and sensory fibers to the kidneys, while the renal capsule and perirenal tissues possess sensory endings of cerebrospinal origin. The pelvis and ureter receive sympathetic fibers from the plexuses along their course and from fibers accompanying their blood supply. The bladder receives sympathetic and parasympathetic fibers from the hypogastric plexuses. It is thus evident that any surface pain below the diaphragm may be of renal origin, and this must be considered in the diagnosis of any backache. So diffuse is the nerve supply of the renal tract that any attempt to pinpoint a urologic diagnosis by the characteristics of the pain is often inaccurate. Much has been written regarding the pain of a ptosed kidney and its relation to faulty body mechanics. While a movable kidney is probably blamed too frequently for backaches, there is the occasional patient with an abnormally mobile kidney, proved by pyelography, who gets relief by change in position or correction of poor posture.

Trigger Areas

A trigger area is a localized spot of deep tenderness with a lowered deep pain threshold. When the portion of a muscle containing the trigger area is rolled under the fingers, a localized twitch may be observed. This may be followed by fasciculation that persists for several seconds and by referred pain to some remote area. The four characteristics of a trigger area—lower deep pain threshold, hyperalgesia, fasciculation, and capacity to set off referred pain (Chart II)— must be appreciated by the examiner in determining the cause of a backache.

Etiology of Back Pain by Systems

The etiology of low back pain and sciatic pain may be divided into the orthopedic causes and the pelvic causes that contribute to the patient's general pelvic discomfort but are not directly responsible for backache. The orthopedic causes are as follows:

A. Strains and sprains
  1. Lumbosacral joint
  2. Sacroiliac synchondrosis
B. Arthritis
  1. Rheumatoid arthritis
  2. Hypertrophic arthritis
C. Trauma
  1. Ruptured intervertebral disks
  2. Fractures
  3. Malunited fractures
D. Congenital anomalies
  1. Spondylolisthesis
  2. Sacralization of the transverse processes
  3. Spina bifida
  4. Supernumerary vertebrae
E. Neoplasms
  1. Primary bone tumors, benign or malignant
  2. Metastatic bone tumors
  3. Spinal cord tumors

CHART II

CHARACTERISTICS OF A TRIGGER AREA

1. A localized spot of deep tenderness with a lowered deep pain threshold
2. A localized twitch which is usually observed as the muscle is rolled under the fingers
3. Fasciculation which may be set off and persist for several seconds
4. Referred pain which can usually be induced by pressure or needle contact

Localization of Involved (Trigger) Areas

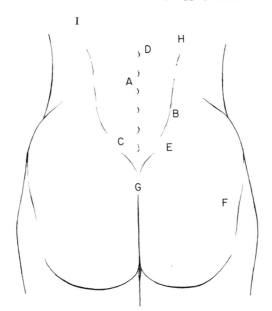

A. Spinous process of L4-L5
B. Iliolumbar ligaments
C. Articular facets L5-S1
D. Interspinous ligaments
E. Sacroiliac ligaments

F. Sacrosciatic notch
G. Tenderness on body of sacrum
H. Transverse process
I. Iliocostalis muscle sprain

This list is incomplete, for many more causes exist. The contributing pelvic causes are as follows:

A. Urinary tract
    1. Pyelonephritis
    2. Nephrolithiasis
    3. Tuberculosis of the urinary tract
    4. Congenital anomalies
    5. Malignant disease with spread to pelvic side-wall
B. Rectum and sigmoid
    1. Diverticulosis and diverticulitis
    2. Malignant disease with local extension
    3. Congenital anomalies and prolapse
C. Gynecologic causes
    1. Chronic cervicitis
    2. Prolapse
    3. Endometriosis
    4. Pelvic inflammatory disease
    5. Pelvic neoplasms

The gynecologic lesions that contribute to the patient's general pelvic discomfort and backache are our primary concern. It is only with due regard for the orthopedic and psychosomatic aspects associated with this symptom complex that the true picture of the patient's complaints can be honestly evaluated. Since this is a book on gynecology the reader will be admonished to look into these factors first, although he should realize that they are of little importance compared with the mechanical findings.

Treatment of Backache by the Gynecologist

Less than 10 per cent of the patients seen by the gynecologist have a backache with other than a mechanical etiology. Less than 10 per cent of women with a mechanical backache need more than some simple but effective treatment for their complaint. Excluding, then, the gynecologic and urologic causes of back pain, the patient is advised, educated, reassured, and treated along this line. She is shown the difference between extension and flexion of the spine if her pain was caused by an extension injury. A parous patient will comprehend how the lordosis of pregnancy exaggerates extension of the spine and causes back pain. She may recall that the backache was relieved post partum by the hospital bed, elevated at the head and broken at the knees. She could be reminded that in performing her kitchen chores she should assume a posture with knees elevated and back flexed. This ideal position stretches the posterior intervertebral ligaments and widens the intervertebral foramina. Irritation of the ligaments, fascia, muscles, synovia, and periosteum and the state of inactivity into which many pregnant women retire can produce back pain, with contraction and splinting of the muscles in the area.

The early control of pain in an acute back strain is important to prevent the complaint from becoming chronic. To bring this about, the pain-spasm syndrome must be interrupted by the use of exercises and a skeletal muscle relaxant. Some analgesic drug, as well as sedation, should also be administered to ensure restful sleep. Mephenesin, 0.25 Gm., combined in a capsule with glutamic acid hydrochloride, 0.30 Gm., is effective in some patients. The dose is 2 to 4 capsules every six hours, with the amount adjusted to the patient's response.

Anti-inflammatory Agents

Recently nonhormonal, anti-inflammatory agents have been introduced in the management of backache associated with rheumatoid and other inflammatory conditions. One of these, Tandearil (oxyphenbutazone), can be used in conjunction with local infiltration of trigger areas.

The initial daily dosage of the drug in adults ranges from 300 mg. to 600 mg. in three or four divided doses. This is continued for one week. If there is no response after this length of time, the patient will receive no benefits from this drug, and it should be discontinued. With a favorable response the drug can be continued for several more weeks with greatly reduced amounts on the order of 100 mg. to 200 mg. with further benefit to the patient. Because of some toxic effects in some patients, the drug is stopped a few days after a satisfactory relief of symptoms.

When taking this drug, the patient should be instructed to report the occurrence of fever,

CHART III

FLEXION AND STRETCHING EXERCISES

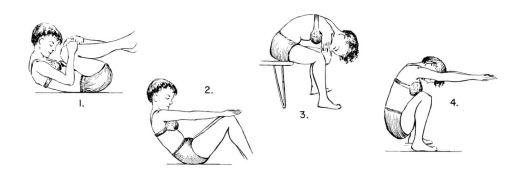

EXERCISE 1

Flex the thighs on the abdomen at a 45-degree angle. Grasp the knees on the outside and rythmically pull them toward the armpits. Arch the back as much as possible and point the head toward the buttocks. Repeat as frequently as prescribed.

Date	Repeat_____times_____times per day	
------	------	------
------	------	------
------	------	------
------	------	------

EXERCISE 2

Assume a position flat on the back with the knees flexed to a 45-degree angle. Extend the arms forward and rise to a sitting position, using the abdominal muscles to pull up. Repeat as frequently as prescribed.

Date	Repeat_____times_____times per day	
------	------	------
------	------	------
------	------	------
------	------	------

EXERCISE 3

Sit on the edge of a chair with the legs well separated. Cross the arms and bend forward, pushing the arms through the legs as far as they can go. Pull the head toward the feet several times and then return to the sitting position and repeat the exercise as frequently as directed.

Date	Repeat_____times_____times per day	
------	------	------
------	------	------
------	------	------
------	------	------

EXERCISE 4

Squat with the feet about a foot apart and the hands extended. Keep the heels on the floor and bend the head forward. Now pull the buttocks toward the floor and bend the head toward the floor at the same time. Come to a standing position at the end of each performance of the exercise. Repeat as directed by your doctor.

Date	Repeat_____times_____times per day	
------	------	------
------	------	------
------	------	------
------	------	------

lesions of the mouth, sore throat, or tarry stools. Blood counts should be taken every three or four days if prolonged therapy is indicated. Nausea, edema, or drug rash may necessitate interruption of the therapy. The drug is contraindicated in the presence of renal disease, cardiac failure, blood dyscrasias, liver disease, and other conditions when a potentially toxic though useful agent might cause serious complications.

Two of the weak and atonic postural muscle groups, the abdominal and gluteal muscles, are seldom used except to get out of bed in the morning. The exercises to strengthen these and other back muscles are well known and have many variations, but all result in the pulling of the head toward the coccyx. The patient is instructed to exercise these muscle groups both systematically and at frequent intervals during the day while at work or play. A bed board may help at night. Chart III shows four of the common flexion and stretching exercises that can be employed. A record should be kept as a matter of discipline, and the number and frequency of the exercise periods should be increased as more tone is acquired in the muscle groups.

Simple infiltration of a trigger area with 1 per cent procaine or its equivalent of other local anesthetic may give relief in acute pain. More complicated nerve blocks are in the province of the orthopedic surgeon and, if they are necessary, one may suspect organic disease or mechanical derangement. The treatment of backache should be aggressive from both the organic and the psychosomatic aspects, for backache may easily lead to chronic disability and fixation on pain.

References

Adlerman, E.: Urologic Origins of Backache, New York J. Med. 55: 1598, 1955.

Bancroft, F., and Marble, H.: Surgical Treatment of Motor-Skeletal System, vol. 2, Philadelphia, 1945, J. B. Lippincott Co.

Davies, J. W.: Man's Assumption of the Erect Posture: Its Effect on the Position of the Pelvis; Gynecologic and Obstetrical Applications, M. Ann. District of Columbia 25: 372, 1956.

Diveley, R. L., Kiene, R. H., and Meyer, P.: Low Back Pain, J. A. M. A. 160: 729, 1956.

Francis, C.: The Human Pelvis, St. Louis, 1952, The C. V. Mosby Co.

Godfrey, J. D.: The Management of Backache, New York J. Med. 54: 2601, 1954.

Goldthwaite, J. E.: A Consideration of the Pelvic Articulations From an Anatomical, Pathological, and Clinical Standpoint, Boston M. & S. J. 21: 22, 1905.

Hunter, R. G., Henry, G. W., and Larsen, I. J.: Stirrups and Post-operative Backache, Obst. & Gynec. 4: 344, 1954.

Jessup, R., Murray, R. J., and Rossi, A.: The Management of Low Back Pain in the Ambulant Patient, Am. Pract. & Digest of Treat. 5: 792, 1954.

Kelly, R. P., and Johnson, J. T.: Acute Low Back Pain, J. A. M. A. 158: 1520, 1955.

Miller, N. F.: The Research Quarterly of the American Physical Education Association, May, 1930.

Miller, N. F., and Kretzschmar, N. R.: Posture of Women. In Davis, C. H., and Carter, B.: Gynecology and Obstetrics, vol. III, Hagerstown, Md., 1953, W. F. Prior Co., Inc., chap. 12.

Miller, N. F., and Kretzschmar, N. R.: Backache. In Davis, C. H., and Carter, B.: Gynecology and Obstetrics, vol. III, Hagerstown, Md., 1953, W. F. Prior Co., Inc., chap. 13.

Rodriguez-Gomez, M., Valdes-Rodriguez, A., and Drew, A.: Effect of Zoxazolamine (Flexin) in Treatment of Spasticity; Preliminary Report, J. A. M. A. 160: 752, 1956.

Steindler, A.: Mechanics of Normal and Pathological Locomotion in Man, Springfield, Ill., 1935, Charles C Thomas, Publisher, page 199.

Sullivan, J. D.: Psychiatric Factors in Low Back Pain, New York J. Med. 55: 227, 1955.

Tebrock, H. E., and others: The Physiologic Potensification of Mephenesin With a Smooth Muscle Relaxant and Analgesic, New York J. Med. 57: 101, 1957.

Travell, J.: Referred Pain From Skeletal Muscle, New York J. Med. 55: 331, 1955.

White House Conference on Child Welfare, Subcommittee on Body Mechanics, New York, 1952, Appleton-Century-Crofts Co., Inc.

Section II · CONGENITAL ANOMALIES AND PSYCHOSOMATIC ASPECTS OF GYNECOLOGIC SURGERY

3 · Congenital Anomalies

General Considerations

Anomalies of the female genitalia seldom lend themselves to a rigid classification. The defects in any one patient commonly overlap any groups that are established. Three basic defects permit a division into major groups: (1) aplasia, or the absence of organs or tissues; (2) hermaphroditism, or the union of elements of the male and female in one person; and (3) inhibition, or developmental retardation. Accurate statistics on the incidence of genital anomalies in the female could scarcely be expected for several reasons. Many anomalies are present among infants dying at birth or in the neonatal period, few are recognized by a cursory examination of the newborn, and a large group are never brought to the attention of the clinician because of modesty or because they do not interfere with the individual's growth and development. The importance of congenital anomalies in clinical medicine is equaled by the emotional impact upon the patient that the discovery of such malformations entails.

Etiology

Two main theories of fetal malformations have been explored by embryologists: (1) the defective germ plasm theory and (2) the unfavorable environment theory. Since studies to substantiate these theories cannot be undertaken in human beings, all interpretations must be based on the results of animal experimentation. It seems probable that grossly abnormal ova do not survive even in the best environment and that normal ova with great vitality succumb in a poor environment. Abnormalities are produced when the conception survives because the balance of both factors is not sufficient to cause death but still is not adequate to produce a normal offspring.

Embryology

Spaulding divides the development of the external genitalia into three stages: (1) the genital tubercle stage, characterized by the appearance of the genital eminence in conical form prior to the formation of the labioscrotal swelling; (2) the phallus stage, during which the labioscrotal swellings separate the genital tubercle from surrounding areas; and (3) the definitive stage, characterized by the transition of the primary external genitalia into their final form.

The anomalies found in the vulval cleft and rectum are the result of some failure in the following sequence of events. The cloaca, a dorsoventrally expanded portion of the hindgut, is already well developed in a 3 mm. embryo. Meanwhile, from the ectodermal elements, the genital tubercle appears as a conical eminence between the umbilical cord and the base of the tail. The urethral groove appears on the caudal slope of this eminence, and the anal pit develops at the basal end of this groove. The urethra and anus are now mere depressions and both are imperforate. The Müllerian ducts, Wolffian ducts, and allantoic stalk all open into the primitive cloaca. The fact that both ectodermal and entodermal elements form the external genitalia and anus must be appreciated in order to understand the anomalies of the structures. During the fifth to seventh weeks of development the rectum migrates backward toward the anal depression. The ventral portion of the cloaca develops further into the larger urogenital sinus. The division between the rectum and urogenital sinus becomes more evident, forming the urorectal septum. The most ventral portion of the urogenital sinus extends outward to the genital tubercle or eminence, and toward the end of the seventh week this extension breaks down and the urogenital sinus then presents a fissurelike opening. This gives direct communication between the phallic (ventral or pubic) part of the urogenital sinus (future bladder and urethra) and the exterior. The ectodermal anal depression and the tissue intervening between the depression and advancing rectum (anal plate) break down and the anal canal is perforate. Meanwhile the clitoris becomes further differentiated by a groove (coronary sulcus) into a glans area and a shaft, and the labioscrotal folds become more prominent (phallus stage). In embryos of 38 to 45 mm. in length the caudal ends of the labioscrotal swellings unite in front of the anus to form the posterior commissure. The labioscrotal swellings form the labia majora, and the urethral folds surrounding the urogenital opening become the labia minora. The development of the vagina which is also taking place at the same time will be described separately, since the greater part of it is formed from the Müllerian ducts, as are the uterus

and tubes—structures of the upper genital tract.

Two common anomalies occur from interruption of this sequence of events: (1) The cloacal septum may be imperfect, resulting in the anal opening continuing into the urogenital sinus. The anus then opens into the vestibule of the vagina. (2) The cloacal anus closes off from the urogenital sinus, but the anal plate is not resorbed and there is an atresia ani or, in more simple form, an imperforate anus with a membrane a few millimeters thick. Defects associated with the vagina are frequently accompanied by anomalies of the external genitalia. Before the hermaphroditic states and other malformations can be understood, the development of the vagina must be described.

The Müllerian ducts appear as invaginations of the celomic epithelium. The lower portions of these ducts fuse in the midline and form a solid cord which tunnels caudally through the mesenchyme and impinges on the posterior wall of the urogenital sinus to form the Müllerian tubercles. The cephalic, unfused portions of these ducts become the Fallopian tubes, while the fused caudal portions give rise to the uterus, cervix, and the greater part of the vagina. Failure to fuse at the proper level gives rise to the varieties of bicornuate uterus. Failure of fusion combined with persistence of the septum between the two ducts causes anomalies ranging from a small septum, as in the uterus subseptus, to complex anomalies, such as uterus didelphys with a double vagina. Arrest of the mechanism of proliferation and canalization can cause atresia at any level.

Investigators differ in their interpretation of the development of the lowermost portion of the vagina and hymen. The studies of Koff on the formation of the human vagina give us a workable explanation of the later clinical findings. His investigations reveal that the lower one-fifth of the vagina and the hymen are derived from the urogenital sinus. Bilateral posterior evaginations of the urogenital sinus occur which obliterate the Müllerian tubercle. These are called sinovaginal bulbs. By proliferation of their epithelial lining and by fusion, they form, together with the lowermost portion of the fused Müllerian ducts, the primitive vaginal plate. The solid primitive vaginal plate grows in all directions, while the central cells break down to form the lumen of the vagina. The hymen is composed of a posterior segment and anterior paired segments. The posterior segment is seen to arise from a bulbous expansion of the primitive vaginal plate. The anterior paired segments are formed from bilateral lips at the point of origin of the sinovaginal bulbs.

Imperforate hymen may be interpreted as occurring because of excessive proliferation and coalescence of the epithelium of the sinovaginal bulbs. Congenital retrohymenal atresia probably arises from noncanalization of the lowermost end of the fused Müllerian ducts.

The ovary develops with the Müllerian duct (tubes, uterus, and vagina), the mesonephros (which degenerates), and metanephros (kidney). The possibilities for concomitant malformations are immediately apparent. The sex gland first appears as a thickening of the peritoneum and subperitoneal tissue over the mesonephros or Wolffian body. The mesonephros degenerates from above downward, and the ovary follows the caudal portion which is growing as the cephalic end is resorbed. The ovary soon becomes outlined as a rounded mass attached to the urogenital fold by a stalk (mesovarium). Meanwhile the ovary is differentiating into superficial, epithelial, and deep layers. The latter is looser in texture and is developing genital cells. At birth the fetal ovary shows the usual connective tissue stroma, blood vessels, primary follicles, and young ova.

Surgical Anatomy

The endless varieties of malformations encountered do not permit a detailed description of the anatomic findings except in the more common types or in those that lend themselves to surgical correction. Little help can be given a patient with small and underdeveloped ovaries and only remnants of Müllerian ducts for tubes. Occasionally excision in conjunction with some other operative procedure is performed.

Clinically, the Jarcho classification of uterine, cervical, and concomitant vaginal anomalies is the most useful since it suggests those types amenable to some degree of surgical correction.

1. Uterus didelphys bicollis (septate vagina)
2. Uterus duplex bicollis (vagina simplex)
3. Uterus bicornis unicollis (vagina simplex)
4. Uterus septus (complete)
5. Uterus subseptus (partial)
6. Uterus arcuatus (concave fundus)
7. Uterus unicornis

Vaginal septa, as well as septa within the uterine cavity, may be excised. The several varieties of uterus didelphys and bicornis lend themselves to a unification procedure if the uterine wall is well developed. Rarely a double uterus will require a double or single hysterectomy, and pregnancies in one or both uteri are constantly being reported.

The lower one-third of the vagina and vulva are commonly involved in abnormalities. Congenital absence of the vagina, female pseudohermaphroditism, vaginal atresias, septate or double vagina, imperforate hymen, rectovaginal fistula, and urethrovaginal fistula are some of the common types.

Concomitant Malformations

In about one-third of the cases with major genital anomalies there is an associated renal anomaly. This is particularly true when the genital anomaly involves an abnormal development or lack of the Müllerian ducts. Other genetic faults frequently occur with the defects involving the urogenital fold, but they involve such distant organs and systems that they cannot be included here. The urologic defects are many and varied. Exstrophy of the bladder with separation of the symphysis in conjunction with a bicornuate uterus, crossed unfused ectopy with absence of the uterus, absence of a kidney with a rudimentary uterine horn on the same side, ectopic kidneys with undescended ovaries, complete absence of uterus and vagina with a solitary ectopic kidney, and horseshoe kidney are the common findings. The complete urologic study that is done on all patients with genital anomalies (major or minor) frequently results in a modification of the treatment or operation. Several representative operations for genital tract anomalies will be described to illustrate the surgical principles involved in these conditions.

CONGENITAL ABSENCE OF THE VAGINA
General Considerations

Congenital absence of the vagina results from the failure of the Müllerian ducts to form their part of the structure. A dimple or slightly deeper invagination at the site of the introitus may represent attempts of the ectodermal elements to provide their part of the tract. While gonads of one or the other sex must be present for the fetus to survive, congenital absence of the vagina provides inferential evidence that the cervix, uterus, and tubes are absent or rudimentary.

Surgical Principles

Many operations have been suggested and successfully performed to provide an artificial vagina. These vaginal reconstructions have ranged in complexity from a prolonged pressure indentation of the perineum by graduated tubes to the use of transplanted bowel. The operations using loops of small intestine or segments of the rectum to form a vagina have been abandoned. The use of the pedicle flaps turned into the space between rectum and bladder has the technical difficulty of fixing the distal end of the flap in the depths of the new vagina. In one such operation performed on a patient after pelvic exenteration, the flaps retracted despite every effort to maintain an adequate depth of the artificial vagina.

Two procedures result in a satisfactory vagina. First, if there is a depression a few centimeters deep between the urethra and rectum, this can be enlarged by sharp and blunt dissection to the peritoneal reflection of the bladder and rectum. This opening can be maintained with an obturator and permitted

to form a mucosal lining. The patient is placed on large doses of estrogens. A lining of epithelium eventually covers the new vagina, and some have insisted that it will be a true vaginal epithelium if buds or remnants of the Müllerian duct are present and provide the basic cells. It is worth biopsying the tract in all these dissections for further study of the problem. The second method is to surface the new vagina with a split-thickness skin graft. This is the most popular at the present time and will be described in detail.

Two-Stage Operation

Sargis and associates suggest a two-stage operation in those patients with a shallow rectovesical septum. The objective is to provide a larger space during the second or perineal stage which is carried out six weeks later.

The first stage consists in mobilizing the bladder base through an adequate laparotomy incision, deperitonealizing the Müllerian remnants which converge toward the midline, and then uniting the tissues (or remnants) by interrupted sutures which places them at a superior level while at the same time the bladder base is elevated out of the cul-de-sac. This provides more space between bladder and rectum for the subsequent vaginal reconstruction.

Preoperative Care and Anesthesia

The proximity of the bowel and bladder during the operation and the disturbance of their functions in the postoperative period require special attention. A bowel preparation is instituted several days before surgery in the event that the rectum is inadvertently entered during the dissection. The plug and graft used will not permit spontaneous evacuation for some time, and enemas may have to be siphoned back. If the lower bowel is well cleansed prior to surgery, the patient will have less discomfort from impacted fecal material.

Steps of the Operation

1. Ureteral catheters are inserted into the kidney pelves and strapped out of the field of operation (Plate 7, *A*). The cystoscope should be kept on

the table so that the interior of the bladder can be observed during the course of the operation if the position of the urethra, bladder neck, and bladder base is not obvious at any time. A redundant prepuce and an enlarged clitoris (Plate 7, *A*) may require some repair, but in most instances these are not unsightly and the eventual cosmetic result of the operation is not improved by attempts to reduce their prominence. Frequently (as in the patient observed for this series of drawings) there is a shallow depression representing the sole contribution of the urogenital sinus (Plate 7, *A*). This depression should be utilized in forming the new introitus and in guiding the surgeon in the dissection to follow.

2. The bladder is now distended and the vaginal depression palpated to indicate the direction of the vesicorectal cleavage plane that must be entered later (Plate 7, *B*). During most of the dissection it is better to have the bladder empty, although it can be filled from time to time if this helps the surgeon. Methylene blue or other dyes should not be added to the solution, for they would hinder cystoscopy during the procedure and usually result only in discoloring the instruments and field of operation.

3. Lateral incisions are now made beginning just below the urethra and curving gently outward and downward toward the rectum (Plate 7, *C*). If there is any suggestion of labia minora (as is the case in the patient demonstrated), the incisions should be inside these structures and they should be preserved for whatever improvement they may give to the ultimate cosmetic result. Clamps should be used discriminately on the edges of the wounds throughout this operation so that unnecessary crushing of tissue is avoided.

4. A transverse incision is now made at about the middle of the two lateral incisions. This connects them to make an H-shaped incision with anterior and posterior flaps of skin that will be inverted into the rectovesical space to line the new vagina distal to the graft. The subcutaneous tissue under these flaps should be disturbed as little as possible in order to preserve their blood supply. The dissection will proceed along the bar of the H incision and laterally as indicated so the anterior and posterior flaps can be inverted without being mobilized in the midline (Plate 7, *D*).

5. The dissection is continued between bladder and rectum (Plate 7, *E*), alternately using the knife and knife handle. At the same time the space is widened by lateral dissection until the connective tissue extensions of the paravesicum and paraproctium offer resistance. The vesical and hemorrhoidal arteries, veins, nerves, and lymphatics are within these connective tissue thickenings but probably with an anomalous arrangement due to the absence of the vagina and its connective tissue supports. I have never seen or read of the prolapse of the vault of an artificially constructed vagina except for the development of a perineal hernia after attempted vaginal reconstruction in a patient who had survived a pelvic exenteration. In visualizing the statics of the pelvic floor in such a patient, it is apparent that the levator muscles are intact and, due to the absence of the vagina, are closer together at their anterior margins. Two sisters who had vaginal reconstructions were observed to have levator function and reported the existence of a vaginal orgasm during intercourse. A vaginal orgasm is reported by many to be dependent, in part, on the existence of pubococcygeal function. It is reasonable to assume that with the levators normally developed they should exert some effect, if not their normal action, on a reconstructed vagina.

6. Preoperative study of the bladder in these patients (in the absence of a bladder anomaly) usually shows it to have a large capacity without retention. If the bladder is distended to 350 to 400 ml., it will be noted on rectal examination to fill the hollow of the sacrum (Plate 7, *F*). It is here that the operator may have some difficulty in determining when he has reached the peritoneal reflection between bladder and rectum. The surgeon will also do well to palpate the ureters (Plate 7, *E*) frequently during the course of the operation and, presuming that they are normal in number, caliber, and insertion into the bladder, they will be displaced somewhat laterally during the dissection and remain there while the vaginal plug and graft are in place. In Plate 7, *F,* is shown the combined technique of performing this dissection. This is indicated only when an exploration of the pelvis, abdomen, or inguinal canals is necessary to clarify the exact diagnosis prior to excision of some anomalous structure. The operator's hand within the abdomen is placed in the most dependent part of the pelvis between the bladder and rectum to serve as a guide during the dissection.

7. The dissection is continued toward the hollow of the sacrum, using sharp and blunt dissection (Plate 7, *G*). The gauze-over-finger technique is useful to the operator in feeling his way between the bladder and rectum. As the vaginal cavity

Text continued on p. 62.

PLATE 7

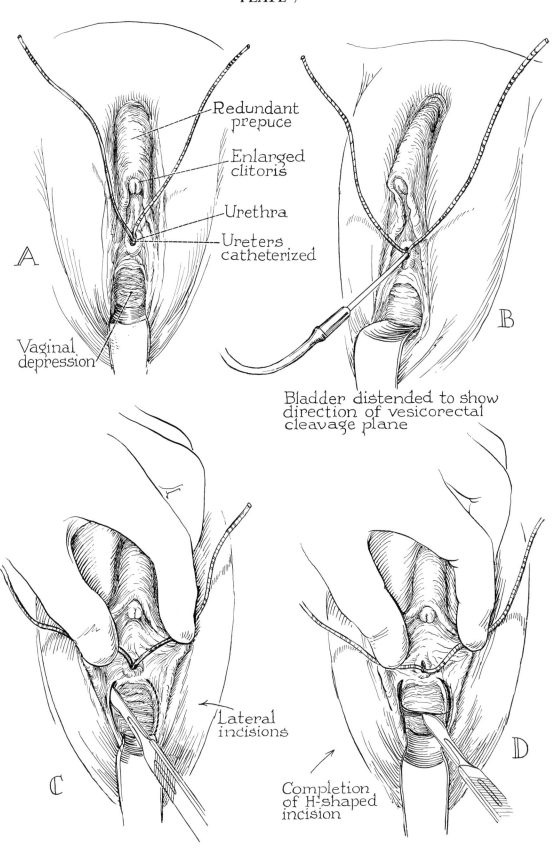

Redundant prepuce

Enlarged clitoris

Urethra

Ureters catheterized

A

Vaginal depression

B

Bladder distended to show direction of vesicorectal cleavage plane

C

Lateral incisions

D

Completion of H-shaped incision

PLATE 7 *(Continued)*

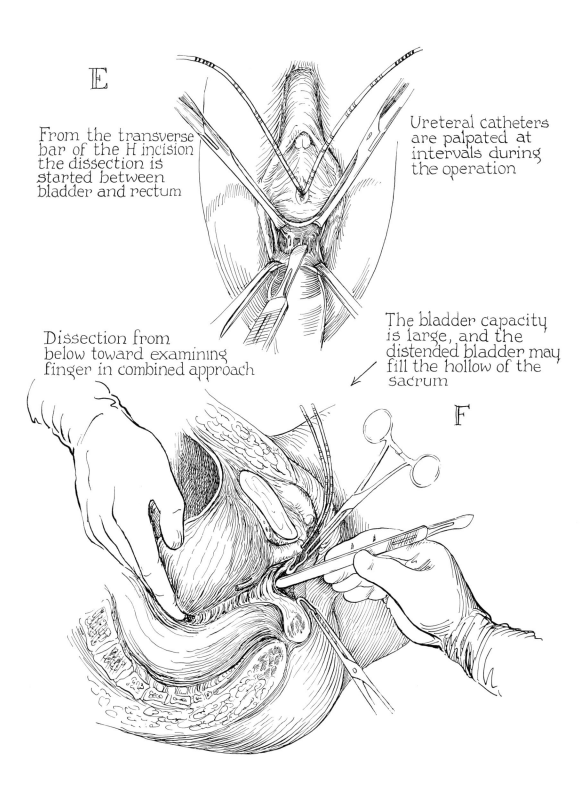

E

From the transverse
bar of the H incision
the dissection is
started between
bladder and rectum

Ureteral catheters
are palpated at
intervals during
the operation

Dissection from
below toward examining
finger in combined approach

The bladder capacity
is large, and the
distended bladder may
fill the hollow of the
sacrum

F

PLATE 7 (Continued)

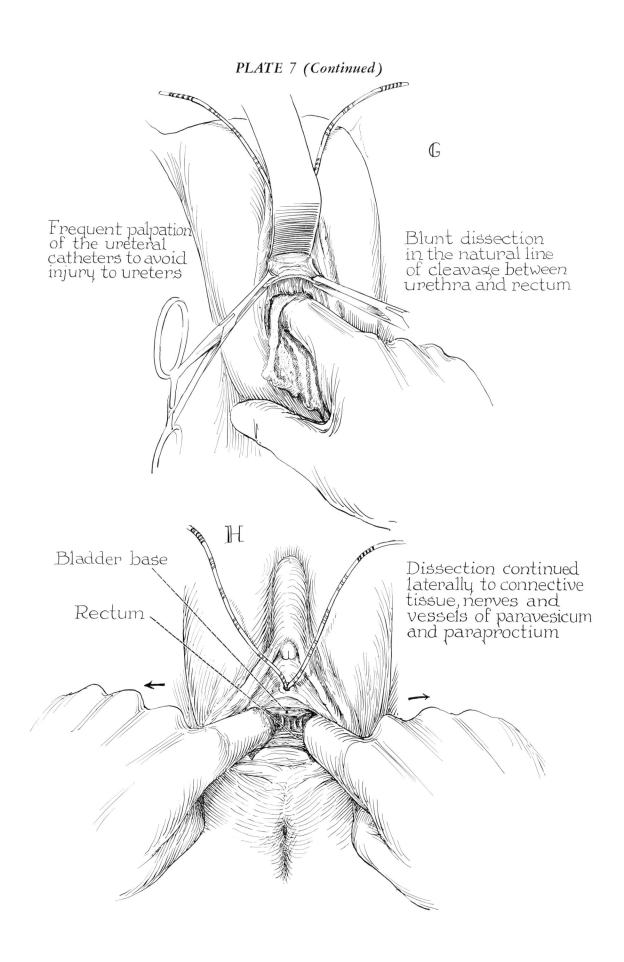

G

Frequent palpation
of the ureteral
catheters to avoid
injury to ureters

Blunt dissection
in the natural line
of cleavage between
urethra and rectum

H

Bladder base

Rectum

Dissection continued
laterally to connective
tissue, nerves and
vessels of paravesicum
and paraproctium

PLATE 7 (Continued)

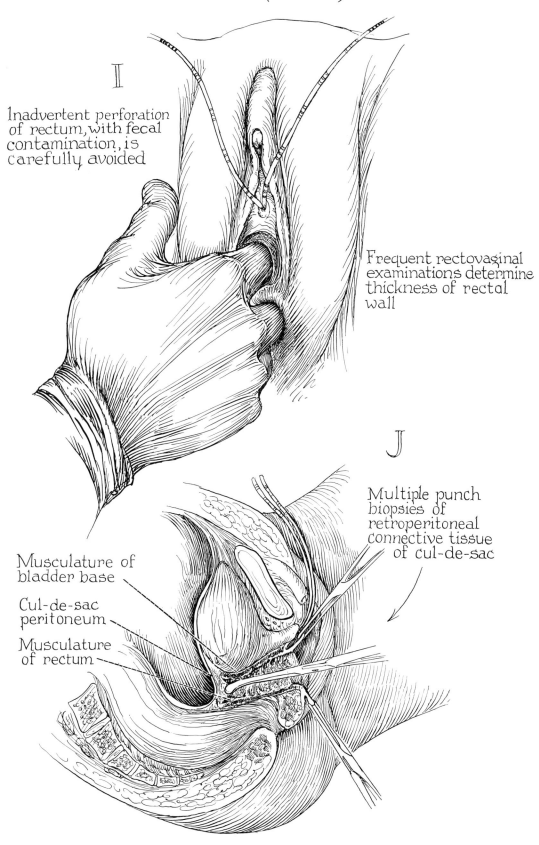

I

Inadvertent perforation of rectum, with fecal contamination, is carefully avoided

Frequent rectovaginal examinations determine thickness of rectal wall

J

Multiple punch biopsies of retroperitoneal connective tissue of cul-de-sac

Musculature of bladder base

Cul-de-sac peritoneum

Musculature of rectum

PLATE 7 (Continued)

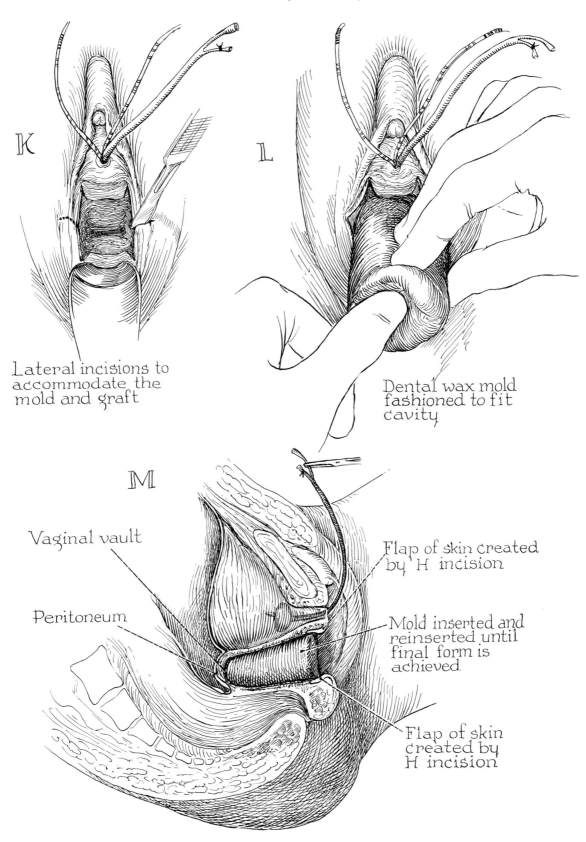

K

Lateral incisions to
accommodate the
mold and graft

L

Dental wax mold
fashioned to fit
cavity

M

Vaginal vault

Peritoneum

Flap of skin created
by H incision

Mold inserted and
reinserted until
final form is
achieved

Flap of skin
created by
H incision

PLATE 7 (Concluded)

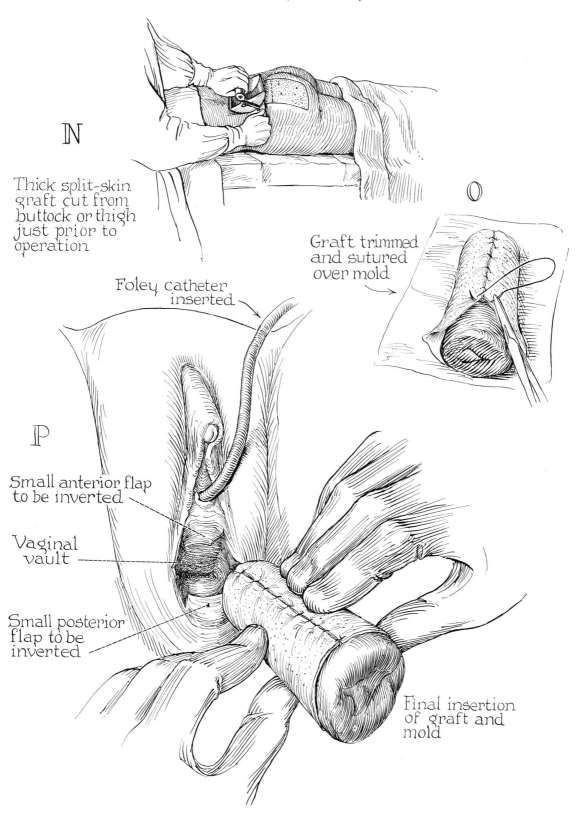

N

Thick split-skin
graft cut from
buttock or thigh
just prior to
operation

O

Graft trimmed
and sutured
over mold

Foley catheter
inserted

P

Small anterior flap
to be inverted

Vaginal
vault

Small posterior
flap to be
inverted

Final insertion
of graft and
mold

61

deepens, it is useful to place Deaver retractors anteriorly and posteriorly to displace the bladder and rectum away from the area of dissection. As shown in Plate 7, *G,* the anterior flap of skin may be drawn away from the field of operation, but strong traction should be avoided so the edges are not necrosed.

8. The characteristic structure of the musculature of the bladder base and rectum soon becomes discernible (Plate 7, *H*). The normal vagina in the collapsed state is in the form of the letter H with lateral sulci that allow for considerable distention in addition to the cavity created by displacement of the bladder and rectum. The fingers can be used to advantage to dissect laterally until the connective tissue, nerves, and vessels of the paravesicum and paraproctium are reached (Plate 7, *H*). A sense of resistance is met laterally that is not found in the midline cleavage plane between the bladder and rectum. The anterior edge of the levator muscles will be felt by this maneuver, and one may obtain further information on the development of the pelvic musculature.

9. Should the rectum be inadvertently entered, the resultant contamination, regardless of the bowel preparation, would complicate the primary union of the graft. During the course of the operation it is useful to palpate the thickness of the rectal wall (Plate 7, *I*) with a gloved hand. The glove should be carefully removed after rectal palpation. The thickness of the bladder base is determined by inserting and palpating a glass catheter. When the position of the ureters or thickness of the bladder is in doubt, cystoscopy is useful, as has been repeatedly suggested.

10. When the cul-de-sac is reached, the areolar tissue underlying the peritoneal reflection is biopsied in several places for study (Plate 7, *J*). If this operation has been done without the insertion of a split-thickness graft, one cannot help being impressed with the rapidity of epithelization of the canal that is created. It has not been established without question just how an epithelial lining is acquired. Some histologists have identified epithelial buds in the retroperitoneal connective tissue which they feel are the primordial remains of cells that might have formed the upper vagina and which, under the circumstances, proceed to develop and form a vaginal epithelium. Other observers insist that the reconstructed vagina is epithelized by a growth of the epithelium upward from the introitus. In any event it is valuable to submit some of the tissue of the vault for histologic section.

11. A dental wax mold is then fashioned by an assistant to the approximate size of the space created between the bladder and rectum. Lateral incisions extending from the original H incision are usually needed to accommodate a mold that allows for an ample introitus (Plate 7, *K*). This mold is needed because of the tendency of the skin of the vulva to contract and cause a stricture at the entrance to the new vagina.

12. Before the wax mold hardens, it is shaped both to the depth and diameter of the new vesicorectal space (Plate 7, *L*). It should be approximately one-third again as large as a normal, pliable, distended vagina. At the same time (and this depends on the size of the pelvis and bony framework of the particular patient) it should not cause excessive pressure on the bladder or rectum from which it must eventually derive its blood supply. The length of the mold should allow for the anterior and posterior flaps of the vulval skin that are turned into the new vagina.

13. In Plate 7, *M,* is shown a lateral view of the mold in place. With the bladder distended there should not be more than gentle pressure against the mold, and with the bladder collapsed by continuous drainage, the opposing surfaces should still be in opposition. This would seem difficult to obtain, but with muscular, distensible, and contractile organs on both sides of the newly fashioned vagina it works out quite well in practice. Again, if there is any doubt, a finger inserted into the rectum and sounding of the bladder will clarify the amount of pressure on the adjacent structures.

14. The site selected as a donor area for the graft should be free of hair, such as the buttock or thigh in most women (Plate 7, *N*). A split-thickness or three-quarter thickness graft is most satisfactory. The surgeon who does not work with skin grafts frequently and who is unable to have the assistance of a plastic surgeon should use a dermatome of the semicircular drum type which permits the cutting of a graft of uniform thickness. This instrument removes an area about 4 by 7¾ inches which may be adequate in itself to cover the mold. The instrument is calibrated to cut a graft to a depth of 0.012 to 0.018 inch for this operation, but this may be varied depending on the donor site. Since it is difficult to forecast the exact size of the mold before operation, elaborate outlining of the graft is not feasible. These patients are in good health and the grafting is an elective procedure so any excess skin can be returned to the donor area if desired. The kind of antiseptic used on the skin

before taking the graft is unimportant so long as a strong solution is not used. The donor area is dressed with silver foil or some type of impregnated gauze for protection while the patient is being moved and then is treated like any primary healing surface or incision. I prefer to use little or no dressing except for such protection as may be necessary to the patient's comfort.

15. The graft is then sutured over the hardened mold with interrupted sutures of 000 plain catgut on French (eyeless) needles (Plate 7, *O*). As few sutures as necessary are used and only where they are essential in keeping the graft on the mold. The total amount of even fine, absorbable suture material to be buried in the wound should be kept to a minimum.

16. The mold and graft are now inserted for a final fitting (Plate 7, *P*). The small anterior and posterior flaps of skin from the vulva will be inverted into the new vagina as the mold is put in place. The distal edge of the graft and these small flaps should not overlap and should be separated by a few millimeters to allow for postoperative swelling and any slight change in the position of the mold and graft after the patient is taken out of the lithotomy position. The indwelling catheter is observed to ensure that it is not compressed, and a sanitary napkin is tied or strapped over the vulva.

Postoperative Care

The indwelling catheter is connected to straight drainage, and urinary antiseptics are administered. The mold and graft are inspected daily for evidence of pressure about the introitus. If a hematoma or seroma has formed which can be recognized near the surface, this unfortunate complication is dealt with by adequate drainage. If the most unfortunate complication of infection is encountered, the mold should be removed and the area drained in the hope that some part of the graft will take. The patient is put on a low residue diet, and on the third or fourth day a low enema can be given and siphoned back if necessary. After several days, when it may be presumed that fibrin has been deposited between the graft and the opposing tissues, the patient may be mobilized, although walking is very uncomfortable. The mold is removed (under anesthesia if necessary) in two

weeks. The graft is gently teased away from the surface of the dental compound and any nonviable tissue débrided from the wound. Lubricated Sims' plugs are inserted by the patient as soon as this can be started without too much discomfort. If she is unmarried, the plug insertions must be continued indefinitely to prevent contracture of the vagina. Preoperatively and postoperatively the patient should be given large doses of estrogens. This therapy should be continued indefinitely or until the surgeon is satisfied that a pliable, functional vagina will be maintained without estrogenic stimulation. In anticipation of an indwelling catheter for several weeks in some cases, urinary antiseptics are started in advance of the surgery and continued until bladder function has returned to normal.

PLASTIC UNIFICATION OF THE UTERUS
Symptoms and Diagnosis

The symptoms of a congenital uterine anomaly are variable and depend on the type of anomaly present.

Probably 50 per cent of patients with minor anomalies of the uterus have no symptoms and have had children without difficulty. Many anomalies are unrecognized because of this fact. Common symptoms attendant upon a uterine anomaly are menometrorrhagia, habitual abortion, and sterility. Dysmenorrhea is not an uncommon symptom, and it is particularly significant in a patient who experiences unilateral dysmenorrhea. In the past history of these patients, many report premature deliveries or an abnormal labor with a transverse or oblique position of the fetus. Others give a history of prolonged labor, and there is a high incidence of retained placentas. Anatomists have observed that patients with a bicornuate uterus tend to have a large transverse diameter of the pelvis. The anomaly may be first discovered during a sterility study. A hysterogram will reveal the presence of a septum or other congenital anomaly. A dilatation and curettage may likewise reveal the same findings. Some anomalies are first discovered when, with the onset of menstruation, a hematocolpos or hematometra develops.

Indications and Surgical Principles

The common indications for this operation are sterility or habitual abortion. The more severe anomalies and the presence of a septum or two small uterine cavities do not permit the normal development of the fetus and placenta. The capacity of the uterus is inadequate. Some patients are operated upon because of the severity of the dysmenorrhea.

Prior to operation, and particularly if the operation is undertaken because of infertility, the patency of the tubes should be determined by air insufflation and a uterosalpingogram. Because of the high incidence of concomitant urologic anomalies, a complete urologic work-up is indicated. The hysterogram should be studied, particularly if the operation is being done for habitual abortion, to determine the possibility of providing a single adequate uterine cavity. If the operation is done because of severe dysmenorrhea, a prelumbar sympathectomy and resection of the infundibulopelvic pedicles are done at the same time. If there is a double cervix or a septum that is identifiable vaginally the operation may be rather simple. The septum can be resected after dilatation of one or both cervices. When there are separate fundi in addition to a septum, a laparotomy is necessary in order to unify the two fundi and construct one large and adequate uterine cavity. The use of vasopressin to control bleeding is recommended.

The use of synthetic vasopressin during unification procedures permits surgery in an almost bloodless field. Formerly, replacement by two to three units of blood was not infrequent during prolonged plastic procedures.

Two to four units of the vasopressin are diluted to 20 ml. One-half of this solution is injected before incising the uterus. Depending on the malformation, the sites of injection should include both horns anteriorly and posteriorly, and a milliliter or two should be injected into the septum. The remainder of the solution is reserved for use later in the procedure, should the initial effects wear off.

Since these operations are usually done on patients in a young age group, coronary artery disease would not contraindicate the use of the drug. Rarely is it necessary to monitor the anesthesia with a continuous electrocardiogram. Cyclopropane is not used for inhalation anesthesia.

Steps of the Operation

1. In Plate 8, *A,* is shown a bicornuate uterus with a partial septum and single cervix. The artist's sketches of the operation in this particular patient are shown in Plate 8, *B* to *F*. The great number of variations in the anomalies that may be encountered do not permit a standard description for any of the operations; however, some of the surgical principles can be illustrated for a particular anomaly.

2. In this type of uterine anomaly a transverse incision is made from the left to the right horn of the uterus (Plate 8, *B*), with care being exercised to remain clear of the intramural portion of the tubes.

3. The incision is carried deep enough until the septum within the uterus is recognized and excised (Plate 8, *C*). Bleeding points in the uterine musculature are clamped and ligated as encountered. The cavity of the uterus is explored, not only to eliminate the possibility of any intrinsic lesions that were overlooked at the curettage, but also to formulate an idea in the mind of the operator as to how the interior of the uterus will appear after unification.

4. The unification of this uterus is done by the incisions shown by dotted lines in Plate 8, *D*. These incisions remove the area from which the septum arises, eliminating the possibility of any contracture or weakening of the wall. After outlining the incision, the wedges are cut anteriorly and posteriorly so that normal uterine wall is approximated.

5. The deep layers of the myometrium are closed with interrupted sutures in the same manner as the closure of the uterine wall after a myomectomy (Plate 8, *E*). The superficial layers of the myometrium and the perimetrium are closed with interrupted sutures (Plate 8, *F*), after which the unified uterus, while still broader transversely than a normal fundus, has a reasonably good appearance. An adequate, single uterine cavity results.

PLATE 8

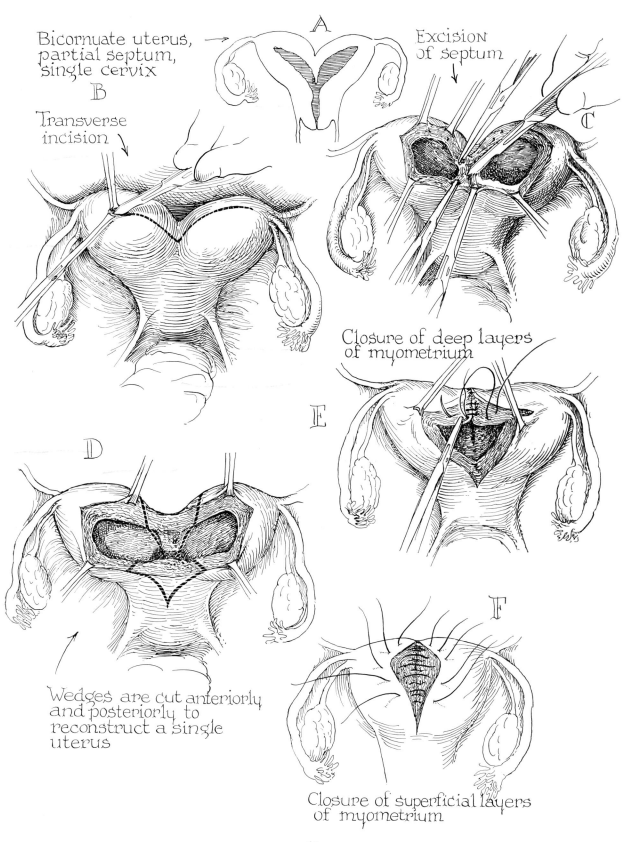

A

Bicornuate uterus, partial septum, single cervix

Excision of septum

B

Transverse incision

C

Closure of deep layers of myometrium

E

D

Wedges are cut anteriorly and posteriorly to reconstruct a single uterus

F

Closure of superficial layers of myometrium

During the procedure the intramural portions of the tubes are carefully avoided to preserve their continuity.

Postoperative Care

Because the uterine cavities are entered from below during the curettage and then subsequently invaded from above, with considerable dissection and resection of the muscular wall of the uterus, the patient is given antibiotic therapy. A combination of penicillin and streptomycin for three days postoperatively is suggested. The postoperative course of these patients parallels that of a simple myomectomy. Urinary antiseptics are given postoperatively if the patient has anomalies or distortion of the urinary tract that would make her susceptible to a urinary tract infection.

HEMATOMETRA AND SIMILAR DISORDERS
General Considerations

Cryptomenorrhea or hidden menstruation may be congenital or acquired. It will occur whenever an obstruction exists in the genital tract below a functional endometrium or a pathologic process that causes bleeding. The obstruction may be complete or incomplete, and the endometrium may menstruate in response to normal stimuli or the bleeding may be secondarily induced by estrogens.

Pathologic Anatomy

Common congenital types are imperforate hymen and congenital retrohymenal atresia. The distinction between these two anomalies is difficult but may often be made by location and histologic study of the occluding membrane. A hymen has stratified squamous epithelium on both sides. Patches of Müllerian duct epithelium may be recognized on the inner surface of the membrane, in a true retrohymenal atresia. The subepithelial layers contain muscle fibers, many blood vessels, and lymphocytes. Atresia of the vagina is a common cause, although collectively more cases involving complex uterine anomalies have been recorded. Lateral hematocolpos and lateral hematometra are seen if a blind side exists in one or another type of didelphic or bicornuate uterus. The acquired disease results from some agent which causes occlusion of the cervix or stricture of the vagina. Infection caused by, or following in the wake of, the primary etiologic agent is an important factor. Agents destroying the epithelial lining of the vagina with subsequent adhesions between granulating surfaces cause some cases. Operative procedures on the cervix and the use of heavy cautery tips may cause subsequent contracture of the cervical canal. Atresias of the cervix after improperly screened radium may cause retention of menstrual blood when castration has not been complete. As an indirect result of pregnancy, cases have been seen after abortion, missed abortion, and lacerations of the cervix or vagina. Fibromyomas may mechanically obstruct the cervical canal and are a common acquired cause. Atrophic changes which occlude the lower genital tract or cervix before the complete cessation of menstruation or subsequently induced estrogen bleeding will result in a retention of blood. In rare cases the labia minora may be completely agglutinated from a vulvitis in childhood. (See Plate 9, *A* to *L*.)

Where the obstruction exists at the outlet, as in congenital retrohymenal atresia and imperforate hymen, the onset of menstruation initiates a sequence of events that may ultimately involve the entire genital tract. Prior to the menarche the secretions of the cervical, uterine, and tubal glands form a hydrocolpometra which may be insignificant in size or contain an appreciable amount of fluid. To this is now added the periodic menstrual flow. Fortunately, the vagina is very distensible and will hold a large amount of fluid before the retrograde distention fills and distorts the upper, more vulnerable uterus, tubes, and ovaries that may be permanently damaged. The contractile powers of the uterus spare this organ until late in the disease, and in the moderately advanced cases the walls show hypertrophy due to the expulsion of the menstrual flow against positive pressure. A laparotomy at this time would reveal the uterus to be located on the dome of the hematocolpos. The tubes and cervix collect menstruum. The isthmic portion of one or both tubes may seal off, causing a hematosalpinx. If it does not seal off, blood will spill onto the peritoneum, causing a hematoperitoneum. Spillage about the ovary results in a hematovarium. Local reaction on the peritoneum seals the fimbriated ends of the tubes which expand and involve the surrounding structures in a tubo-ovarian tar cyst. The cervix effaces and dilates, causing a hematotrachelos. The uterus dilates and its walls become thinner and the glands compressed. Secretions and menstrual flow become less as the glands throughout the tract become atrophic and functionless. The process would be self-limited were it not symptomatic long before reaching such an advanced state.

Where obstruction exists at a higher level, multiple abnormalities of the genital tract are common. Above a vaginal or cervical atresia or in the blind horn of a bicornuate uterus, a functioning endometrium will menstruate and present exceedingly bizarre findings. Not infrequently one uterus and one vagina of a didelphic uterus are blind.

The acquired cases rarely reach the large size of the congenital types since the disease is treated earlier and the level of obstruction is higher. The process becomes a pyohematocolpos or pyohematometra when partial obstruction allows an ascending infection from the vagina. An intermittent hematometra or hematocolpos exists when an obstruction such as a cervical fibroid gives way periodically and drains.

Urinary Tract Complications

The urinary tract is so commonly involved in this disease that urologic studies should be done in each case. In low obstructions the expanding pelvic lesion may elevate and compress the bladder. With further increase in the size of the hematocolpos, the ureters are spread wider apart as they course through the pelvis, and the angle at which they enter the bladder is more obtuse. The pressure soon becomes sufficient to cause a hydroureter and a hydronephrosis. The urethra may be compressed against the symphysis in addition to being angulated at the bladder neck. Complete obstruction can take place with enormous dilation of the bladder. In high obstruction, concomitant anomalies of the urinary tract are frequent. Duplication and malformation in the course of the ureters, ectopic kidney, bladder anomalies, and the absence and duplication of the urethra have been reported. It is important in each case to demonstrate by cystoscopy and urography the course, number, and relationships of the ureters.

The membranes seen in imperforate hymen and retrohymenal atresia are thick and tough and obviate spontaneous rupture. Diverticulum formation or rupture into the rectum, bladder, or ischiorectal fossa is possible. Spontaneous amputation and rupture of a dilated blind horn are reported. Rupture of a large hematosalpinx with hemorrhage causes an abdominal catastrophe.

Symptoms and Diagnosis

Periodic pelvic pain, failure to menstruate, and dysuria form a triad of symptoms suggesting an expanding pelvic lesion, such as hematocolpos, caused by obstruction at the outlet. The failure of the menarche to appear is not the most common primary complaint that brings the patient to the doctor, for many mothers just consider their daughters late. Occasionally the urinary symptoms dominate the picture and are the primary complaint. The pain due to vaginal distention is a dull ache in the perineum and sacrum which is increased by sitting and defecation. Painful hemorrhoids may occur from pressure on the rectum. Menstrual molimina often recur at monthly intervals associated with nausea, vomiting, and vertigo. At cyclic intervals an acute hypogastric pain, as in severe dysmenorrhea, may be added. Acute lower abdominal pain, as in pelvic peritonitis, suggests a hematoperitoneum.

Rare is the patient who has not had an appendectomy prior to definitive treatment of the real cause of her difficulty. Many case histories reveal the patient placed in the lithotomy position for her first vaginal examination at the conclusion of a fruitless exploratory laparotomy.

Dysuria is the most common urinary complaint. With increasing obstruction the patient may complain of frequency, and the stream becomes progressively smaller and less forceful. Abdominal pressure may be used to start the flow. An attack of complete retention first brings the patient to the physician in a surprising number of cases. With the development of a hydronephrosis, flank pain may be a symptom.

In cases of high obstruction of congenital origin, no set pattern of complaints is discernible. Primary amenorrhea, vague pelvic pain, attempts at coitus in cases of vaginal atresia, urinary complaints, unilateral dysmenorrhea in cases of lateral hematocolpometra, sterility, or the appearance of an abdominal swelling prompt the patients to seek medical advice. The symptom complex in a given case depends on the extent, duration, and location of the expanding lesion.

The patients with acquired lesions are seen early because they have usually been under treatment for a pelvic complaint prior to the development of an obstructive lesion. Secondary amenorrhea, pelvic pain, and intermittent passage of old blood and pus are the common complaints. The urinary tract is not involved as a rule and does not give rise to symptoms. Patients frequently date the onset from some treatment or operation that reveals the cause.

In a patient with a large hematocolpometra from obstruction at the outlet a tender suprapubic mass can be palpated. This mass frequently rises to the umbilicus or above. An imperforate hymen spreads the labia minora and presents a bulging, dusky membrane. An impulse created by percussion of the abdominal tumor is transmitted to the hymen and perineum. This abdominoperineal fluid wave is pathognomonic of a large hematocolpos. Coughing also produces an impulse on the bulging membrane. Rectal examination reveals the distended, tense vagina filling the pelvis. Following aspiration, the thickness of the occluding membrane can be roughly estimated by palpation between a finger in the rectum and an external finger. On combined rectoabdominal examination an outline of the pelvic organs may be obtained. It is of primary importance to determine the extent of involvement of the uterus and tubes. With the vagina alone involved, the uterus may at times be felt atop the dome of the distended vagina. With advanced adnexal involvement, boggy, painful masses may be felt in one or both adnexal regions.

The membrane of retrohymenal atresia may frequently be distinguished from an imperforate hymen on gross inspection. The former is thinner and the hymen itself may often be seen exterior to, and stretched on, the anterior perimeter of a bulging retrohymenal membrane.

Palpation and inspection will disclose atresias of the vagina and cervix with a pelvic mass above. A bulging mass can be felt on the affected side of the vagina with a lateral hematocolpos. Under strictly aseptic conditions an exploratory needle may be passed into the fluctuant mass and the characteristic fluid withdrawn. The latter may now be replaced with an equal amount of radiopaque media and x-rays taken to give further information on the anomaly.

Acquired atresias are seen in the upper one-third of the vagina. Probing may reveal a partial atresia and allow the escape of blood and pus. Acquired, complete cervical atresias present a bulging, fluctuant tumor of the vaginal vault. The cervix is effaced, and careful inspection reveals a dimple or linear depression at the location of the external os. The exploring needle should enter at this point. Where partial obstruction exists, probing will usually reveal the nature of the disease. The amenorrhea and a pelvic mass frequently lead to a diagnosis of ovarian neoplasm. Appendicitis and ruptured ectopic pregnancy can be closely simulated by a hematoperitoneum. The symptom complex of recurrent monthly pelvic pain together with amenorrhea will alert one to the possibility of hidden menstruation and prompt a search for a source of obstruction or the presence of genital anomalies.

Surgical Principles and Treatment

The obscure findings in these diseases not infrequently lead to surgical exploration before a diagnosis is made. During such an exploration, certain principles should be followed:

1. Do not remove any organs unless convinced they are injurious to the patient.

2. Withhold any definitive surgery until the urinary tract is studied, even if this means terminating the exploration.

3. If definitive surgery is indicated, then the anatomy of the urinary tract should be explored by dissection and retrograde catheterization of the ureters.

4. Blind sacs containing endometrium must be removed or peritoneovaginal fistulas and a pyohematometra may result.

5. Studies by uterograms or the injection of aqueous dyes into tracts, uteri, or blind horns will guide the surgeon in the subsequent management and can be done on the operating table in emergencies.

6. Planning of the operation may require the insertion of a Foley catheter or other tube into the blind sac or horn from the vagina. This allows ready identification from the abdominal approach.

The treatment of imperforate hymen and retrohymenal atresia is identical. The patient is prepared for both perineal and abdominal operations, and a rectoabdominal examination under anesthesia is performed to determine if a hematosalpinx exists.

The evacuation of a large hematocolpos and hematometra is full of dangers. An hematosalpinx (adherent to the pelvic sidewall) may be torn away by the decompressed vagina and uterus as they contract and attempt to assume their normal shape. For the future fertility and preservation of the female organs it is necessary that the gynecologist treat these rare problems by a combined procedure when such

an approach will disclose and preserve a functioning genital tract.

Where a mass is palpable below as well as above, the operation is best performed with one surgeon operating vaginally and one abdominally. Hasty resection of organs that may be saved is prevented by caution and knowledge of the exact extent of the disease by this combined technique. Ingenuity in this type of surgery is endless. Catheters are placed in the urethra and tubes or large catheters in the rectum for orientation. If no adnexal involvement is evident at this examination, a few cubic centimeters of old blood are aspirated by needle and syringe to confirm the diagnosis (Plate 9, M). Further procedures are deferred until the following day since it is desirable to have the patient awake for the hymenotomy. Local anesthesia is used so that the patient may report any signs of intraperitoneal hemorrhage from an undetected small hematosalpinx. A cruciate incision is made in the membrane, the quadrants excised, and the edges approximated with sutures of fine catgut. This prevents future closure or rigidity of the hypertrophic membrane. Suprapubic pressure is not used to hasten drainage nor is the cervix visualized at this time. The prophylactic use of antimicrobials is recommended prior to operation and for several days postoperatively until the profuse drainage of old blood ceases. Irrigation of the vagina or the use of drains can only be condemned as inviting infection. The patient is placed in Fowler's position and can be mobilized early if her course is normal. Frequent vaginal examinations are avoided until after the first menstrual period unless indicated earlier by persistence of symptoms or other developments. Involution of the tract requires several months, and the first few menstrual periods may be abnormal. No douches, coitus, or swimming should be allowed until the involution is complete. The uterus and tubes are studied several months postoperatively by uterosalpingograms, by using a small quantity of contrast material. Residual damage and tubal patency are determined.

The examination under anesthesia may reveal adnexal involvement. In this event laparotomy is performed prior to hymenotomy in order to observe the drainage abdominally. The dangers of an intra-abdominal hemorrhage are very real. The sudden release of pressure with contraction of the uterus can tear adherent tubes away from the pelvic wall or rupture vascular adhesions. All bleeding is controlled and only hopelessly diseased organs are removed. The tubes are milked of old blood and the adhesions at the fimbriated ends gently separated. While many tubes might empty spontaneously, it is not believed that expectant treatment is indicated in cases with hematosalpinx. (Plate 9, N.)

Atresias of the vagina and cervix are explored from below, and a canal is created from the apex of the blind vaginal vault to the lower pole of the pelvic mass. An assistant's finger in the rectum and a sound in the bladder serve as guides. The combined approach is indicated when exploration from below is unsuccessful or the pyelograms indicate an anomaly of the ureters in the field of operation. While the preoperative care and study include a complete urologic study, it is advisable to insert catheters in the ureters, normal or abnormal, before surgery. This ensures rapid identification deep in the pelvis where there may be multiple adhesions or spillage of old blood in the resection of blind sacs. A hysterotomy is performed, the old blood evacuated, and the anomalous ureters visualized. A finger is then placed in the cervix or lower pole of the uterus and used as a guide for an assistant to dissect on from below. Alternately, dissection may be done from above on the assistant's finger below. The newly formed canal is kept open by insertion of glass dilators or a formed balsa wood plug beginning in the early postoperative period.

Lateral hematocolpos is treated by complete excision of the septum between the blind and patent vaginas if such an anomaly exists. Simple incision should not be done, for secondary closure is common. A laparotomy is performed for the anomalies that do not lend themselves to vaginal drainage. A hemi-hysterectomy, excision of an atretic horn, or rarely a hysterectomy may be indicated.

Treatment of acquired cryptomenorrhea involves the re-establishment of the continuity of the vagina or cervix and subsequent measures to ensure patency. The dissection is easier than in the congenital types since the relationships of the bladder and rectum are normal. Infection will respond to adequate drainage but is resistant to treatment if partial obstruction remains. The denuded areas of the vaginal cases are separated daily while healing. The cervix is dilated as often as necessary to assure a patent canal. Further surgical procedures, indicated because of the etiologic agent, are preferably deferred until the infection is controlled.

Psychosomatic Aspects

Patients with congenital cryptomenorrhea require special guidance to prevent the normal psychic trauma of the menarche from becoming pathologic. The anxiety connected with the onset of menstruation is exaggerated when the adolescent girl finds her menstrual function is abnormal. The patients with uncomplicated hematocolpos should be reassured and given an adequate explanation of the amenorrhea. Should pregnancy fantasies exist these are dispelled. As optimistic a prognosis as is compatible with the findings should be given regarding menstruation and reproduction.

Those patients with abnormalities having a poor prognosis may react acutely to the discovery of an anomaly. The questions of marriage, sexual compatibility, and sterility will arouse marked anxiety in a young woman normally much concerned with these events. The tendency to devaluate herself after becoming aware of her affliction may cause serious conflicts. A profound neurotic disturbance may threaten, requiring prolonged psychotherapy for which a psychiatric consultant should be sought.

Common Anomalies Requiring Surgery

The endless combinations of anomalies do not permit a step-by-step description of opera-

PLATE 9

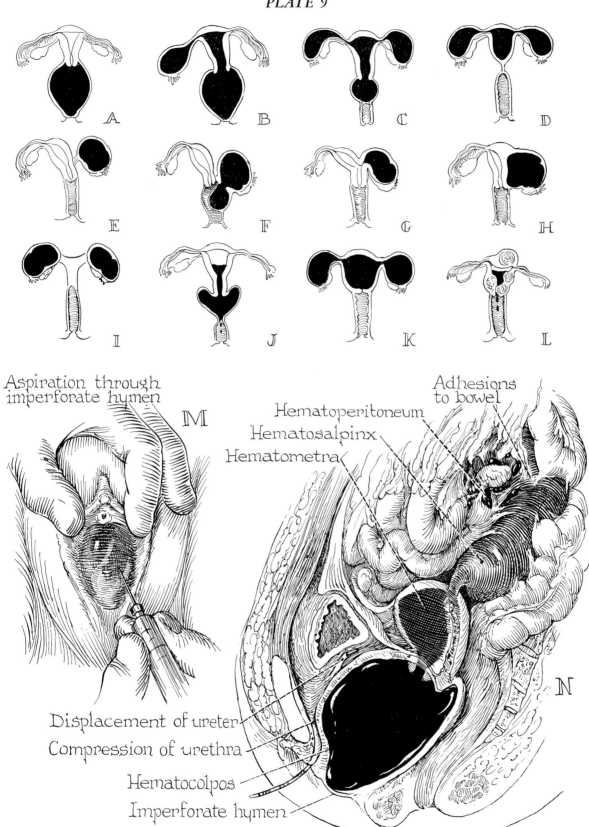

A   B   C   D

E   F   G   H

I   J   K   L

Aspiration through
imperforate hymen
M

Adhesions
to bowel
Hematoperitoneum
Hematosalpinx
Hematometra

N

Displacement of ureter
Compression of urethra
Hematocolpos
Imperforate hymen

tions for cryptomenorrhea. Some of the more common malformations are shown in Plate 9, A to L. These frequently observed surgical problems only serve as a guide in deciding on the approach to a specific anomaly.

A, Imperforate hymen, hematocolpos.

B, Imperforate hymen, hematocolpometra, right hematosalpinx.

C, Congenital atresia of the vagina, hematocolpometra, bilateral hematosalpinx.

D, Congenital atresia of the cervix, hematometra, bilateral hematosalpinx.

E, Uterus bicornis unicollis, lateral hematometra in a blind rudimentary horn.

F, Uterus didelphys, lateral hematocolpometra due to a blind left vagina.

G, Uterus bicornis unicollis, lateral hematometra in a blind left horn.

H, Uterus septus duplex, lateral hematometra in a blind left uterine cavity.

I, Uterus didelphys, two rudimentary horns, hematometra due to gynatresia.

J, Acquired atresia of the cervix, intermittent hematocolpometra.

K, Acquired atresia of the cervix, hematometra, bilateral hematosalpinx.

L, Cervical fibromyoma, intermittent hematometra.

The first step is accurately to determine the extent of the disease and prepare for a combined vaginal and abdominal approach. A hematocolpos, as well as any accumulations of menstrual blood in blind horns or other structures that are accessible, should be aspirated (Plate 9, M). The ureters are catheterized, especially when large accumulations of blood or a known anomaly in the course or number of the ureters is present. As previously described under Surgical Principles and Treatment, the uterus should be evacuated under direct vision at laparotomy if there is any suspicion that the tubes are involved and adherent to the surrounding structures (Plate 9, N). Every case is different, but the guiding principle in young women is to save all useful and functional structures.

Prognosis

The uncomplicated hematocolpos is cured by hymenotomy, with return of the genital and urinary tracts to normal. Menstrual difficul-ties usually do not occur after the first few periods, and the urinary tract suffers no permanent damage. Later pregnancies have been regularly reported when the disease has been confined to the vagina. The prognosis is not good when a large bilateral hematosalpinx is found, for the salpinges suffer permanent damage. Many patients reported as sterile in later life had some form of irrigation or packing used in the treatment of a cryptomenorrhea.

Individual prognostication, based on the structures that can be spared at operation, must be made in the case of the various anomalies. The anomalies of duplication with unilateral involvement lend themselves to operations that spare some healthy ovarian and endometrial elements. In general, the prognosis is good regarding the relief of symptoms but poor in regard to pregnancy. The acquired disease responds favorably when the infection is controlled. Recurrences must be guarded against by periodic examinations.

References

Allen, B. D.: The Embryonic Development of the Ovary and Testis of the Mammals, Am. J. Anat. 3: 89, 1904.

Baldwin, J. F.: The Formation of an Artificial Vagina by Intestinal Transplantation, Ann. Surg. 40: 398, 1904.

Ball, T. L., and Douglas, R. G.: Cryptomenorrhea: Congenital and Acquired, Am. J. Surg. 78: 40, 1949.

Barrett, J. E., Peer, L. A., and Walia, L. S.: Tissue Transplant for Vaginal Reconstruction: The Buried Dermal Graft, Obst. & Gynec. 11: 70, 1958.

Bell, W. B.: The Nature of Haematocolpos Fluid, and the Character of the Obstructing Membrane, Lancet 1: 1269, 1911.

Benjamin, H.: Transsexualism and Transvestism as Psychosomatic and Somato-Psychic Syndromes in Transsexualism and Transvestism—A Symposium, Am. J. Psychotherapy 8: 219, 1954.

Benson, R. C., Kolb, F. O., and Traut, H. F.: Hirsutism, Defeminization, and Virilization, Obst. & Gynec. 5: 307, 1955.

Bisca, B. V.: Mesonephric Remnants in the Adult Female, Obst. & Gynec. 8: 265, 1956.

Bradbury, J. T., and Bunge, R. G.: Male Intersex With Ambiguous External Genitals and Well-Developed Mullerian Elements, Am. J. Obst. & Gynec. 80: 76, 1960.

Chapple, C. C.: Possible Mechanisms of Some Congenital Defects, Am. J. Obst. & Gynec. 70: 711, 1955.

Corner, G. W.: Abnormalities of the Mammalian Embryo Occurring Before Implantation, Contrib. Embryol. 13: 63, 1921.

Counseller, V. S., and Flor, F. S.: Congenital Absence of the Vagina; Further Results of Treatment and a New Technique, S. Clin. North America 37: 1107, 1957.

Deutsch, H.: The Psychology of Women, vol. 1, New York, 1944, Grune & Stratton, Inc.

Dougherty, C., and Thompson, J.: Adrenal Cortical and Leydig Cell Nodules in Dysgenetic Ovaries, Am. J. Obst. & Gynec. 80: 317, 1960.

Evans, T. N., and Riley, G. M.: Pseudohermaphroditism, Obst. & Gynec. 2: 363, 1953.

Fisher, J. J.: Surgical Unification of a Double Uterus; Case Report, Am. J. Obst. & Gynec. 81: 807, 1961.

Frank, R. T.: Formation of an Artificial Vagina Without Operation (Intubation Method), New York J. Med. 40: 1669, 1940.

Frazier, T. M.: A Note on Race-Specific Congenital Malformation Rates, Am. J. Obst. & Gynec. 80: 184, 1960.

Frost, I. F.: Case Report of a Patient With a True Unicornuate Uterus With Unilateral Renal Agencies, Am. J. Obst. & Gynec. 75: 210, 1958.

Genell, S., and Sjovall, A.: The Strassmann Operation, Acta obst. et gynec. scandinav. 38: 477, 1959.

Gerbie, A. B., Greene, R. R., and Reis, R. A.: Heteroplastic Bone and Cartilage in the Female Genital Tract, Obst. & Gynec. 11: 573, 1958.

Goldman, J. A., and Eckerling, B.: An Unusual Case of Rupture of a Pregnant Rudimentary Horn of a Bicornuate Uterus, Am. J. Obst. & Gynec. 78: 1205, 1959.

Gutheil, E. A.: The Psychologic Background of Transsexualism and Transvestism in Transsexualism and Transvestism—A Symposium, Am. J. Psychotherapy 8: 231, 1954.

Haddad, H. M., and Wilkins, L.: Congenital Anomalies of Gonadal Aplasia, Pediatrics 23: 885, 1959.

Hamburger, C., Sturup, G. K., and Dahl-Iversen, E.: Transvestism; Hormonal, Psychiatric, and Surgical Treatment, J. A. M. A. 152: 391, 1953.

Hervet, E.: Uterine Malformation; New Observations of Reparative Surgery (Malformation uterine; nouvelle observation d'operation reparatrice), Gynéc. et obst. 9: 504, 1957.

Hunter, W.: The Rectovesical Ligament in Association With Double Uterus, J. Obst. & Gynaec. Brit. Emp. 67: 429, 1960.

Jackson, G. W.: Primary Carcinoma of an Artificial Vagina, Obst. & Gynec. 14: 534, 1959.

Jarcho, J.: Malformations of Uterus, Am. J. Surg. 71: 106, 1946.

Johnston, G.: Vaginal Reconstruction After Radical Surgery for Rectal Carcinoma, Bull. Vancouver M. A. 35: 450, 1958.

Jones, H. W., and Jones, G. E. S.: The Gynecological Aspects of Adrenal Hyperplasia and Allied Disorders, Am. J. Obst. & Gynec. 68: 1330, 1954.

Jones, I. D.: Hematocolpos Simulating Acute Appendicitis, Lancet 1: 88, 1935.

Kiefer, J. H., and others: Management of the Intersex Patient, Illinois M. J. 112: 7, 1957.

Koff, A. K.: Development of the Vagina in the Human Fetus, Contrib. Embryol. 24: 61, 1933.

Mall, F. P.: On the Frequency of Localized Anomalies in Human Embryos and Infants at Birth, Am. J. Anat. 22: 27, 1917.

Merckel, G. C., Sucoff, M. C., and Sender, B.: The Syndrome of Dysmenorrhea and Unilateral Gynatresia in a Double Uterus, Am. J. Obst. & Gynec. 80: 70, 1960.

Meyer, R.: Lateral Hematocolpos With Incipient Engorgement of Uterine Horn and Tubes; Origin and Pathology of Congenital Occlusion, Zentralbl. Gynäk. 62: 1810, 1938.

Miller, N. F., and Stout, W.: Congenital Absence of the Vagina, Obst. & Gynec. 9: 48, 1957.

Miller, N. F., Wilson, J. R., and Collins, J.: Surgical Correction of Congenital Aplasia of the Vagina, Am. J. Obst. & Gynec. 50: 735, 1945.

Mitchell, J. S.: Some Aspects of the Chemistry of Hematocolpos Fluid, J. Obst. & Gynaec. Brit. Emp. 41: 390, 1934.

O'Sullivan, D.: Spontaneous Rupture of the Uterus Bicornis Unicollis Complicating Missed Abortion, J. Obst. & Gynaec. Brit. Emp. 65: 428, 1958.

Philipp, E., and Staemmler, H. J.: Geschwister und Zwillinge als männliche Scheinzwitter mit intersexuellem ausseren Genitale, Acta obst. et gynec. scandinav. 38: 645, 1959.

Pilkington, J. W.: Pregnancy and Spontaneous Delivery

Following Operation for Congenital Atresia of the Vagina, Am. J. Obst. & Gynec. 78: 804, 1959.

Pommerenke, W. T., and Benjamin, J. A.: Coexistence of Malformations of the Genital and Urinary Tracts in Women, New York J. Med. 47: 996, 1947.

Ramirez, D.: Vaginal Atresia: Its Treatment by the Use of Heteroplastic Homologous Transplant, Personal Technique of the Author, Ginec. y obst. México 8: 22, 1953.

Ricci, J. V.: The Genealogy of Gynaecology, Philadelphia, 1943, The Blakiston Co., pp. 227, 364, 399.

Riva, H. L., and Harding, R. L.: Vaginal Reconstruction, Obst. & Gynec. 4: 517, 1954.

Sargis, H., and others: Construction of a Functional Vagina; a New Surgical Approach in Congenital Absence of the Vagina, Am. J. Obst. & Gynec. 79: 67, 1960.

Semmens, J. P.: Uterus Didelphys and Septate Vagina; Review; Report of a Case With Gynatresis Right Vagina and Associated Hematoceles, Obst. & Gynec. 8: 620, 1956.

Sheares, B. H.: Congenital Atresia of the Vagina. A New Technique for Tunnelling the Space Between Bladder and Rectum and Construction of the New Vagina by a Modified Wharton Technique, J. Obst. & Gynaec. Brit. Emp. 67: 24, 1960.

Sosnowski, J. R.: Factors to Be Considered in the Treatment of Ovarian Agenesis, Am. J. Obst. & Gynec. 78: 792, 1959.

Southern, E. M.: Combined Strassmann Metroplasty and Bilateral Tuboplasty; Report of a Case Resulting in Normal Pregnancy, Obst. & Gynec. 17: 501, 1961.

Spaulding, M. K.: The Development of the External Genitalia in the Human Embryo, Contrib. Embryol. 13: 67, 1921.

Stange, H. H.: Gonadal Malformations and Their Relation to Tumor Formation (Ueber Fehlbildungen der Gonaden und ihre Bezeihung zur Geschwulstbildung), Geburtsh. u. Frauenh. 17: 63, 1957.

Steenstrup, O. R.: Congenital Uterine Anomalies and Pregnancy, Acta obst. & gynec. scandinav. 38: 143, 1959.

Stockard, C. R.: The Artificial Production of One-Eyed Monsters and Other Defects, Which Occur in Nature, by the Use of Chemicals, Anat. Rec. 3: 167, 1909.

Stoeckel, W.: Handbuch der Gynäkologie 5: 10, 1930.

Strassmann, E. O.: Plastic Unification of Double Uterus, Am. J. Obst. & Gynec. 64: 25, 1952.

Teter, J., and Tarlowski, R.: Tumors of the Gonads in Cases of Gonadal Dysgenesis and Male Pseudohermaphroditism, Am. J. Obst. & Gynec. 79: 321, 1960.

Wharton, L. R.: Congenital Malformations Associated With Developmental Defects of the Female Reproductive Organs, Am. J. Obst. & Gynec. 53: 37, 1947.

Wharton, L. R.: Congenital Absence of the Uterus and Associated Developmental Defects, Surg., Gynec. & Obst. 40: 31, 1925.

Wharton, L. R.: Two Cases of Supernumerary Ovary and One of Accessory Ovary, With an Analysis of Previously Reported Cases, Am. J. Obst. & Gynec. 78: 1101, 1959.

Wilkins, L.: The Diagnosis and Treatment of Endocrine Disorders in Childhood and Adolescence, Springfield, Ill., 1950, Charles C Thomas, Publisher.

Wilkins, L., and others: Further Studies on the Treatment of Congenital Adrenal Hyperplasia With Cortisone, J. Clin. Endocrinol. 12: 1015, 1952.

Wilson, T. M.: Retained Placenta Incarcerated in the Rudimentary Horn of a Double Uterus, Am. J. Obst. & Gynec. 70: 669, 1955.

Woolf, R. B., and Allen, W. M.: Concomitant Malformations. The Frequent, Simultaneous Occurrence of Congenital Malformations of the Reproductive and Urinary Tracts, Obst. & Gynec. 2: 236, 1953.

Worden, F. G., and Marsh, J. T.: Psychological Factors in Men Seeking Sex Transformation, J. A. M. A. 157: 1292, 1955.

Zuspan, F. P.: Testicular Feminizing Syndrome in Male Pseudohermaphroditism; a Report of Its Occurrence in Successive Siblings, Am. J. Obst. & Gynec. 80: 454, 1960.

4 · Psychosomatic Aspects of Gynecologic Surgery

"To a greater degree than any other physician the gynecologist is forced to be acquainted with the psychosomatic being of the woman instead of the pathological anatomy of the female genitalia. Departing from the usual cauterization, douching, and curetting which by focusing attention on the genital only makes the condition worse, we must come more and more to see and treat in many gynecological disturbances the expression of psychic disharmonies, especially of an erotic-sexual nature. Gynecologists, who for a long time were remarkable for their small knowledge of these things, show today a most decided revolution in their concepts of their discipline. A gynecologist who fails to see the effects of psychic disturbances in each situation is blind indeed."

—Dr. G. R. Heyer*

General Considerations

In gynecologic surgery the psychologic importance of the genital area cannot be overemphasized. This holds to almost the same extent for rectal and elective plastic surgery. Triebel, of the Westchester Division (Psychiatry) of the New York Hospital–Cornell Medical Center, has reported an excellent study of 300 emotionally disturbed women and the surgery to which they had been subjected. He found that the surgical rate among the disturbed women was 43 per cent as compared with 28 per cent in the carefully selected control group. The psychoneurotic group had had operations of all types at the rate of 65 per cent as compared with 23 per cent in matched controls. Furthermore, the psychoneurotic group tended to have multiple procedures. In each diagnostic category (that is, surgical specialty) the emotionally disturbed patients had a surgical rate significantly higher than the controls with the exception of the patients diagnosed as schizophrenics. More significant, however, was Triebel's finding that gynecologic and rectal procedures made up 44 per cent of the operations performed on the emotionally disturbed women, while these procedures constituted only 20 per cent of the surgery performed on the control group!

Symptoms from a gynecologic illness are invariably modified by a woman's emotional reaction to trouble in the genital area. The psychiatrically oriented gynecologist determines the extent to which a complaint is frankly on a psychoneurotic basis before he ever considers surgery. If this is not done he will find that many of the patients will have an increase in their symptoms postoperatively or will transfer their complaints to another organ system. Triebel offers several hypotheses to explain the higher rate of surgical procedures among women with emotional problems: (1) Emotionally ill individuals may have more disease as a result of some constitutional inferiority, or the organic lesions may arise from the somatic effects of psychic events. (2) Disturbed patients may have an increased response to the organic disease that would be of little concern to a more stable person. (3) The emotionally ill patient may expect more from a surgical procedure, or the meaning of the operation in the psychosexual sphere may have an interpretation far removed from that of her better-oriented sister.

The dynamisms involved may operate in

*From Heyer, G.: Das korperlich-seelische Zusammenwirken in den Lebensvorgangen. An Hand klinischer und experimenteller Tatsachen dargestellt, München, 1935, J. F. Bergmann. (Grenzfragen d. Nerven- und Seelenlebens, Heft 121.)

several ways. Women like to blame their complaints on a socially acceptable organic disease. They may want to regress and be cared for. On a deeper psychologic level there may be some masochistic factor in a genital operation. The preference for gynecologic and rectal operations points out the symbolic meaning of this surgery.

Psychotherapy by the Gynecologic Surgeon

Initial rapport is established with the patient during the interview prior to examination. Preconceived ideas that she has come to the gynecologist for surgery should be considerately dismissed pending the examination and the results of other studies. Ventilation of her feelings about the genital complaints is left until after the examination so that the surgeon can weigh the organic findings against the psychosexual aspects. The surgeon then prompts the patient to discuss the development of her symptoms, which is a means of allowing her to ventilate freely. Most patients respond to this technique with information the extent of which is limited only by the gynecologist's time. One's suspicions regarding the importance of the emotional factors are easily aroused at this point, and the time for reassurance has arrived. A few additional appointments with inquiry into the patient's life history may suggest that psychotherapy should be tried before any suggestion of surgery for the illness is made. The greatest satisfaction awaits the gynecologic surgeon who recommends surgery only after psychosomatic evaluation of the patient's complaints. Postoperative management is easier and the patient will be more appreciative of her physician's studied surgical judgment.

Psychosomatic Aspects of Spontaneous and Missed Abortions

Many women do not want a pregnancy for a variety of reasons and react by becoming tense and resentful. Study of patients who habitually abort has reawakened interest by obstetricians and psychiatrists in the psychopathologic mechanisms by which a deeply resentful woman manages to induce an abortion or cause the death of the fetus in utero. Pregnancy, delivery, and post-partum period, which consume a year of the patient's life and involve possible complications, have psychologic significance to the normal woman. The implications to the psychoneurotic woman have a correspondingly greater effect. Conscious and unconscious reasons determine the psychoneurotic patient's attitude toward a pregnancy, but most frequently a combination of situations exists. The conscious reasons are often economic, fear of responsibility or disfigurement, and fears based on misinformation and superstitions. Illegitimacy has been indicted by many, but this cause does not stand critical analysis, for few unwed mothers spontaneously abort. There must be deeply hidden reasons for this observation made by many of us. The unconscious reasons for a woman not wanting a pregnancy are usually related to the phobic and compulsive-obsessive tendencies in her psychoneurotic illness. She may subject herself to numerous examinations and treatments in order to conceive as soon as possible—and then promptly abort. The combination of sterility and habitual abortion, without organic cause, should alert the obstetrician to the possibility of a deeply disturbed patient. Resentment of and hostility to the husband are commonly found. Fear of harming the infant after birth and the husband's reaction to the child are ideas often expressed. The role of the husband and his resentment of the pregnancy should not be forgotten. I have delivered a patient, however, where just the opposite was true in regard to the husband. He had a severe psychoneurosis with a history of suicides among the male members of his family for many generations. He was infanticidal and quietly announced he would destroy the child and himself. On the advice of the director of a large psychiatric clinic, the child was carefully secluded after delivery and given out for adoption. The mother, who did not resent the pregnancy, was in the latter years of the childbearing span and had multiple large fibroids, yet carried to term without incident!

The inference is not to be drawn that all psychoneurotics abort and that patients who habitually abort are all psychoneurotics. Nor should it be inferred that psychoneurotics cannot have organic disease that causes the abortion. What is important is that we evaluate the emotional problems of pregnancy in both the well-adjusted and the psychoneurotic woman so that we can treat the minor problems and help the psychiatrists manage the severe disturbances.

Emotional Reaction to Hysterectomy

The genital organs are so highly invested with symbolic meaning that disease or injury to the genital tract causes more anxiety than disorders in organs not concerned with childbearing. Many patients who have had a full and active sexual life, with several children, are not distressed by the loss of the uterus or any of their reproductive organs. Women have peculiar ideas relative to the intensity of sexual life after hysterectomy. Patients necessitating this operation should be educated in this regard. Sturgis and associates at The Peter Bent Brigham Hospital have an excellent study in progress among posthysterectomy patients. They are examined daily by a psychologist who limits his questioning to several fields. Sociability is studied by observation and by questioning the patient regarding the desire to be left alone or her enthusiasm for visits from relatives and friends. The patient's interest in the progress of other hysterectomy patients is noted. The activity-passivity of the convalescent is evaluated by observations and by inquiry into her desire to try to do things for herself or, on the contrary, to assume a condition of helplessness. Her interest in radio and television, in activities on the ward, and in volunteering for duties to help the more critically ill patients is noted. Her general morale is observed. Simple questions regarding the patient's progress are significant in revealing her attitude toward this emotionally laden surgical procedure. Some patients reveal outright anxiety and are tense, worried, and unrelaxed with the usual postoperative care.

They may or may not have been prepared for this assault on their genital organs and, more important, their sexuality. The reaction of some patients is that of anger and resentment toward the entire surgical procedure.

Patients whose postoperative course was complicated by abnormal physiology reacted to discussions in several fields of study with a statistically significant lower rating. Some patients were reported to be so stunned by the significance of the operation as to become confused. It must be presumed that they were not properly oriented preoperatively. A patient who manifested paranoid behavior on the sixth postoperative day provided some studies into the primitive fantasies that may accompany operations on the uterus or other genital organs. Examinations, operation, anesthesia, and medications were perceived as annihilation of her genital organs and sexual attacks. The operation was regarded as a successful attempt to change her sex. Some of the preoperative examinations were regarded as impregnation or actual childbirth. As a result of therapy she gained control of her panic but became depressed over her future inability to have children. While the postoperative depression is disappointing, it is better than the original paranoid reaction.

The female genitalia, rectum, and breasts are the areas most frequently involved in female surgical addicts. The pelvic bandits of a different era have not all been brought to law and order. There are still too many women being subjected to gynecologic surgery without being sick organically. Innumerable complaints are in the realm of wish fulfillment. The examination and incidental manipulations are closely related in these patients to repressed wishes such as exhibitionism. Women are free under the cover of surgery to use this self-deception to break through the normal taboos on such conduct. These patients are readily recognized, and a short interview will usually reveal them to be seriously disturbed. They frequently require extensive psychotherapy or psychoanalysis.

Sequence and Management of Emotional Reactions in Gynecologic Cancer

The worst possible approach in the psychosomatic management of the cancer patient is to permit a curtain of silence to fall between the gynecologist and the patient. The frankness with which one can deal with different patients varies considerably. It is here that the psychiatrically oriented gynecologist can relieve much mental anguish. Sutherland divides the sequence of emotional reactions to cancer into three phases: (1) the anticipatory phase, (2) the operative phase, and (3) the reparative phase. In the anticipatory phase he points out that you cannot have a standard doctor, a standard cancer, a standard patient, a standard operation, a standard postoperative course, and a standard prognosis. Each patient must be told of her condition on an individual basis. The case for the deliberate, cultivated lie in incurable cancer has been debated many times. Regardless of how stoic a patient may seem during the first interview, certain stress situations may be brought out during subsequent examinations that will make it questionable whether in best judgment a patient should be informed of the extent of the disease and the inevitable outcome. The morale of some patients will always suffer if they are told frankly that they have cancer. For these patients, one learns to talk around the truth, and most persons appreciate the surgeon's consideration in this game of deception. However, the patient's common sense and courage should not be underestimated, and certainly her personal affairs need to be in order when the terminal phase of her illness becomes evident.

The significance of the female genital organs and the necessity for mutilating surgery to attack the primary cancer often result in very serious emotional disturbances. Frequently there is a feeling of guilt and punishment since an organ whose use was frequently forbidden in early life is to be removed. A woman who was well adapted to her feminine role may now find that her basic patterns are disrupted and that she must adopt some other patterns, even though they are frankly neurotic, in order to restore her emotional equilibrium. Interpretive psychotherapy will reveal whether the patient is going to accept her illness realistically. Her activity is directed in general toward the attainment of pleasure and the avoidance of pain (the pleasure-pain principle of dynamic psychiatry). Patients attempt to avoid psychic trauma by delaying treatment. Seriously disturbed patients avoid facing their illness realistically by denying the existence of illness or the necessity of treatment. They are most difficult to handle postoperatively. The patient's anxiety can be relieved to some extent by a sympathetic surgeon who has established good rapport and minimizes the mutilating aspects of the operation so far as is consistent with what has to be done. Even before operation patients are prepared and encouraged to resume their usual life activities in the face of what inconveniences the surgery may create. The patient's anxiety reaches a peak during the preparation for the operation and in the immediate postoperative period. It is at such times that the patient should be seen frequently by the surgeon so she senses his protective attitude toward her. Postoperatively the patient naturally reviews the physical alterations and wonders how she can resume her former life.

In visiting the patient the gynecologist encourages the free expression of the patient's impulses and continues to minimize any feelings of guilt. Despite this, some patients will react beyond the usual anxiety associated with genital surgery and go on to a depressive, hypochondriacal, compulsive, or paranoid reaction. In some of these patients it will not be feasible to continue the nonspecific psychotherapy that does not inquire deeply into the patient's emotional substructure. Specific psychotherapy may be required if the severe reaction persists or shows signs of becoming frankly psychotic.

The security a patient may obtain from her family depends on the relationship they had prior to her illness. Sutherland divides the type of family support into three groups: supportive, ambivalent, and hostile. Where the family relationship, particularly between the wife and her husband, has been warm and trusting, the patient will return to an atmosphere where she is well tolerated. If the partners in the marriage have been indifferent to each other, the patient returns home to an atmosphere where she can expect little help from her husband. If the marital union has degenerated to the point where there is a frankly hostile relationship, the woman will return to a home where her husband immediately tries to transfer the responsibility for her care to some other person or to an agency and will have as little as possible to do with her. The gynecologist evaluates the environment into which the patient is going to return. When the patient is not going to have much support from the family, agencies and other means are utilized to help provide for the patient. The gynecologist's responsibility in the management of genital cancer never ceases, and he must continue to support the patient even should her disease progress to death. The patient should never be avoided or abandoned, and all of the skill and wisdom of the surgeon should be brought to her support by relieving pain through the skillful use of drugs and other methods of palliation.

References

Abramson, M., and Torghele, J. R.: Weight, Temperature Changes, and Psychosomatic Symptomatology in Relation to the Menstrual Cycle, Am. J. Obst. & Gynec. 81: 223, 1961.

Bard, M.: The Sequence of Emotional Reactions in Radical Mastectomy Patients, Pub. Health Rep. 67: 1144, 1952.

Bennett, A.: Prevention of Suicide, California Med. 81: 396, 1954.

Benson, R. C., and Hanson, K. H.: Atypical Pelvic Pain in Women: Gynecological-Psychiatric Considerations, Am. J. Obst. & Gynec. 77: 806, 1959.

Blaikley, J. B.: Psychogenic Menorrhagia, J. Obst. & Gynaec. Brit. Emp. 66: 786, 1959.

Blumberg, E., West, P., and Ellis, F.: A Possible Relationship Between Psychological Factors and Human Cancer, Psychosom. Med. 16: 277, 1954.

Bozeman, M., Orbach, C., and Sutherland, A.: Psychological Impact of Cancer and Its Treatment. III. The Adaption of Mothers to the Threatened Loss of Their Children Through Leukemia, Parts I and II, Cancer 8: 1, 1955.

Cantor, A., and Fox, A. (editors): Psychosomatic Aspects of Surgery, New York, 1956, Grune & Stratton, Inc.

Cohen, H.: Psychiatric Aspects of Childbearing, Yale J. Biol. & Med. 16: 77, 1943.

Deutsch, H.: Psychology of Women; a Psychoanalytic Interpretation, vol. 2, New York, 1945, Grune & Stratton, Inc.

Deutsch, H.: Some Psychoanalytic Observations in Surgery, Psychosom. Med. 4: 105, 1942.

Diddle, A.: Emotional Stress and Female Disorders. Sociologic Influences, Obst. & Gynec. 2: 353, 1953.

Diethelm, O.: Treatment in Psychiatry, ed. 3, Springfield, Ill., 1955, Charles C Thomas, Publisher.

Donovan, J.: Psychologic Aspects of the Menopause, Obst. & Gynec. 6: 379, 1955.

Dunbar, F.: Emotions and Bodily Changes, ed. 4, New York, 1954, Columbia University Press.

Ebaugh, F.: Psychosomatic Medicine; A Review, International Forum, vol. 2, No. 3, March, 1954, Parke, Davis & Co.

Engel, George L.: Medical Psychology and Psychopathology, Lectures at the University of Rochester, School of Medicine and Dentistry (mimeographed outline), Rochester, N. Y., 1954 (revised).

Foundeur, M., Fixsen, C., and Triebel, W. A.: Postpartum Mental Illness: A Controlled Study, A. M. A. Arch. Neurol. & Psychiat. 77: 503, 1957.

Frankl-Hochwart and Zuckerkandl, O.: Die nervosen Erkrankungen der Harnblase, Vienna, 1906, Alfred Hölder.

Geijerstam, G. A.: The Psychosomatic Approach in Gynaecological Practice, Acta obst. et gynec. scandinav. 39: 346, 1960.

Gengerelli, J., and Kirkner, F.: The Psychological Variables in Human Cancer, Los Angeles, 1954, University of California Press.

Gerard, R. W.: Anxiety and Tension, Bull. New York Acad. Med. 34: 429, 1958.

Gidro-Frank, L., Gordon, T., and Taylor, H. C., Jr.: Pelvic Pain and Female Identity, Am. J. Obst. & Gynec. 79: 1184, 1960.

Giffin, M.: Psychosomatic Aspects of Gynecology, Obst. & Gynec. 5: 382, 1955.

Greaves, D. C., Green, P. E., and West, L. J.: Psychodynamic and Physiologic Aspects of Pseudocyesis, Psychosomat. Med. 22: 24, 1960.

Heiman, M.: Psychological Aspects of Uterine Bleeding, Obst. & Gynec. 7: 234, 1956.

Heiman, M., and Shapiro, W.: Postmenopausal Uterine Bleeding of Psychogenic Origin, Am. J. Obst. & Gynec. 79: 11, 1960.

Henry, G.: Essentials of Psychopathology, Baltimore, 1935, William Wood & Co.

Heyer, G.: Hypnose und Hypnotherapie. In: Die psychischen Heilmethoden, Hrsg. von Karl Birnbaum, Leipzig, 1927, Georg Thieme, pp. 73-135.

Hollender, M.: A Study of Patients Admitted to a Psychiatric Hospital After Pelvic Operations, Am. J. Obst. & Gynec. 79: 498, 1960.

Johnson, A. M., and Robinson, D. B.: The Sexual Deviant (Sexual Psychopath)—Causes, Treatment and Prevention, J. A. M. A. 164: 1957.

Johnstone, J. W.: Psychogenic Amenorrhea, J. Obst. & Gynaec. Brit. Emp. 66: 774, 1959.

Kraines, S.: Treatment of Psychiatric States Following Pregnancy, Illinois M. J. 80: 200, 1942.

Kroeger, W.: Psychosomatic Aspects of Obstetrics and Gynecology, Obst. & Gynec. 3: 504, 1954.

Kroger, W., and Freed, S.: Psychosomatic Gynecology, Philadelphia, 1951, W. B. Saunders Co.

Mackay, R., and others: The Year Book of Neurology, Psychiatry and Neurosurgery, Chicago, 1955-1956, The Year Book Publishers, Inc.

Mann, E.: Psychiatric Investigation of Habitual Abortion, Obst. & Gynec. 7: 589, 1956.

Menninger, K.: Polysurgery and Polysurgical Addiction, Psychoanalyt. Quart. 3: 173, 1934.

Montassut, M., Chertok, L., and Aboulker, P.: De quelques investigations psychiatriques en urologie, Semaine hôp. Paris 27: 3002, 1951.

Orbach, C., and Sutherland, A.: Acute Depressive Reactions to Surgical Treatment for Cancer. In Hoch, P., and Zubin, J. (editors): Depression; the Proceedings of the Forty-Second Annual Meeting of the

Psycho-pathological Association, held in New York City, June, 1952, New York, 1954, Grune & Stratton, Inc.

Ordway, M., and McIntire, A.: Mental Disorders Associated With Pregnancy and the Puerperium, New England J. Med. 226: 969, 1942.

Patterson, R. M., and others: Social and Medical Characteristics of Hysterectomized and Nonhysterectomized Psychiatric Patients, Obst. & Gynec. 15: 209, 1960.

Piker, P.: Psychoses Complicating Childbearing, Am. J. Obst. & Gynec. 35: 901, 1938.

Pleshette, N., Asch, S., and Chase, J.: A Study of Anxieties During Pregnancy, Labor, the Early and Later Puerperium, Bull. New York Acad. Med. 32: 436, 1956.

Rangell, L.: Psychiatric Aspects of Pain, Psychosom. Med. 15: 22, 1955.

Robbins, F.: Psychosomatic Aspects of Dysmenorrhea, Am. J. Obst. & Gynec. 66: 808, 1953.

Schwarz, O.: Psychogene Miktionsstorungen. In Schwarz, O.: Psychogenese und Psychotherapie korperlicher Symptome, Vienna, 1925, Julius Springer, p. 273.

Smalldon, J.: A Survey of Mental Illness Associated With Pregnancy and Childbirth, Am. J. Psychiat. 97: 80, 1940.

Solomon, H.: Psychiatric Implications of Cancer, Rocky Mountain M. J. 44: 801, 1947.

Stephenson, J., and Grace, W.: Life Stress and Cancer of the Cervix, Psychosom. Med. 16: 287, 1954.

Sturgis, S., and others: Anesthesia Recovery Patterns After Elective Hysterectomy, Obst. & Gynec. 7: 363, 1956.

Sturgis, S., and others: Gynecologic-Psychiatric Unit, Peter Bent Brigham Hospital, Third Annual Report, Boston, 1955, The Commonwealth Fund.

Sutherland, A.: Psychological Impact of Cancer Surgery, Pub. Health Rep. 67: 1139, 1952.

Sutherland, A.: The Sequence of Emotional Reactions in Cancer and Its Treatment. (Personal communication and lectures in the Sloan-Kettering Division, Cornell University Medical College.)

Triebel, W.: A Survey of General Surgical Procedures in a Group of Emotionally Disturbed Women Patients, New York J. Med. 55: 2188, 1955.

Ulett, P., and Gildea, E.: Survey of Surgical Procedures in Psychoneurotic Women, J. A. M. A. 143: 960, 1950.

Von Felsinger, J., Lasagna, L., and Beecher, H.: Drug-induced Mood Changes in Man, J. A. M. A. 157: 1113, 1955.

Wolf, H., and Wolf, S.: Pain, Springfield, Ill., 1948, Charles C Thomas, Publisher.

Worden, F., and Marsh, J.: Psychological Factors in Men Seeking Sex Transformation, J. A. M. A. 157: 1292, 1955.

Yaskin, J.: Some Psychiatric Problems in Obstetrics and Gynecology, M. Clin. North America 29: 1508, 1945.

Zilboorg, G.: The Clinical Issues of Postpartum Psycho-pathological Reactions, Am. J. Obst. & Gynec. 73: 305, 1957.

Section III · INFECTIOUS, TROPHIC, and DERMATOLOGIC CONDITIONS

5 · Venereal Diseases

General Considerations

Because of the alarming increase of venereal diseases among the teen-age group now being reported by several public health agencies, a new look must be taken at this problem. Statistics being compiled reflect the lack of diligence by many groups within the profession that was engendered by the effectiveness of antimicrobial therapy. In addition to specific treatment, we must return to the tested methods of case finding to bring the problem under control.

Specific surgical procedures are not applicable to the treatment of the venereal diseases, but their complications may require anything from a simple incision and drainage to extensive bowel surgery. The recognition of the various lesions and the diagnosis of the venereal diseases after they are masked by inadequate therapy are of increasing importance.

SYPHILIS
General Considerations

Syphilis is an infectious disease that is first generalized, then localized, and finally dispersed to involve many organs of the body. The period of blood stream invasion is without severe systemic symptoms and is followed by a slow progression of the localized lesions.

Etiology and Pathologic Anatomy

Treponema pallidum, an actively motile, thin, spiral organism, is the cause of syphilis. It is distinguished from other spiral organisms by its characteristic motility patterns in a wet-field preparation. Fixed tissue specimens can be used for identification only by inference. The lesions with which the gynecologist is concerned from a surgical point of view are the primary chancres, regional lymphadenopathy, the secondary skin lesions, and condyloma lata. Lymphadenitis due to syphilis does not go on to suppuration unless it occurs in conjunction with some other disease. There is nothing so characteristic about the chancre that permits its positive identification from similar lesions. It is indurated, circumscribed, and usually painless. There tend to be multiple lesions in the female genitalia, and these are believed to be metastatic. The breasts may be the site of the primary infection. Secondary involvement of the mucous membranes of the genitalia may give rise to the hypertrophic, papular, or more often flat, raised nodule called condyloma latum. It must be distinguished from the condyloma acuminatum or genital wart, and about the anus such papules may simulate hemorrhoidal tabs or other minor rectal pathologic conditions. The many other lesions of infectious, early and late latent, and late syphilis are beyond the scope of a text of gynecologic surgery. At no time, however, in the diagnosis of pelvic lesions should this disease be dismissed as the cause or source of complications without appropriate study.

Symptoms and Diagnosis

The diagnosis of infectious syphilis, regardless of how characteristic the lesions appear, can be done only by dark-field microscopy. A persistently positive serologic test in the presence of a suspicious lesion that responds promptly to antisyphilitic treatment is presumptive evidence that the patient is syphilitic. The many tests used by syphilologists in the diagnosis and management of the disease beyond the infectious stage do not concern the surgeon.

Treatment of Infectious Syphilis

The intramuscular injection at multiple sites of a total dose of 2.4 million units of benzathine penicillin G fortified with procaine penicillin G is considered adequate therapy and relapses are uncommon. The extraordinary sensitivity of *Treponema pallidum* to penicillin is so well established that other drugs are considered only for penicillin-sensitive patients. The lesions in the female genitalia promptly respond, with some scarring and contracture about the larger ones. Some types of hypertrophic vulvitis and proliferative lesions about the vulva that have been vaguely related to syphilis require excision for cosmetic reasons. It is probable that these lesions are the result of uncleanliness or chronic skin infections, although the number of patients with positive serologic reactions is unusually high.

GONORRHEA
General Considerations

Gonorrhea is the most prevalent of the venereal infections. Robbed of its former terror by the advent of penicillin and wide-spectrum antibiotics, fear has been replaced by disdain, and apparently an increase in sexual promiscuity by the youth of the nation is resulting in an increase in the disease among the younger age groups. This fact has been recently revealed in studies by the United States Public Health Service, the World Health Organization, American Social Hygiene Association, and state and local public health agencies.

Etiology and Pathologic Anatomy

Gonorrhea is caused by the gonococcus *(Neisseria gonorrhoeae)*, a gram-negative, kidney-shaped diplococcus seen both extracellularly and intracellularly within the cytoplasm of polymorphonuclear leukocytes. The primary foci in the female are in the cervix and urethra. From these sites the disease may spread to involve other organs, particularly those with serosal or synovial surfaces. The extragenital complications of the disease are rare because of the availability of penicillin and other antibiotics.

The internal os serves as the dividing line between lower and upper genital tract gonorrhea. The infection in the lower tract involves those structures with columnar epithelium and particularly glands with poor drainage. In acute lower tract disease the cervix is most commonly involved, followed by the terminal urethra, Bartholin's glands, and the anus. The tenacious secretion of the cervix, together with its compound tubuloracemose glands and small ducts, makes it the natural site for acute and chronic involvement of the lower genital tract. Acute gonorrheal cervicitis is manifested by an enlarged, inflamed, and tender cervix exuding a profuse purulent discharge. Acute urethritis is characterized by a purulent discharge, swelling, and a granular appearance of the external meatus. Skene's glands are subsequently involved, with reddish macules appearing about the duct openings. Acute bartholinitis is accompanied by swelling, fluctuation, and regional lymphadenopathy. Gonorrheal proctitis involves only the lower 4 to 6 cm. of the anorectum. It is manifested by a diffuse reddening and swelling, with subsequent localization in the anal crypts. Chronic lower genital tract gonorrhea persists in glands and ducts with inadequate drainage. Skene's ducts, the paraurethral glands, the cervix uteri, Bartholin's gland and duct, and the anal crypts may harbor chronic foci of infection. Most of the chronic abscesses of Bartholin's glands are not gonorrheal in origin, although they may have been infected at some previous time by the specific organism. Mediolateral episiotomies, infected lacerations of the perineum, and occlusions of the ducts by a perineorrhaphy probably cause more cysts and abscesses of these glands than does venereal infection.

Prompt treatment has reduced the incidence of upper tract gonorrhea. Particularly have the antibiotics reduced the amount of probing, examining, douching, heating, and other means formerly employed in the treatment of the lower tract disease. These only increased the chances of dissemination to the upper tract. A transitory gonorrheal endometritis occurs that does not go beyond the endometrium unless the uterus is invaded or a combined pyogenic and specific inflammation occurs with a parametritis. Gonorrheal salpingitis is almost always bilateral and follows the lower tract infection in a few weeks. The part played by regurgitation of endometrial debris into the tube can only be surmised from the observation that many acute gonorrheal pelvic infections immediately follow a menstrual period. The infection involves the endosalpinx, which becomes reddened, congested, and swollen. The muscular layers are also involved, and a perisalpingitis develops. The tube does not remain a reservoir of gonorrhea for long, as repeated cultures at surgery have shown. If the fimbria becomes swollen and closed early in the disease, a pyosalpinx develops that readily falls into, and becomes adherent in, the cul-de-sac. Pus pouring out of the open end of a tube involves the ovary and adjacent peritoneum, and as the abscess is walled off, the typical tubo-ovarian mass develops. Secondary organisms replace the gonococcus in the chronic phase of the infection. The acute exacerbations of the disease are more often due to nonspecific pyogenic organisms. Attempts at abortion, uterine manipulation, dilatation and curettage, cauterization of the cervix, sterility studies and hysterosalpin-

gography, and operative interference may result in an acute pelvic inflammatory disease. With each attack the adhesions become more dense, until the uterus and adnexa are adherent to the bowel, omentum, and bladder. The finding of adhesions in the upper abdomen (proof of a generalized gonorrheal peritonitis) has become rare since the advent of specific and effective therapy.

Symptoms and Diagnosis

An initial attack of gonorrhea is characterized by the discharge of thick, yellow pus from the cervix and urethra. The terminal urethra becomes swollen and edematous, and pus can be expressed from the paraurethral glands. In some patients there is an acute bartholinitis or proctitis, with pain referred to the affected areas. Smears taken from the cervix, urethra, Skene's glands, or Bartholin's glands are individually spread and cultured. Cultures are more reliable than a spread, and fermentation tests are done if there are medicolegal aspects to the case.

Upper tract gonorrhea in the acute phase or during an acute exacerbation causes lower abdominal pain, chills and fever, and nausea and vomiting. Frequently there are vaginal discharge and painful urination. Examination reveals bilateral lower abdominal tenderness. Involvement of the parietal peritoneum causes rebound tenderness and rigidity. More extensive peritonitis is characterized by distention and a paralytic ileus. Movement of the cervix causes pain, and the fornices are tense. A tubo-ovarian mass may be palpable on one or both sides and is exceedingly tender. The degree of fixation of the uterus and adnexa depends on the number and severity of the attacks. A large abscess or bilateral tubo-ovarian abscesses may point in the cul-de-sac or lower abdomen. Involvement of the pelvic ureter results in a periureteritis, pyelonephritis, or obstruction with the usual symptoms of these complications.

Chronic pelvic inflammatory disease is not due to the gonococcus but to secondary invaders. Acute exacerbations are due to reinfection by the gonococcus rather than to organisms that subsist in the tube or in other chronic foci of infection. Recurrent lower abdominal pain is the common complaint, although the degree of pain reported by the patient does not necessarily parallel the extent of the disease. Menstruation may be prolonged or irregular and may be accompanied by an increase in pelvic discomfort. Vesical and rectal symptoms occur but are related with difficulty to specific findings in the pelvis. Endometriosis is frequently superimposed on pelvic inflammatory disease and makes the symptomatology even more bizarre. Sterility or an ectopic gestation may bring the patient to the gynecologist. Physical examination during the quiescent phases of the disease reveals the adnexa to be adherent in the cul-de-sac, irregular in outline, and tender. In advanced disease, the uterus, vesicouterine reflection of the peritoneum, sigmoid and small bowel, peritoneum of the cul-de-sac, omentum, cecum, and appendix are bound together with the adnexa to form a tender fixed mass that simulates the frozen pelvis of extensive pelvic malignancy.

Treatment

A single dose of 600,000 units of benzathine penicillin G fortified with procaine penicillin G will cure 95 per cent of the patients in the acute phase of the disease. Cultures and smears are repeated at weekly intervals to confirm the effectiveness of the therapy. Patients sensitive to penicillin are treated with one of the wide-spectrum antibiotics. Tetracycline or one of its derivatives, 0.5 Gm. every six hours for two days, results in a comparable response. Patients with acute upper tract gonorrhea require hospitalization so that general supportive measures as well as specific therapy can be instituted. Complete bed rest in a low Fowler's position is advised for several days until the acute phase is over and the temperature curve flattens out. Sedation and analgesics are given and hot packs are applied to the abdomen.

Chronic pelvic inflammatory disease requires surgery when the pelvic discomfort or menstrual difficulties become incapacitating. Intes-

tinal obstruction and rupture of a tubo-ovarian abscess are surgical emergencies. Operations to restore tubal patency in patients with chronically infected tubes are still done by those not discouraged by the futility of these procedures. Various operations, such as cornual resection, salpingectomy, salpingo-oophorectomy, release of adhesions, and hysterectomy, can be performed. The age of the patient and degree of incapacity will determine whether ovarian and menstrual functions can be preserved by conservative surgery.

Surgical Principles

1. A long and intensive course of antibiotic therapy is given prior to surgery. A combination of penicillin and one of the wide-spectrum antimicrobials can be given for ten to fourteen days before operation unless there is a surgical emergency.

2. The ureters are catheterized, and No. 6 ureteral catheters are left in place during the operation.

3. The blind and inept scooping out of tubo-ovarian masses adherent in the cul-de-sac is surgically unsound. Whenever possible, the adhesions are lysed by sharp dissection under direct vision and with positive identification of the surrounding structures (Plate 10, *A*).

4. Culdoscopy is done preoperatively in the less advanced cases or where the feasibility of a tubal plastic procedure is in doubt. The culdoscopic views seen in a patient with extensive tube involvement are shown in Plate 10, *B* and *C*. The tubes were hopelessly involved for any type of procedure except, perhaps, a snorkel-type of operation, where the cornual end of the tube is allowed to project into the uterine cavity after the rest of the tube is resected and the ovary sutured to the cornu of the uterus.

5. In advanced disease the ureters are mobilized and positively identified at the brim of the pelvis (Plate 10, *D*) before attempting the dissection of fixed and firm masses of inflammatory tissue deep in the pelvis. Injury to the ureter is avoided since it can be followed during the operation until it enters the bladder.

CHANCROID
General Considerations

Chancroid (soft chancre, ulcus molle) is a venereal disease involving the external genitalia and lymph nodes. It is seen most frequently

PLATE 10

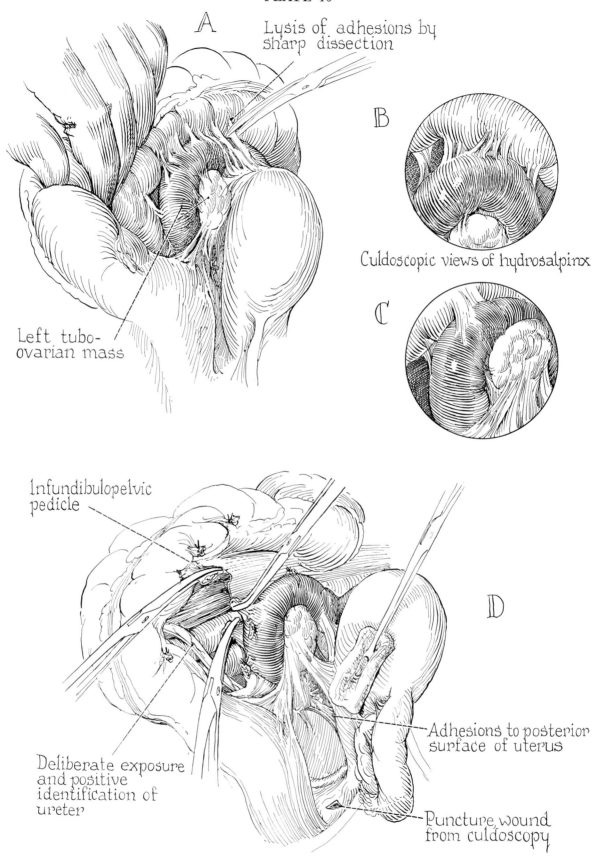

A

Lysis of adhesions by sharp dissection

B

Culdoscopic views of hydrosalpinx

C

Left tubo-ovarian mass

Infundibulopelvic pedicle

D

Adhesions to posterior surface of uterus

Deliberate exposure and positive identification of ureter

Puncture wound from culdoscopy

among persons with poor personal hygiene. Its differential diagnosis from syphilis is the most important consideration since it responds to many antimicrobial agents and abundant use of soap and water.

Etiology and Pathology

Chancroid is caused by the *Hemophilus ducreyi,* a minute gram-negative bacillus, 1 to 2 microns in length. The organisms are arranged in pairs, chains, or "fish school" formations as seen in stained material from the chancre. It can be grown on special media (Dienst's media) provided the lesion has not been contaminated by many secondary invaders. The histologic picture is used to distinguish the lesion from tuberculosis, syphilis, and cancer. The typical lesion develops from two to fourteen days after exposure and begins as a small, red papule on the vulva. The papule enlarges, becomes purulent and then necrotic, and finally ulcerates, with surrounding erythema and edema. The edges of the ulcer are undermined. The regional nodes are enlarged and matted, become secondarily invaded, and may go on to suppuration and abscess formation.

Symptoms and Diagnosis

The patient complains of a swollen and tender ulceration on some part of the genitalia. The inguinal lymph nodes may be involved and are swollen, tender, and matted together. Smears and cultures of the primary lesion are done. Dark-field examinations are performed to exclude syphilis. The bacillary antigen of Sanderson and Greenblatt is useful, particularly if the test is negative. An intradermal injection of 0.1 ml. is given on the skin of the forearm. An indurated area of at least 7 mm., surrounded by an area of erythema again as large, is considered positive. This reaction may take several weeks to develop, so its usefulness is limited since some type of specific treatment will have been initiated.

Treatment

Sulfonamides are used if syphilis cannot be positively excluded. The wide-spectrum anti-biotics are spirocheticidal and would further confuse the diagnosis of syphilis—the important consideration. Sulfadiazine or Gantrisin, 1 Gm. four times a day for ten days, cures almost all cases. When syphilis is excluded the wide-spectrum antibiotics can be given in doses of 500 mg. four times a day for ten days. The vulva and inguinal regions are kept clean with soap and water to prevent autoinoculation. Fluctuant buboes are aspirated when they become tense and painful. They should not be incised or drained. Streptomycin and penicillin have not been as consistently effective as the drugs mentioned.

LYMPHOGRANULOMA VENEREUM
General Considerations

Lymphogranuloma venereum (lymphopathia venereum, climatic bubo) is a virus disease of venereal transmission characterized by a vulval lesion associated with inguinal adenitis and proctitis. It is less frequent among females than males, and it is not limited to, nor does it have a predilection for, the Negro. Esthiomene and elephantiasis vulvae are probably manifestations of this disease and not separate entities as previously thought.

Etiology and Pathologic Anatomy

Lymphogranuloma venereum is transmitted by sexual contact. The agent is intermediate between a virus and rickettsial body and is tentatively placed with the psittacosis-lymphogranuloma group. The antigenic interrelationships and common susceptibility to certain antimicrobial agents warrant this assumption pending further clarification. After an incubation period of three to twenty days the initial lesion appears as a macule, papule, or ulcer. It is noticed by accident if in the upper vagina. Vulval lesions may be disregarded by the patient, and it is not until the local lymph nodes are involved, swollen, and tender that most patients are seen. This may be several months after the initial infection. The location of the primary lesion determines the group of lymph nodes involved. Lesions in the upper third of the vagina involve the pelvic and perirectal lymphatics which may subsequently result in the anorectal syndrome and rectal stenosis. Multiple small abscesses are formed in the nodes, and the surrounding tissues become swollen and edematous. The nodes may suppurate and break down, with the formation of secondarily infected chronic abscesses. The disease may be systemic as well as local, and the organisms have been isolated from the peripheral blood. Involvement of the supraclavicular nodes and isolation of the organisms from the cerebrospinal fluid attest to the constitutional nature of the disease. The rectal involvement may progress to complete obstruction, requiring a temporary colostomy. Multiple fistulas may be formed between the rectum and perineum. The rectovaginal septum may be extensively involved with multiple rectovaginal fistulas.

Symptoms and Diagnosis

The invasion of the lymphatic system occurs ten to thirty days after the initial infection. With this there may be systemic symptoms common to any infection, such as headache, sweats, chills, fever, anorexia, weakness, and general muscular soreness. In the female the involvement of nodes of the inguinal chain may be minimal if the lesion is in the upper vagina. Painful glands appear in the inguinal region, and the pain is relieved if the gland drains spontaneously. As the lymphatic drainage is impaired by infection, the labia and clitoris become swollen and brawny. Ulcers about the urethra or in the urethra itself cause a discharge and burning on urination. The rectal symptoms of stricture develop much later, but an acute proctitis is manifested by a bloody, purulent discharge that irritates the perianal skin, causing pain and pruritus.

The diagnosis is confirmed by the Frei test, while serologic and dark-field tests are done to exclude syphilis. Smears and cultures are done to exclude gonorrhea, chancroid, and granuloma inguinale. Biopsy may be indicated to exclude a malignancy of the vulva. The Frei antigen is given by an intradermal injection of 0.1 ml. in the skin of the forearm. A cor-

responding area on the other arm should be injected with the same amount of normal saline as a control. The results are read in forty-eight to seventy-two hours. An inflammatory nodule or papule 5 to 6 mm. in diameter and at least twice as large as any reaction about the control is considered positive. It indicates that the patient has or has had the disease. A complement fixation test is under study and, when refined, may provide another reliable test. Elevation of the total serum proteins and the development of hyperglobulinemia occur with the infection but are not specific for disease.

Treatment

The treatment is the same as in any acute infection, with bed rest, a diet adequate in protein, minerals, and vitamins, and other general supportive measures. The management of the bowels requires individualization, depending on the degree of proctitis. The chemotherapy and wide-spectrum antibiotics prescribed sterilize the bowel and probably reduce the secondary infection of the anorectal lesions. It is not known whether a potent antibiotic such as neomycin (which reduces the intestinal flora to a marked degree) should be used in conjunction with the specific therapy. The routine use of cortisone, especially in Negro patients who develop scar tissue extensively, is under observation. I have given cortisone in moderate doses, together with specific therapy, to recurrent cases with existing strictures of the rectum. A remission resulted with significant softening of the strictures. One patient who had required daily enemas and dilatations with a large rectal tube was able to have spontaneous bowel movements for the first time in eleven years after having taken a mild laxative the preceding night. She had been advised on several occasions to submit to a permanent colostomy.

Specific therapy with sulfadiazine or a comparable sulfonamide is given for three to six weeks, depending on the response. The dose is 2.0 Gm. three times daily for three weeks, after which it can be reduced if a prolonged course of therapy is indicated. Tetracycline therapy (chlortetracycline or oxytetracycline) is given in the dosage of 500 mg. four times daily for three to six weeks, depending on the response of the lesions. Combined therapy with a sulfonamide and tetracycline derivative is indicated for lesions that fail to respond to a single agent. Fluctuant buboes are aspirated periodically but are not incised. Rectal strictures are gently dilated to prevent further contracture. Surgery should be conservative since complete obstruction of the rectum is rare and the results of therapy with cortisone have yet to be assessed.

GRANULOMA INGUINALE
General Considerations

Granuloma inguinale (venereum) is a chronic venereal disease affecting the skin and subcutaneous tissues of the lower genital tract. It rarely spreads to the upper genital tract. While it is most common among Negroes, the disease is not limited to them.

Etiology and Pathologic Anatomy

This specific granulomatous disease is characterized by the presence of Donovan bodies in smears taken from the lesion. Donovan bodies are probably protozoa. They appear as small, pink bodies with a blue coccoid structure in the center and are found in the cytoplasm of large mononuclear plasma cells. The disease has been transferred from person to person by exudate containing the Donovan bodies, and it is possible that pubic lice may be responsible for carrying the organism from the infected person.

The disease starts as a small nodule or ulcer on the vulva and spreads by the development of contiguous lesions which eventually merge with the original lesion. The soft, red granulation tissue characteristic of the disease spreads in the groin, vagina, and about the rectum. The lesions become secondarily infected with pyogenic organisms, with swelling and occasional suppuration of the regional lymph glands. The cervix may become involved, the lesions simulating a malignancy.

Symptoms and Diagnosis

The patient's complaints depend on the extent of the lesion, the degree of contracture, and the amount of swelling of the labia. The typical, red beefy granulation tissue is biopsied, and smears are taken from the depths of one or more of the lesions to be stained for Donovan bodies. Tests for the other venereal diseases are run concurrently.

Treatment

One of the tetracyclines, 0.5 Gm. four times daily, is given for three weeks. As healing takes place the lesions become epithelized and the Donovan bodies are no longer seen on smears. Streptomycin, 2 Gm. daily for two to three weeks, results in a high cure rate. Recurrences are common with any treatment routine used. Fuadin, a trivalent compound of antimony and sodium, is effective against the organism; 1.5 ml., gradually increased to 5.0 ml., is injected deep in the gluteal muscles three times a week for three months. Seven- to ten-day rest periods from the drug are allowed each time the patient receives a total of 45 ml. in any one course. The local lesions can be reduced in size by the application of podophyllin, 20 per cent in olive oil, for twenty minutes. The surrounding tissues must be protected. Surgical or electrosurgical excision may be necessary, with subsequent skin grafting. Severe dyspareunia due to constriction of the introitus may require plastic repair. Advanced scarring and contracture of the vagina and outlet may necessitate cesarean section in the event of a term pregnancy.

References

Arean, V. M.: Manson's Schistosomiasis of the Female Genital Tract, Am. J. Obst. & Gynec. 72: 1039, 1956.
Campbell, C. G., and Bowman, J.: Enterobius Vermicularis Granuloma of Pelvis; a Case Report, Am. J. Obst. & Gynec. 81: 256, 1961.
Collins, C. G., Nix, F. G., and Cerha, H.: Ruptured Tuboovarian Abscess, Am. J. Obst. & Gynec. 72: 820, 1956.
Eiseman, B., and Muller, C.: A New Operative Approach to Inflammatory Strictures of the Rectum and Rectosigmoid, Surgery 30: 448, 1951.
Grace, A., Frank, L., and Wyse, R.: Effect of Cortisone Upon Hypersensitivity Due to Lymphogranuloma Venereum, Arch. Dermat. & Syph. 65: 348, 1952.
Greenblatt, R.: Management of Chancroid, Granuloma In-

guinale and Lymphogranuloma Venereum in General Practice, ed. 2, 1953, United States Department of Health, Education, and Welfare, Publication No. 255.

Kalstone, B. M., Howell, J. A., and Cline, F.: Granuloma Inguinale With Hematogenous Dissemination to the Spine, J. A. M. A. 176: 530, 1961.

Ledbetter, R. K.: The Treponema Pallidum Immobilization Test, a Diagnostic Aid to the Clinician, J. A. M. A. 160: 1392, 1956.

Lighter, A. G., Syphilis in Pregnancy, With Special Emphasis on Serologic Problem Cases, Am. J. Obst. & Gynec. 74: 139, 1957.

Sedlis, A.: Manson's Schistosomiasis of the Fallopian Tube; A Case Report, Am. J. Obst. & Gynec. 81: 254, 1961.

Sunden, B.: The Results of Conservative Treatment of Salpingitis Diagnosed at Laparotomy and Laparoscopy, Acta Obst. et Gynec. 38: 286, 1959.

Thomas, E.: Recent Developments in the Treatment of Syphilis, New York J. Med. 56: 1918, 1956.

Thomas, E. W.: Current Status of Therapy in Syphilis, J. A. M. A. 162: 1536, 1956.

6 · Pelvic Tuberculosis

General Considerations

The management of pelvic tuberculosis has been greatly altered by the advent of specific antituberculosis drugs. It may be expected to change constantly as additional drugs are discovered and studied. The biologic characteristics of the tubercle bacillus, with its great faculty for survival in the tissues of the body and the unique lesions it causes, and the complex anatomic and physiologic nature of the female pelvic organs together create many situations which will require much study and investigation. An understanding of the behavior of the disease in parenchymatous organs such as the lung and kidney as contrasted with its behavior on mucous and serous membranes will clarify many findings in genital tuberculosis. In the female anatomy the ovary represents a parenchymatous structure, the uterus and tubes present a serous surface, the tubes also offer a mucous membrane, while the endometrium presents a medium that sheds itself monthly. An additional consideration is the intimate association of the urinary tract with the genital organs and the possibility of involvement of both.

Incidence

Reliable data on the incidence of tuberculous salpingitis in the general population in this country are not available. The incidence of the disease has usually been expressed in terms of chronic salpingitis from all causes, with tuberculosis being responsible for about 5 per cent or less. It is most common in the childbearing age group, with a peak in the 25- to 30-year age group. This refers to the time at which the diagnosis is made, although it is quite probable the infection occurred many years before and quite likely within a year or so after the primary lung complex. Since tuberculosis is more prevalent in young diabetic patients and is more likely to be active, one might expect a slightly higher incidence of pelvic disease in this group.

Etiology

With a few exceptions pelvic tuberculosis is secondary to pulmonary disease. It is caused by the human type, not the bovine, although the latter has been reported in a small percentage of patients. The route to the genital organs is by hematogenous seeding after a lesion in the lung or lymph node has eroded. It is possible that bacilli may be spilled into large lymphatic channels and from there find their way into the blood stream. However, the evidence points to the fact that lymphatic dissemination commonly stops in the regional nodes and that bacilli enter the lymphatic channels phagocytosed by migrating leukocytes. Enough attention has not been given to this aspect of pelvic tuberculosis and its lymphatic spread in the abundant channels draining the genital organs. These lympho-hematogenous disseminations would surely cause widespread disease were it not that many organs are unsuited for survival of the bacillus and its propagation. In some organs where the bacillus survives for a long time, progressive or clinical disease does not develop, although the possibility of such disease is always present. An extrapulmonary foci, such as bone or meninges, could erode a vessel and spread the disease, but proved instances of this are rare.

Pathology

The mucosa of the tube is the site of the earliest lesions. If the tubal mucosa is not involved, the suspicion of an etiologic agent other than the tubercle bacillus arises. In over 90 per cent of patients the infection is bilateral. The progress of the disease depends to some extent upon the number of bacilli that survive the process of necrosis and disseminate to the local lymphatics. First there is a tuberculous endosalpingitis, and as the tubercles coalesce there are the same necrosing, liquefying, and sloughing features that characterize the disease in the lungs. The tube becomes thicker and nodular, and as tubercles rupture into the lumen, further dissemination of the process takes place. Next, extension into the muscularis occurs, with a tuberculous myosalpingitis and further thickening of the wall. Finally, a perisalpingitis develops which may seal off the fimbriated end of the tube. If the disease continues to progress, the tube becomes distended with a caseous, purulent material—a tuberculous pyosalpinx.

The involvement of the ovary is less striking. The surface may show some tubercles, but the parenchyma of the ovary resists destruction until the disease is far advanced. Frequently only a few tubercles will be found in the substance of the ovary, while the tube is practically destroyed.

Tuberculous peritonitis assumes two forms: exudative and dry. In the exudative type the preperitoneal connective tissue is edematous, and there may be free or encapsulated ascites. There is clear, yellow fluid with multiple, but yielding, adhesions. Miliary nodules stud the pelvic organs, peritoneum, and bowel. Fibrinous deposits mat the structures together. In the dry form there are massive, dense, thick adherences. The genitalia, together with bowel and bladder, form a compact mass with an indistinct outline of the individual structures. As the peritoneum is destroyed, the retroperitoneal fat and serosa are replaced by granulation tissue with central caseation. The entire mass has the feel of a frozen pelvis and forms a pseudotumor filling the true pelvis.

Dissemination to the regional lymph nodes probably occurs early in the disease and, as in pulmonary tuberculosis, the nodes are effective in containing the disease. I have done a lymphadenectomy on a patient with large, caseous nodes straddling the ureters on both sides and causing a mild hydronephrosis. Since the excisional treatment of cervical lymph node tuberculosis is so effective, it seemed reasonable to excise such pelvic foci completely. Nodes often may be felt along the hypogastric, common iliac, and para-aortic chains and are firmly adherent to the adjacent structures.

Tuberculous endometritis is present in more than half of the patients with known adnexal disease. The route of infection is from the infected tube, from which bacilli are spilled into the lumen and thence into the uterine cavity. Frequently a thorough curettage or repeated diagnostic curettages are needed to demonstrate tubercles in the endometrium. It is improbable that infection is transmitted by intercourse, and it is most unusual to find a patient with tuberculous endometritis with normal tubes. The repeated discharge of the endometrial lining with menstruation is an important factor in the healing of tuberculous endometritis. The myometrium is infected by direct spread from the endometrium. The perimetrium is involved from the tubes as part of the tuberculous peritonitis.

Tuberculosis of the cervix is secondary to the process in the endometrium and myometrium. It has never been demonstrated that an infected sexual partner could provide the source of infection, nor has it been possible to cultivate the tubercle bacillus from the endocervical secretions of patients whose husbands are known to have genitourinary tuberculosis. The cervical lesions are ulcerative and on biopsy show the usual picture of granulation tissue and tubercles.

Tuberculosis of the vulva is seen in two forms: ulcerative and hypertrophic. This rare lesion is seen during the active sex life of the patient, and almost always there is active pulmonary tuberculosis or a recently active lesion. The possible means of infection is through infected sputum with inoculation of the vulva by clothing, masturbation, or abnormal sexual practices. However, the source of infection is difficult to prove, and it may well be that vulval tuberculosis is again just a rare manifestation of a general infection. The inguinal nodes are metastatic sites for dissemination of the infection and again are excellent barriers until caseation ensues, with the possibility of erosion into a major vessel. The ulcerative type is the more serious since it has been known to cause widespread dissemination. The hypertrophic type probably represents a massive blockage or containment by the lymphatics and is less likely to spread and also lends itself better to excision.

Symptoms

The symptoms of tuberculous salpingo-oophoritis are not characteristic. Most patients complain of lower abdominal pain, and the presence of a fever of undetermined origin is suggestive of the disease. Menstrual disturbances are common, with menorrhagia the usual abnormality, although patients are seen with amenorrhea. Weight loss is common, and at the same time the patient may complain of swelling of the abdomen. A considerable number of patients are first seen because of infertility, and the diagnosis is established during studies for this problem. The disease will be discovered in other patients when they fail to respond to the usual therapy for pelvic inflammatory disease of gonorrheal or nonspecific bacterial origin. A fistula or colpotomy wound that heals poorly should alert the gynecologist to the possibility of tuberculosis. The initial symptoms may be of renal origin if the urinary tract is involved or the bladder disturbed by a tuberculous peritonitis.

Diagnosis

On bimanual examination, hard adnexal swellings, as well as nodules in the cul-de-sac, are felt. These findings are particularly sug-

gestive when found in a young girl or virgin not in the age group in which endometriosis is common. A low-grade fever is not uncommon, and the white cell count may be elevated with a lymphocytosis. Culture of representative curettings is reliable when endometritis exists. The culture of the menstruum (which theoretically should be ideal since it would contain material from the entire uterine cavity as well as the tubes) has been unsatisfactory. Hysterosalpingography with injection of the contrast material at very low pressures may show fistulous tracts and dilated and irregular tubes. The x-ray appearance is not characteristic enough to permit a positive diagnosis by this means. Culdoscopy or exploratory colpotomy with biopsy of the lesion will render a positive diagnosis, and with adequate preoperative drug therapy there is little risk of developing a chronic peritoneovaginal fistula. Vulvar tuberculosis must be distinguished from granuloma venereum, lymphopathia venereum, chancre, chancroid, carcinoma, and gumma. Serologic examinations, smears and cultures for the Ducrey bacillus, Frei tests, dark-field examinations, biopsy, smears, and cultures may all have to be done to diagnose the nature of a vaginal ulceration. Tubercle bacilli may be distinguished from smegma bacilli and other nonpathogenic acid-fast bacilli by means of culture and guinea pig inoculations.

Surgical Anatomy and Principles

When surgery is required in female genital tuberculosis the bowel and lymphatic system of the pelvis are invariably involved in the process. Separation of the bowel from the uterus, tubes, and ovaries is difficult and in the past caused a high mortality from perforation and peritonitis. The bowel should be gently separated and any lacerations meticulously repaired. In this regard it is a good surgical principle to prepare the bowel for resection if tuberculosis is suspected. Even though the bowel may be perforated during the operation, drains should not be used since they may be the cause of fecal fistula.

The extent of the operation to be done is an

all-or-none matter. With advanced disease the tubes, as well as the ovaries, are hopelessly involved. The uterus and cervix should not be left if a bilateral salpingo-oophorectomy is performed. Since the excisional treatment of lymph node tuberculosis is so effective in other locations, it seems logical to excise large caseous nodes found in the pelvis, particularly if they surround and compress the ureter. There is little precedent to follow in this matter, but it would seem reasonable that a pelvic node dissection would not disseminate the disease any more than a dissection of tuberculous nodes in the neck. It seems illogical to leave known caseous foci behind.

The bladder and ureters may be intimately bound to the uterus by the tuberculous process. Care is exercised to prevent perforation of the bladder. Should any accidental lacerations occur, the bladder wall should be closed in layers and an indwelling catheter left. A suprapubic cystotomy is to be avoided. If the bowel has been thoroughly prepared, the appendix should be removed if it is bound down to the right adnexa or is involved in a tuberculous peritonitis. This will avoid confusion later should the patient present any acute right lower quadrant symptoms. If the bowel is not prepared and the appendix is normal or atrophic, it is more conservative to avoid the contamination incidental to the prophylactic appendectomy.

Preoperative Care and Anesthesia

The ideal time for operation is when the maximum effects of the drugs have occurred. This would be about four months in the average patient. By that time the persistence of symptoms or evidence of spread will provide convincing evidence that surgery is necessary. During this time repeated pelvic examinations help in following the course of the disease. Repeated curettages may also be done to follow the response of a tuberculous endometritis. It is difficult to say how much tissue may be in the prenecrotic stage at the beginning of medical treatment. Such tissue should heal during the preoperative period, but necrotic elements may go on to liquefaction in spite of the drugs. An

ascites will frequently clear up with the decrease in activity of the lesions under drug therapy. During this period the urinary tract is thoroughly examined by pyelograms and urine cultures. Retrograde studies are done as indicated. Five days prior to operation the bowel is prepared by saline catharsis at night and enemas the following morning. Neomycin, 1.0 Gm. every six hours, is given for three or more days prior to surgery. At the present time it is our most effective agent for sterilizing the bowel. There is seldom any contraindication to general anesthesia in patients with pelvic tuberculosis. If they have had extensive collapse therapy, a spinal anesthetic could be used.

Treatment

Conservative treatment is indicated in early lesions and especially in young patients. An early lesion would be the accidental discovery of a tuberculous endometritis as a result of an existing mild tuberculous salpingitis. An early lesion might be found at laparotomy and the conservative plan of therapy carried out subsequently. The important point is to institute a long course of drug and rest therapy.

Three major drugs have gained wide acceptance in the treatment of tuberculosis: isoniazid, streptomycin, and para-aminosalicylic acid (PAS). Two other antituberculous drugs, viomycin and pyrazinamide, have a limited usefulness. Numerous other drugs are under investigation at the present time, but their efficacy in the pulmonary form of the disease has not been adequately appraised and trials in pelvic tuberculosis have been few. The patient should be treated with the best current combined drug therapy over an extended period of time, and a decision as to the necessity of surgery based on their response to such therapy.

There is no unanimity of opinion as to a single regimen of chemotherapy superior to all others. Three principles of chemotherapy on which most would agree are as follows: (1) therapy must be prolonged at least twelve to eighteen months; (2) isoniazid is the most potent single drug; (3) as a rule two drugs should be administered simultaneously. The three most generally used regimens are isoniazid-PAS, isoniazid-streptomycin, and streptomycin-PAS, in the order given. Tompsett recommends starting off with the isoniazid-PAS regimen in the average patient with pelvic tuberculosis and no previous chemotherapy. The dose of isoniazid is 5 mg. per kilogram of body weight per day in divided doses. The average adult would receive about 300 mg. per day. Streptomycin is given twice each week in the dosage of 40 mg. per kilogram of body weight or higher by some therapists. Half of this may be given as streptomycin and the other half as dihydrostreptomycin. Thus a patient weighing 50 kilograms would receive 1 Gm. of streptomycin and 1 Gm. of dihydrostreptomycin on each of two days each week. The dosage may have to be modified in the course of treatment. PAS is administered by mouth in four divided doses for a total of 12 Gm. per day. With early genital tuberculosis one of these regimens is continued for a year; repeated curettages are done to help note the response to therapy. In advanced disease the response to therapy dictates whether surgery is necessary and when. If, in the course of six to twelve months of intense therapy, the adnexal lesions show no further regression or a tuberculous endometritis persists, then laparotomy may be indicated and usually results in a complete hysterectomy, bilateral salpingo-oophorectomy, and excision of obviously involved large, caseous nodes. It is important that a long course of isoniazid therapy precede surgery since this drug prevents tuberculous meningitis even though large masses of caseous tissues are disturbed at operation. Postoperatively the patient should be maintained on combined antituberculosis therapy for a year or more by any of the drugs tolerated and to which the tubercle bacillus has not become resistant. Should the findings at laparotomy prove more favorable than expected, cultures and biopsies may be done and the abdomen closed. As in pulmonary tuberculosis, post-treatment relapse is common unless a long course of therapy is imposed on the patient.

In the rare instances in which pregnancy has occurred in the presence of pelvic tuberculosis or in which the adnexal infection appears to have taken place after an intrauterine conception, the pregnancy has been a very dangerous complication. Cases have been reported of an acute spread in the pelvis and abdomen and of hematogenous spread with fatal termination. Before the advent of the antituberculosis drugs, if one were fortunate enough to diagnose such a rarity, the termination of the pregnancy was indicated. We have no precedent to rely on at the moment, but it would appear that more conservative therapy would be justified.

The use of low dosage x-ray therapy to induce a temporary or permanent amenorrhea has had its exponents in the past, but at present chemotherapy has replaced this form of therapy. The effect of artificial pneumoperitoneum for pulmonary tuberculosis on the normal female genitalia has been observed. Most frequently it causes dysmenorrhea and an increase in the flow. That this is a direct cause-and-effect relationship is dubious since the patient is usually getting drug therapy at the same time or undergoing major pulmonary surgery, and too many events are occurring simultaneously.

Vulval tuberculosis is treated by the same antituberculosis regimen as upper genital tract disease. In addition, local therapy is instituted. Ulcerated areas are bathed several times a day with a 5 per cent solution of PAS. Large, swollen labia or the hypertrophic form of the disease requires wide excision, after which healing usually takes place by granulation.

The diagnosis of genital tuberculosis results in an anxiety-producing situation for the patient in two ways: (1) in regard to her health and (2) in regard to the psychosexual implications. The management of both situations requires that the patient be allowed to ventilate and talk about the disease, herself, and her sex life. Avoid specifically giving her overenthusiastic reassurance based on the possibilities of modern therapy when first informing her of the nature of her disease. Such reassurance will only cause the patient to bury her concerns and later may make her a difficult patient to deal with when the length and extent of treatment become apparent. After ventilation, a careful explanation of the nature of the disease and of the rationale of treatment should be given to prevent a revolt from therapy. Reassurance is then given after considerable study and thought and must not go beyond what is reasonable to expect of present-day therapy. It is unwise to promise specific dates at which the patient may reach certain treatment goals. Sexual activity is proof to many women that they are really loved, and residential treatment denies them contact with their husbands. More significant is the emotional impact of frigidity on the part of the husband when he learns the nature of the disease. The nontransmissibility by sexual contact of genital tuberculosis in either partner is explained to husband and wife. Except where advanced disease or lower genital tract lesions contraindicate it, sexual intercourse may be permitted as long as it does not seem to cause a relapse. Certainly, where the psychosexual aspects of a woman's illness may cause her to take flight from the physician's treatment and confidence, it is better to take a risk on any unproved harmful effects of the sexual act on the disease.

References

Amberson, J. B.: Current Methods in the Treatment of Tuberculosis, Bull. New York Acad. Med. 31: 20, 1955.

Asplund, J., and Ryden, A. B. V.: The Diagnosis of Tuberculosis of the Cervix, Acta obst. et gynec. scandinav. 32: 186, 1952.

Barbour, E.: Post-Menopausal Endometrial Tuberculosis, J. Obst. & Gynaec. Brit. Emp. 67: 1008, 1960.

Barclay, W. R.: Distribution and Excretion of Radioactive Isoniazid in Tuberculous Patients, J. A. M. A. 151: 1384, 1953.

Bobrow, M., Posner, C., and Friedman, S.: A Successful Pregnancy After Endometrial Tuberculosis; a Case Report, Am. J. Obst. & Gynec. 74: 1136, 1957.

Bobrow, M. L., Winkelstein, L. B., and Friedman, S.: Streptomycin in Advanced Pelvic Tuberculosis; Evaluation; Report of Six Cases, Obst. & Gynec. 8: 299, 1956.

Chalmers, J. A.: Coincident Carcinoma and Tuberculosis of the Uterine Cervix, J. Obst. & Gynaec. Brit. Emp. 65: 438, 1958.

Coletta, S.: A Case of Primary Tuberculosis of the Cervix (Su di un caso di tuberculosi primitiva del collo dell' utero), Arch. ostet. e gin. 63: 83, 1958.

Denniss, R. G.: Successful Pregnancy Following Treatment for Pelvic Tuberculosis, J. Obst. & Gynaec. Brit. Emp. 67: 434, 1960.

Eckerling, B., and Goldman, J. A.: Coexisting Adenomyosis and Tuberculosis; Report of a Case, Obst. & Gynec. 16: 461, 1960.

Halbrecht, I.: The Relative Value of Culture and Endometrial Biopsy in the Diagnosis of Genital Tuberculosis, Am. J. Obst. & Gynec. 75: 899, 1958.

Hedberg, G. A.: Changing Concepts in the Treatment of Tuberculosis, M. Clin. North America 38: 1161, 1954.

Henderson, D. N., Harkins, J. L., and Stitt, J. F.: Pelvic Tuberculosis, Am. J. Obst. & Gynec. 80: 21, 1960.

Hunt, B., and Wassersug, J. D.: Effects of Isoniazid on Patients With Tuberculosis and Mental Illness, New England J. Med. 249: 1051, 1953.

Kika, K.: A Clinical Analysis of the "Angiograms" Found in the Course of Hysterosalpingography With Special Reference to Tuberculosis of the Female Genitals, Am. J. Obst. & Gynec. 67: 56, 1954.

Malkani, P. K., and Rajani, C. K.: Pelvic Tuberculosis, Obst. & Gynec. 14: 600, 1959.

Molthan, L., Cohen, R. V., and Zarafonetis, C. J. D.: Clinical Use of Potassium Para-Aminosalicylic Acid, Am. Rev. Tuberc. 71: 220, 1955.

Muschenheim, C.: The Treatment of Tuberculosis Lymphadenitis, Tuberculosis Abstracts, National Tuberculosis Association, vol. 28, no. 4, April, 1955.

Nogales, F., and Vilar, E.: The Clinical Management of Tuberculosis of the Uterine Cervix (Klinik und Behandlung der Tuberkulose des Gebaermutterhalses; Studie gestuetzt auf 112 Faelle), Geburtsh. u. Frauenh. 17: 677, 1957.

Nokes, J. M., Claiborne, H. A., Thornton, W. N., and Yiu-Tang, H.: Extrauterine Pregnancy Associated With Tuberculous Salpingitis and Congenital Tuberculosis in the Fetus, Obst. & Gynec. 9: 206, 1957.

Rothstein, E., and Bruce, T. H.: Management of Isoniazid Intolerance, J. A. M. A. 155: 745, 1954.

Ryden, A.: Treatment of Tubercular Salpingitis, Acta obst. et gynec. scandinav. 37: 114, 1958.

Salzer, H. M., and Lurie, M. L.: Anxiety and Depressive States Treated With Isonicotinyl Hydrazide (Isoniazid), A. M. A. Arch. Neurol. & Psychiat. 70: 317, 1953.

Schaefer, G.: Treatment of Female Genital Tuberculosis, Am. J. Obst. & Gynec. 68: 1333, 1955.

Schaefer, G.: Tuberculosis in Obstetrics and Gynecology, Boston, 1956, Little, Brown & Co.

Schaefer, G., Douglas, R. G., and Silverman, F.: A Reevaluation of the Management of Pregnancy and Tuberculosis, J. Obst. & Gynaec. Brit. Emp. 66: 990, 1959.

Schaupp, K. L.: Genital Tuberculosis in Women, Am. J. Obst. & Gynec. 81: 1126, 1961.

Segovia, S., Bunster, E., and Parrochia, E.: Genital Tuberculosis; Management With Antibiotic Therapy and Surgery, Obst. & Gynec. 7: 665, 1956.

Shapiro, W. J.: Pregnancy Following Treated Pelvic Tuberculosis, Obst. & Gynec. 12: 148, 1958.

Snaith, L.: Surgery for Female Genital Tuberculosis, Obst. & Gynec. 12: 135, 1958.

Suranyl, S.: Fatal Tuberculous Generalization of Genital Origin in Women (Les generalisations tuberculeuses mortelles a point de depart genital chez la femme), Rev. Franc. Gynec. Obst. 55: 447, 1960.

Sutherland, A. M.: Tuberculosis of the Endometrium: A Report on 250 Cases With the Results of Drug Treatment, Obst. & Gynec. 11: 527, 1958.

Sutherland, A.: Genital Tuberculosis in Women, Am. J. Obst. & Gynec. 79: 486, 1960.

Vago, T., Rikover, M., and Reif, A.: Ectopic Pregnancy Associated With Tuberculous Salpingitis, Obst. & Gynec. 16: 360, 1960.

Weiss, W., Eisemberg, G. M., and Flippin, H. F.: Impact of Isoniazid on Tuberculous Meningitis, J. A. M. A. 164: 947, 1957.

Ylinen, O.: Genital Tuberculosis in Women; Clinical Experiences With 348 Proved Cases, Acta obst. et gynec. scandinav. (Suppl. 2) 40: 1, 1961.

Zummo, B. P., Sered, H., and Falls, F. H.: The Diagnosis and Prognosis of Female Genital Tuberculosis, Am. J. Obst. & Gynec. 70: 34, 1955.

7 · Surgical Management of Anovulval Pruritus

UNDERCUTTING OPERATIONS
Etiology, Pathologic Anatomy, or Mechanism of Disease

Anovulval pruritus is not a specific disease but a wretched symptom that plagues the patient relentlessly. The general causes such as moniliasis associated with diabetes, jaundice from various causes, allergic reactions, drug reactions, and many other causes are not relieved by surgery. The common skin diseases, bacterial and parasitic infections, and itching associated with edema and congestion from various causes are treated medically. The psychogenic factors in each patient should not be overlooked, and guilt complexes from marital infidelity or the desire to avoid intercourse where there is marital disharmony may be elicited from the patient.

Denervation of the vulva is indicated for intractable pruritus after all other efforts have failed to give the patient relief. Lichen sclerosis, leukoplakic vulvitis, and kraurosis vulvae with unbearable itching provide some indications for surgery. Occasionally, a specific diagnosis cannot be made, and the vulva is denervated because of the severity of the complaint.

Indications and Surgical Principles

Gynecologists more frequently see a combination of vulval and anal pruritus rather than a lesion restricted to one area or the other. For this reason vulval and anal pruritus are discussed together since an undercutting operation for one condition may be combined with a similar procedure for the other. Undercutting operations are indicated after all measures, including psychotherapy, have failed to relieve an intractable pruritus of the anus or vulva. The situation should have reached the stage where the itching is intolerable to the patient and the skin of either the anus or the vulva is starting to show irreversible changes. The principle of both operations is to interrupt the cutaneous nerve supply for a period of six to eight months, during which time the scratch-itch syndrome is interrupted and the skin permitted to heal. Both operations are relatively simple and may be combined by extending the vulval incision to the region of the anus in order to continue the undercutting posteriorly.

Surgical Anatomy of the Sensory Nerves Supplying the Vulva, Perineum, and Perianal Skin

The vulva, perineum, and perianal skin are supplied with ample sensory fibers approaching their terminal areas from multiple sources. Afferent sensory fibers supply the area with terminal branches that approach from the abdomen, from the posterior aspect of the thigh, from the depths of the pelvis, and finally from the sacrum. Denervation of the area can only be done successfully by systematically undercutting all the avenues of approach with a thorough knowledge of the nerve supply.

Plate 11, A, shows the sensory nerves that supply the area. The iliohypogastric nerve provides branches to the mons pubis and the anterior portion of the labia majora and adjacent skin. The ilioinguinal nerve and genital branches of the genitofemoral nerve follow the course of the round ligament and then, penetrating into the superficial fascia and skin, fan out towards the anterolateral aspect of the labia majora and adjacent skin of the thigh.

The perineal branch of the posterior cutaneous nerve of the thigh gives off many branches to the labia and adjacent skin of the leg subject to many secretions irritative to the vulva itself. The extension of the undercutting operation to the skin of the thigh is necessary to interrupt these sensory nerve fibers.

The pudendal nerve contains both sensory and motor fibers. The division that runs in the superficial perineal compartment gives off the major sensory nerves to the vulva, perineum, and perianal skin. As the pudendal nerve emerges from Alcock's (pudendal) canal and proceeds anteromedially toward the vulva, the sensory branches are distributed to the skin of the area. The inferior rectal nerve passes medially toward the perianal area as the first major branch (Plate 11, *A*). It provides branches to the skin of the perineum, anterior and lateral aspects of the perianal area, and adjacent skin of the buttocks.

The perineal branch of the pudendal nerve and the dorsal nerve of the clitoris are the terminal branches of the pudendal nerve. The dorsal nerve of the clitoris passes almost directly to the skin and mucous membrane of this structure. Atrophic changes in the several diseases that cause intractable pruritus frequently start in the anterior fourchette. The number of nerves that send fibers to this area serves to emphasize the necessity for a complete and systematic dissection.

The perineal nerve then divides into two main branches, named after the areas of the labia they innervate. The medial posterior labial nerve passes to the posterior portion of the labia, with fibers extending to the skin over the perineal body. The lateral posterior labial nerve supplies the skin of the labia somewhat more lateral and more anterior. Since the operation is not designed to specifically interrupt each nerve by positive identification in its peripheral course, the location of the main trunk and its approach to the vulva is more important.

Finally, the perineal branch of the fourth sacral nerve innervates a small area of skin posterior to the anus and over the coccyx. This is frequently involved in a generalized vulval and anal pruritus. The blood supply in this area is not so abundant as in the areas previously described, so that the interruption of the nerve fibers, if this area is involved, will have other considerations in surgical technique described later.

Steps of the Operation

1. Incisions are made just outside the labia majora from above the level of the clitoris to a point about midway between the introitus and rectum (Plate 11, *A*). If the operation is to be combined with denervation of the perirectal skin, three cloverleaves of skin are excised. They are placed to the right of the anus, to the left of the anus, and posterior to the anus (Plate 11, *A*). If the denervation can be confined to the vulva, the perineal skin can be undercut from the paralabial incisions.

2. A Metzenbaum scissors or knife is used to undercut the subcutaneous tela for a distance of 8 to 10 cm. out on the thigh. This will interrupt the medial posterior labial branch and lateral posterior labial branch of the perineal nerve, the dorsal nerve of the clitoris, and the perineal branch of the posterior cutaneous nerve of the thigh (Plate 11, *A* and *B*).

3. Anteriorly the skin is undercut 10 to 12 cm. or more up on the lower abdominal wall. This will interrupt fibers of the iliohypogastric, the ilioinguinal, and genital branches of the genitofemoral nerves. The operator should attempt to identify the external inguinal ring and thoroughly dissect this area to lyse all the fibers of the ilioinguinal nerve emerging at this point (Plate 11, *B*).

4. The abundant blood supply to the vulva precludes a completely dry field. After each area of undercutting is completed, gauze squares or miniature laparotomy pads are packed in the area after the major bleeding points have been clamped and ligated (Plate 11, *C*).

5. The dissection is then completed on the other side before undermining the skin of the perineal body and proceeding to the perianal areas if this is to be done.

6. Plate 11, *C*, shows the three cloverleaves of skin excised and the dissection on the patient's left completed. Undermining of the skin of the perineum interrupts sensory fibers going to the area from the

Plate 11

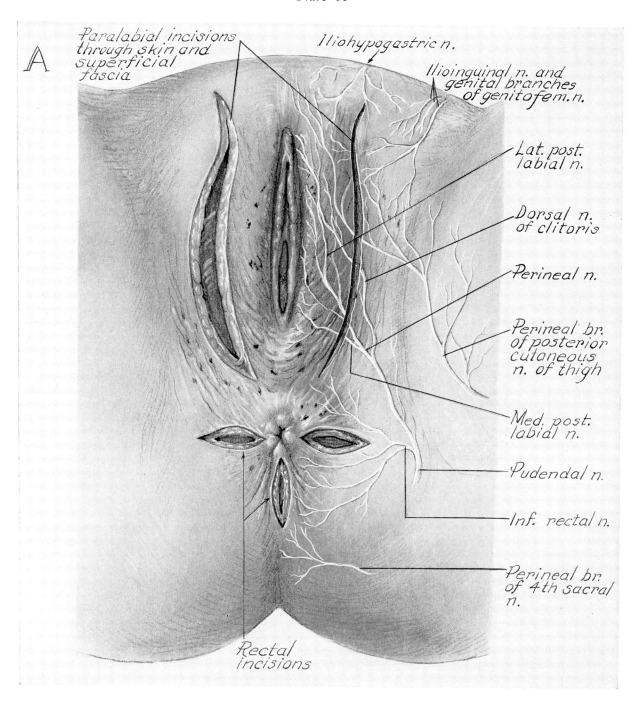

A

Paralabial incisions
through skin and
superficial
fascia

Iliohypogastric n.

Ilioinguinal n. and
genital branches
of genitofem. n.

Lat. post.
labial n.

Dorsal n.
of clitoris

Perineal n.

Perineal br.
of posterior
cutaneous
n. of thigh

Med. post.
labial n.

Pudendal n.

Inf. rectal n.

Perineal br.
of 4th sacral
n.

Rectal
incisions

97

Plate 11 (Continued)

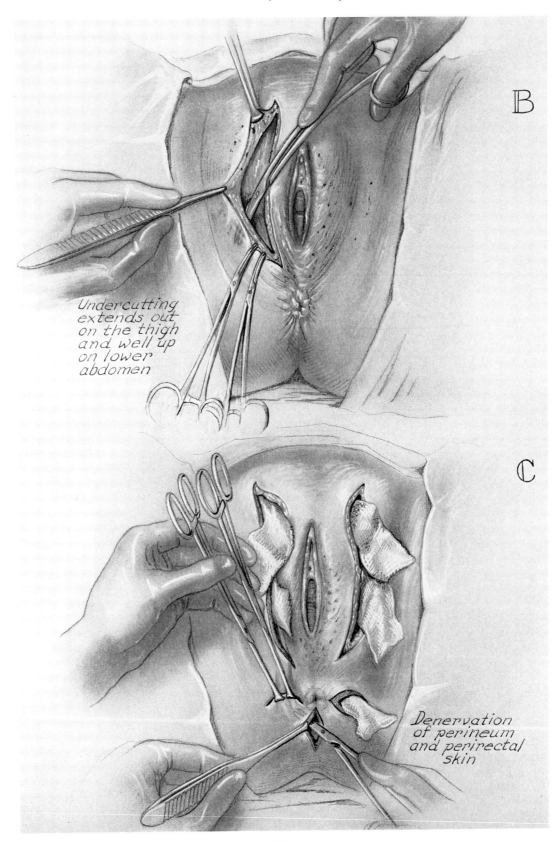

B

Undercutting extends out on the thigh and well up on lower abdomen

C

Denervation of perineum and perirectal skin

Plate 11 (Concluded)

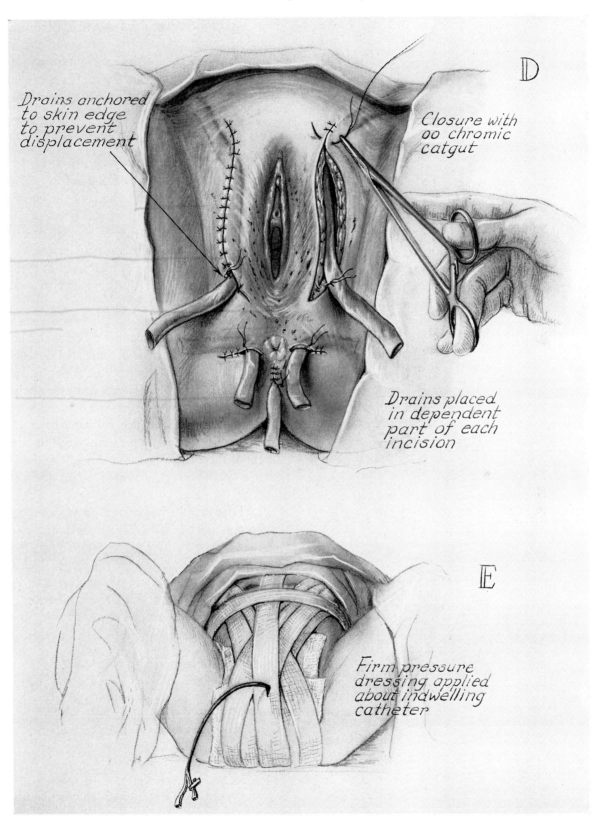

Drains anchored to skin edge to prevent displacement

Closure with oo chromic catgut

Drains placed in dependent part of each incision

Firm pressure dressing applied about indwelling catheter

inferior rectal branch of the pudendal nerve (Plate 11, *A*).

7. The denervation of the perianal skin is then completed. The edges of the skin of each cloverleaf are elevated by Allis clamps while Metzenbaum scissors are used to cut the subcutaneous tela (Plate 11, *C*).

8. Care should be exercised during this dissection to protect the external anal sphincter since trauma to this muscle results in considerable postoperative pain.

9. The nerves to the perianal skin from the inferior rectal branch of the pudendal nerve and fibers from the perineal branch of the fourth sacral nerve are resected by this technique (Plate 11).

10. The skin edges, except for the sites of the drains, are then closed with interrupted sutures of 00 chromic catgut (Plate 11, *D*).

11. The placement of the drains is a most important phase of the operation to prevent accumulations of serum that might cause a wound breakdown or febrile postoperative course. They should emerge from the most dependent portions of the incisions and extend far enough to ensure drainage of the most distant areas that have been undermined. The drains for each paralabial incision extend up on the lower abdominal wall. The drainage of the perianal area is shown in Plate 11, *D*. Two lateral drains extend out to the skin over the ischiorectal fossae. The posterior drain emerges from the lowermost (posterior) area that has been undercut. The drains are anchored to the skin edges to prevent displacement (Plate 11, *D*).

12. An indwelling catheter is inserted. Abundant dressings are used after which elastoplast is used to exert firm pressure over the entire operative field. The adhesive strips may be criss-crossed from the buttocks to the patient's shoulders if necessary. The catheter is observed to ensure that the method of dressing the wound has not constricted it and blocked urine drainage (Plate 11, *E*).

Postoperative Care

The pressure dressings are removed forty-eight hours later. The wound is dressed at this time, the sutures holding the drains are cut, and the drains are advanced 6 to 8 cm. This permits the drainage of a great deal of lymph and serum. The use of an indwelling catheter requires that a urinary antiseptic drug be administered. The choice of drug may depend on previous cultures taken by the surgeon.

The drains should be removed as soon as the amount of drainage decreases on the third or fourth postoperative day. At this time sitz baths, after observation of the wound, may be started and add to the patient's comfort. Principles of postoperative care for benign anorectal disease are observed if the denervation of the perianal skin was necessary.

SIMPLE VULVECTOMY
Indications and Surgical Principles

A simple vulvectomy is frequently done in patients with leukoplakia because of the known predilection of these patients to develop carcinoma of the vulva. It may be used as a treatment for intractable pruritus in older patients who are no longer active sexually and in many conditions of the skin of the vulva such as vitiligo, kraurosis, and lichen sclerosus et atrophicus. It has been advocated for Bowen's disease and some forms of specific chronic vulvitis. Occasionally it is indicated for the hypertrophic types of the specific venereal diseases, lymphopathia venereum and granuloma inguinale. A rare case of the hypertrophic form of tuberculosis of the vulva may require local excision. The operation consists of the removal of the labia majora, the labia minora, and the structures making up the clitoris.

Not infrequently the perianal area is involved in the preceding lesions. This is especially true with the patients who have intractable pruritus associated with kraurosis of the vulva, leukoplakia of the vulva, and lichen sclerosus et atrophicus. In these patients the perianal skin that is involved is excised together with the vulva.

Steps of the Operation

1. Depending on the extent of the lesion, the incision is started anteriorly 3 to 5 cm. above the clitoris. This is continued lateral to the labia majora to the midline of the perineum or, as illustrated, around the anus when this is involved in the disease (Plate 12, *A*).

2. Periurethral and perivaginal incisions are made. Obviously, one must stop during the procedure to obtain hemostasis since the area is vascular, even

Plate 12

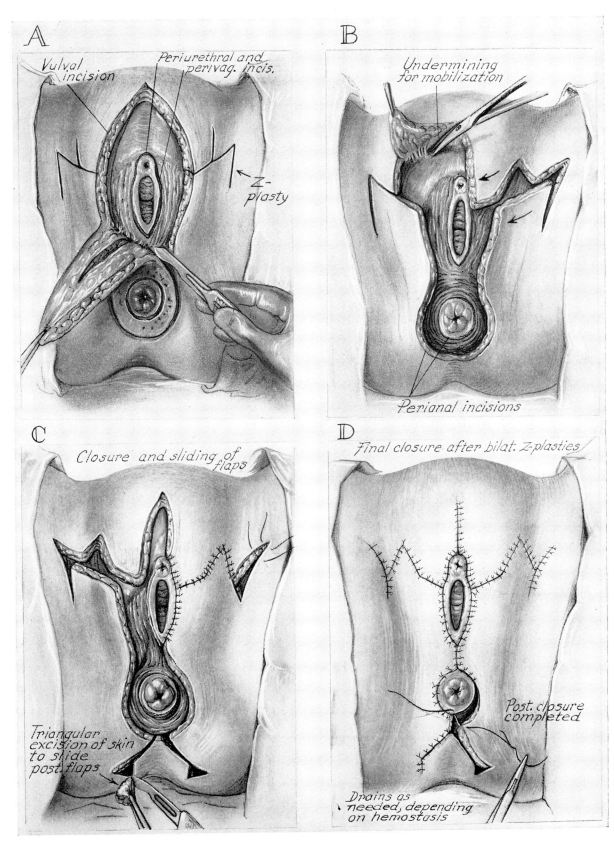

A — Vulval incision; Periurethral and perivag. incis.; Z-plasty

B — Undermining for mobilization; Perianal incisions

C — Closure and sliding of flaps; Triangular excision of skin to slide post. flaps

D — Final closure after bilat. Z-plasties; Post. closure completed; Drains as needed, depending on hemostasis when dealing with an atrophic lesion in an elderly patient (Plate 12, *A*).

3. Since these operations frequently break down because of a combination of the original disease plus the tension placed on the suture lines to effect the closure, a simple bilateral Z-plasty permits approximation without tension about the area of the external urethral meatus (Plate 12, *A*).

4. All of the skin and subcutaneous tissues are undermined and mobilized to the extent that approximation of these normal tissues may be approximated to the urethra and vagina without tension (Plate 12, *B*). The perianal area is also resected when this area is involved, and some simple expedients of plastic surgery are used to slide normal skin to the affected area.

5. Closure of the incisions is done with 00 chromic catgut. If the patient has urinary incontinence or if it appears that the operation and subsequent contracture of the tissues will displace the urethra and bladder neck and result in urinary stress incontinence, a prophylactic plication of the bladder neck is done. Plate 12, *C,* shows a method of triangular excision of skin about the anus to slide flaps of skin.

6. Plate 12, *D,* shows the final closure of the operative area. Other improvizations may have to be made, depending on the areas involved in the primary disease.

7. Drains may be placed in the dependent areas of the operative field if hemostasis does not provide a completely dry field. They are withdrawn one-half of their length the first postoperative day and removed the second day.

Postoperative Care

The area is kept dry by the use of astringent solutions and a heat lamp. Healing is usually rapid despite the fact that the area is contaminated. An indwelling catheter is left together with a vaginal pack. The pack is removed the following day. The catheter may be left an additional few days if the operation has been very extensive. Prophylactic urinary antiseptics are given when the catheter is permitted to remain more than twenty-four hours. The patient may be up and about immediately postoperatively. No special diet is required.

References

Alexander, R. M., and Manheim, S. D.: The Effect of Hydrocortisone Acetate Ointment on Pruritus Ani, J. Invest. Dermat. 21: 223, 1953.

Anderson, R. E., Pontius, G. V., and Witkowski, L. J.: Complications Following Surgery for Benign Anorectal Lesions, J. A. M. A. 159: 9, 1955.

Berkow, S. G.: A Replacement for the Vaginal Douche, Obst. & Gynec. 15: 773, 1960.

Cockerell, E. G., Knox, J. M., and Rogers, S. F.: Lichen Sclerosis et Atrophicus, Obst. & Gynec. 15: 554, 1960.

Collins, D., and Osment, L. S.: Lichen Sclerosis et Atrophicus of the Vulva, Obst. & Gynec. 14: 60, 1959.

Ensey, J. E.: Treatment of Vulvovaginitis With a New Combination of Nitrofurans, Am. J. Obst. & Gynec. 77: 155, 1959.

Frykman, H. M.: Anal Pruritus, Minnesota Med. 38: 19, 1955.

Kayser, H. L., Eisenberg, G. M., Shapiro, J., and Flippin, H. F.: The Use of Nystatin in the Treatment of Vaginal Candidiasis in Pregnancy, Am. J. Obst. & Gynec. 74: 139, 1957.

Lawrence, W. D.: Lichen Sclerosus et Atrophicus of the Vulva, Obst. & Gynec. 14: 65, 1959.

Mering, J. H.: Some Further Observations on Wide Skin Undercutting for Intractable Pruritus Vulvae, Am. J. Obst. & Gynec. 71: 386, 1956.

Norburn, L. M., and Coles, R. B.: Recurrent Erysipelas Following Vulvectomy, J. Obst. & Gynaec. Brit. Emp. 67: 279, 1960.

Parker, R. T., Jones, C. P., and Thomas, W. L.: Causes and Therapy of Pruritus Vulvae, North Carolina M. J. 16: 570, 1955.

Pickhardt, W. L., and Breen, J. L.: Identification of and Therapy of Vaginal Candidiasis, Am. J. Obst. & Gynec. 74: 42, 1957.

Vanbreuseghem, R.: Mycoses of Man and Animals, Springfield, Ill., 1958, Charles C Thomas, Publisher.

Zachariae, F.: Vaginitis Emphysematosa, Acta obst. et gynec. scandinav. 35: 393, 1956.

Section IV · RELAXATIONS and PROLAPSE

8 · The Statics of the Female Pelvic Viscera

"And this is the reason why the cure of many diseases is unknown to the physicians of Hellas, because they are ignorant of the whole, which ought to be studied also; for the part can never be well unless the whole be well."

—Plato

The Musculature and the Pelvic Parietal and Visceral Connective Tissues That Support the Pelvic Organs

The musculature that bears the brunt of all stresses from the abdominal cavity is the levator ani. Understand its mechanics—understand the surgery of the pelvic floor! It consists of three parts in the living anatomy: the most posterior and least well-developed portion, the iliococcygeus; a middle portion, the pubococcygeus; and the much thicker anterior portion, anatomically and functionally recognized as the puborectalis (Plate 13, *A*). The puborectalis originates from the posterior aspect of the pubic bones, more or less horizontally, within half an inch of the symphysis. The bilaterally paired puborectalis muscles pass backward in a gentle curve and blend into the sides of the vagina and rectum. The thickened anterior edges of these muscles are readily palpable in the living subject. Their combined action pulls the rectum, vagina, and bladder neck upward toward the inferior border of the symphysis in an effort to close the pelvic aperture. The pubococcygeus and iliococcygeus arise from the posterior aspects of the pubic bones above the puborectalis and along the

white line of the obturator fascia. They insert into the anococcygeal raphe and coccyx. Contraction of these muscles pulls the coccyx forward. This action can be palpated vaginally and, in contrast to the action of the puborectalis, contributes little to the closure of the pelvic aperture.

The classic studies of Paramour show that the pelvic fascia consists of the visceral extensions of the parietal connective tissue of the pelvis (Plate 13, *A* and *C*). In no instance are true ligaments formed on the pelvic floor for the purpose of supporting the pelvic viscera. The magnitude and extensions of the pelvic connective tissue form the basis of plastic surgery of the pelvic floor. The connective tissue thickens along the course of vessels and nerves. Such thickenings have inadvertently been described as ligaments, such as the cardinal, uterosacral, and broad ligaments, by anatomists who described these things in the dehydrated, shriveled corpse. In living anatomy, with the structures pliable and resilient, with blood coursing through them, and with forces applied against them, they seem to stand out as distinct formations.

In terms of anatomic descriptions the uterus would appear to have more ligaments than any comparable human organ, while at the same time it is easily the most frequently herniated. The round ligaments are identifiable as such but are not responsible for any suspension of the organ, for if this were so, the vagina and

Plate 13

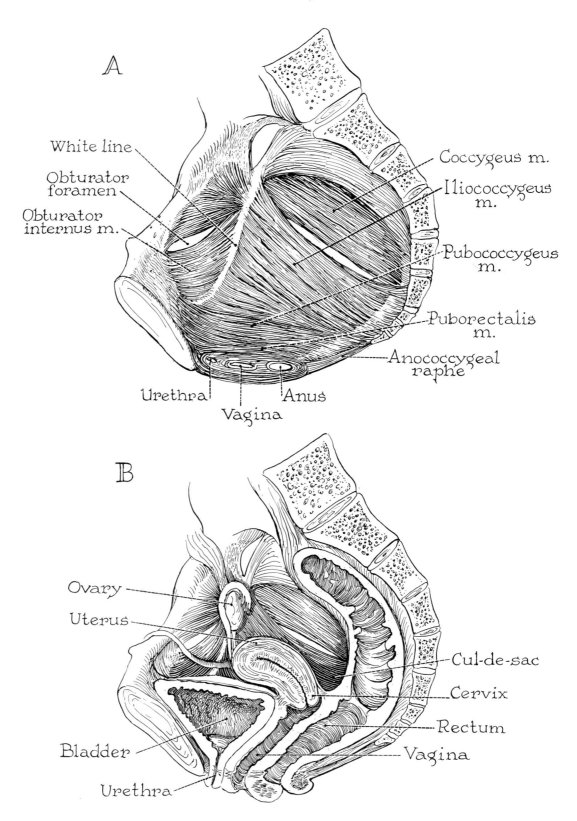

A

White line

Obturator
foramen

Obturator
internus m.

Coccygeus m.

Iliococcygeus
m.

Pubococcygeus
m.

Puborectalis
m.

Anococcygeal
raphe

Urethra

Vagina

Anus

B

Ovary

Uterus

Cul-de-sac

Cervix

Rectum

Vagina

Bladder

Urethra

Plate 13 (Concluded)

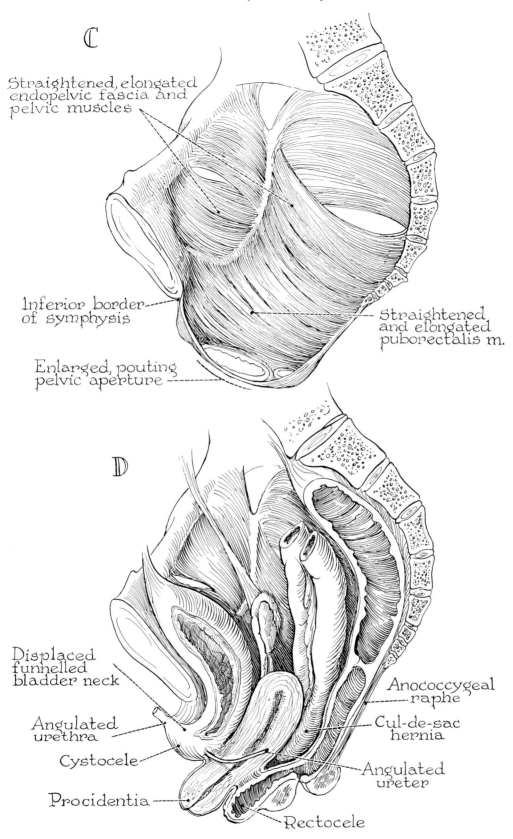

C

Straightened, elongated
endopelvic fascia and
pelvic muscles

Inferior border
of symphysis

Straightened
and elongated
puborectalis m.

Enlarged, pouting
pelvic aperture

D

Displaced
funnelled
bladder neck

Angulated
urethra

Cystocele

Procidentia

Anococcygeal
raphe

Cul-de-sac
hernia

Angulated
ureter

Rectocele

cervix should prolapse and elongate while the fundus stayed in the pelvic cavity. The para-colpium and suspensory ligaments of the rectum likewise represent the same process of thick-ening of the visceral connective tissue surround-ing vessels and nerves passing to the vagina and rectum.

The suspension of the uterus by the round ligaments as part of an operation for prolapse is ridiculous. Regardless of the type of opera-tion performed, it has only the effect of in-creasing the depth of the cul-de-sac for a period following the procedure and aids the forces that may initiate a herniation of the pelvic floor.

The Shape and Closure of the Pelvic Floor Aperture and the Forces Confronting the Levator Sling

The pelvic cavity is basinlike in form rather than a true funnel. The gentle curve which the levators make as they merge into the sides of the urethra, vagina, and rectum becomes straight and funneled only when the pelvic floor is relaxed. Whereas the bony hiatus of the outlet may measure 10 cm. in the antero-posterior dimension and 13 cm. in the trans-verse, the pelvic floor aperture of the soft parts measures much less. Resembling in the nullip-ara an elongated droplet, the diameter of the pelvic aperture at the fourchette is about 2.5 cm. and its length from the inferior border of the symphysis to a point just behind the anus is about 4 cm. The obturators that close this aperture are the urethra, vagina, and rectum (Plate 13, B). These organs, while concerned with three different and special functions, de-pend on the pelvic floor musculature and con-nective tissue for support. Fortunately the total visceral impact is not directed at the pelvic aperture; part impacts upon the sacrococcygeal platform, the anococcygeal raphe, and the promontory of the sacrum.

These obturators that close the pelvic floor outlet must be pressure-resisting structures. Their strong muscle coats in the healthy state fulfill this requirement. What happens when the levators contract? The anteroposterior and transverse dimensions of the aperture are de-creased and together they make more firm the obturators seated in their outlets. The uterus, al-though sitting on the pelvic floor and receiving connective tissue thickenings along the course of its vessels and nerves, nevertheless floats in equilibrium with the liver, spleen, bowel, and other viscera and, like them, would be in sorry shape if it had to depend on its so-called liga-ments for support.

The abdominal and pelvic viscera filling and floating in the peritoneal cavity are subjected to two forces: (1) the upward suction of the diaphragm and (2) the hydrostatic pressure of the viscera themselves. These forces oppose each other with a zero level about 10 cm. be-low the cupola of the diaphragm. These pres-sures fluctuate with changes in position, pos-ture, and respiratory movements. Studies of vaginal pressures by Stegmann show that hydro-static pressures are greater in the sitting than in the standing position since the former posi-tion compresses the viscera and adds the ele-ment of strain to the hydrostatic force. This difference is relatively slight and unimportant compared with sudden stresses such as coughing or sneezing, where the sucking action of the diaphragm is temporarily voided by its sudden descent. The application of this knowledge to postoperative early ambulation suggests that we mobilize early but pay more attention to the avoidance of severe stresses such as post-operative coughing and vomiting.

An Understanding of the Pathologic Physiology in the Event of a Pudendal Hernia

The speciousness of diagnosing a single, iso-lated vaginal lesion such as a cystocele without consideration of all the musculature and the ab-dominal as well as the pelvic viscera is ap-parent as one learns more about the pelvic floor. The size of the abdominal panniculus must be noted with as much interest as the bulge of the cystocele. In the course of prolapse the obtura-tor fascia, the parietal connective tissue with its thickenings (ligaments), and the perivascular connective tissue all respond with some degree of hypertrophy, but, unable to withstand the visceral thrust, they become elongated and incompetent (Plate 13, *C*). If the so-called ligaments of the uterus were alone responsible for its position, then a complete prolapse of the vault should occur after every radical hysterectomy, in which all of these ligaments are systematically severed as close to their presumptive origins as possible. Likewise, if the principal support of the vaginal vault were ligamentary, then an artificially created vagina should invert from lack of ligaments. As we all know, these things do not occur. What happens then? First, in a radical hysterectomy the posterior thickenings (uterosacral ligaments) far from the uterus, together with the peritoneum of the cul-de-sac, are resected, resulting in a partial obliteration of the posterior portion of the aperture. Next, the lateral thickenings are removed together with most of the vagina down to the superior aspect of the levator basin, and this is closed, with perhaps a drain. But subsequently in healing, the vaginal vault frequently admits only a fingertip and its depth is but a few centimeters. The anterior aspect of the aperture is now decreased. Then, the bladder falls over the remains of the vaginal musculature to become adherent to the rectum either by suture or in the healing process to form an additional bridge of muscle, connective tissue, and mucous membrane across this postoperative genital hiatus. Remember that the levators are not removed in this operation. In contrast, one does see perineal hernias of large dimensions after a pelvic eviscerectomy where the levators are hemisected and the bladder, vagina, and rectum (the normal obturators) are removed.

Two things happen in prolapse: (1) the pelvic floor is wounded or is congenitally incompetent and (2) the visceral downthrust is too much for it. If the pelvic floor, even though injured or relaxed, can contract with sufficient strength to resist the visceral downthrust, an asymptomatic relaxed outlet results. Prolapse is an extrusion, and the bearing down caused by inequality of the visceral downthrust and its opposition by the pelvic floor and obturators results in progressive anatomic changes diagnosed as varying degrees of relaxation and prolapse (Plate 13, *D*). Whether the uterus is anteverted, retroverted, or in a formalin jar has no bearing on the mechanics of this hernia. Who has not seen prolapse after a uterine ventrofixation? The cervix shows some of the end results of prolapse in the form of hypertrophy of its anterior lip and general elongation probably as a result of lymph stasis and nature's attempt to compensate. The uterus is only part of the visceral mass, and changes are simultaneously occurring in the other organs that form the pelvic obturator. In fact, the constriction of the prolapsed mass in the pelvic aperture may be the only thing that prevents a procidentia. The weight alone of the uterus has nothing to do with causing prolapse. I have observed a large, fibroid uterus filling the genital hiatus and preventing a prolapse. This same patient's pelvic floor was completely relaxed and atonic from a cord transection. Pregnancy in a prolapsed uterus results in temporary relief when the uterus forms a larger mass.

What happens in prolapse to the bladder neck, ureters, and rectum? The bladder neck is displaced downward and forward into the anterior portion of the hiatus. The ureters must elongate if the region of the interureteric ridge is displaced. They may be compressed by the damming effect of the obturators pressing in the hernial ring. With procidentia they may be occluded by the uterine artery and its connective tissue thickenings that pull on them as they make their way to the better supported trigone of the bladder. When viewed cystoscopically, the ureteral orifices become more and more perpendicular to the urethra and closer and closer to the cystoscopist while a larger retroureteric recess or bas-fond is forming. In rectocele the pouchlike extrusion may impede the dilatation of the rectal sphincters by the advancing fecal column.

Principles of Surgery in the Restoration and Permanent Sufficiency of the Pelvic Floor

The concept of the role of the levator muscles and the importance of providing a smaller aperture with an adequate obturator form the basis of modern vaginal surgery. In this way the connective tissue thickenings may be shortened or plicated when this method decreases the pelvic aperture. Correction of a cystocele or rectocele strengthens the muscular wall of the bladder and rectum. A cul-de-sac hernia imposes a sac between the vagina and rectum in the course of prolapse. This must be reduced so the vagina and rectum are again in opposition to function as adequate obturators. All this makes it imperative in vaginal plastic surgery to take into account all the structures in the pelvis in addition to the factors responsible for the visceral downthrust.

The retroperitoneal obliteration of the cul-de-sac has been practiced by Watson of New Zealand for many years in dealing with procidentia. His technique requires complete deperitonization of the cul-de-sac, obliteration by suturing together the uterosacral thickenings, and fixation of the vaginal vault to the uterosacral thickenings. The technique described later varies somewhat from his original description but the principle is the same.

The old concept of the importance of ligaments seems impossible of application to the living body. The habitual imperfection of plastic repair has resulted from piecemeal surgery. Whatever the operation, *decrease the aperture and strengthen the obturators!* Whatever the operation, *attack the pelvic floor and the visceral mass in its functional entirety!*

References

Bailey, K. V.: A Clinical Investigation Into Uterine Prolapse With Stress Incontinence; Treatment by Modified Manchester Colporrhaphy, J. Obst. & Gynaec. Brit. Emp. 63: 663, 1956.

Berglas, B.: Die Anatomie des Beckenbindegewebs bei Prolaps, Arch. Gynäc., Berl. 137: 1077, 1929.

Berglas, B., and Rubin, I.: Histologic Study of the Pelvic Connective Tissue, Surg., Gynec. & Obst. 97: 277, 1953.

Bissel, D.: A Vaginal Hysterectomy Technique for the Cure of Prolapse of the Uterus When the Removal of the Uterus Is Necessitated; With Special Reference to Lapping of the Vaginal Fascia in All Forms of Vaginal Prolapse, Surg., Gynec. & Obst. 28: 138-145, 1919.

Fothergill, W. E.: The Supports of the Pelvic Viscera; A Review of Some Recent Contributions to Pelvic Anatomy, With a Clinical Introduction, Proc. Roy. Soc. Med., Lond. 1: 43-60, 1907.

Friedman, E. A., and Little, W. A.: The Conflict in Nomenclature for Descensus Uteri, Am. J. Obst. & Gynec. 81: 817, 1961.

Goff, B. H.: Histological Study of Perivaginal Fascia in a Nullipara, Surg., Gynec. & Obst. 52: 32-42, 1931.

Halban, J.: Operative Behandlung des weiblichen Genitalprolapse unter Berüksichtigunger der Anatomie und Aetiologie, Vienna, 1919, Wilhelm Braumueller.

Kocks, J.: Die normale und pathologische Lage und Gestalt des Uterus sowie deren Mechanik, Bonn, 1880, Max Cohen & Son.

Koster, H.: On Supports of Uterus, Am. J. Obst. & Gynec. 25: 67-74, 1933.

Lewin, P.: Belt for Back Strain, J. A. M. A. 157: 38, 1955.

Mackenrodt, A.: Ueber die Ursachen der normalen und pathologischen Lagen des Uterus, Arch. Gynäk., Berl. 48: 303-421, 1895.

Mengert, W. F.: Mechanics of Uterine Support and Position; Factors Influencing Uterine Support; Experimental Study, Am. J. Obst. & Gynec. 31: 755-782, 1936.

Paramore, R. H.: The Statics of the Female Pelvic Viscera, London, 1918, H. K. Lewis & Co.

Ricci, J. V., Lisa, J. R., Thom, C. H., and Kron, W. L.: Relationship of Vagina to Adjacent Organs in Reconstructive Surgery; Histologic Study, Am. J. Surg. 74: 387-410, 1947.

Savage, H.: The Surgery, Surgical Pathology and Surgical Anatomy of the Female Pelvic Organs, London, 1870, J. Churchill & Sons.

Sederl, J.: The Operative Treatment of Prolapse of the Blind-Ending Vagina (Zur Operation des Prolapses der blind-endigen Scheide), Geburtsh. u. Frauenh. 18: 824, 1958.

Stegmann, H.: The Strain on the Pelvic Floor Before and After Gynecologic Operations and Its Significance for Early Post-operative Ambulation, Geburtsh. u. Frauenh. 14: 52, 1954.

Stoddard, F. J.: The Anatomy and Etiology of Genital Prolapse in Women, Obst. & Gynec. 15: 790, 1960.

Tandler, J.: Anatomie und topographische Anatomie der weiblichen Genitalien. In Stoeckel: Handbuch der Gynaecologie, vol. I, part 1, Munich, 1930, J. F. Bergmann.

Uhlenhuth, E., and Nolley, G. W.: Vaginal Fascia, a Myth? Obst. & Gynec. 10: 349, 1957.

Varco, S.: New Method of Pelvic Traction for the Relief of Low Back Pain, Surg., Gynec. & Obst. 98: 760, 1954.

Watson, A. L.: Technique of Vaginal Hysterectomy for Uterine Prolapse, Tr. Internat. & 4th Am. Cong. Obst. & Gynec. 61A: 191, 1951 (supp. Am. J. Obst. & Gynec.).

9 · Reconstructive Surgery of the Female Pelvic Floor

ANTERIOR AND POSTERIOR REPAIR
General Considerations

The simplest problem presented to the pelvic surgeon is the correction of a cystocele and rectocele that are symptomatic. Some of the most atrocious results in the surgery of pelvic relaxations and prolapse are seen when a surgeon performs a simple plastic procedure on a patient in need of more extensive surgery. The indications for a simple anterior and posterior repair become rare indeed as one learns more of the mechanics of prolapse. This operation has been combined in the past with a laparotomy to tie the round ligaments to something to suspend the uterus. Few students of the anatomy and the physiology of the female pelvic floor would be capable of commenting with restraint upon such a procedure.

Symptoms, Diagnosis, and Psychosomatic Aspects of Disease

The symptoms of a minor pelvic relaxation most frequently concern urinary control. While the relaxation of the anterior vaginal wall is not conspicuous, it nevertheless may represent an anatomic arrangement that permits rather severe stress incontinence. Some patients are annoyed with urinary urgency and frequency or rectal pressure. They may vaguely describe the entire feeling as a bearing-down sensation.

First observe the size of the abdominal panniculus. Note the depth of the symphysis and bony architecture. Carefully test for inguinal and femoral hernias. Note the presence of varicosities. All of these reflect the fascial make-up of the patient and add to your understanding of the pelvic floor.

Palpate the outlet and determine the status of the levator sling. The "loose, gaping introitus," as described by Emmet, "appears like the mouth of a bag without its drawstring." Observe that the cleft of the buttocks is flattened and broad. Now place two or more fingers in the fourchette and draw out and down. Note the laxity and thinness. At the same time, the anus is everted and displaced backward and the sphincter ring is evident under the skin. Have the patient strain down and note to what degree the anterior and posterior walls roll out with characteristic circumferential gaping. Study the enlargement of the pelvic aperture in relationship to the size of the obturators. Measure the descent of the cervix, using the nearest palpable point to the internal os as a guide.

Now palpate the levator ani by the following method and steps:

The anterior thickened portion, the puborectalis, is normally U shaped with short arms arching to the midline and blending into the sides of the vaginal and rectal walls to support the vagina and rectum. Place one index finger just inside the labium minus and press inward and anteriorly close to the pubic rami. Place the other index finger within the vagina in opposition. The puborectalis or its remains are now between your fingers, covered by the lateral vaginal wall of that side. You can see that the direction of the muscle with a relaxed outlet is now almost vertical and parallels the lateral vaginal wall instead of curving to the midline. It is this enlarged levator loop, often more distorted on the left than the right, that causes the bulging introitus. Above this we must diagnose other supporting structures equally compromised.

Have the patient strain down, and observe the endwise descent and mobility of the urethra. With the patient holding back as if to restrain urination, palpate the puborectalis for function and presence of scarring and injury. Palpate the remainder of the levator ani. With a single-bladed speculum, bring the posterior fornix into view and have the patient strain and cough. A cul-de-sac hernia is diagnosed this way above the rectocele. The features of the pelvic floor are now studied with the patient in the standing and knee-chest positions. If you still have your head mirror from your student days in ophthalmology, it is ideal to view the introitus with the patient in the standing-straddle position. The knee-chest position allows for inspection of the urethra and anterior wall with the pelvic and abdominal viscera gravitating toward the diaphragm rather than the pelvic basin.

Kegel has divided the pubococcygeus into segments: the supportive, the sphincteric, and the sexual. It is not clear how this muscle with a common motor innervation can individualize the diverse functions of its various segments. From his description the anterior supportive segment would seem to correspond to the attachments of the urethra to the remnants of the urogenital diaphragm, the sphincteric segment to the bladder neck, and the sexual segment to the iliococcygeus plus the vaginal musculature of the upper vagina that gives origin to the vaginal orgasm. While Kegel may simplify the origin of the vaginal orgasm, his observations are not amiss, and his perineometer has transformed many an inert sexual partner (devoid of feeling and complaining of frigidity) into a more energetic companion, though many an older patient with a scarred, contracted urethra has never been rejuvenated. The astute gynecologist will seldom be naive enough to promise any improvement in sexual gratification because the sagging perineum has

been sutured. The seat of the problem is in the psychosexual sphere.

Surgical Principles

The surgical principles involved in this operation concern the bladder and rectum. An early stage of the total picture of prolapse is to be corrected. The normal obturators are giving way, everting the pelvic aperture slightly, and giving rise to minor symptoms. To correct this, the bladder is restored to its normal position, the herniation of the rectum corrected, and the vaginal walls resected so as to strengthen the vagina. The full thickness of the vaginal wall is utilized in this operation rather than a denudation technique, which creates artificial layers often described as a fascia. This operation, while representing the most elementary of the vaginal plastic procedures, should be done thoroughly from vaginal fornices to the introitus lest it only set the stage for future surgery.

A common surgical pitfall in an anterior colporrhaphy is the plication of the bladder neck at the urogenital diaphragm at or near its middle third. Frequently the middle third of the urethra is mistaken for the true bladder neck. If an adequate urethrolysis has been done, the bladder neck will stand out within a centimeter or less. It is identified by the level at which the operator can see the anterolateral walls of the bladder passing laterally away from the bladder neck. Identification by an indwelling catheter of the Foley or other type is often deceptive, and the ideal is for the operator to positively identify the anatomic landmarks before proceeding with a plication of the bladder neck. An adequate dissection and release of all adhesions about the urethra and bladder neck will make the identity of the bladder neck simple and accurate.

Steps of the Operation

1. The labia are sewn back and traction sutures placed on the anterior and posterior lips of the cervix. Crushing instruments are not used for traction since the cervix is to be preserved. An incision is made at the bladder reflection (Plate 14, *A*). The knife handle is used to locate the

Text continued on p. 118.

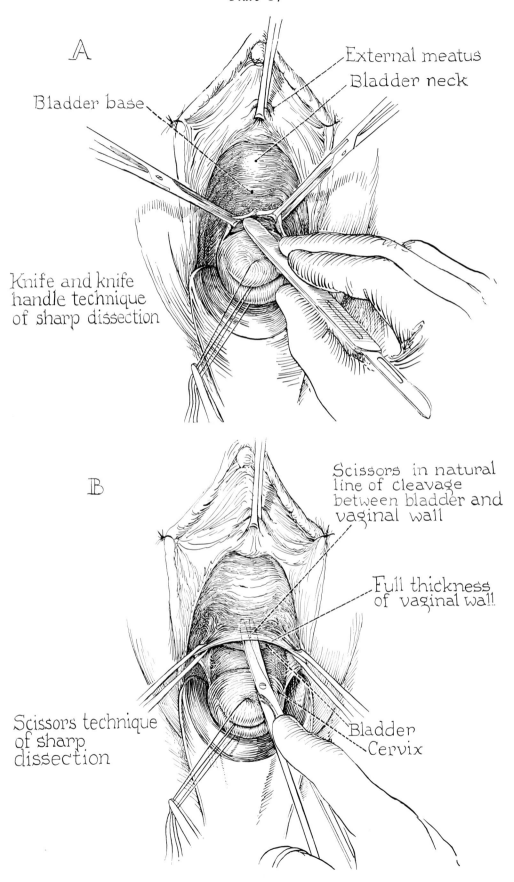

Plate 14

A

External meatus
Bladder neck

Bladder base

Knife and knife
handle technique
of sharp dissection

B

Scissors in natural
line of cleavage
between bladder and
vaginal wall

Full thickness
of vaginal wall

Scissors technique
of sharp
dissection

Bladder
Cervix

Plate 14 (Continued)

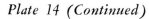

C

Sharp dissection
about trigone,
bladder neck, and
urethra

Urethra
Bladder neck
Region of trigone

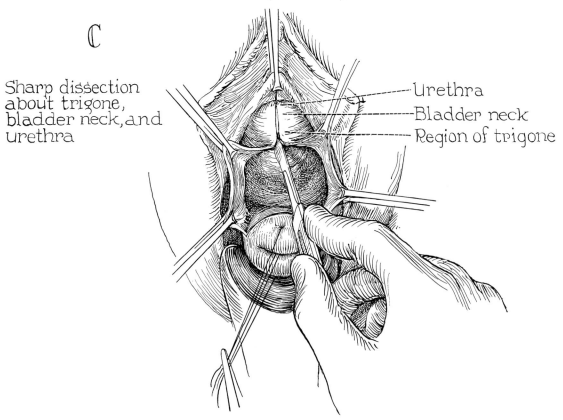

D

Mobilization of
urethra and
bladder neck

Fragile areolar tissue
of paravesicum

Lateral recess of
space of Retzius

Paravesicum and
branches of the
inf. vesical artery

Straight posterior
urethrovesical angle

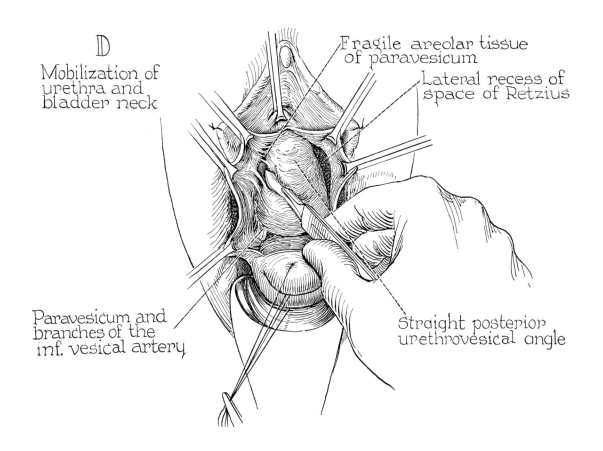

Plate 14 (Continued)

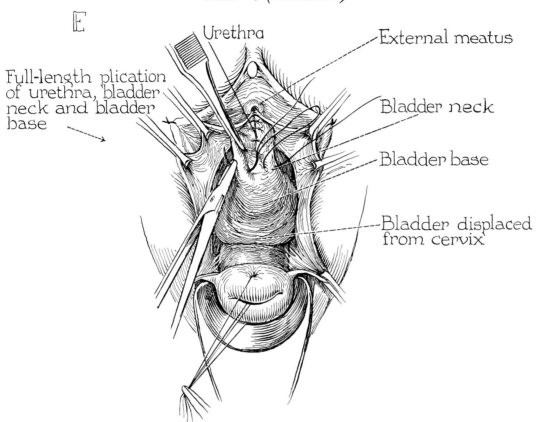

E

Urethra

External meatus

Full-length plication of urethra, bladder neck and bladder base

Bladder neck

Bladder base

Bladder displaced from cervix

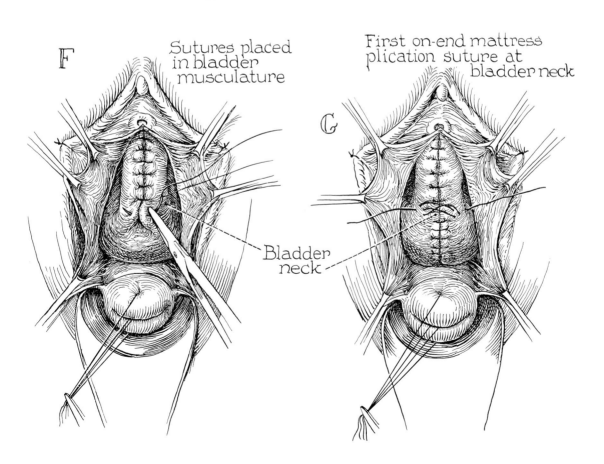

F

Sutures placed in bladder musculature

First on-end mattress plication suture at bladder neck

G

Bladder neck

Plate 14 (Continued)

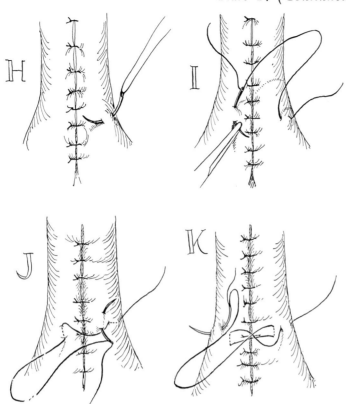

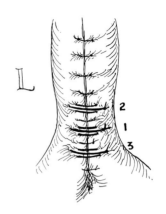

Technique of bladder neck plication

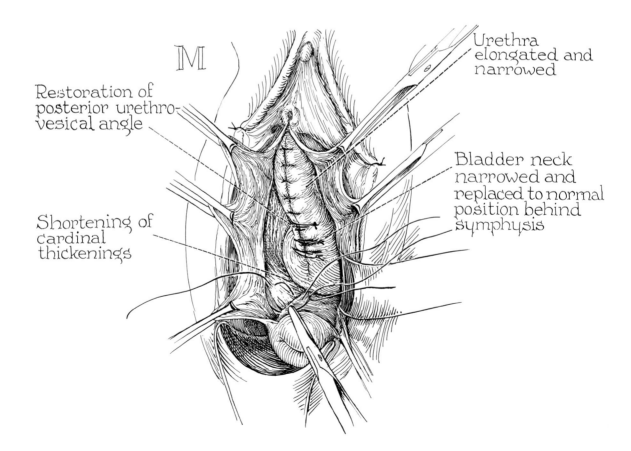

Restoration of posterior urethro-vesical angle

Shortening of cardinal thickenings

Urethra elongated and narrowed

Bladder neck narrowed and replaced to normal position behind symphysis

Plate 14 (Continued)

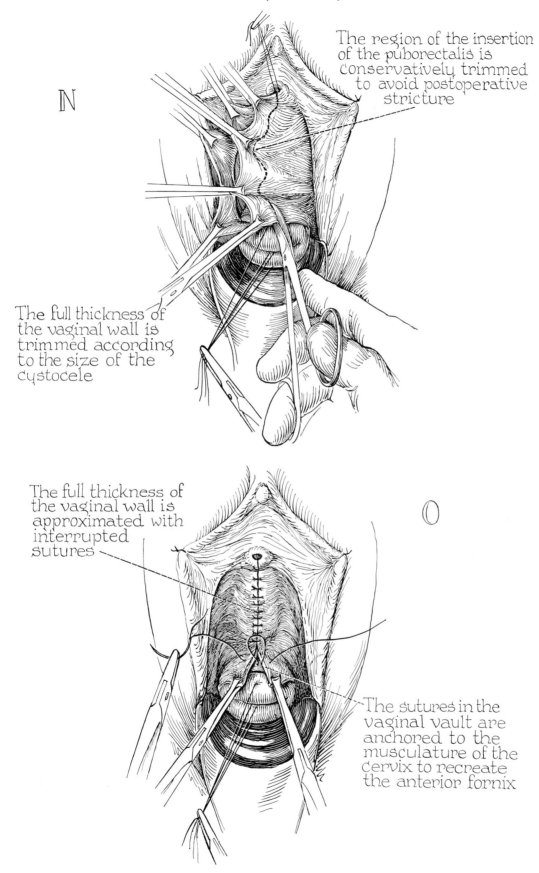

N

The region of the insertion
of the puborectalis is
conservatively trimmed
to avoid postoperative
stricture

The full thickness of
the vaginal wall is
trimmed according
to the size of the
cystocele

The full thickness of
the vaginal wall is
approximated with
interrupted
sutures

O

The sutures in the
vaginal vault are
anchored to the
musculature of the
cervix to recreate
the anterior fornix

Plate 14 (Continued)

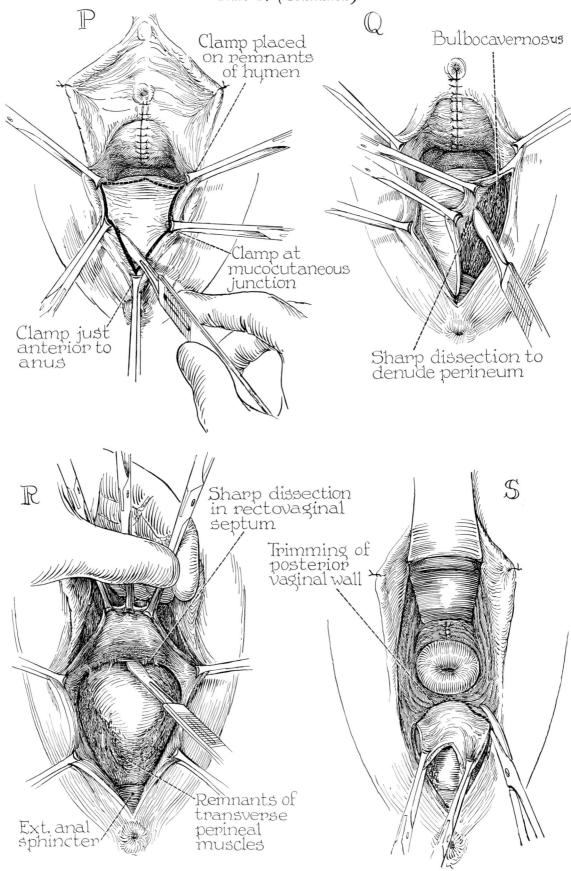

P

Clamp placed
on remnants
of hymen

Clamp at
mucocutaneous
junction

Clamp just
anterior to
anus

Q

Bulbocavernosus

Sharp dissection to
denude perineum

R

Sharp dissection
in rectovaginal
septum

Ext. anal
sphincter

Remnants of
transverse
perineal
muscles

S

Trimming of
posterior
vaginal wall

Plate 14 (Concluded)

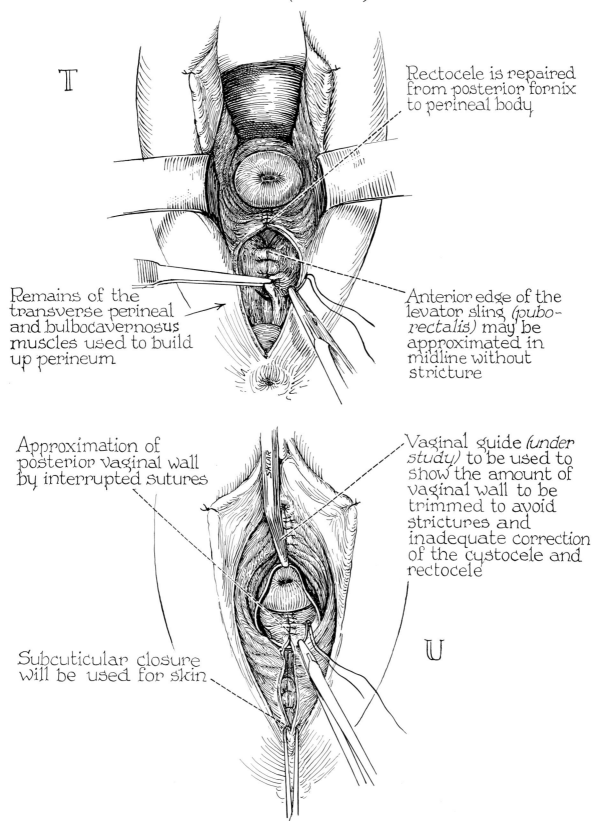

T

Rectocele is repaired
from posterior fornix
to perineal body

Remains of the
transverse perineal
and bulbocavernosus
muscles used to build
up perineum

Anterior edge of the
levator sling *(pubo-
rectalis)* may be
approximated in
midline without
stricture

Approximation of
posterior vaginal wall
by interrupted sutures

Vaginal guide *(under
study)* to be used to
show the amount of
vaginal wall to be
trimmed to avoid
strictures and
inadequate correction
of the cystocele and
rectocele

U

Subcuticular closure
will be used for skin

thin layer of areolar tissue between the bladder and vagina, and the full thickness of the vaginal wall is separated up to the bladder neck. In Plate 14, B, is shown the method of doing this dissection with curved dissecting scissors.

2. Since the urethra, bladder neck, and trigone are more intimately attached to the anterior vaginal wall than to the bladder base, the next dissection is best done with a knife. It is preferable to start at the external meatus and incise the wall retrograde to meet the first incision (Plate 14, C).

3. The urethra and bladder neck are now freely mobilized by alternately using knife blade and handle (Plate 14, D). Dissection with several thicknesses of gauze over the index finger is helpful for any fragile tissue once the firm bands of scar tissue have been incised and the proper line of cleavage entered. The mobilization of the bladder neck is the critical point of the dissection. Whether or not the patient has urinary incontinence, the urethra and bladder neck must be freely mobilized for either a necessary or prophylactic plication of the bladder neck. The anatomic landmarks are now evident (Plate 14, D).

4. On each side the connective tissue thickenings along the vaginal and cervical branches of the uterine arteries and branches from the inferior vesical arteries blend into the sides of the bladder base (Plate 14, D). These have been referred to as bladder pillars by many writers. The bladder is now advanced a few centimeters on the cervix. The extent to which this is done depends on the size of the cystocele, but it should be remembered that there is a normal angulation between the bladder neck and the bladder base. If the bladder base is too extensively mobilized (bladder advancement operations) and pushed up in line with the bladder neck and urethra, the anatomic derangement characteristically found in stress incontinence is created.

5. A full-length plication of the urethra, bladder neck, and bladder base is done, using 00 chromic catgut (Plate 14, E). The sutures penetrate the superficial layers of the muscular wall and can be tied without tension after such a complete mobilization (Plate 14, F). The degree of narrowing effected by the plication should conform to the normal anatomy. Less tissue is encompassed at the urethra than at the broader bladder base. After the full-length plication is completed, the specific on-end mattress sutures at the bladder neck are placed (Plate 14, G).

6. The technique of placing the bladder neck sutures is shown in Plate 14, H to L. The first suture (point 1, Plate 14, L) is placed directly at the bladder neck. The needle first passes into tissue quite far laterally on the left side of the bladder neck. It then takes a bite into the muscularis just across the midline on the right side, then passes back across to the left side, and then far laterally on the right side. When tied, this has the effect of doubly inverting the tissue, and it distinctly narrows the bladder neck and delineates the posterior urethrovesical angle. The second and third sutures are then placed in the same manner (points 2 and 3, Plate 14, L). When all three are placed, the assistants relax any traction on the flaps or cervix and they are tied in the order 3, 1, 2 and the ends cut.

7. The connective tissue thickenings on the lateral aspect of the cervix are now sutured into the cervix closer to the midline with 0 chromic catgut (Plate 14, M). This, as well as its variations, is called parametrial fixation. It has the effect of shortening the cardinal thickenings slightly and strengthening the support afforded by these structures.

8. Allis clamps are applied to the edges of the incision, and the left flap of vaginal wall is drawn across the midline (Plate 14, N). It is trimmed so that the new edge reaches to the midline without tension. The new anterior vaginal wall should conform to the changes effected in the bladder plication. In the healing process it is again attached to the bladder and urethra. The same process is repeated for the right flap of the vaginal incision.

9. The anterior vaginal wall is now closed with interrupted sutures of 00 chromic catgut. Interrupted sutures, in contrast to a continuous suture, do not shorten the vagina. The suture nearest the cervix is anchored to the anterior aspect of the cervix in order to recreate an anterior vaginal fornix (Plate 14, O).

10. Allis clamps are now placed posterolaterally at the mucotaneous junction on each side; two more are placed at the hymenal ring, and one is placed just above the anus (Plate 14, P). The bilaterally placed clamps are then brought together in the midline over two fingers as a guide to estimate the circumference of the new introitus and the height of the new perineum. Some simple mechanical guide can be used in this outline such as shown in Plate 14, U. When a functional introitus which also adequately reduces the posterior aspects of the genital hiatus has been outlined, the skin and mucosa are incised and dissected from the musculature tissue beneath (Plate 14, Q).

11. Three or more clamps are then placed on the full thickness of the posterior vaginal wall and drawn sharply anteriorly. By sharp dissection any scar tissue is lysed and the dissection continued to the posterior vaginal fornix (Plate 14, R). The extent of the dissection laterally is determined by the size of the rectocele and redundancy of the vaginal walls. The tissue removed should leave a functional vagina without stricture. The vagina should be, in the final reconstruction, a firm muscular tube and adequate obturator. Likewise, the rectocele is reduced and the competency of the rectum as an obturator restored. If successive wedges of tissue are removed as shown in Plate 14, S, a stricture will rarely result. Further trimming can be done later as indicated during the closure.

12. The thinned-out rectal wall proximal to the puborectalis is strengthened by several sutures. These sutures grasp the connective tissue thickenings laterally, bringing them to the midline. Bleeding is frequently encountered since the connective tissue accompanies vessels and nerves. The vaginal wall is then closed from above downward to the anterior edge of the puborectalis.

13. The reduction of the size of the pelvic aperture is mainly effected by approximating the leading edge of the puborectalis in the midline. The perineal body is made thicker, higher, and stronger by the midline approximation of the transverse perineal muscles, ischiocavernosi, and the bulbocavernosi. This also helps to close the pelvic aperture and fixes the vaginal and rectal obturators in their places.

14. The closure is done with interrupted sutures of 0 chromic catgut without any routine as to number of sutures. The individual anatomy and the amount of scarring and relaxation are the important factors. The build-up is begun in the deeper layers, placing sutures which approximate but do not strangulate and cut through the tissues. The size of the introitus is continuously observed to avoid a stricture (Plate 14, T). The leading edge of the puborectalis is approximated in the midline until an adequate pelvic aperture results (Plate 14, T).

15. The mucosa and skin are then trimmed further if necessary. The remaining closure is effected by interrupted sutures down to the mucocutaneous junction and the skin closed with a subcuticular suture of 00 chromic catgut (Plate 14, U).

16. A two-inch vaginal pack is inserted in the vagina and a fine catheter (No. 12 or No. 14 Fr.) left in the bladder.

In Plate 14, U, is shown an instrument under study to be used in an attempt to take some of the guesswork out of the repair of the pelvic floor when a functional vagina is desirable. Some of our predecessors sensed the need for such a device if only to impress upon operators the importance of preoperative study in this surgery. Its inclusion in a text of this type is justified when one realizes that in describing a vaginal plastic operation writers find themselves without some standard object that could be used to tell the reader how big to make the vagina. One wonders how long it may take for the vagina to come into its rightful place among the organs upon which plastic surgery is performed. While moulages are made of future noses, while artists draw ears to guide plastic surgeons, and even simple grafts are planned and plotted days in advance, vaginal plastic surgery is undertaken with a shameful lack of study. Habitually the operators' fingers are unceremoniously poked into the field of operation to determine the ultimate dimensions of the organ. Fat fingers, thin fingers, big fingers, or small fingers—this technique has yet to be replaced by something more esthetic and reliable. While constrictions and dyspareunia, recurrent relaxations and gaping, and scarring and abnormal fixation have been all too frequent results in vaginal surgery, the same postoperative appearance would scarcely be tolerated elsewhere. Should not the guesswork be taken out of this surgery?

While the vaginal surgeon may passionately desire faithfully to restore the virginal dimensions, axis, contour, and markings of his subject, this is not possible. In place of this the objective is resolutely to reconstruct a functional, pain-free, pliable, distensible, and well-supported structure. The dimensions of the instrument under study are based on the studies of Dickinson, who has made some of the most memorable contributions to the human sex anatomy. He insisted on distinguishing the anatomy of the "quick from the dead," a philosophy vaginal surgeons should devoutly embrace.

The anterior vaginal wall measures 7 cm. or

better, while the posterior wall is 1.5 to 2.0 cm. longer. The distal two-fifths of the vagina forms a 55-degree angle with the horizontal with the patient in the lithotomy position. The central two-fifths dips farther posterior to narrow the angle to 10 degrees. The proximal one-fifth is modified by the cervix and the position of the uterus—whether anterior or retrodisplaced. The average, erect penis measures 16 cm. in length from its bony insertion. Less than this is functional in coitus. It is 3 to 4 cm. wide and has a total circumference of about 10 cm. While these measurements were considered in the construction of the guide, the results obtained by use of the instrument modified its final construction. One must remember that the collapsed vagina assumes the form of the letter H, with a rather long transverse bar. Our surgery modifies the anterior and posterior walls of this H-shaped structure since the lateral walls, while they may be damaged, are not employed in the standard operations.

The instrument consists of a V-shaped mold whose dimensions have been found to result in a functional vagina when used as described. To this mold is attached a shank which is angulated to follow the contour of the symphysis or perineum. The handle allows continuous positioning by an assistant without fatigue. The V-shaped mold is 2.5 cm. wide and 2 cm. in height. The shank is ruled in centimeters for convenience in measuring the depth of the vagina, the degree of prolapse, and other factors.

After dissection of the anterior wall is completed, the instrument is inserted to judge the amount of excess tissue that must be removed. The anterior horizontal bar of the instrument as seen in this position measures 2.5 cm. Using this as a guide, the wall is trimmed so that the horizontal bar snugly reaches to each anterolateral fornix. This measurement is particularly useful in preventing too enthusiastic trimming at the point of insertion of the pubococcygeus, which is a common place of constriction.

The guide is next placed at the introitus and the skin and mucous membrane of the four-chette are stretched about it to determine the extent, trimming, and build-up of the perineal body. The incisions are made and the remainder of the posterior wall is opened. The guide is then inserted to the vault, handle up, and the final and most important phase of the colporrhaphy begun. Starting from the vault, the mucosa is trimmed to fit snugly about the circumference of the guide, and one can successively place sutures in the posterior wall as the assistant moves the instrument. When the mid-vagina is reached, sutures are placed in the levator ani and bulbocavernosus and the effect on the vaginal circumference is noted. The remainder of the wall can then be closed as was the upper vagina without fear of a constriction. With practice, the speed with which a plastic operation can be done is aided by this instrument.

Several other uses for such an instrument have come to mind as it is being studied to determine whether its primary purpose is worth while. The guide may be inserted into the vagina prior to abdominal hysterectomy to identify the vaginal vault. The handle is manipulated through the drapes. During suprapubic fixation of the bladder or other operations in the space of Retzius, it can be used to elevate the bladder base through the vagina. As an office instrument it can be used in mensuration, searching for high inaccessible fistulous tracts, and in the study of constrictions. In the study of stress incontinence the instrument is useful in that successive areas of the bladder base and neck can be elevated and the effect on the degree of incontinence noted.

General Postoperative Care in Vaginal Plastic Surgery

At the conclusion of the vaginal operation, a fine catheter (No. 12 or No. 14 Fr.) is inserted. A small retention catheter may also be employed. The catheter is attached by rubber tubing to a receptacle at floor level. A two-inch gauze pack is inserted. The pack is removed in twenty-four hours and the catheter in four days.

Urinary antiseptics are given in the infusion and continued by mouth as soon as tolerated. Sulfadiazine, 0.5 Gm. four times a day, with sodium bicarbonate, 1.0 Gm. four times a day, is adequate prophylactic therapy. Aureomycin, Terramycin, Chloromycetin, Achromycin, and erythromycin, 250 mg. every six hours, can be used. Where a resistant organism such as *Proteus vulgaris* or *Pseudomonas aeruginosa* is cultured or the infection is long standing, combinations of antibiotics and sulfonamides are used. The wide-spectrum antibiotics every six hours and streptomycin, 500 mg. I.M., every twelve hours seem to complement each other. The emphasis is on prophylaxis rather than treatment of a postoperative pyelocystitis that may have been avoided. Patients are mobilized early, and a full diet is ordered.

Postoperative retention frequently complicates the operation. Despite every measure from tidal drainage to hypnosis, some patients will not void for several weeks. The following measures are instituted on the sixth postoperative day for those "who have not passed a drop":

Day 6—Urge the patient not to strain violently and reassure her that the inability to void means that the repair is holding up well and she will soon start, even though the quantities are small. Instill 30 ml. of 1 per cent aqueous Mercurochrome twice a day after catheterization.

Day 7—Start therapy with the parasympathomimetic drugs. Methacholine chloride, U.S.P. (Mecholyl chloride) may be given by subcutaneous injection in a test dose of 2.5 to 5.0 mg. Atropine sulfate, 0.5 mg., is immediately available as an antidote. If well tolerated, the dosage is increased to as high as 50 mg. every four hours under careful observation. Mecholyl chloride can be given by mouth, adjusting the dose between 0.2 and 0.6 Gm. three times a day. Many similar drugs are available and may be substituted. Furmethide is used in the dosage of 3.0 mg. every six hours subcutaneously or 10 to 30 mg. twice a day per os. Stigmonene bromide can be given intramuscularly, 1 to 2 mg. Urecholine,

5 mg. subcutaneously or 10 to 30 mg. twice a day per os, may be given for its bladder-stimulating effect in retention.

Day 10 and subsequently—Dilate the urethra with a local anesthetic, such as Xylocaine, 2.5 per cent, and continue reassurance and suggestive therapy. A slow dilatation up to about a No. 8 Hegar dilator or a No. 24 Fr. sound after administering one of the tranquilizing drugs (Miltown, Equanil, 400 mg.) is the latest nonspecific psychotherapy for urinary retention. The patient will start to void of her own accord in due course from cause or causes unknown.

Early ambulation is desirable in pelvic surgery. The following instructions should be given patients and nurses:

1. The patient should report immediately any desire to cough or sneeze, and drugs to depress these reflexes are freely given.

2. When ambulated, the patient should walk with the legs together to minimize danger of hematomas or dehiscence.

3. Thoracic breathing is taught and encouraged in the erect posture to reduce the hydrostatic pressure on the pelvic diaphragm and site of operation.

FOTHERGILL-HUNTER OPERATION
Indications and Surgical Principles

The Fothergill-Hunter operation has its most clear indication in young women with prolapse who desire preservation of the child-bearing function. In others, the retention of a symptom-producing organ that may have served its purpose is illogical in modern gynecology that strives to be definitive and final in the first operation. The operation should be performed with due regard for an anatomic reconstruction of the pelvic floor, using the full thickness of the vaginal walls and disregarding artificial fascias created by stripping the vaginal mucosa from its muscularis. It has been done by this stripping technique of superficial dissection and amputation of the cervix, suggestive of the "iron chink"—that peculiar machine of the Alaskan canneries that skins salmon and cuts off their heads at the same time. Such a technique fails to completely correct the pelvic floor and may fall short of relieving the patient's symptoms and prolapse. Failure to recognize and correct a cul-de-sac hernia during the operation is common if the posterior vaginal wall is not completely opened from the introitus to the posterior fornix. The technique shown here eliminates this possibility by starting the rectocele repair from above downward toward the vulva. The patency of the cervical canal must be assured, and all of the surgical principles outlined for a simple anterior and posterior repair must be incorporated in this operation.

Steps of the Operation

1. A dilatation and curettage are done. The cervix should be dilated to a No. 10 Hegar dilator and the length of the cervical canal measured.

2. The full thickness of the vaginal wall is opened from the bladder reflection with an inverted V incision, and then the incision is continued to the urethral meatus in the same manner as illustrated for a simple anterior repair (Plate 14, A to D). The bladder is pushed off the cervix at its natural line of cleavage and the urethra mobilized for future plication. Bleeding points are ligated, and then attention is directed to the cervical amputation.

3. The inverted V incision at the bladder reflection is now extended around the cervix (Plate 15, A). The degree of hypertrophy of the cervix, the extent of the prolapse, and the elongation of the visceral connective tissue determine the site of amputation of the cervix. The internal os is the guiding landmark in describing descensus. In general, a distance of 3 cm. from the internal os to the point of amputation will allow for shortening of the ligaments and correction of the cystocele and rectocele, both of which strengthen the vagina as an obturator and contribute to correction of the prolapse.

4. The flaps are now developed laterally and posteriorly to demonstrate the cardinal and uterosacral ligaments. The extent of this dissection is governed by the amount of cervix to be amputated. The ligaments should be cut, clamped, and tied close to the cervix in order to permit suture in the midline (Plate 15, B). By suture of these thickenings, anterior to the amputated cervix for the cardinal structures and posterior for the

uterosacral thickenings, the vagina is restored as a competent obturator.

5. The cardinal ligaments, which at this level contain the descending branch of the uterine artery, are secured with two suture ligatures of 0 chromic catgut (Plate 15, B). They are mobilized to a sufficient length to be brought together in the midline after the cervical amputation (Plate 15, C).

6. The posterior thickenings, the uterosacral ligaments, are cut, clamped, and tied (Plate 15, D). In these thickenings are vaginal branches of the inferior vesical arteries, and failure to respect this fact can give rise to postoperative bleeding and a hematoma of the rectovaginal septum.

7. The cervix is amputated and coned (Plate 15, E). Active bleeding points are secured and ligated. A bullet tenaculum is attached to the anterior lip of the cervix, which is drawn anteriorly (Plate 15, F).

8. Following the principle of correcting the pelvic floor as a whole, attention is now directed to obliteration of the cul-de-sac since some degree of herniation inevitably exists because of the nature of uterine prolapse (Plate 15, E and F). This is done by dissecting the full thickness of the vaginal wall from the cul-de-sac peritoneum and subsequently from the rectum in retrograde fashion. It is continued until the posterior thickenings (uterosacral ligaments) fan out and lose their identity as their vessels approach their origins from the hypogastric artery. Hemostasis is important as the ligaments are approximated. Realize the proximity of the ureters so that they are not ligated nor distorted.

9. The uterosacral ligaments are now united in the midline (Plate 15, F). If a definitive hernial sac is evident, the peritoneum is opened prior to this and the neck of the sac transfixed and amputated. Retrograde dissection is continued, stopping periodically to unite the uterosacral thickenings and control bleeding.

10. Depending on the size of the cul-de-sac herniation, the rectovaginal septum is soon reached. The dissection goes remarkably well if it is in the right plane. Simultaneous correction of the upper portion of the rectocele is started. No part of the composite picture of the pathologic anatomy of prolapse is thus neglected (Plate 15, F and G).

11. Plate 15, G, shows this retrograde method of dissection. Consecutive wedge-shaped sections of the posterior vaginal wall are removed, the utero-

Plate 15

A

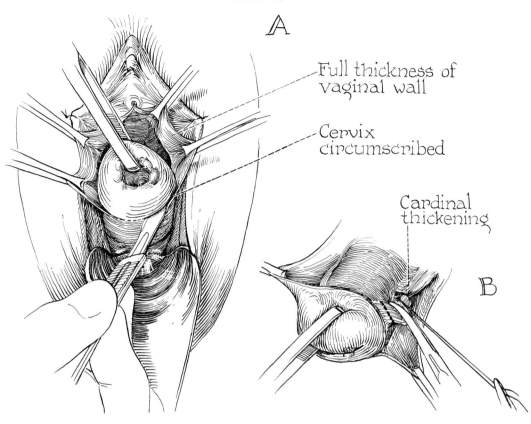

Full thickness of
vaginal wall

Cervix
circumscribed

Cardinal
thickening

B

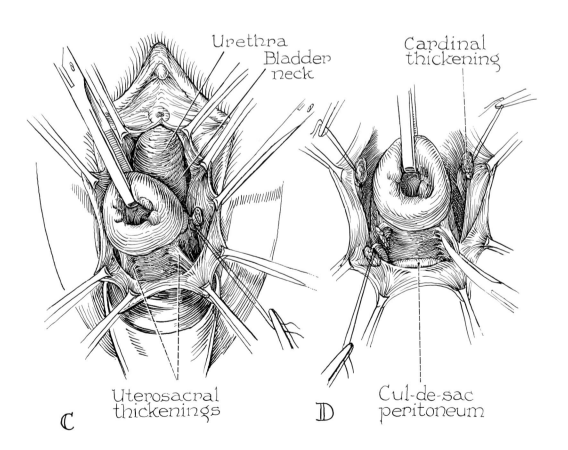

Urethra
Bladder
neck

Cardinal
thickening

Uterosacral
thickenings

C

D

Cul-de-sac
peritoneum

Plate 15 (Continued)

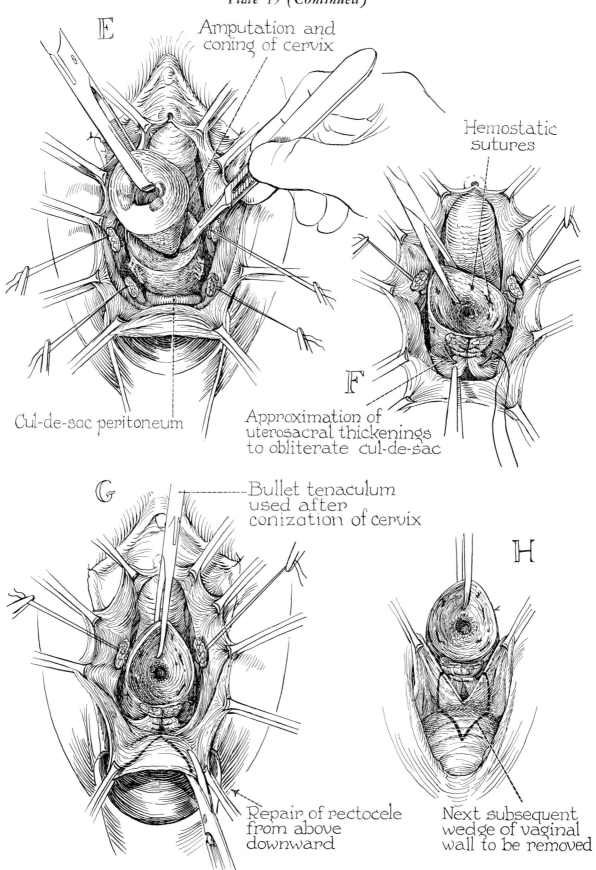

E

Amputation and coning of cervix

Hemostatic sutures

Cul-de-sac peritoneum

F

Approximation of uterosacral thickenings to obliterate cul-de-sac

G

Bullet tenaculum used after conization of cervix

H

Repair of rectocele from above downward

Next subsequent wedge of vaginal wall to be removed

sacral thickenings are approximated, and the field is kept free of active bleeding. The connective tissue fanning out toward the sacrum gradually thins out and its identity is lost in the perirectal connective tissue.

12. Plate 15, *H,* shows the appearance of this dissection and line of trimming if folded back and seen from the vaginal aspect. This line of incision will be met from below upward when the perineorrhaphy is done and the lower part of the rectocele is corrected.

13. An inverting suture, commonly known as a Sturmdorf, is used to slide the flaps of the vagina over the raw fibromuscular tissue of the cervix (Plate 15, *I*). As illustrated, this has the effect of drawing the edges into the new external os and recreating the posterior fornix.

14. Interrupted sutures of 00 chromic catgut are now inserted to approximate the posterior wall. The last suture is left long and is tagged as a landmark to be used later when the reconstruction of the perineal body and completion of the rectocele repair are done from below upward (Plate 15, *J*).

15. A full-length plication of the urethra, bladder neck, and bladder base is done in the same manner as illustrated for a simple anterior repair (Plate 14, *E* to *L*). This plication is done regardless of the pre-existence of stress incontinence. The anatomic arrangement that results in incontinence can easily be fabricated in repair of the anterior wall by the surgeon intent upon curing the protuberances of a cystocele and rectocele but neglecting a prophylactic plication of the bladder neck. Once again, the importance of attacking the herniation as a whole is apparent (Plate 15, *J*).

16. The cardinal thickenings are then sutured in the midline by several interrupted sutures (Plate 15, *K*). This feature of the operation has the effect of shortening these extensions of the parietal connective tissue and enhancing their contribution to the support of the pelvic floor.

17. An anterior Sturmdorf-type suture is placed and left untied pending a study of the flaps of the anterior wall (Plate 15, *L*). The original inverted V incision will have reconstructed a few centimeters of the anterior vaginal wall comprising the anterior fornix. The remainder of the walls are developed by the following method: Push the cervix toward the sacrum with the bullet tenaculum and observe the flaps of the anterior vaginal wall. Cross the Allis clamps so that one flap overlaps the other. Observe the amount of

vaginal wall to be resected on each side and then do the resection with the Metzenbaum scissors as it is done in a simple anterior repair.

18. The anterior vaginal wall is now closed with interrupted sutures of 00 chromic catgut, beginning at the anterior fornix. As the walls are approximated, more vaginal wall can be resected if this seems indicated. The anterior Sturmdorf suture, when tied, will complete the reconstruction of the anterior vaginal wall (Plate 15, *M*).

19. The lateral or crown sutures which bring together the vaginal wall in the lateral fornices are placed as shown in Plate 15, *M*. These sutures should include some of the superficial layers of the fibromuscular structure of the cervix since their purpose is to epithelize all raw areas.

20. As in the posterior repair previously illustrated for a simple vaginal plastic operation (Plate 14, *P* to *U*), a butterfly section of skin and mucous membrane is outlined on the perineum (Plate 15, *M*). The landmarks are the skin just anterior to the anus, the mucocutaneous junction laterally, and above this the hymenal ring or its remnants (Plate 15, *M*). The genital hiatus must now be closed at one of its crucial areas. Its anteroposterior length must be decreased and the width of its transverse slit narrowed. This cannot be done by a routine method of placing sutures in the hiatus. Descriptions of the placing of "levator sutures" are as unrealistic as the frequent illustrations of this anatomic forgery. The levator muscles (specifically, the puborectali) are centimeters away from the perineum. One should not place heavy sutures and forcibly draw the insertions of a group of paired, laterally placed muscles to an abnormal position in the midline. The plastic reconstruction of the genital aperture requires more selective surgery if a functional vagina is desired.

21. From the hymenal ring the butterfly pattern is advanced by incisions up to the traction suture left from the retrograde dissection and repair of the rectocele (Plate 15, *M*). This proceeds without the usual difficulty in locating the proper line of cleavage between vagina and rectum since this has already been identified from above (Plate 14, *Q* to *S*).

22. The last phase of this operation, the formation of a strong obturator and a narrow hiatus, is now begun. By using interrupted sutures of 0 chromic catgut, the musculature of the perineum is built up. Multiple sutures are placed without strangulation to build up the perineum so that the

Plate 15 (Concluded)

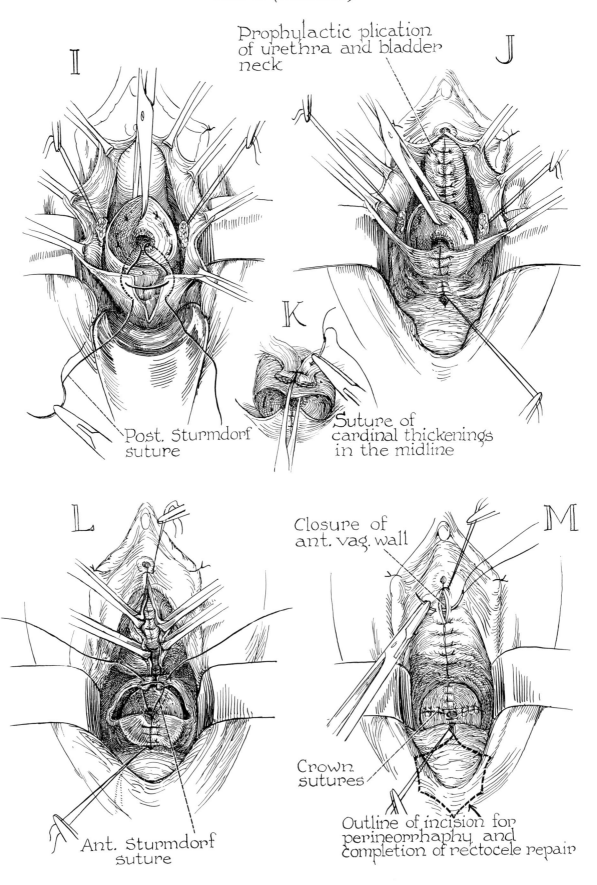

Prophylactic plication of urethra and bladder neck

I

J

K

Post. Sturmdorf suture

Suture of cardinal thickenings in the midline

L

M

Closure of ant. vag. wall

Ant. Sturmdorf suture

Crown sutures

Outline of incision for perineorrhaphy and completion of rectocele repair approximation of the bulbocavernosi and remnants of the transverse perineal muscles decreases the genital aperture and adds to the support of the pelvic viscera (Plate 14, *T*). The anterior edges of the puborectalis may be drawn to the midline to decrease the pelvic aperture, but this must be done with caution or a stricture will result despite the fact that adequate vaginal wall remains. Repeated palpation of the lower third of the vagina is necessary during the reconstruction of the perineum. Individualize with each operation, for the depth of the pelvic floor varies and the extent of the musculature support remaining varies in each patient. The vaginal wall is closed with interrupted sutures of 00 chromic catgut (Plate 14, *U*).

Postoperative Care

The postoperative care is the same as that described under Anterior and Posterior Repair (page 127).

VAGINAL HYSTERECTOMY
Indications and Surgical Principles

The indications of yesteryear for a vaginal hysterectomy are disappearing as gynecologic surgery is again finding its place among the surgical disciplines. Treatment of gynecologic conditions is preferably managed by the vaginal route when the operation can be done just as adequately and exploration of the upper abdomen is not indicated. Vaginal hysterectomy is accompanied by a lower morbidity, fewer postoperative complications, and less discomfort than abdominal hysterectomy. It permits vaginal plastic work at the same time. Many of the contraindications to vaginal hysterectomy disappear as the skill of the operator increases. Thus, prolapse is not necessary, for the skillful operator delivers the uterus by section of the connective tissue supports. Fixation of the uterus by endometriosis, inflammatory disease, ventrofixation, or some previous bizarre operation may tax the ingenuity of the vaginal surgeon. The vaginal approach is contraindicated in pelvic malignancy except for the rare indication for a Schauta procedure. Large uteri can be removed vaginally by morcellation or bisection of a large fibroid uterus and separate removal of each half. The question of removal of

the ovaries at the time of hysterectomy has produced some of the most inconsistent statistical reports to be found in clinical literature. Surgeons advocating a bilateral salpingo-oophorectomy at a specified age during an abdominal hysterectomy fail to remove the normal ovaries of a patient during a vaginal hysterectomy because of the technical difficulties. The technical difficulties of vaginal salpingo-oophorectomy are much exaggerated and will be less insurmountable if the surgeon will equip himself with the proper instruments. The use of long Deaver retractors, long Babcock clamps, long angle clamps, long Heaney and Kelly clamps, and long needle holders soon dissipates the reputed hazards of the vaginal approach to adnexal disease.

Steps of the Operation

1. The labia are sewn back and a dilatation and curettage performed. In the absence of any suspicious tissue, Jacobs clamps are placed on the anterior and posterior lips of the cervix. Any suitable tenaculum may be substituted that will permit strong traction without tearing and its subsequent annoying bleeding. Single 0 chromic catgut is used for hemostatic ligatures. Simple approximation of vaginal wall or ties on bleeding points are accomplished with 00 chromic catgut.

2. An inverted V incision is made anteriorly through the full thickness of the vaginal wall and extended laterally around the cervix for a short distance. The bladder is pushed off the cervix by the knife handle entering the fragile areolar tissue between these organs. The vesicouterine reflection of the peritoneum appears between the bladder and upper part of the cervix. Any active bleeding is controlled by ties. The remainder of the anterior vaginal wall will be opened retrograde after the hysterectomy. This sequence in the steps of the operation avoids unnecessary bleeding from the incised anterior vaginal wall during the hysterectomy. The extent of this first incision is shown in Plate 16, *A*.

3. Plate 16, *B*, shows the dissection carried farther and the landmarks of importance. The bladder base, vesicouterine peritoneal fold, and cervix should be clearly evident if the correct tissue plane was entered. Previous surgery or scarring may make this difficult at times. A sound placed in the bladder can help differentiate the tissue of the

Text continued on p. 134.

Plate 16

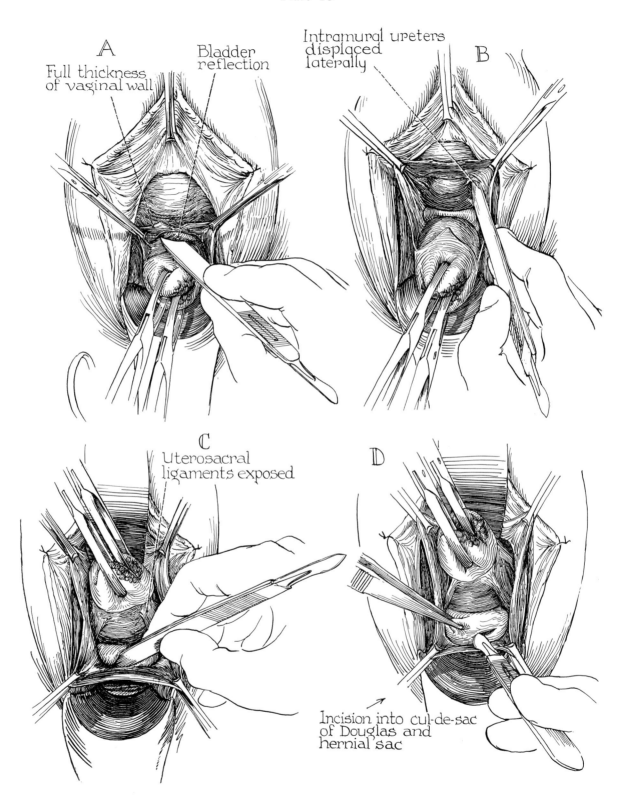

A

Full thickness of vaginal wall

Bladder reflection

B

Intramural ureters displaced laterally

C

Uterosacral ligaments exposed

D

Incision into cul-de-sac of Douglas and hernial sac

Plate 16 (Continued)

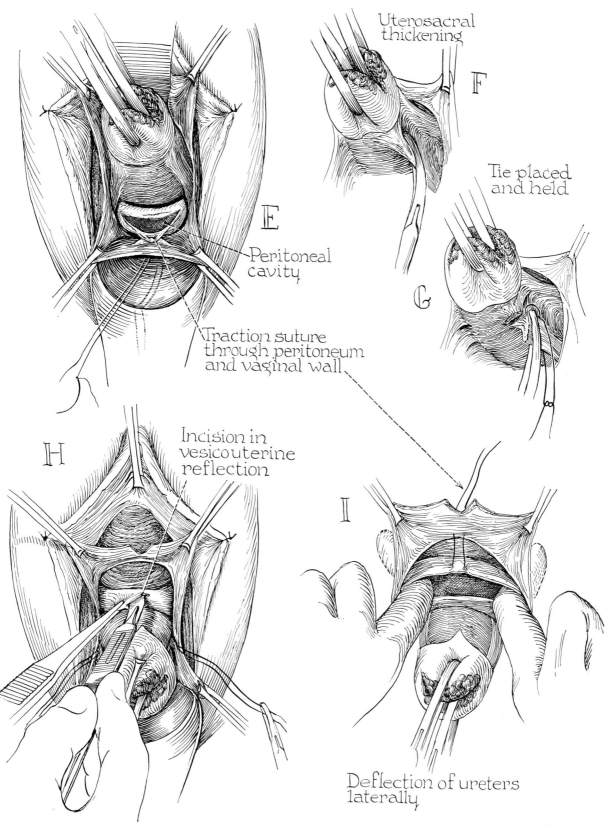

Uterosacral
thickening

F

Tie placed
and held

G

E

Peritoneal
cavity

Traction suture
through peritoneum
and vaginal wall

H

Incision in
vesicouterine
reflection

I

Deflection of ureters
laterally

Plate 16 (Continued)

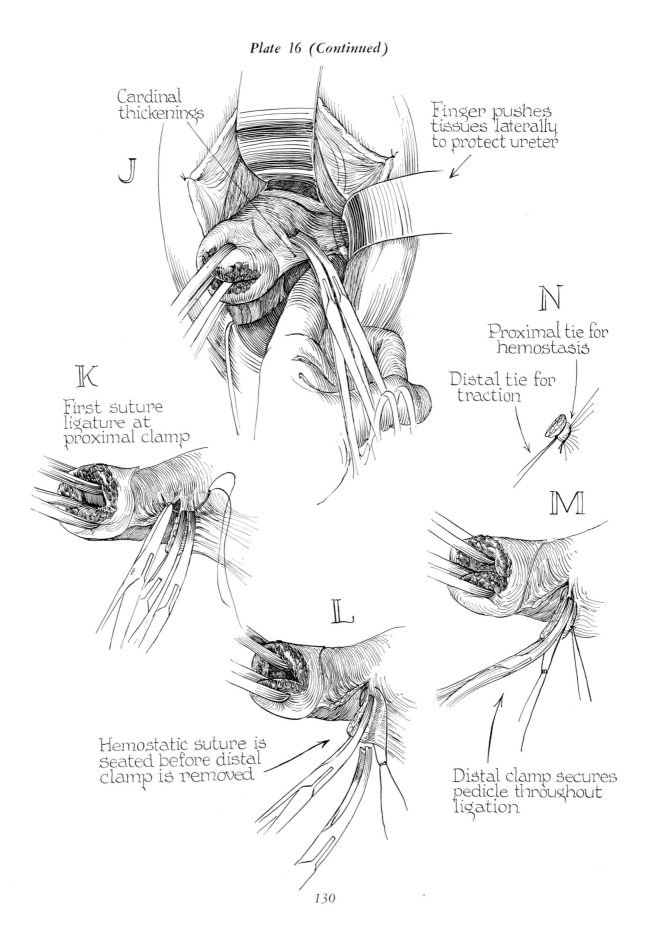

Cardinal thickenings

Finger pushes tissues laterally to protect ureter

J

N

Proximal tie for hemostasis

Distal tie for traction

K

First suture ligature at proximal clamp

M

L

Hemostatic suture is seated before distal clamp is removed

Distal clamp secures pedicle throughout ligation

Plate 16 (Continued)

Bladder

O

Clamps on uterine
a., v.

Strong traction
to opposite side

Finger deflects
tissues away
from clamps

P

Delivery of fundus in the
cul-de-sac

Clamps on ovarian a., v.
and round lig.

Q

Clamps on tube
and ovarian lig.

Plate 16 (Continued)

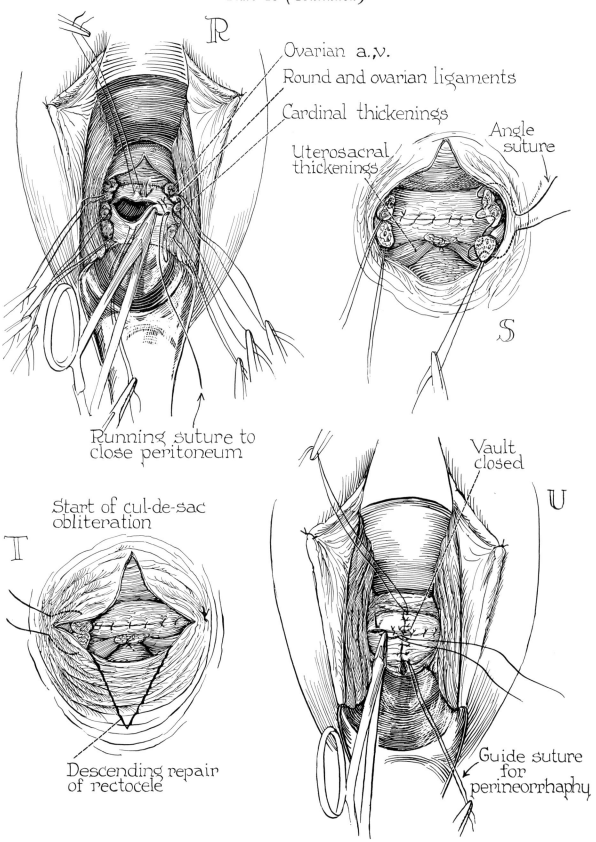

R

Ovarian a.,v.

Round and ovarian ligaments

Cardinal thickenings

Uterosacral thickenings

Angle suture

S

Running suture to close peritoneum

Start of cul-de-sac obliteration

T

Vault closed

U

Descending repair of rectocele

Guide suture for perineorrhaphy

Plate 16 (Concluded)

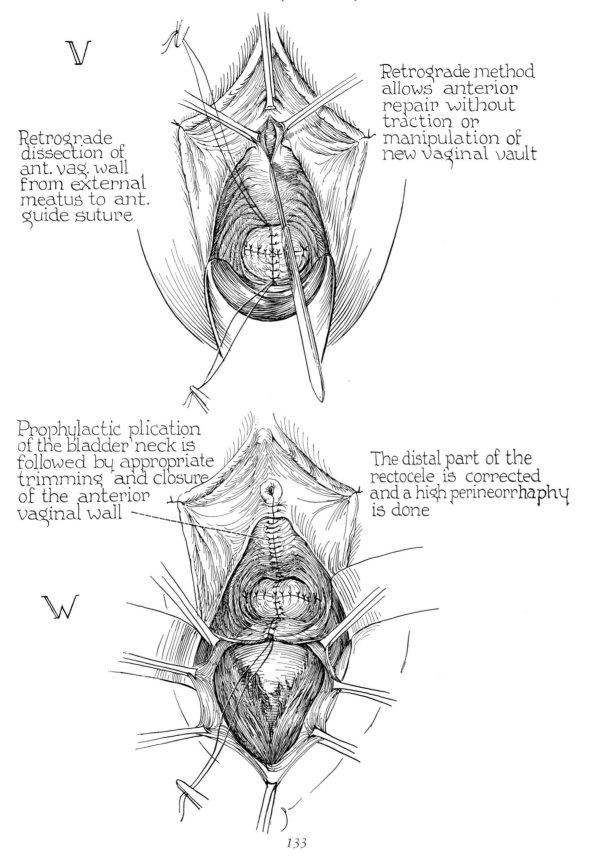

V

Retrograde
dissection of
ant. vag. wall
from external
meatus to ant.
guide suture

Retrograde method
allows anterior
repair without
traction or
manipulation of
new vaginal vault

Prophylactic plication
of the bladder neck is
followed by appropriate
trimming and closure
of the anterior
vaginal wall

The distal part of the
rectocele is corrected
and a high perineorrhaphy
is done

W

bladder base from the cervix when they are unusually adherent.

4. The incision is now carried completely around the cervix, and the posterior vaginal wall is grasped with Allis clamps. The uterosacral ligaments are identified, and the dissection is continued until the peritoneum of the cul-de-sac is evident. The degree of herniation of the cul-de-sac will vary but must inevitably exist coincident with prolapse. The larger the herniation, the more extensive the dissection and exposure at this time (Plate 16, C).

5. The cul-de-sac peritoneum is now picked up with a thumb forceps and the peritoneal cavity entered (Plate 16, D). An exploration of the pelvis is carried out with one finger while strong traction is made on the uterus in an anterior direction. The status of the ovaries and tubes, as well as the presence of any bowel or omentum adhesions to the uterus, is determined.

6. A suture of 00 chromic catgut is used to tag the peritoneum to the posterior vaginal wall (Plate 16, E). The posterior thickenings or uterosacral ligaments contain blood vessels that can be a troublesome source of bleeding from the posterior flap. These vessels should be systematically ligated. They are vaginal branches of the hypogastric artery which, in the male, are called the inferior vesical arteries. Furthermore, if the cul-de-sac hernia is large, the dissection must be more complete and the vessels originating from the superior and middle hemorrhoidal vessels may be encountered.

7. The uterosacral thickenings are cut close to the cervix. This connective tissue is useful in re-establishing the vaginal obturator, obliterating the cul-de-sac, and suspending the vaginal vault. As with any hernia, tissue useful in the herniorrhaphy should not be sacrificed. A curved Kocher clamp is used to grasp the tissue close to the cervix (Plate 16, F).

8. The uterosacral ligaments are ligated and the ends of the ligatures left long and tagged. The method of resecting this connective tissue close to the cervix is shown in Plate 16, G. Resection of the uterosacral thickenings permits further descensus of the uterus. Palpation of the cul-de-sac can be carried higher in the pelvis and the size of the fundus more accurately determined. The operator may start planning for the correction of the cul-de-sac hernia and resection of excess peritoneum that will be part of the posterior repair.

9. Attention is directed toward opening into the peritoneal cavity anteriorly. To this end the uterus is now drawn strongly downward. Assistants who can anticipate and sense the steps of this operation make matters easy by drawing the uterus in just the right direction. A Deaver retractor may be used to retract the bladder if it seems to facilitate the exposure of the peritoneum.

10. The bulge of the vesicouterine fold of peritoneum is picked up with thumb forceps and sharply incised (Plate 16, H). Frequently this is not as simple as illustrated, and the surgeon finds himself too close to the cervix and lower uterine segment of the uterus, with the cleavage plane entering the superficial layers of fibromuscular tissue. An excessive amount of bleeding indicates that the wrong cleavage plane has been entered and the surgeon should try dissecting closer to the bladder. In elderly patients the bladder wall is thin and in a procidentia the musculature is further attenuated. In such patients the bladder may be inadvertently entered. This is not a serious complication. If it does happen, the bladder should be closed in two layers with interrupted sutures of 0000 chromic catgut and the operation continued. Filling the bladder with dye to avoid this is useless and untidy. A finger placed through the cul-de-sac (which has already been opened into the peritoneal cavity) and directed medially alongside the uterus will aid in locating the vesicouterine reflection.

11. The vesicouterine reflection of the peritoneum is now tagged by a suture passing through the anterior vaginal wall. Both index fingers are passed within the peritoneal cavity, and, with a lateral rolling motion, the opening is enlarged, while at the same time the ureters, together with their surrounding areolar tissue, are displaced laterally (Plate 16, I). This maneuver aids in keeping the ureters out of the field of operation and simulates the same method used to displace the ureters during an abdominal hysterectomy.

12. In performing a simple total abdominal hysterectomy for benign disease the clamping of vessels near the ureters is preceded by displacement of the latter away from the uterus. This is done by traction on the uterus to the opposite side and pushing the connective tissue surrounding the vessels and ureters laterally. The clamps can then be placed close to the uterus. The same principles apply in removing the uterus vaginally.

13. The left index finger of the operator is introduced into the peritoneal cavity preparatory to clamping the patient's left cardinal thickening (Plate 16, J). The base of the cardinal thickening

is first doubly clamped, cut, and doubly ligated. The assistant makes traction on the cervix to the right and downward while the operator's index finger pushes the connective tissue and ureter laterally. This minimizes the chance of the ureter being included in the clamps. The same thing is done on the right side, reversing the direction of traction and the placing of the clamps.

14. The course of the pelvic ureter has been outlined in the background of Plate 16, *J*. It is always within a few centimeters of the field of operation. If damage is suspected, the most simple expedient is to pass a catheterizing cystoscope and insert a catheter in the ureter. The point of obstruction or torsion is readily determined and the sutures compromising the ureter are released. Diagnosis and correction of this serious complication at the operating table prevents an inevitable fistula coursing through its necrotic and infected tract.

15. The technique of the ligation of pedicles is shown in Plate 16, *K*. Ligatures nearest the origin of a vessel are not used for traction, which may unseat them. A ligature distal to a truly hemostatic suture can be used for identification of a pedicle. Major vascular structures are doubly clamped and the first or hemostatic ligature is seated in the bed created by the clamp nearest the vessel's origin. The distal clamp is flashed as the tie is seated to assure a tight ligature (Plate 16, *L* and *M*). The base of the broad ligament or thickest portion of the visceral extensions of the pelvic fascia is shown in Plate 16, *L* and *M*. The uterine arteries are just above this and are specifically identified.

16. While the distal clamp holds the pedicle (Plate 16, *M*), a second ligature is placed distal to the first and this is left long to facilitate identification later (Plate 16, *N*). Obvious shortcuts are apparent: one clamp instead of two, one ligature instead of two, and disregard of isolating pedicles and specific vessels. The technique described assures an operation free of lost vessels, oozing pedicles, and general consternation while adding little or no time to the duration of the procedure.

17. The same technique is followed on the right side, and one can now observe the uterus to prolapse even farther as the obturator is detached, the genital hiatus broadened, and a most unusual visceral downthrust exerted in the form of strong traction by the assistant.

18. The uterine arteries are now doubly clamped as shown in Plate 16, *O*. The index finger in the

peritoneal cavity pushes laterally as the clamps are applied. Double suture ligatures are placed around the vessels, and the distal ligature is left long and tagged. This procedure is repeated for the right uterine artery and veins.

19. The vesicouterine reflection of the peritoneum is smaller in all dimensions than the rectovaginal reflection or pouch of Douglas. The fundus of the uterus is thus more easily delivered posteriorly than by forcibly extracting it through a hiatus artificially created between the vagina and bladder. Some local pathology may cause a variation in this rule. In this type of surgery one does not create bigger openings when such can be avoided. The basic objectives (namely, to decrease the size of the genital hiatus and to strengthen the obturators filling this outlet) make logical the delivery of the uterus posteriorly.

20. The uterus is now mobile except for the resistance offered by the round ligaments, tubes, and infundibulopelvic vessels and their connective tissue thickenings. The fundus is now delivered through the posterior route by applying bullet tenaculi alternately along the posterior aspect of the uterus. This sometimes is accomplished by a finger alone (Plate 16, *P*). If it does not come out without difficulty, make traction on the fundus and push the cervix back up under the symphysis; this has the effect of rotating the organ about its last remaining attachments. This maneuver is usually successful unless abnormal attachments exist. In this event the anterior Deaver retractor is manipulated to see the reason for resistance and any structures adherent to the uterus or adnexa. Failure to deliver the uterus by this technique is rare.

21. When the ovaries are to be left, clamps are placed as shown in Plate 16, *Q*. Two Kocher clamps from below and two from above ensure an adequate grasp of the pedicles. These can be wide, vascular, and substantial in size in younger women. The use of two Kocher clamps or similar instruments ensures the operator against the loss of the pedicle. Time is not lost in this operation by safety devices but by bleeding pedicles, the result of failure to clamp, cut, and ligate major pedicles systematically. Again two suture ligatures of 0 chromic catgut are used to secure these vessels and pedicles. The same technique is used on the right side and the uterus removed. The reward of this cautious technique is a relatively short operation.

22. The peritoneum between the rectum and vagina is now approximated with a running suture (Plate 16, *R*). Should a large cul-de-sac

hernia exist, this is isolated, the neck defined, and the hernial sac ligated. When the herniation is not so complete, a retroperitoneal obliteration of the cul-de-sac is done. The prevention of enterocele and prolapse of the vaginal vault (irrespective of the technique of the original operation for prolapse, whether hysterectomy, Fothergill-Hunter, or some other operation) depends on the surgeon's deliberate and thorough obliteration of the cul-de-sac by approximation of the uterosacral thickenings.

23. Plate 16, S, shows the method of placing the angle sutures in conjunction with the obliteration of the cul-de-sac technique. The suture passes from the vaginal wall through the infundibulopelvic ligament and round ligament, through the cardinal ligament, and out through the vagina wall about a centimeter from its point of entrance. It is then tied on the vaginal aspect of the new vault. The uterosacral ligaments are sutured in the midline after exposing them further by a retrograde dissection of the rectovaginal septum.

24. When this operation is done in the absence of prolapse and cul-de-sac hernia, the uterosacral thickenings are treated in the same manner. This follows logically the principle of always strengthening the obturator (in this instance the new vaginal vault) while at the same time reducing the genital aperture.

25. Successive wedge-shaped sections of the vaginal wall are removed after dissection from the rectum. This can be continued as long as it proceeds easily (Plate 16, T). The uterosacral ligaments are approximated in the midline as long as these thickenings are substantial enough to contribute to the support of, and do not constrict, the rectum.

26. The last interrupted suture is left long. The lowermost portion of the rectocele and the perineum are approached from below upward to meet this incision. Sutures are placed to close the remainder of the vaginal vault laterally. A few sutures are placed anteriorly to close the wedge removed at the start of the operation (Plate 16, U).

27. In order not to disturb the new vaginal vault the anterior vaginal wall is opened retrograde, beginning at the urethral meatus (Plate 16, V). Some operators consider the major part of the operation done after the uterus is removed. This is a misconception when performing a vaginal hysterectomy for prolapse, since the reconstruction of the pelvic floor has just begun. If the repair of the cystocele is started at the vault and con-

tinued to the external urinary meatus, traction on the new vault is inevitable and results in disturbing a recent operative field, which, in itself, is a violation of surgical technique. The attendant bleeding may result in a hasty repair and neglect of the posterior vaginal wall and other structures. The retrograde method of repair permits a dissection of the anterior vaginal wall and region of the bladder neck with traction on tissues previously undisturbed. Following this dissection the bladder neck is plicated prophylactically and the vaginal wall appropriately resected to correct the cystocele (Plate 16, W).

28. The posterior repair is completed as illustrated (Plate 14, P to U) and described under Anterior and Posterior Repair. However, since the upper half or more of the rectocele may have been corrected already by the retrograde technique, this proceeds rapidly. The incision is carried toward the vault to meet the upper incision that was previously tagged (Plate 16, W). A high perineorraphy is done to complete the reconstruction of the pelvic floor.

Postoperative Care

The postoperative care is the same as that described under Anterior and Posterior Repair (page 120).

VAGINAL HYSTERECTOMY WITH MORCELLATION AND BISECTION OF THE UTERUS
Indications and Surgical Principles

The common indication for this operation is a uterus that is too large to deliver between the pubic rami during a vaginal hysterectomy. Delivery of a large uterus is further complicated in an obese patient with a narrow subpubic angle. Hysterectomy by this method is elected when a laparotomy is contraindicated for other reasons and repair of the pelvic floor is necessary. The technique is useful in performing a vaginal salpingo-oophorectomy, for it allows for better visualization and exposure of the infundibulopelvic pedicles prior to clamping and ligation. Seldom is the problem of previous laparotomies a contraindication to vaginal hysterectomy as has been taught in the past. Adhesions of omentum or bowel to the fundus of the uterus, with adequate exposure and the proper instruments to perform the operation, are readily released.

Plate 17

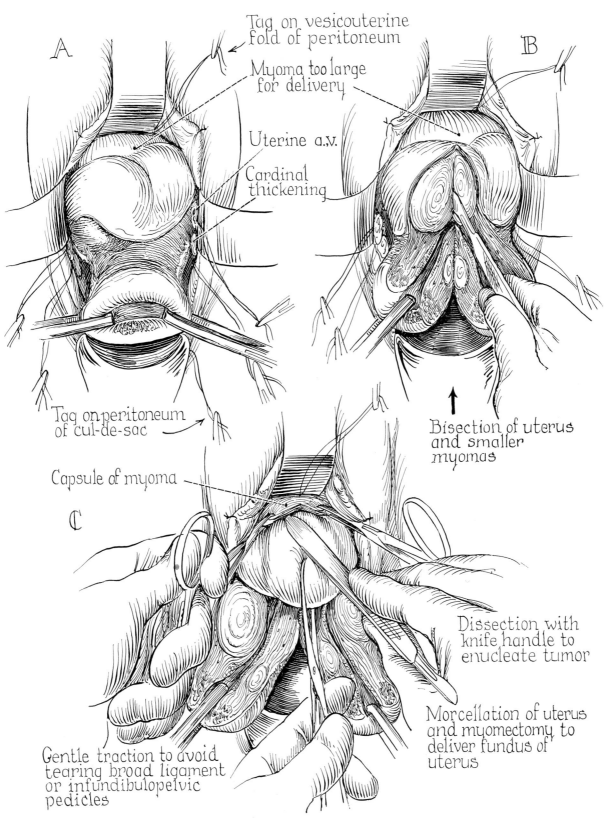

A

Tag on vesicouterine fold of peritoneum

Myoma too large for delivery

Uterine a.v.

Cardinal thickening

Tag on peritoneum of cul-de-sac

B

Bisection of uterus and smaller myomas

Capsule of myoma

C

Dissection with knife handle to enucleate tumor

Morcellation of uterus and myomectomy to deliver fundus of uterus

Gentle traction to avoid tearing broad ligament or infundibulopelvic pedicles

137

Plate 17 (Continued)

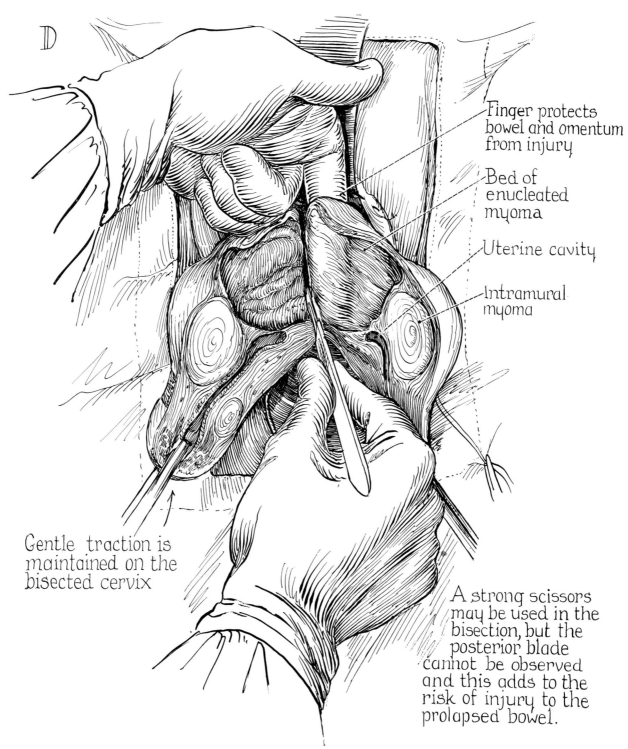

D

Finger protects
bowel and omentum
from injury

Bed of
enucleated
myoma

Uterine cavity

Intramural
myoma

Gentle traction is
maintained on the
bisected cervix

A strong scissors
may be used in the
bisection, but the
posterior blade
cannot be observed
and this adds to the
risk of injury to the
prolapsed bowel.

The myomectomized uterus can now be delivered
and the bisection completed

Plate 17 (Concluded)

The two halves of the bisected uterus,
together with the tubes and ovaries,
are delivered out of the pelvis

Collapsed capsule
of enucleated
myoma and
overlying uterine
wall

Double suture
ligature placed
on ovarian a.,v.

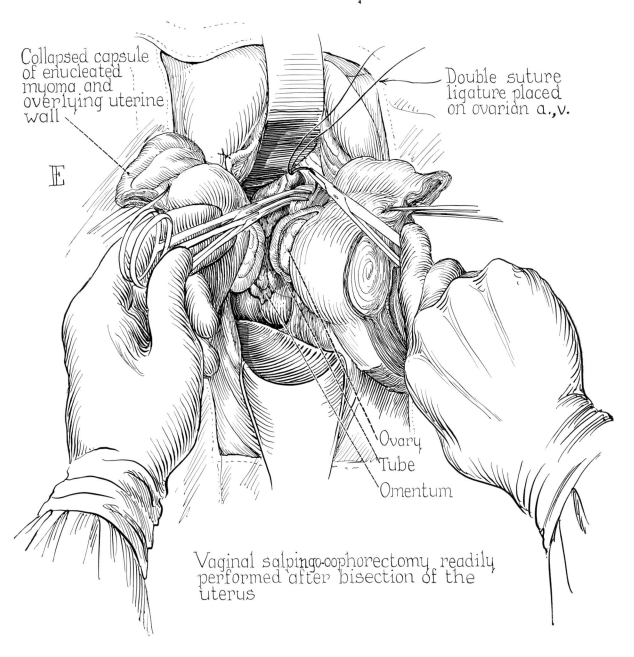

Ovary
Tube
Omentum

Vaginal salpingo-oophorectomy readily
performed after bisection of the
uterus

Steps of the Operation

1. The operation proceeds as in any vaginal hysterectomy until the uterine artery and veins have been identified, doubly clamped, cut, and ligated. At this time the vesicouterine fold of peritoneum, as well as the peritoneum of the cul-de-sac, will have been entered. Both of the peritoneal reflections have been tagged with a suture ligature. The cardinal thickenings and the uterosacral thickenings will have been cut, clamped, and ligated and appropriately identified for closure of the vaginal vault at the conclusion of the operation. Two Jacobs tenaculi are placed on the cervix at the lateral angles in preparation for bisecting the uterus (Plate 17, *A*).

2. Strong traction is made downward and outward, and a knife is used to bisect the cervix in the mid-sagittal plane. Small fibroids that are encountered may be bisected together with the uterus itself (Plate 17, *B*) rather than a myomectomy performed.

3. As shown in Plate 17, *C*, a large myoma that could not be delivered under the symphysis is grasped with a bullet tenaculum. A vaginal myomectomy is performed by grasping the capsule of the myoma with Allis clamps. The operator cautions his assistants to exert only gentle traction from now on, since with the delivery of the uterus, considerable strain is placed on the infundibulopelvic pedicles. They may be torn and the ovarian vessels ruptured. The myoma is enucleated either by the knife handle technique (Plate 17, *C*) or by the use of scissors, leaving the capsule intact. After removal of the large myoma the remainder of the uterus is delivered to the outside and the bisection continued.

4. The bisection is continued by cutting through the remainder of the posterior portion of the capsule of the myoma that was removed. As shown in Plate 17, *D*, a finger should be placed behind the uterus to protect bowel or omentum from injury. Small laparotomy pads are used to pack off the bowel and omentum. In performing the bisection a strong scissors may be used; a crushing instrument, particularly when the posterior blade cannot be observed, adds to the risk of injury to prolapsed bowel or omentum.

5. The two halves of the bisected uterus, together with tubes and ovaries, are delivered out of the pelvis. Traction is made on the capsule of the enucleated myoma and, together with gentle traction on the cervix, the infundibulopelvic pedicles are visualized. Angle clamps are used to clamp the infundibulopelvic pedicle, and this is doubly ligated with 0 chromic catgut (Plate 17, *E*). The round ligament is doubly clamped, cut, and ligated and the left half of the uterus is removed together with the tube and ovary on that side attached to the specimen. An identical procedure is carried out on the right side, completing the removal of the uterus, tubes, and ovaries. The surgeon further explores the pelvis for other pelvic pathology. The closure of the vaginal vault and the anterior and posterior colporrhaphies are completed in the same manner as a routine vaginal hysterectomy.

Postoperative Care

The postoperative care is the same as that described under Anterior and Posterior Repair (page 120).

PARTIAL COLPOCLEISIS (LE FORT OPERATION)
Indications and Surgical Principles

A partial colpocleisis has rather limited indications in modern gynecologic surgery. Rarely are the advantages of this operation superior to a quickly performed vaginal hysterectomy and subsequent repair of the pelvic floor. A one-finger introitus that gives excellent support with a nonfunctional vagina can be left. In fact, the vaginal hysterectomy can be followed by a complete colpocleisis that eliminates all the disadvantages of leaving a uterus with all its cancer-bearing potentialities. Further, should an elderly patient require female hormones in the management of breast malignancy, arthritis, osteomalacia, or other constitutional diseases, it is an advantage to know that the uterus has been removed. In isolated instances of prolapse where a basal local anesthetic is preferable to an inhalation anesthesia, the partial colpocleisis operation may be the simplest repair of the pelvic floor. A patient with prolapse who has had a ventrofixation of the fundus of the uterus that might prove annoying during a vaginal hysterectomy would provide a rare indication.

Preoperative Care and Anesthesia

Ulcerations of the vagina or cervix (often from the use of a hard pessary) are healed by local therapy before surgery. Estrogenic cream

Plate 18

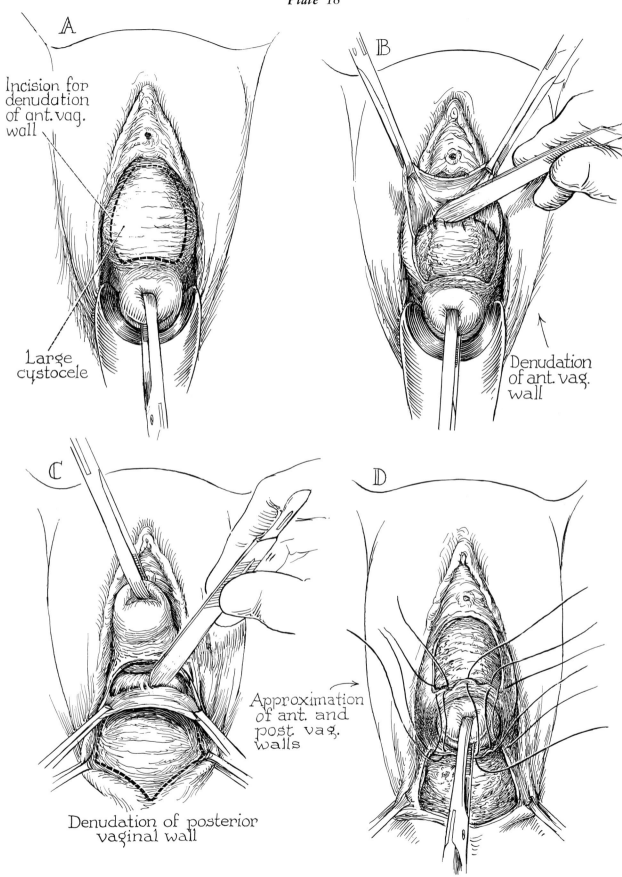

A

Incision for
denudation
of ant. vag.
wall

Large
cystocele

B

Denudation
of ant. vag.
wall

C

Denudation of posterior
vaginal wall

Approximation
of ant. and
post. vag.
walls

D

Plate 18 (Concluded)

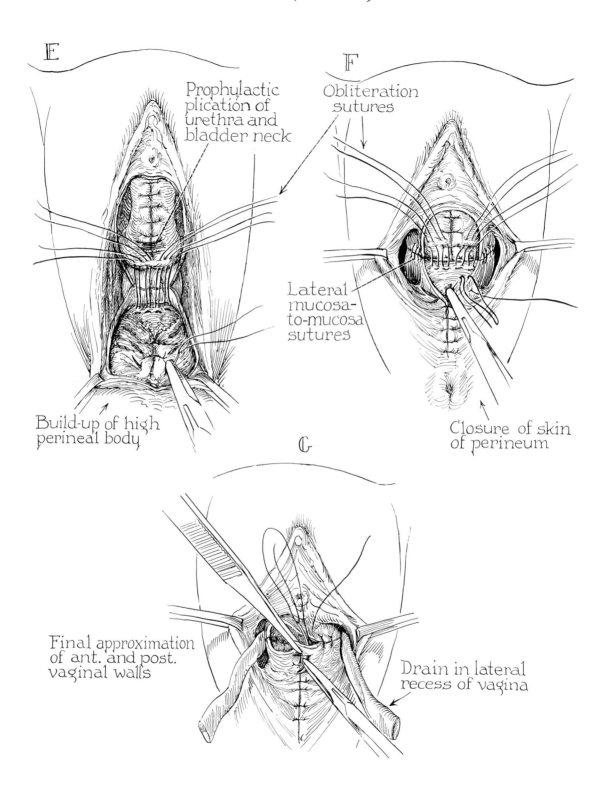

E

Prophylactic
plication of
urethra and
bladder neck

Build-up of high
perineal body

F

Obliteration
sutures

Lateral
mucosa-
to-mucosa
sutures

Closure of skin
of perineum

G

Final approximation
of ant. and post.
vaginal walls

Drain in lateral
recess of vagina

and astringent douches are used several weeks before admission. Most anesthetists prefer a general anesthetic in geriatric surgery over a depressing basal anesthetic used in conjunction with local infiltration.

Steps of the Operation

1. An area to be denuded is outlined from the external urinary meatus to the bladder reflection on the cervix (Plate 18, *A*). Along the outline an incision is made which extends through the mucosa and superficial musculature of the vaginal wall.

2. The area is now denuded of mucosa, leaving as much of the muscular wall as is possible while dissecting in this unnatural line of cleavage (Plate 18, *B*). Considerable general oozing may be encountered despite the fact that patients subjected to this procedure are postmenopausal.

3. A similar area is denuded posteriorly but also including a triangular area of the skin of the perineum (Plate 18, *C*). Bilateral strips of mucosa will now be left.

4. Using interrupted sutures of 00 chromic catgut, the mucosa of the vault is approximated over the cervix. After the anterior wall has been united to the posterior wall, the lateral edges on each side are approximated (Plate 18, *D*).

5. The denuded vaginal wall is approximated anteroposteriorly by a series of mattress sutures in conjunction with the mucosal closure (Plate 18, *E*). When the area of the bladder neck is reached, this is plicated not only in the event of stress incontinence, but also for prophylactic purposes (Plate 18, *E*).

6. The musculature of the perineal body is then built up with interrupted sutures to aid in the obliteration of the genital aperture (Plate 18, *E*).

7. Successive rows of mattress sutures continue the obliteration of the vaginal canal. The skin of the perineum is approximated in the midline by interrupted sutures (Plate 18, *F*).

8. The remainder of the anteroposterior approximation is then done, and drains are placed in both of the lateral tunnels of the vagina that result (Plate 18, *G*).

Postoperative Care

Measures previously described for postoperative care under Anterior and Posterior Repair (page 120) are instituted. The patient can usually be ambulated the same day, and this is important in the elderly group. The drains usually fall out but otherwise are removed in forty-eight hours. An indwelling catheter is left in place for several days, and urinary antiseptics are continued for a course of ten days.

OTHER OPERATIONS FOR PROLAPSE
WATKINS INTERPOSITION OPERATION

The Watkins interposition operation was first done in the United States by Thomas J. Watkins in 1898. It had been done by Schauta and Wertheim of Vienna. The principle of the operation is to draw the fundus of the uterus through the uterovesical fold of peritoneum and suture it to the descending rami of the pubis. It should not be done in young women who might become pregnant, unless the tubes are tied. It should not be done in elderly women in whom the atrophic uterus will not form an adequate obturator to subsequent prolapse. It should not be done when the uterus is diseased. It should not be done when there is adnexal disease. It should not be done when the cervix is diseased or hypertrophied. It should not be done if the patient wishes to be continent since it obliterates the all-important posterior urethrovesical angle. It should not be used for closure of large fistulas since the gracilis muscle has a much better blood supply. The operation exaggerates the depth of the cul-de-sac, subjecting it to further pressure and the development of a hernia. This violation of the basic principles in the repair of the pelvic floor alone obviates its usefulness. Many adequate operations for prolapse are available without this bizarre procedure.

OPERATION FOR PROLAPSE OF THE VAGINAL VAULT WITH RESULTANT FUNCTIONAL VAGINA
Indications and Surgical Principles

A prolapse of the vaginal vault results from failure of the operator to strengthen the obturators (bladder, vagina, and rectum) and reduce the size of the pelvic aperture during his first operation. The most common mistake is the failure to recognize and reduce a cul-de-sac hernia that later initiates all the forces that caused the prolapse originally. The illogicality of attempting to correct this condition from the abdominal route is apparent to anyone with the simplest knowledge of the mechanics of the female pelvic floor. The technique of the operation to follow incorporates the repair and strengthening of all elements concerned with the prolapse with special attention directed toward the correction of the cul-de-sac hernia and the obliteration of its sac.

Steps of the Operation

1. The prolapsed vault is reposed after the induction of anesthesia and the insertion of No. 6 ureteral catheters. A small, indwelling catheter (No. 14 or No. 16 Fr.) is left in place at this time. If the bladder is sounded later to help in the dissection, the bladder catheter is removed.

2. The vault is now inverted again by traction on Allis clamps. The landmarks are identified. A ridge of attenuated scar tissue usually marks the bladder base where it merges into the cul-de-sac hernia. This was the original vaginal vault which is now prolapsed (Plate 19, A).

3. The inverted vagina is now studied to determine the line of incision. By placing Allis clamps at varying distances and then reposing the vault, an idea of the amount of vaginal wall to be removed is gained. The vagina can now be opened by making the incision shown in Plate 19, A, or the incision can be outlined on the prolapsed vault and the dissection begun in the midline. The method which permits the finding of a good plane of cleavage will vary. The dissection may be tedious but must be thorough and extend far laterally. Posteriorly the importance of exposing the bulbocavernosi and puborectali is obvious if the aperture of the pelvic floor is to be restored to normal dimensions.

4. Plate 19, B, shows the landmarks after the dissection of the vaginal walls off the bladder and cul-de-sac hernia. The dissection is carried laterally to locate the remains of the cardinal and uterosacral thickenings that will be used later to help strengthen the vagina as an obturator. The ureteral catheters are indispensable in this lateral dissection since the position of the ureter as the result of previous surgery and the prolapse is uncertain. The ureter is palpated frequently during this dissection.

5. The peritoneal sac of the cul-de-sac hernia is now dissected free (Plate 19, C). It invariably has a wide neck. Bowel or omentum may be adherent to it and these are dissected free. This is one of the most important steps of the operation, and with the ureters catheterized the cul-de-sac can be obliterated without fear of inadvertently kinking or ligating the ureters which are close by. The ureters can, in fact, be pushed to the side in order to perform a complete dissection.

6. Plate 19, D, shows the technique of ligating the hernial sac with a double, medium, silk suture ligature. Bowel or omentum is pushed back while the figure-of-eight ligature is placed at the neck of the sac. While the hernial sac is opened wide, the ovaries are palpated and inspected. They are readily removed through the hernial sac since they are prolapsed deep in the pelvis by the herniation of the pelvic floor. The surgeon will have to be guided here by his own convictions regarding the removal of ovaries in the various age groups. Again it should be stated that if a gynecologist removes ovaries in certain age groups when performing an abdominal hysterectomy, he should remove them during a vaginal hysterectomy on a patient the same age or in the course of a procedure such as this.

7. Any tissues useful in the formation of a more firm obturator or capable of reducing the pelvic aperture are studied. The remnants of the uterosacral and cardinal thickenings are palpated for the proximity of the ureters. A prophylactic plication of the urethra, bladder neck, and bladder is then done (Plate 19, E).

8. The remnants of the cardinal and uterosacral thickenings are now systematically plicated with 0 chromic catgut. The ends are left long and passed through the vaginal wall at the angles of the new vaginal vault. Connective tissue, representing the remnants of the paracolpium and so-called suspensory ligaments of the rectum, is likewise plicated where this can be done without tension or stricture. The two sutures that will anchor the new vault are then tied. They are shown in Plate 19, F, prior to tying. The rectocele is reduced by suture and inversion of its wall.

9. If a wedge of vaginal wall was cut out in the original dissection, this is now inspected to see if further trimming is necessary. If the redundant vaginal wall was only outlined, then the wall is trimmed to leave a functional vagina. The perineum is built up by layers of interrupted sutures of 0 chromic catgut. This is carried up until the edges of the puborectalis are seen, and this tissue

Plate 19

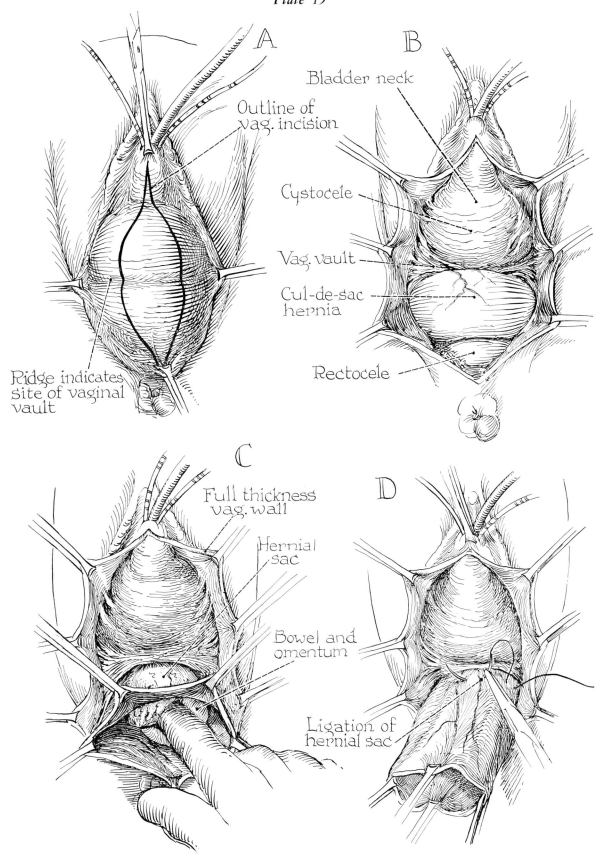

A

Outline of
vag. incision

Ridge indicates
site of vaginal
vault

B

Bladder neck

Cystocele

Vag. vault

Cul-de-sac
hernia

Rectocele

C

Full thickness
vag. wall

Hernial
sac

Bowel and
omentum

D

Ligation of
hernial sac

Plate 19 (Concluded)

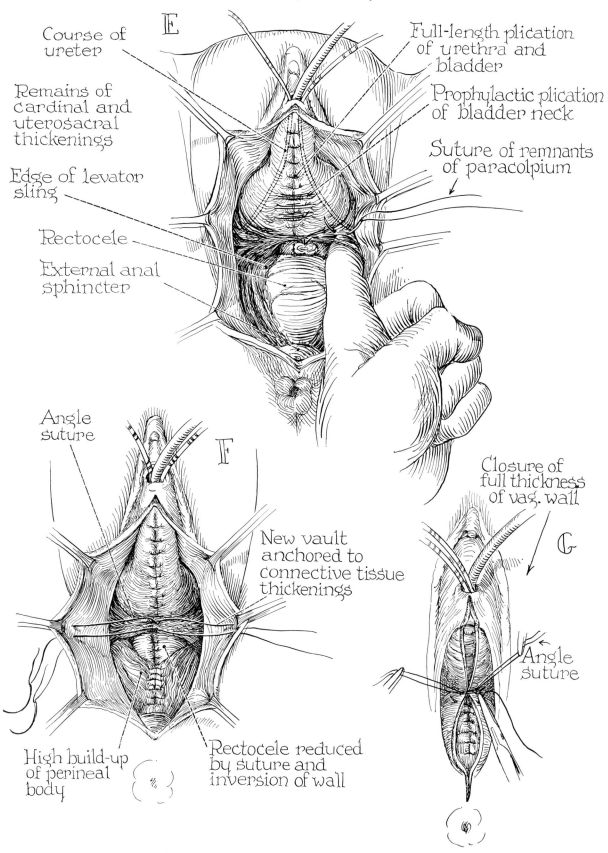

E

Course of ureter

Remains of cardinal and uterosacral thickenings

Edge of levator sling

Rectocele

External anal sphincter

Full-length plication of urethra and bladder

Prophylactic plication of bladder neck

Suture of remnants of paracolpium

F

Angle suture

New vault anchored to connective tissue thickenings

High build-up of perineal body

Rectocele reduced by suture and inversion of wall

Closure of full thickness of vag. wall

G

Angle suture

is used to narrow the pelvic aperture so long as it does not result in a stricture. It must be remembered that these muscles do not insert in the midline and their approximation there is an artifact. Since this condition necessitates the utilization of any tissues available, the lower edges of the puborectalis or its remnants may be approximated in the midline to narrow the pelvic cleft. The unclosed portions of the vaginal and rectal walls and the skin of the perineum are then closed with interrupted sutures of 00 chromic catgut (Plate 19, *G*).

Postoperative Care

The postoperative care is the same as that described under Anterior and Posterior Repair (page 120).

COMPLETE RESTORATION OF THE DECOMPENSATED PELVIC FLOOR
COMPOSITE OPERATION TO CORRECT UTERINE PROCIDENTIA, PROLAPSE OF THE VAGINAL VAULT, PROLAPSE AND PROCIDENTIA OF THE RECTUM, AND REPAIR OF A CUL-DE-SAC HERNIA

The artist drew the following operation of a patient with a prolapse of the vaginal vault combined with a procidentia of the rectum and the inevitable cul-de-sac hernia. This was selected to cover most of the surgical principles involved in vaginal plastic surgery. With minor changes, such as an incidental hysterectomy or excision of a prolapse of a cervical stump, the technique and principles of operation may be adapted to the various combinations the surgeon might find among the herniations of the pelvic viscera.

Preoperative Care and Anesthesia

Ulcerations of the mucous membrane of the vaginal vault, or cervix if the uterus or cervical stump is present, are treated before the patient is scheduled for surgery. Douches, estrogenic cream, and replacement of the prolapse followed by extended periods of bed rest will restore the vaginal mucosa to a healthy state. The patient should have an intravenous pyelogram and barium enema to exclude intrinsic disease of the urinary and lower intestinal

tracts. Urinary antiseptics, known to be effective by sensitivity tests, against any organisms cultured from the bladder during study of the patient are started forty-eight hours prior to the operation.

Bowel preparation is begun three days before surgery. One routine is to give 240 ml. of citrate of magnesia at night with an enema of tap water in the morning for the first two days. The patient is placed on clear liquids during the preparation. Neomycin, 1.0 Gm. three times a day, is ordered. The enema on the morning of operation should be returned clear. This method may be exhausting to older patients or those with a poor nutritional status and should be appropriately modified by the surgeon. Since this composite operation starts with the vaginal approach, has a major portion concerned with the rectum and its contents, and then returns to the vagina as the final operative area, the cleansing of the lower bowel is mandatory.

General anesthesia is commonly employed. A spinal anesthesia would be satisfactory where inhalation anesthesia is contraindicated. Vasopressin to reduce blood loss may be employed, and the anesthesiologist may wish to exclude the use of cyclopropane. The antihypertensive drugs, that some patients may be receiving, are discontinued ten days to two weeks before surgery. I have never had the occasion to resort to local anesthesia for such an extensive plastic repair, but it certainly is possible although it probably extends the operating time.

Steps of the Operation

1. The procidentia of the vaginal vault and the procidentia of the rectum are examined under anesthesia. The attenuation of the supports of the pelvic floor are further studied. The scar in the vaginal vault which will be the dividing line between the bladder base and cul-de-sac hernia is identified (Plate 20, *A*).

2. The rectal procidentia may be covered by sterile drapes or replaced before the cystoscopy. The position of the ureteral orifices, although only slightly modified by the reposition of the vault prolapse, are observed in all positions. Previous surgery may have altered the course of either ureter in the vaginal vault before entering the

bladder. Many variations from the normal anatomic course or distorted course of the ureters should be anticipated. Ureteral catheters are inserted. Technically, this may be possible only if the vault prolapse is replaced or the trigone of the bladder held up (anteriorly) by an assistant's hand in the vagina in order to elevate the trigone into the view of the cystoscopist (Plate 20, *A*).

3. The procidentia of the rectum may herniate again from the anesthesia room to the operating room. This is replaced and carefully excluded from the field of operation by sterile drapes (Plate 20, *B*).

4. The angles of the vaginal vault are identified by sutures bilaterally (Plate 20, *B*). This is particularly important when, in a young patient, a functional vagina with sufficient depth must be achieved. A maximum length of anterior vaginal wall is preserved.

5. Allis clamps are placed at the angles of the prolapsed vault. Beginning just beyond the external urethral meatus, an incision is made through the full thickness of the vaginal wall (Plate 20, *C*). Sharp dissection is the preferred technique. The use of scissors is blind and blunt, less likely to find the normal tissue plane between the bladder and vagina, and more likely to enter the bladder although this may happen regardless of the skill and patience of the surgeon.

6. Plate 20, *D*, shows the dissection further advanced to find the transverse line of division between the bladder base and the cul-de-sac hernia. With the uterus or cervix present, they would have been removed first and this landmark easily recognized. Alternate sharp dissection combined with the use of the knife handle is the preferred technique. The initial stages of the dissection are the most difficult. As the lateral aspects of the cul-de-sac hernia and the bladder base are mobilized, cleavage planes free of scar tissue from previous surgery are encountered, and the operator finds the dissection proceeding without difficulty. The index finger of the left hand (for right-handed operators) can be conveniently placed behind the vaginal wall to help in developing the exact line of cleavage (Plate 20, *D*).

7. The isolation of the bladder base from the cul-de-sac hernia requires dissection under direct vision and good hemostasis (Plate 20, *E*). Metzenbaum scissors with retraction by gauze over the left index finger can be used to advantage here. The tips of the scissors are directed toward the cul-de-sac, for the most part, to avoid an incidental

perforation of the bladder. This is one of the common hazards of plastic repairs on patients with operative failures. If it happens, the bladder is closed in layers with fine plain catgut for the deep layer and fine chromic catgut for the second layer in the bladder musculature.

8. The neck of the sac of the cul-de-sac hernia is further delineated (Plate 20, *F*). Vessels encountered near the neck of the sac are the vaginal arteries which may be terminal branches of the hypogastric artery or arise from the inferior vesical arteries. Complete mobilization of the hernial sac may require ligation of these vessels.

9. The sac will now be composed of an outer layer of retroperitoneal connective tissue (counterpart of the transversalis fascia in the anterior abdominal wall) and an inner layer of peritoneum. The sac is carefully opened after being tented by elevating the dome with smooth forceps (Plate 20, *G*). Injury to small bowel, sigmoid, or omentum is avoided by this technique.

10. Allis clamps are placed on the edges of the peritoneum while a finger explores the interior of the sac to determine its contents (Plate 20, *H*). Any structures adherent to the peritoneum lining the hernia are dissected free and replaced in the peritoneal cavity. In Plate 20, *H*, omentum was encountered. This can be released or resected at the surgeon's discretion.

11. With the index finger in the peritoneal cavity, further dissection of the neck of the sac is done by sharp and blunt dissection. Failure to obliterate the sac in this, as well as the common varieties of inguinal and femoral hernias, is a major factor in recurrence. It is even more important here where the pelvic floor must subsequently bear the brunt of all the intra-abdominal forces. Posteriorly the peritoneum is dissected beyond the neck of the sac in order to remove an additional amount of the cul-de-sac peritoneum (Plate 20, *I*).

12. With the sac opened and a finger inserted into the peritoneal cavity, the bladder base can be completely freed from the hernial sac (Plate 20, *J*). When the cervix and uterus have been removed, as is the case in the operation sketched by the artist, the line of closure of peritoneum over the vaginal vault at the time of hysterectomy or stump removal is eventually encountered Further dissection will only result in perforations in the neck of the sac, and dissection of the peritoneum off the bladder beyond the line of the old vesicouterine reflexion of peritoneum toward the dome of the bladder does not contribute anything to the support of the pelvic floor. Anteriorly

Text continued on p. 160.

Plate 20

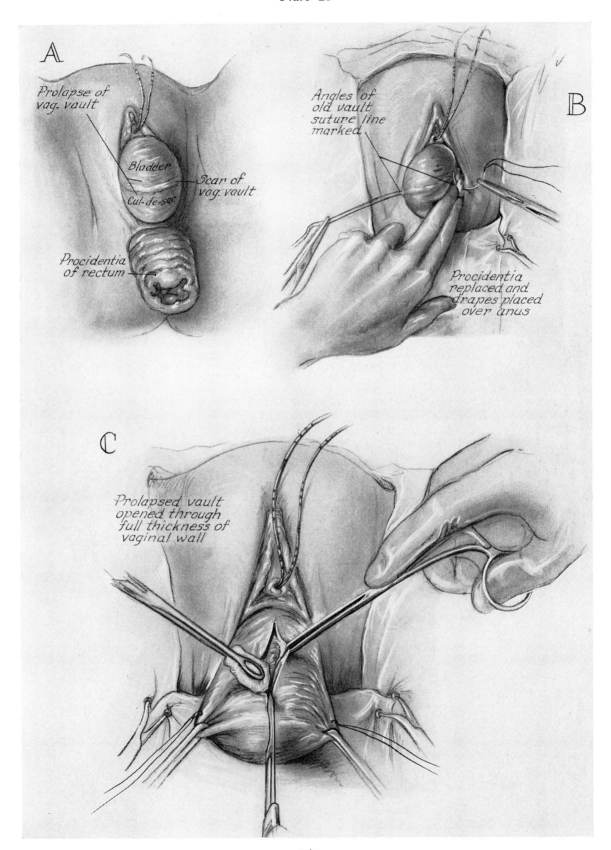

A — Prolapse of vag. vault
Bladder
Scar of vag. vault
Cul-de-sac
Procidentia of rectum

B — Angles of old vault suture line marked
Procidentia replaced and drapes placed over anus

C — Prolapsed vault opened through full thickness of vaginal wall

Plate 20 *(Continued)*

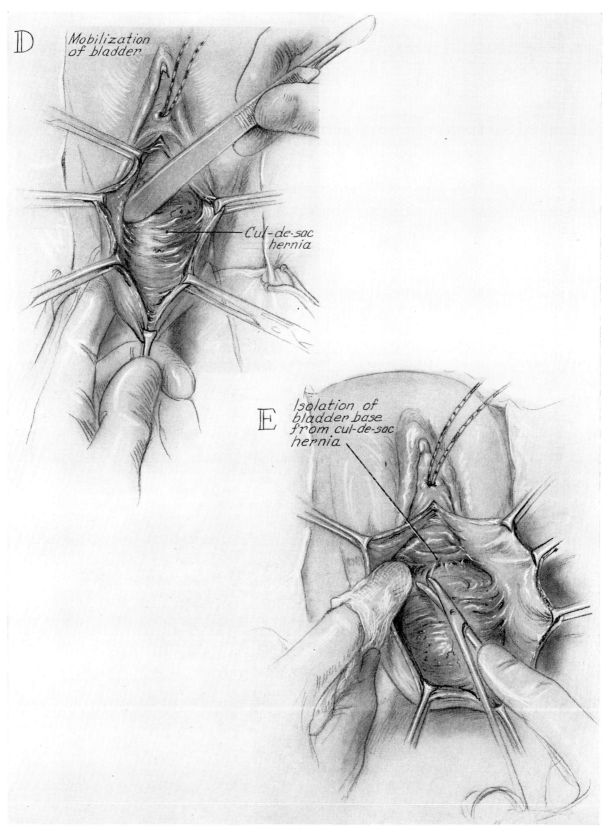

D   *Mobilization of bladder*

Cul-de-sac hernia

E   *Isolation of bladder base from cul-de-sac hernia*

Plate 20 (Continued)

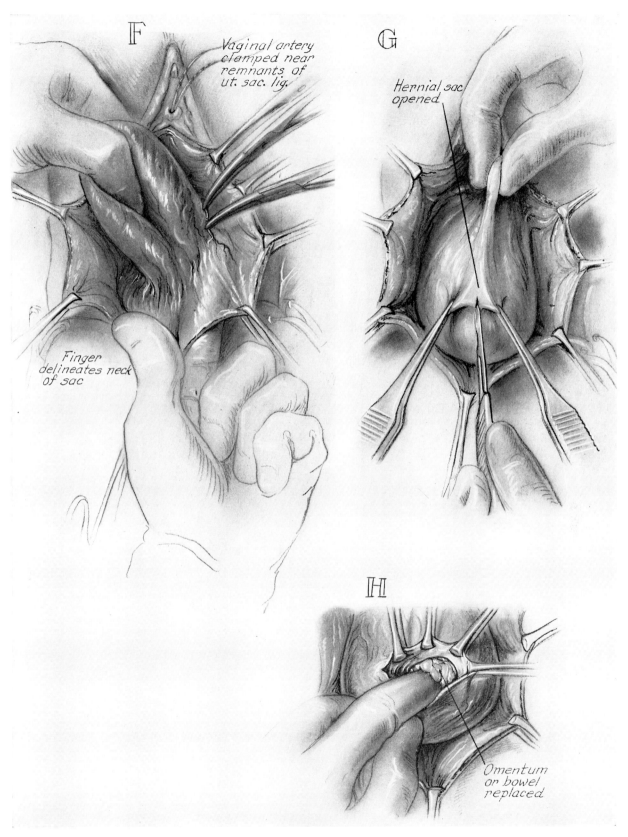

F

Vaginal artery
clamped near
remnants of
ut. sac. lig.

Finger
delineates neck
of sac

G

Hernial sac
opened

H

Omentum
or bowel
replaced

Plate 20 (Continued)

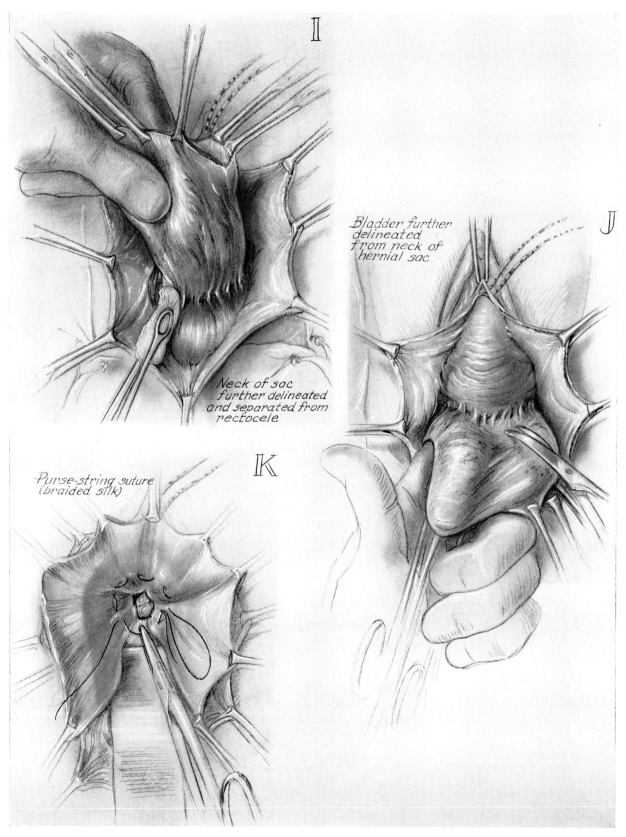

I

Neck of sac
further delineated
and separated from
rectocele

Bladder further
delineated
from neck of
hernial sac

J

K

Purse-string suture
(braided silk)

Plate 20 (Continued)

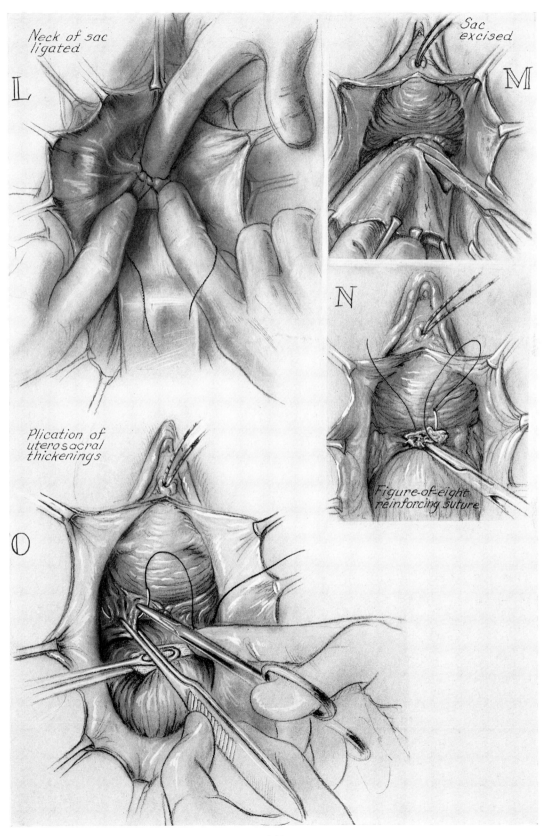

Neck of sac
ligated

L

Sac
excised

M

N

Figure-of-eight
reinforcing suture

Plication of
uterosacral
thickenings

O

Plate 20 *(Continued)*

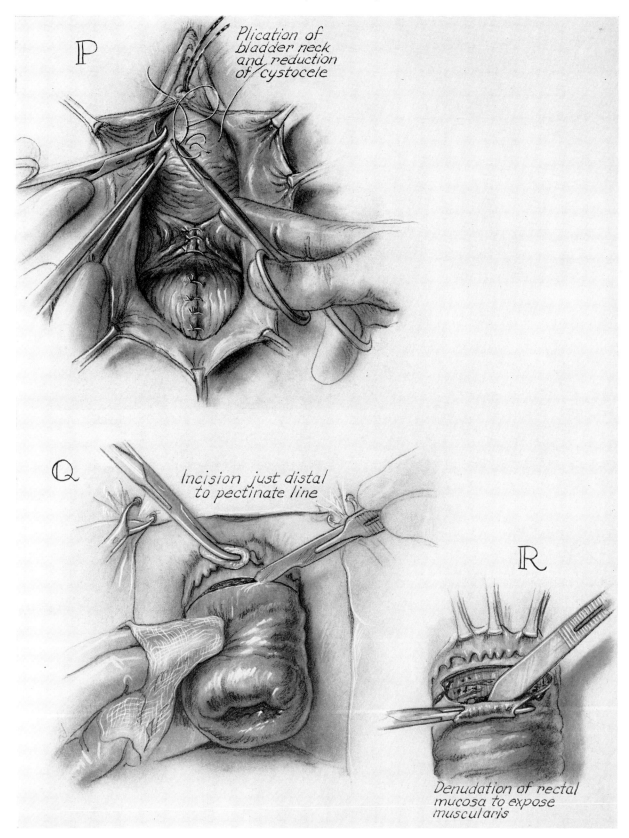

P Plication of bladder neck and reduction of cystocele

Q Incision just distal to pectinate line

R Denudation of rectal mucosa to expose muscularis

Plate 20 (Continued)

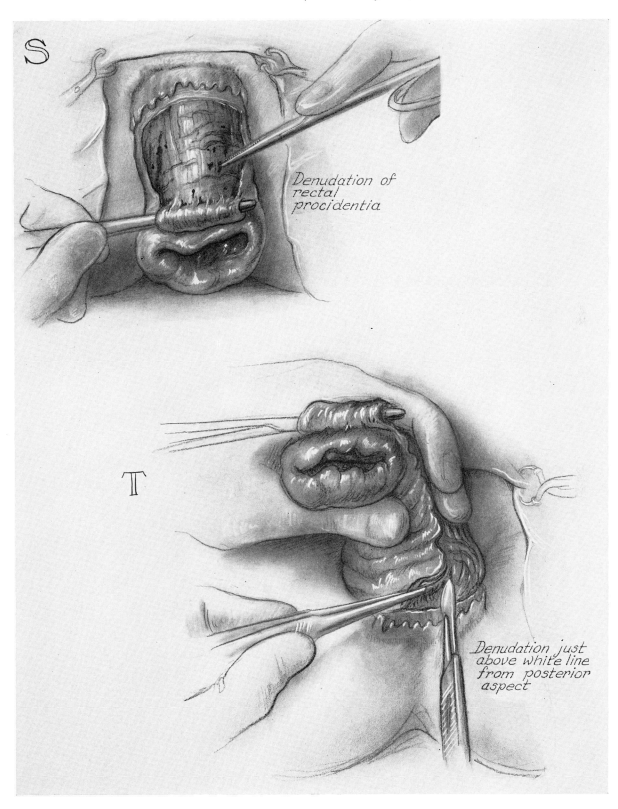

S

Denudation of
rectal
procidentia

T

Denudation just
above white line
from posterior
aspect

Plate 20 (Continued)

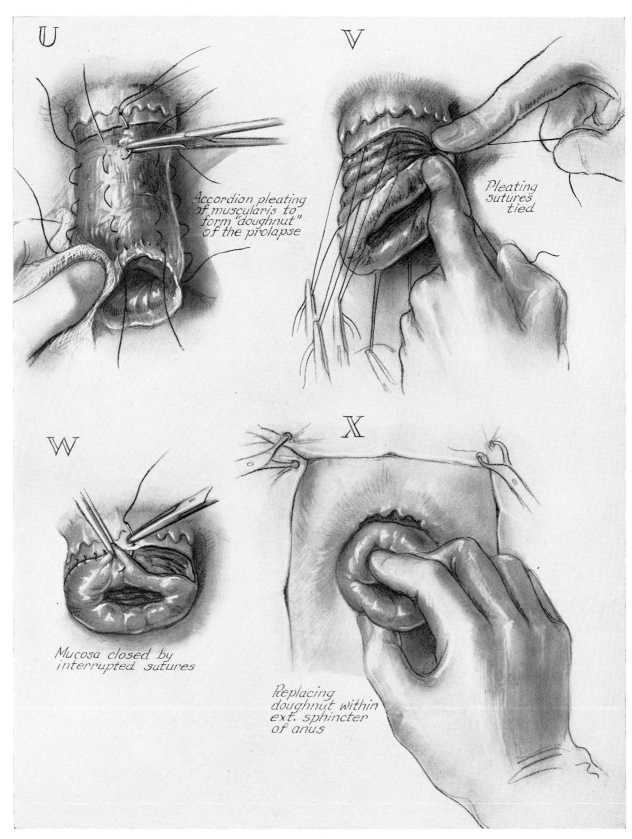

U

Accordion pleating
of muscularis to
form "doughnut"
of the prolapse

V

Pleating
sutures
tied

W

Mucosa closed by
interrupted sutures

X

Replacing
doughnut within
ext. sphincter
of anus

Plate 20 (Continued)

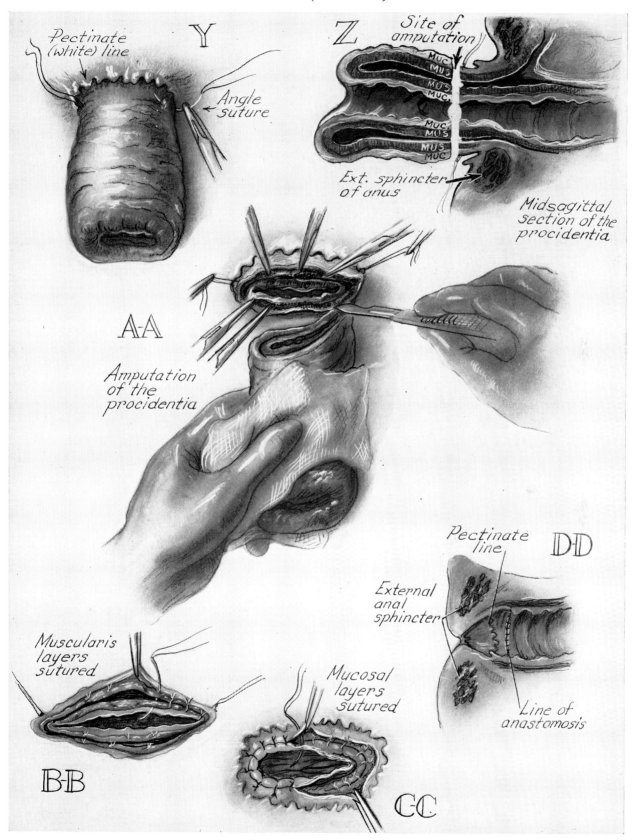

Pectinate (white) line

Y

Angle suture

Z

Site of amputation

MUC
MUS
MUS
MUC

MUC
MUS
MUS
MUC

Ext. sphincter of anus

Midsagittal section of the procidentia

A-A

Amputation of the procidentia

Pectinate line

DD

External anal sphincter

Line of anastomosis

Muscularis layers sutured

BB

Mucosal layers sutured

CC

157

Plate 20 (Continued)

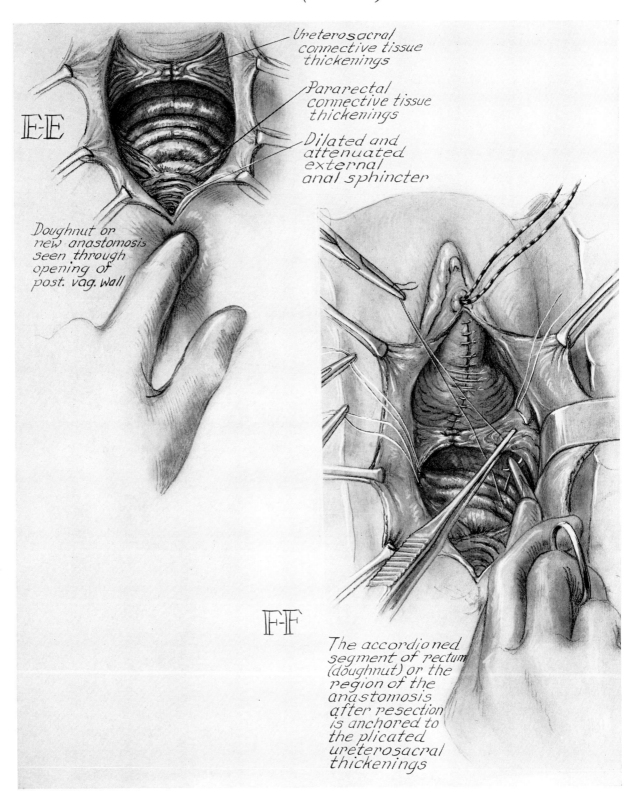

E-E

Ureterosacral
connective tissue
thickenings

Pararectal
connective tissue
thickenings

Dilated and
attenuated
external
anal sphincter

Doughnut or
new anastomosis
seen through
opening of
post. vag. wall

F-F

The accordioned
segment of rectum
(doughnut) or the
region of the
anastomosis
after resection
is anchored to
the plicated
ureterosacral
thickenings

Plate 20 (Concluded)

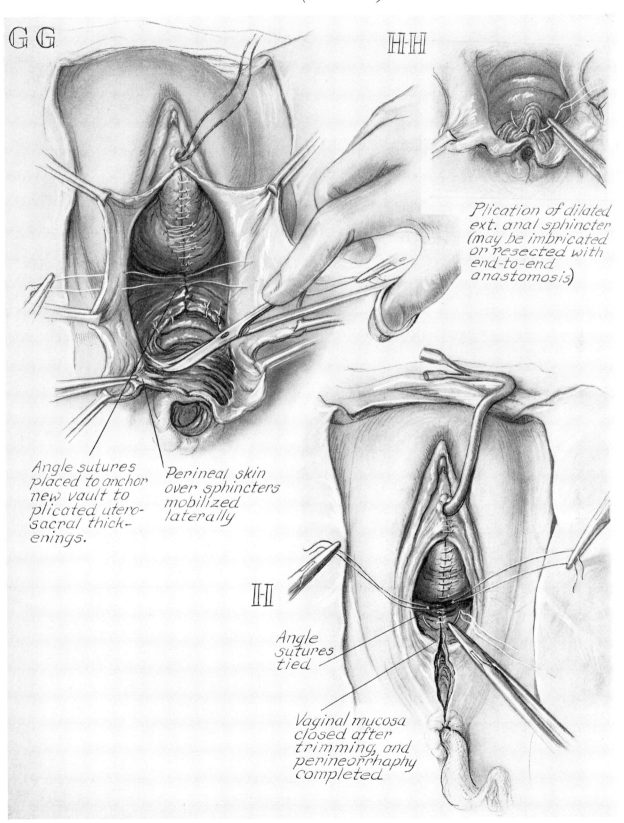

G G

H-H

Plication of dilated ext. anal sphincter (may be imbricated or resected with end-to-end anastomosis)

Angle sutures placed to anchor new vault to plicated utero-sacral thick-enings.

Perineal skin over sphincters mobilized laterally

I-I

Angle sutures tied

Vaginal mucosa closed after trimming, and perineorrhaphy completed this is the farthest point of mobilization of the sac that is necessary.

13. A purse-string suture of braided silk is now placed as high as possible on the peritoneal aspect of the sac (Plate 20, K). Anteriorly this will be at or slightly above the old vesicouterine reflexion of peritoneum. Posteriorly, as indicated in Plate 20, K, this may be well up in the cul-de-sac toward the sacrum, and an additional wedge of peritoneum may be removed to complete the obliteration.

14. Plate 20, L, illustrates the method of tying this important suture. The assistant's finger is placed in the peritoneal cavity to displace bowel or omentum prolapsed into the neck of the sac. This is really a stylized and traditional technique since the operator, with such a complete dissection, is fully aware of the contents of the operative field. Nevertheless, it does ensure exclusion of bowel within the purse-string suture.

15. The hernial sac is excised 1 cm. from the purse-string suture (Plate 20, M). With the dissection previously described that extends high in the cul-de-sac peritoneum, the surgeon will find that this now retracts deep toward the sacrococcygeal junction. This now places the restored vaginal vault in the proper anatomic position to act as an effective obturator above the levator sling which will be subsequently strengthened.

16. A reinforcing suture of medium silk is placed in figure-of-eight fashion in the neck of the sac just distal to the purse-string suture (Plate 20, N). This may be left long and retracted anteriorly during the plication of the uterosacral thickenings which, in effect, places these all-important supports in a retroperitoneal position.

17. Attention is now directed to the plication of the uterosacral thickenings (ligaments). This so completely outweighs any other factors in support of the pelvic floor that a detailed and sometimes repetitious description follows of the technique. Just laterally and slightly posterior to the ligated hernial sac, the remnants of the uterosacral thickenings where they formerly inserted into the region of the internal os of the uterus or into the cervical stump are identified (Plate 20, O).

18. A suture of 0 chromic catgut is placed to unite this tissue in the midline. It may be necessary in those patients with a prolapse of the vaginal vault to extend the dissection laterally to positively identify this connective tissue. Although we have always described the subsequent sutures used to obliterate the cul-de-sac as further plication of the

uterosacral thickenings, the extensions of the parietal connective tissue from the pelvic sidewall as they approach the rectosigmoid junction gradually merge with the pararectal connective tissue (sometimes called the suspensory ligament of the rectum) and this is the tissue used to augment the support of the pelvic floor.

19. The profuse anastomosis of the vessels of the vagina and rectum results in the perforation of vessels during this plication. It is rarely disturbing, but specific bleeding points of arterial origin are clamped and tied by ligature or suture ligature. I prefer to place all of the cul-de-sac sutures, obtain hemostasis, and then tie the obliteration sutures.

20. The number of sutures placed in the pararectal connective tissue is determined by the caliber of the rectosigmoid and rectum. Four sutures, placed 2 cm. apart including the original suture in the uterosacral thickenings, should obliterate the area of herniation in the cul-de-sac without constricting the rectum. This will vary depending, for the most part, on the configuration of the pelvis and the curvature of the sacrum.

21. If it is felt that the rectum may be constricted by the last sutures which are now distal to the cul-de-sac hernia and reducing the upper part of the rectocele, a finger can be inserted into the rectum to determine its caliber and the constricting sutures cut if necessary.

22. Plate 20, P, shows the sutures in the uterosacral thickenings and the pararectal connective tissue after they are tied and these tissues approximated in the midline. Distal to these sutures, several sutures are taken in the perirectal connective tissue and superficial layer of the rectal wall to reduce the remainder of the rectocele down to the level of the insertion of the levator muscles. The remainder of the repair will be concerned with the perineal body beyond this level.

23. A plication of the bladder neck and reduction of the cystocele is then done to restore the posterior urethrovesical angle (Plate 20, P). The details of this plication have been described with the operation of anterior colporraphy (pages 113 and 114).

24. The remaining steps of the vaginal plastic reconstruction must now await the management of the rectal procidentia. The vaginal introitus is protected with towels, and the rectal intussusception delivered into the operative field (Plate 20, Q).

25. An incision is made just distal to the pectinate line down to the superficial layers of the muscu-

laris. This is the first of two techniques of reducing the rectal procidentia. First is the accordion type of plication. Since the peritoneal sac from the cul-de-sac has already been reduced and retracted upward during the reduction of the hernia vaginally, it is not necessary to locate and deal with the hernial sac as it would be were this an isolated operation for rectal procidentia alone (Plate 20, Q).

26. The surgeon will encounter a general ooze of blood from the operative area during this dissection. Distinct bleeding points are clamped and ligated. Final hemostasis is obtained when the longitudinal plication sutures are tied.

27. Plate 20, R, shows a method of denuding the mucosa and underlying muscularis mucosa from the rectal procidentia. Four or five longitudinal segments are selected, and, as the mucosa is separated by sharp dissection, it is rolled upon a Halstead clamp. Specific arterial bleeding points are ligated during this denudation.

28. As the denudation is continued distally, the terminal end of the intussusception is reached. This dissection is continued until a small edge of mucosa at the distal end of the prolapse is left for anastomosis (Plate 20, S).

29. Plate 20, T, shows the denudation of the mucosa from the posterior aspect. The blood loss during this dissection is carefully estimated, and one or more units may be needed for replacement.

30. Accordion pleating sutures are placed longitudinally about 2 cm. apart. These should penetrate the muscular coats of the rectal wall but preferably avoid going deep enough to pass through the full thickness of the rectum (Plate 20, U). The preferred material is 0 chromic catgut on a fine Ferguson needle.

31. After all the pleating sutures have been placed, they are tied by the operator while his assistants gradually draw up on the untied sutures and reduce the prolapse (Plate 20, V).

32. The mucosal edges should now approximate each other without tension. A few additional sutures in the muscularis may be needed at some points to permit approximation. Sutures of 00 chromic catgut are used to close the mucosa (Plate 20, W).

33. The doughnut formed by the accordion method of pleating is then replaced in the pelvis through the dilated rectal sphincter (Plate 20, X). Attention is then directed to further support of the rectum by the transvaginal approach.

Alternate Method

34. The rectal prolapse may be amputated as an alternate method. This is preferred in the younger patients where the doughnut resulting from the plication technique may impinge on the posterior vaginal wall and cause a constriction. This is unimportant when the vagina need not be a functional organ. Plate 20, Y, shows angle sutures placed just above the white line (distal to the white line as seen with the rectum inverted). These should be placed through all layers to prevent retraction when the procidentia is amputated.

35. Plate 20, Z, shows the layers in midsagittal section. The layers to be approximated are shown since the intussuscipiens (outer layers) and intussusceptum (inner layers) are best delineated in midsagittal section. Note that the hernial sac of peritoneum that would prolapse between the two anterior layers is missing. This is because it was dissected out and reduced during the mobilization of the cul-de-sac hernia transvaginally.

36. The prolapsed rectum is then amputated (Plate 20, A-A). The bleeding points are clamped and tied. If the mucosa of the bowel tends to retract, it can be grasped with Allis clamps.

37. The muscularis of the rectum is then anastomosed with interrupted sutures of 00 chromic catgut (Plate 20, B-B). A clamp technique, continuous sutures, or the use of other suture materials may be elected according to the preference of the surgeon.

38. The angle sutures are removed if they distort the approximation of either the mucosal or muscular layers during the anastomosis.

39. Plate 20, C-C, shows the approximation of the muscularis of the bowel. This is done with 00 chromic catgut, but other suture materials may be used, depending on the surgeon's preference.

40. The line of anastomosis is then inverted behind the external sphincter of the anus. Its position, in midsagittal section, is shown in Plate 20, D-D.

41. Attention is now directed toward the suspension of the rectum to the support provided by the plicated uterosacral thickenings (Plate 20, E-E). The connective tissue accompanying the hemorrhoidal vessels and nerves from the pelvic sidewall to the rectal ampulla is utilized in the suspension. Sometimes called the suspensory ligament of the rectum, it is in fact made up of condensations of connective tissue that extend with the middle hemorrhoidal vessels to the lateral aspect of the

ampulla. It is better described as pararectal connective tissue.

42. Plate 20, *E-E,* will either show the accordioned segment of the rectum or the line of anastomosis, depending on which technique was used. Here the "doughnut" is illustrated to show the method of suspension.

43. The fibers of the dilated and attenuated external anal sphincter are visible (Plate 20, *E-E*). They are carefully preserved although the surgeon has his choice of pleating, imbricating, or shortening with an end-to-end anastomosis to reduce the caliber of the anal aperture.

44. After replacement of the "doughnut" or line of suture, it is best to change gowns and gloves before returning to the vaginal approach.

45. Sutures of 0 chromic catgut are then placed from the lateral aspect of the plicated uterosacral thickenings to the lateral side of the rectum and its pararectal connective tissue. The strength and thickness of the remaining connective tissue supports both to the vagina and to the rectum determines the number of sutures that can be placed on each side. Usually two or more sutures can be placed. The first suture is the most lateral, and the others are placed closer to the midline (Plate 20, *F-F*).

46. Each of the paired sutures should be placed so as not to angulate the vagina by drawing it more to one side than the other. At the same time, where a functional vagina must result, the operator estimates the decrease in diameter caused by all the plication so that a midvaginal constriction does not result.

47. Before trimming the redundant vaginal wall the length of the lateral vaginal wall just necessary to reach to the angle of the new vaginal vault is measured. The new vaginal vault at its greatest depth is at the level of the most proximal plication suture in the uterosacral thickenings. On each side an angle suture is passed from the vaginal aspect through the full thickness of the vaginal wall, anchored to the uppermost uterosacral plication suture, and returned through the vaginal wall (Plate 20, *G-G*).

48. The anterior half of the dilated rectal sphincter is now exposed from the vaginal aspect. To do this, the lower vaginal wall and perineal skin is mobilized laterally over the circular muscle fibers until enough of the sphincter is free for plication, imbrication, or resection (Plate 20, *G-G*).

49. The external sphincter is now plicated as shown in Plate 20, *H-H*. The number of sutures will vary but should be sufficient to reduce the caliber of the anal canal so that an average-sized index finger passes with ease. The surgeon should remember that the patient is under anesthesia and the sphincter dilates with greater ease. If a simple plication will not adequately reduce the caliber of the anal canal, the surgeon may elect to section the sphincter and imbricate the ends to achieve the desired result. If parturition has caused the anterior segment of the external sphincter to be scarred and thin, this segment may be resected and an end-to-end anastomosis done without impairing the patient's rectal continence.

50. The angle sutures can then be drawn taut but not tied while the surgeon studies the amount of vaginal wall that must be trimmed. The need for a functional vagina will determine the amount of vaginal wall that is resected. The angle sutures are tied (Plate 20, *I-I*). The vaginal wall is closed with interrupted sutures of 00 chromic catgut. A high perineorrhaphy is done, and the skin of the perineum is closed with interrupted sutures. An indwelling catheter is placed as well as a light vaginal pack. A plug of Vaseline gauze is placed in the anal canal (Plate 20, *I-I*).

Postoperative Care

The vaginal pack and Vaseline gauze plug in the rectum are removed in twenty-four hours. The patient's diet is modified, depending on whether the rectal procidentia was accordion-pleated or resected. With a bowel resection, even though it is retroperitoneal, the patient is maintained on intravenous fluids for the first two days. Vitamins and milliequivalents of potassium as indicated are added to the infusions. Blood chemistry studies to include serum potassium and chlorides are made for the first few days. The diet is then progressed to clear liquids, then a soft diet as tolerated, and finally to a regular diet by the eighth day or sooner. This is modified, depending on the postoperative course of the individual patient. If the rectal procidentia is accordion-pleated, the patient can proceed to a regular diet much sooner. Intubation is seldom necessary, but the usual indications may necessitate this on some occasions.

With a thorough bowel preparation prior to surgery and the preceding dietary routine, a warm mineral oil enema of 240 ml. can be administered about the sixth postoperative day.

If the patient is not uncomfortable, a tap water enema can be deferred until the eighth or ninth day. All this must be adapted to the individual patient and situation.

The patient is progressively ambulated, beginning by being out of bed the day following operation. Urinary antiseptics are administered. Because of the extent of the operation, I prefer to give combined therapy consisting of one sulfonamide preparation and one wide-spectrum antibiotic. The selection of drugs may be guided by the cultures and sensitivity tests if a bactiuria was found. The catheter is removed on the fifth postoperative day and residuals measured. An average hospital stay would be fourteen days.

References

Amar, A. D.: Comparison of Furadantin and Tetracycline in Prevention of Experimental Pyelonephritis, J. Urol. 85: 89, 1961.

Anselmino, K. J.: Surgical Treatment of Vaginal Prolapse After Total Extirpation of the Uterus, Geburtsh. u. Frauenh. 17: 501, 1957.

Bauer, A. W., Perry, D. M., and Kirby, W. M. M.: Drug Usage and Antibiotic Susceptibility of Staphylococci, J. A. M. A. 173: 475, 1960.

Benson, R. C.: Surgical Complications of Vaginal Hysterectomy, Surg., Gynec. & Obst. 106: 527, 1958.

Berglas, B., and Rubin, I.: Histologic Study of the Pelvic Connective Tissue, Surg., Gynec. & Obst. 97: 277, 1953.

Bowers, J. E., and others: A Study of Bladder Function Following Vaginal Hysterectomy, Surg., Gynec. & Obst. 104: 287, 1957.

Bunn, P., Knight, R., and Amberg, J.: Some Notes About a New Synthetic Penicillin for Staphylococcal Disease, New York J. Med. 60: 3074, 1960.

Cariker, M., and Dockerty, M. B.: The Retained Uterine Cervix, Am. J. Obst. & Gynec. 74: 379, 1957.

Carroll, G., and Mallette, W. F.: The Use of Colymycin in Chronic Urinary Infections Due to Pseudomonas Aeruginosa, J. Urol. 85: 86, 1961.

Castro, A.: Procidentia of the Rectum, Dis. Colon & Rectum. 1: 97, 1958.

Clabaugh, G. F., and Rhoads, P. S.: Efficacy of Urethral Catheterization for Determination of Urinary Tract Infection; Results With a New Technique, J. A. M. A. 165: 815, 1957.

Conger, G. T., and Keettel, W. C.: The Manchester-Fothergill Operation, Its Place in Gynecology: A Review of 960 Cases at University Hospitals, Iowa City, Iowa, Am. J. Obst. & Gynec. 76: 634, 1958.

Conill, V.: Ambulatorische Kolpoepisiokleisis bei senilem Prolapsus, Ztschr. Geburtsh. u. Gynäk. 136: 113, 1952.

Cronk, G. A., and Naumann, D. E.: The Use of Tetracycline Phosphate Complex in the Treatment of Infections, Antibiotic Med. & Clin. Ther. 4: 166, 1957.

Dannreuther, W.: Vaginal Dyspareunia, Am. J. Obst. & Gynec. 74: 747, 1957.

Dickenson, R. L.: Human Sex Anatomy, ed. 2, Baltimore, 1949, Williams & Wilkins Co.

Dillon, T. F.: Vasopressin as a Hemostatic in Gynecologic Surgery, Am. J. Obst. & Gynec. 78: 1285, 1959.

Dillon, T. F., and others: Vasopressin as a Hemostatic in Gynecologic Surgery; a Preliminary Report, Obst. & Gynec. 11: 363, 1958.

Emmett, T. A.: The Principles and Practice of Gynaecology, Philadelphia, 1879, H. C. Lea.

Fainstat, T.: Cortisone-Induced Prolapse and Inversion of the Uterus in Mice, Am. J. Obst. & Gynec. 76: 53, 1958.

Falk, H. C.: Uterine Prolapse and Prolapse of the Vaginal Vault Treated by Sacropexy, Obst. & Gynec. 18: 113, 1961.

Falk, H. C.: The Technique of Vaginal Hysterectomy, Harlem Hosp. Bull. 1: 45, 1948.

Falk, H. C., and Kaufman, S. A.: Partial Colpocleisis: The Le Fort Procedure, Obst. & Gynec. 5: 617, 1955.

Faulkner, J. W., and Morrison, A. F.: The Use of Sulfadimethoxine in the Treatment of Urinary Tract Infections, J. Urol. 83: 181, 1960.

Fleming, A. R.: Complete Perineotomy, Obst. & Gynec. 16: 172, 1960.

Fothergill, W.: Anterior Colporrhaphy and Amputation of the Cervix Combined as a Single Operation for Use in the Treatment of Genital Prolapse, Am. J. Surg. 29: 161, 1915.

Frank, R.: A Second Case of Irreducible Prolapse of the Uterus, J. Mt. Sinai Hosp. 14: 299, 1947.

Gibson, G. B.: The Repair of Genital Prolapse, Am. J. Obst. & Gynec. 78: 1275, 1959.

Gordon, C. A., and Gordon, R. E.: A Discussion of the Manchester Operation, Am. J. Obst. & Gynec. 74: 392, 1957.

Hawksworth, W., and Roux, J. P.: Vaginal Hysterectomy, J. Obst. & Gynaec. Brit. Emp. 65: 214, 1958.

Hayden, R. C., and Levinson, J. M.: Total Vaginectomy, Vaginal Hysterectomy, and Colpocleisis for Advanced Procidentia, Obst. & Gynec. 16: 564, 1960.

Heaney, N. S.: Report of 565 Vaginal Hysterectomies Performed for Benign Pelvic Disease, Am. J. Obst. & Gynec. 28: 751, 1934.

Herrold, R. D., and Karabatsos, N.: Current Status of Anti-infective Therapy in Urology, J. A. M. A. 172: 771, 1960.

Herrold, R. D., and Karabatsos, N.: Kanamycin in Chronic Urinary Infections, J. Urol. 82: 165, 1959.

Hill, E. C., and Hoag, R. W.: Experience With the Manchester Operation, Surg., Gynec. & Obst. 104: 167, 1957.

Hunter, J.: The Manchester-Fothergill Operation, Progr. Gynec. 111: 645, 1957.

Hunter, J. W. A.: Conservation of the Cervix Uteri in Operations for Prolapse, Brit. M. J. 2: 991, 1939.

Hunter, J. W. A.: The Conduct of Delivery Following Pelvic Floor Repair. J. Obst. & Gynaec. Brit. Empire 62: 809, 1955.

Ingram, J., Withers, R., and Wright, H.: Vaginal Hysterectomy After Previous Pelvic Surgery, Am. J. Obst. & Gynec. 74: 1181, 1957.

Israel, S.: Vaginal Sequelae of Vaginal Hysterectomy, Am. J. Obst. & Gynec. 69: 87, 1955.

Johnson, C. G.: Giant Calculus in the Urinary Bladder Associated With Complete Uterine Prolapse, Obst. & Gynec. 11: 579, 1958.

Kaplan, M. A., and others: A New, Rapidly Absorbed, Complex Salt of Tetracycline, Antibiotic Med. & Clin. Ther. 4: 99, 1957.

Kegel, A.: Progressive Resistance Exercise in Functional Restoration of Perineal Muscles, Am. J. Obst. & Gynec. 56: 238, 1948.

Kempers, R. D., Hunter, J. S., and Welch, J. S.: Indications for Vaginal Hysterectomy, Obst. & Gynec. 13: 677, 1959.

Kinzel, G. E.: Enterocele; a Study of 265 Cases, Am. J. Obst. & Gynec. 81: 1166, 1961.

Kuharic, H., Roberts, C., and Kirby, W.: Tetracycline Resistance of Group A Beta Hemolytic Streptococci, J. A. M. A. 174: 1779, 1960.

Lazar, M. R., and Krieger, H. A.: Blood Loss in Vaginal Surgery: A Comparative Study, Obst. & Gynec. 13: 707, 1959.

Lazar, M. R., Ottaway, J. P., and Offen, J. A.: Controlled Blood Loss in Vaginal Surgery, Obst. & Gynec. 10: 198, 1957.

Lee, J. H.: Management of Postpartum Urinary Retention, Obst. & Gynec. 17: 464, 1961.

Leff, W. A.: A Clinical Study With a New Sulfonamide (Madribon) in Cystitis Associated With Paraplegia, Read at New Jersey Chapter, American Federation for Clinical Research, Sept. 17, 1958.

Le Fort, L.: Nouveau procede pour la guerison due promaternal, Lisboa 4: 23, 1952.

Levi, P.: Vaginal Hysterectomy, Am. J. Surg. 85: 683, 1953.

McCall, M. L.: Posterior Culdeplasty: Surgical Correction of Enterocele During Vaginal Hysterectomy, Obst. & Gynec. 10: 595, 1957.

Meleney, F., and Prout, G.: Some Laboratory and Clinical Observations on Coly-Mycin (Colistin) With Particular Reference to Pseudomonas Infections, Surg., Gynec. & Obst. 112: 211, 1961.

Mulla, N.: Indwelling Catheter in Gynecologic Surgery, Obst. & Gynec. 17: 199, 1961.

Naidu, P., and Reddy, U.: Irreducible Prolapse and Its Treatment; With a Report on Two Cases, J. Obst. & Gynaec. Brit. Emp. 67: 994, 1960.

Neugebauer, L.: Einige Worte über die mediane Vaginalnaht als Mittel zur Beseitigung des Gebarmuttervorfalls, Zentralbl. Gynäk., No. 1-2, pp. 3 and 25, 1881.

Nigro, N.: Restoration of the Levator Sling in the Treatment of Rectal Procidentia, Dis. Colon & Rectum 1: 123, 1958.

Paterson, M. L., and Barr, W.: Urinary Infection After Colporrhaphy: Its Incidence, Causation and Prevention, J. Obst. & Gynaec. Brit. Emp. 67: 394, 1960.

Phaneuf, L.: The Place of Colpectomy in the Treatment of Uterine and Vaginal Prolapse, Am. J. Obst. & Gynec. 30: 544, 1935.

Pratt, J. H.: Sigmoidovaginostomy: A New Method of Obtaining Satisfactory Vaginal Depth, Am. J. Obst. & Gynec. 81: 535, 1961.

Pratt, J. H., and others: Blood Loss During Vaginal Hysterectomy, Obst. & Gynec. 15: 101, 1960.

Pulaske, E. J., and Isokane, R. K.: Tetracycline Concentrations in Blood Serum, Bile, and Prostatic and Spinal Fluids Following Oral Administration of Tetracycline Phosphate Complex and Tetracycline Hydrochloride, Antibiotic Med. & Clin. Ther. 4: 408, 1957.

Putnam, L. E.: Treatment of Common Infections With Tetracycline Phosphate Complex in Office Practice, Antibiotic Med. & Clin. Ther. 4: 470, 1957.

Radman, H. M., Campbell, C., and Coplan, R. S.: Antiinflammatory Drugs in Obstetrics and Gynecology, Am. J. Obst. & Gynec. 81: 344, 1961.

Ricci, J.: Gleansins and Technical Details From 500 Vaginal Hysterectomies for Prolapse, Am. J. Surg. 79: 377, 1950.

Ross, S., Puig, J. R., and Zaremba, E. A.: Sulfadimethoxine —a New, Long-Acting Sulfonamide; Some Preliminary Clinical and Laboratory Observations in Infants and Children, Read at Sixth Annual Symposium on Antibiotics, Washington, D. C., Oct. 15-17, 1958.

Seneca, H., Lattimer, J., and Zinsser, H.: Chemotherapy of Urinary Tract Infections Past and Current, New York J. Med. 60: 3630, 1960.

Seneca, H., Zinsser, H. H., and Lattimer, J. K.: Relation of Drug Resistance to Enzyme Activity Among Coliform Bacteria, J. A. M. A. 172: 1015, 1960.

Sexton, G. L.: Urinary Tract Infection Following Use of Indwelling Catheter, Obst. & Gynec. 17: 739, 1961.

Smith, I. M, and Soderstrom, W. H.: Clinical Experience With a New Erythromycin Derivative; Report of 105 Cases, J. A. M. A. 170: 184, 1959.

Sohn, H., and Persky, L.: Sulfadimethoxine Use in Chronic Urinary Drainage, A. M. A. Arch. Surg. 82: 719, 1961.

Speert, H.: Leon Lefort and His Operation for Uterine Prolapse, Surg., Gynec. & Obst. 104: 121, 1957.

Stegmann, H.: The Strain on the Pelvic Floor Before and After Gynecologic Operations and Its Significance for Early Postoperative Ambulation, Geburtsh. u. Frauenh. 14: 52, 1954.

Svennerud, S.: Prolapse of the Uterus and Vagina: A Review of 539 Cases, Acta obst. et gynec. scandinav. 37: 416, 1958.

Symmonds, R. E, and Pratt, J. H.: Vaginal Prolapse Following Hysterectomy, Am. J. Obst. & Gynec. 79: 899, 1960.

Tauber, R.: The Stump-Stitch Technique for Vaginal Hysterectomy, Am. J. Obst. & Gynec. 65: 1111, 1953.

Townsend, E. H., and Borgstedt, A.: Preliminary Report of Clinical Experience With Sulfadimethoxine, a New, Long-Acting Sulfonamide, Read at Sixth Annual Symposium on Antibiotics, Washington, D. C., Oct. 15-17, 1958.

Turner, S.: Complete Prolapse of Female Genital Organs: Repair With Vaginal Conservation, Obst. & Gynec. 17: 69, 1961.

Vartan, C. K.: Le Fort's Operation, J. Obst. & Gynaec. Brit. Emp. 67: 470, 1960.

Waters, E. G.: Culdoplastic Technique for Prevention and Correction of Vaginal Vault Prolapse and Enterocele, Am. J. Obst. & Gynec. 81: 291, 1961.

Watkins, J.: Treatment of Cystocele and Uterine Prolapse After the Menopause, Am. J. Obst. & Gynec. 15: 420, 1899.

Watson, A.: Technique of Vaginal Hysterectomy for Uterine Prolapse, Am. J. Obst. & Gynec. (supp.) 61A: 206, 1951.

Welch, H., and others: Blood Concentrations of Three Tetracycline Capsule Preparations Following a Single Oral Dose in Man, Antibiotic Med. & Clin. Ther. 4: 215, 1957.

Whapham, E. M.: Extended Use of the Le Fort Operation for Vaginal Prolapse in the Elderly, J. Obst. & Gynaec. Brit. Emp. 67: 473, 1960.

Section V · URINARY INCONTINENCE, FISTULAS, and BLADDER SURGERY

10 · Stress Incontinence

Introduction

The distressing affliction of stress incontinence challenges the ingenuity and operative skill of the gynecologist so frequently that an orderly method for study of these cases is needed. For the psychic well-being of the patient, as well as the chance of a successful operation, an exhaustive preoperative work-up is indicated. This alone gives some comfort to these unfortunate women who may be leading the life of a recluse because of their urinous odor. During this period of preparation much can be done to help them regain the confidence and bearing which they lose from living with a malady that threatens them with embarrassment at every turn. The psychologic trauma of one or more operative failures is intense. Thorough and systematic evaluation of each case with a carefully planned, individualized, operative procedure will result in fewer failures.

The bladder neck is the focal point in the investigation of incontinence. There exists but a narrow line between a bladder whose function is efficient enough to preserve continence and one that functions with only slightly less efficiency to permit incontinence and is therefore worthless. All of the factors, anatomic, physiologic, and pathologic, that hinder the action of this structure should be uncovered. In this way, accessory as well as principal causes of the incontinence are recognized and an intelligent formulation becomes possible. It is important to determine what part true stress incontinence and what part the frequency-urgency syndrome of chronic urethrotrigonitis is playing in a patient. Central nervous system disease may coexist with anatomic defects, and the responsibility of each in the disability should be evaluated. There is some function preserved in almost every bladder neck and pelvic floor. The task is to determine not only how well the bladder can function, but also all the other defects that in summation cause it to fail.

Normal micturition depends on a finely co-ordinated group of voluntary and involuntary movements. The operative procedure should be so planned as to restore anatomically as many of the structures concerned as is possible. Should this not promise success, then an operation is planned that attains continence by the creation of a somewhat abnormal mechanism. In any event it is necessary to individualize the operative procedure. The objective in the usual case is to make easier the performance of a dislodged and exhausted bladder neck. Since little can be done to improve its function as an isolated organ, each supporting structure the operator can restore or create to aid the closure of the bladder neck will enhance the operative result.

165

Symptoms and Diagnosis

The preoperative work-up for incontinent patients usually requires three or more visits. Complicated cases with multiple operative failures require even more extensive study and preparation. During the first visit the history is taken and a bimanual examination and a urine culture are done. The second visit is devoted to cystoscopy and urethroscopy. A course of sulfadiazine therapy is given prior to cystoscopy if the urine culture is positive for a pathogenic organism or there is a pyuria. It is not possible to get the urine bacteria-free before proceeding with cystoscopy in some cases. The third visit is for trigone tests, cystourethrography as indicated, and recommendations for the operative procedure.

A general outline for history taking is presented in Chart IV. The number of years since the onset and the progression of the incontinence are some index of the attenuation and atrophy of fascia and muscle. Where there is a childhood history of enuresis and delayed control, an occult spina bifida may exist. The details of the patient's deliveries yield information regarding the injuries sustained by the supporting structures. A history of pyelitis of pregnancy may require further investigation of the upper urinary tract prior to operation. A few patients note the onset of incontinence in the wake of post-partum retention, tenesmus, or hematuria.

A neurologic history must not be neglected since many cord and central nervous system lesions may cause cystometric disturbances resulting in retention and overflow incontinence. With sensory interruption the bladder is stretched and atonic. Tabetic patients may present a complaint of dribbling, difficulty in initiating the urinary stream, and a feeling of incomplete emptying. Spina bifida occulta may cause incontinence by defective innervation of the bladder and bladder neck. It may exist with continence until the addition of the trauma of an ordinary childbirth relaxes the bladder neck beyond its threshold for maintaining continence. Advance combined degeneration of the cord results in loss of control, with distention and overflow. Trauma is a common cause of a transverse myelitis and neurogenic bladder. Brain tumors, spinal cord lesions, and arteriosclerosis cause bladder dysfunction. Lesions of the motor nerves cause small, rhythmic, contraction waves in the detrusor muscle as seen in cystograms. Such contractions are inefficient in emptying the bladder, and the pressure is slightly raised due to delayed accommodation of the fluid increments. Spina bifida occulta, radical operations on the rectum or bladder, motor pathway lesions, multiple sclerosis, syphilis, and many other neurologic lesions may interrupt the motor nerves.

The influence of psychic factors on the bladder musculature is profound. Emotional upsets, sexual problems, and menstruation all may aggravate bladder symptoms. The mechanism is not clearly understood. The widespread and well-known symptom of "weak bladder" in young girls during childhood and puberty is an example. While many patients acknowledge having had slight incontinence during childhood when under stress or during laughing "fits," it is not known whether the incidence is greater among those who develop incontinence in later life. During periods of emotional stress it would appear that the detrusor becomes tonic and may aggravate existing lesions.

The degree of incontinence may be roughly graded from 0 to 4 plus (Chart IV). This gives some idea as to the extent of impairment of function and elicits some of the odd provocations causing incontinence, especially among the patients who have had multiple previous operations. When a patient loses urine on stress while at the same time making a determined effort with her voluntary muscles to hold the urine, the anatomic defect is usually quite extensive.

The usual range of genitourinary symptoms is reviewed to determine whether, in addition to bladder symptoms, any upper urinary tract disease coexists. At this time one may start to evaluate the part played by chronic urethrotrigonitis in the patient's complaints. Unless this is fully appreciated, many patients whose primary disease is inflammatory will be subjected to useless surgery. Treatment with radium or deep x-ray to the pelvis should be noted. Lastly it is necessary that the patient be treated for any accessory complaints together with her chief complaint of stress incontinence.

The force, caliber, and direction of the stream may suggest fistulas, aberrant ureters, and a distorted urethra and meatus from previous surgery. Posturinary dribbling can be caused by soft strictures of the urethra. The small amount of urine behind the stricture dribbles out when the patient relaxes and stands up. Tenesmus during the course of micturition has a variety of causes. Strictures, prolapse with angulation of the urethra, postoperative edema, polyps, and tumors cause straining. Any symptoms of pelvic relaxation should be inquired about. A chronic urethrotrigonitis is often found in conjunction with a chronically infected cervix.

A detailed history of previous pelvic operations is an important part of the work-up. Scarring and distortion, with displacement of the bladder neck to an unfavorable position for proper function, are frequently found after operative failures. Overcorrection or distorting sutures in the bladder base may cause ridges and false diverticula. Tenesmus, pain, and frequency after a vaginal hysterectomy may result from a tight midline plication of the round ligaments in the closure. This causes a pelvic sling across the base of the bladder. Postoperative fistulas and soft strictures must always be suspected. An operative failure is always a signal to investigate the patient for some of the more obscure factors contributing to the failure.

Special emphasis is placed on the pelvic supporting tissues during the bimanual examination. The anterior wall is inspected to determine whether the cystocele is posterior to Mercier's bar with good anterior fixation or whether an anterior cystocele exists also. The depth and scarring of the perineal body are noted. Then, with the patient making a conscious effort to hold her urine, the strength and tone of the paired levator ani muscles are estimated. Rectal examination reveals the size of a rectocele and the state of the rectal sphincter. The lumbosacral area should be examined for signs suspicious of spina bifida such as dimples, pigmentation, and hypertrichosis. (Chart IV.)

The vaginal aspect of a urethrocele presents itself as a pouching of the urethra posteriorly which causes the meatus to look upward while the mucosa shows transverse folds. The increase in the caliber of the urethra is not marked, but the suburethral tissues, glands, and spongiosa become hypertrophic, while at the same time the inner half of the urethra is dislodged and moves downward and forward. The meatus may gape or be otherwise distorted. Strictures are most common at the external meatus, with the inferior margin higher and more prominent than any point in the circumference. An olive-tipped bougie is recommended for measuring the caliber of the urethra. A sound or a cystoscope will dilate a soft stricture in passing. To give figures for the normal caliber and length of the urethra is misleading since this would infer that the organ is a symmetrical, afunctional, geometric cylinder. The converse is true since age, parity, previous surgery, position, attachments, inflammation, and method and point of measurement modify any criteria usually designated as normal. With this in mind any portion of the urethra with a caliber of 20 Fr. or less should be evaluated and its effect upon urination determined before diagnosing a stricture. The "point of hang" of a light bougie is the best method of sounding the urethra. The total length of the urethra is not so important as the "effective proximal length" of the inner third. Continent patients are seen with as little as a few millimeters of the inner third of the urethra present. A urethra 4 cm. in length has been measured as average. The direction that a glass catheter in the urethra makes with the horizontal roughly indicates the displacement of the urethra and gives some idea of its mobility. In the normal state the external meatus descends endwise about 1 cm. out of the pelvis when the patient strains. The

167

Text continued on p. 172.

CHART IV
INCONTINENCE STUDY

Name _____ Age_____ History Number_____ Date_____

ONSET OF INCONTINENCE

Age_____ Number of years since onset_____ Progressively   worse_____
Unchanged_____ Improving_____ Tendency to remissions_____

CHILDHOOD HISTORY

Defective or delayed control_____
Enuresis_____ Age_____ How cured_____

OBSTETRIC HISTORY

Relation of onset to deliveries_____

Pregnancies

YEAR	DURATION OF LABOR	WEIGHTS	OPERATIONS	LACERATIONS	REMARKS
----	-----------------	-------	----------	-----------	-------
----	-----------------	-------	----------	-----------	-------
----	-----------------	-------	----------	-----------	-------
----	-----------------	-------	----------	-----------	-------
----	-----------------	-------	----------	-----------	-------
----	-----------------	-------	----------	-----------	-------

Urinary Complications of Pregnancy

Pyelitis of pregnancy: Onset_____ Duration _____
    Severity_____ Treatment_____
    Recurrence with subsequent pregnancies_____
    Chronic pyelitis_____
    Remarks _____
Post-partum retention: Number of days and frequency of catheterizations if occurring with a pregnancy
_____
    Remarks _____
Post-partum tenesmus: Duration and severity if occurring with a pregnancy_____
_____
    Remarks _____
Post-partum hematuria: Duration and amount if occurring with a pregnancy_____
_____
    Remarks _____

NEUROLOGIC HISTORY

Weakness or paralysis of legs_____ Incontinence of feces_____
Ulcers of legs_____ Girdle pains_____
Spinal cord or back injury_____
    Remarks _____

DEGREE OF INCONTINENCE (0 to 4 plus)

Coughing _____	Running _____	Passing flatus _____
Sneezing _____	Bending _____	Heavy lifting _____
Laughing _____	Climbing stairs _____	Recumbent _____

Other _____
Remarks _____

CHART IV (Continued)
INCONTINENCE STUDY

Estimation of the Degree of Incontinence

0   No incontinence

1 plus   Feeling of moisture after stress or other provocation

2 plus   Dribbles small amount of urine with stress or other provocation but requires no constant hygienic device

3 plus   Squirts considerable stream of urine on stress or other provocation and requires constant hygienic device

4 plus   Complete incontinence; urine overflows on slightest provocation; stress incontinence when recumbent

GENITOURINARY SYMPTOMS

Dysuria: Mild_____ Moderate_____ Severe _____
        Initially_____ Terminally_____ Throughout urination_____

Hematuria: Amount_____ Frequency_____ Remarks_____
_____

Nocturia: _____ per night Frequency _____ times every _____ hours

Urgency: Mild_____ Moderate_____ Severe_____

Oliguria: _____ Pyuria: _____ Chills and fever: _____

Pain: Sharp or stablike, dull or aching, constant or intermittent, and any characteristic radiation
          Costovertebral _____
          Course of ureters _____
          Suprapubic _____
          Urethral _____

URINATION

Stream: Force_____ Caliber_____ Direction_____ Posturinary dribbling_____
        Remarks _____

Tenesmus: Straining delay_____ Terminal tenesmus_____

Strangury: Remarks _____

Sensation of incomplete emptying_____

PELVIC RELAXATION

Vaginal protrusion_____ Bearing-down sensation _____

Low back pain_____ Leukorrhea_____ Pruritus_____

FACTORS RELATED TO OR INFLUENCING INCONTINENCE

Respiratory infections_____ Cold weather_____

Full bladder only_____ Emotional upsets_____

Attitudes or devices used to: Prevent incontinence_____
         Initiate stream_____

Social limitations_____

Remarks _____

PREVIOUS GYNECOLOGIC OPERATIONS

Type_____ If for incontinence: Improved _____ Worse _____

Remarks _____

Change in symptoms after operation_____ _____

Remarks _____

CHART IV (Continued)
INCONTINENCE STUDY

BIMANUAL EXAMINATION

Vaginal mucosa: Atrophic_____ Vaginitis_____ Edematous_____

Anterior wall

      Posterior cystocele_____ Small_____ Moderate_____ Large_____

      Anterior cystocele_____ Small_____ Moderate_____ Large_____

      General relaxation_____ Small_____ Moderate_____ Large_____

Uterus

      Cervix: Lacerations_____ Hypertrophy_____

             Elongation of anterior lip_____ Cervicitis_____

             Descensus_____ Remarks_____

      Fundus: Position_____ Size_____

             Mobility_____ Pressure on bladder_____

             Remarks _____

      Adnexa: Right_____ Left_____

Posterior wall

      Perineal body: Depth_____ Scarring_____

      Levator tests: Defects_____ Sagging of posterior wall_____

             Remarks _____

      Rectocele: Small_____ Moderate_____ Large_____

      Enterocele: Small_____ Moderate_____ Large_____

Rectal examination: Sphincter_____ Tone_____ Remarks _____

Back: Dimple, pigmentation, or hypertrichosis over lumbosacral spine_____

_____ Remarks_____

Neurologic, if indicated_____

_____

URETHRA

Urethrocele: Small_____ Moderate_____ Large _____

Meatus: Gaping_____ Distorted_____

      Stricture_____ Caruncle_____ Skeneitis_____

Length: cm._____ Caliber_____ Strictures_____

      Location_____ Congenital _____

Direction catheter makes with horizontal_____ approximate degrees

      Hold_____ Strain_____

      Endwise descent of urethra on straining_____approximate centimeters

      Normal _____ Abnormally mobile _____

TRIGONE TESTS   Degree of incontinence

1. Tenaculum on anterior lip of cervix
      Traction   _____
      Replacement   _____

2. Allis clamp near interureteric ridge
      Traction   _____
      Replacement   _____
      Behind symphysis   _____

CHART IV (Concluded)

INCONTINENCE STUDY

3. Using both clamps

    Traction on trigone; cervix replaced   _____

    Traction on cervix; trigone replaced   _____

    Traction on both clamps   _____

    Replacement of both clamps   _____

4. Depression and spreading of perineal body

    Traction on trigone   _____

    Replacement of trigone   _____

5. Patient standing

    Traction cervix   _____

    Replacement cervix   _____

    Traction trigone   _____

    Replacement trigone   _____

    Replacement behind symphysis   _____

6. Patient walking

    Traction trigone   _____

    Replacement trigone   _____

CYSTOSCOPY

Residual _____ ml.   Scope _____

Bladder capacity

    Urge to void _____ ml.

    Fullness   _____ ml.

    Pain   _____ ml.

Bladder wall

    Cystitis _____ Atrophy _____

    Diverticula _____ Pseudodiverticula _____

    Trabeculations _____ Postoperative deformities _____

    Describe _____

    _____

Trigone

    Trigonitis _____

    Interureteric ridge: Intact_____ Divided_____

    Bell's muscles: Intact_____ Divided _____

    Ureteral orifices: Describe_____

            Movement on straining_____

            Movement on hold_____

    Bas-fond: Describe_____

URETHROSCOPY

Sphincter: Gaping_____ Normal_____ Symmetry_____

    Sluggish_____ Normal action_____

    Closure on hold_____ % of normal_____

    Descent and funneling when urged to strain_____

           Describe _____

    Bar deformity: Describe_____

Urethra

    Urethritis _____Polyps _____

    Diverticula _____Strictures _____

    Scarring and deformities_____

    Remarks _____

endwise descent is noted for abnormal mobility, scarring, and adhesions to the pubic rami. The latter fix the outer third of the urethra at a lower level than normal and by continuity retract the bladder neck downward and forward to an unfavorable position.

Urethroscopy

Local inflammatory lesions in the urethra are common and require both preoperative and postoperative treatment. Rarer findings are aberrant ureters and fistulas. Urethroscopy provides direct observation of the function of the bladder neck and is a critical part of the work-up. The Fulkerson urethroscope or universal Brown-Buerger cystourethroscope with water distention is used to advantage in this clinic to provide a direct view without magnification of funneling of the inner one-third of the urethra (Plate 21, *A* to *C*). The action of the bladder neck is studied with the patient straining and holding. Regardless of the scope used, consistent positioning is necessary so the distortion of the region of the bladder neck by the cystoscope itself is made common to the normal and the abnormal: The scope is always drawn an estimated 1 cm. from the bladder neck while performing the tests of bladder function as viewed from within the bladder. A method of drawing or demonstrating this other than on the individual patient requires high-speed intravesical motion pictures. I have, therefore, been able to teach this only to the residents and visiting surgeons who have observed the normal and then watched the incontinent patient attempt to close the bladder neck. Typical drawings of the configuration of the bladder neck done by this method are shown in Plate 21, *D* to *F*. Patients with no incontinence have a muscular mechanism that closes the internal orifice almost completely and promptly when the patient holds. It opens the orifice quickly and moves it down and slightly forward on straining. A characteristic finding in the incontinent patients is a gaping internal orifice that reacts sluggishly. With the patient making a forceful effort to hold back the urine, the closure is noted in terms of the diameter of the com-

pletely open bladder neck. Cases have been observed where the sphincter contracted slowly and reduced the diameter of the internal orifice as viewed in water by only 10 per cent. Viewed several weeks after an operation that successfully restored continence, almost complete closure is seen but with a distorted outline. One sees occasionally a spastic, irritable bladder neck usually associated with chronic urethrotrigonitis and the frequency-urgency syndrome. This bladder neck is more or less sheared off from the trigone, raising the sphincter above the floor of the bladder. The detrusor becomes more and more irritable, giving rise to the frequency and urgency. The bladder is routinely catheterized for residual urine and a repeat urine culture is taken if indicated.

Cystometric studies are limited in the routine work-up to noting at what volume of distention the patient has the urge to void, the sense of fullness, and finally pain. When a neurologic factor is suspected, more careful evaluation of the detrusor tonus is done by cystometry. An observation cystoscopy reveals the status of the bladder mucosa. This eliminates patients whom surgery could not benefit because of advanced bladder disease. Carcinoma of the bladder, tertiary radiation cystitis, and chronic cystitis with fibrotic contracted bladder and ureteral reflux are seen, but only palliative treatment is possible when incontinence exists. Trabeculation with cellule formation, true diverticula, and dilatation of ureteral orifices may indicate obstruction at the bladder neck. Postoperative deformities are not uncommon. The interureteric ridge and Bell's muscles are observed while the patient holds and strains. With an effort to initiate micturition, Bell's muscles stand out and the ureteral orifices move medially and slightly downward toward the internal orifice. The converse happens when a conscious effort is made to restrain urination. Defects in Bell's muscles from trauma are occasionally observed, but their importance, if any, is not manifest. The type and size of a cystocele as seen intravesically are of importance. The limits of the relaxation are noted, with particular emphasis on the presence of relaxa-

PLATE 21

URETHROSCOPIC TESTS IN URINARY STRESS INCONTINENCE

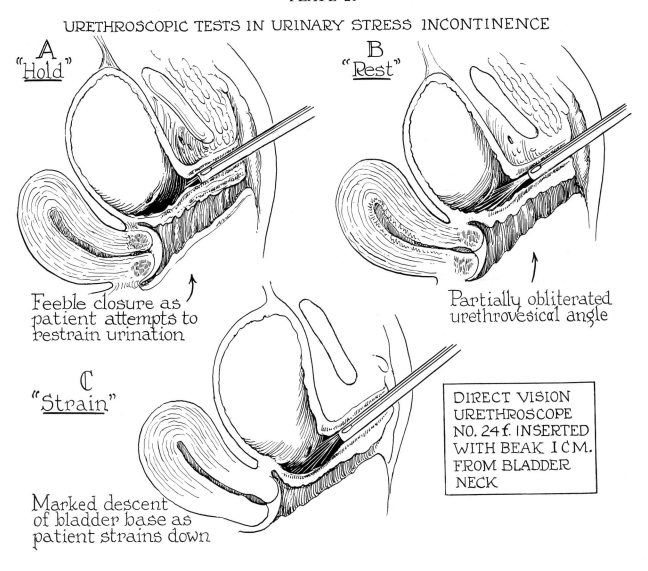

A "Hold"

Feeble closure as patient attempts to restrain urination

B "Rest"

Partially obliterated urethrovesical angle

C "Strain"

Marked descent of bladder base as patient strains down

DIRECT VISION URETHROSCOPE NO. 24 f. INSERTED WITH BEAK 1 CM. FROM BLADDER NECK

URETHROSCOPIC VIEWS

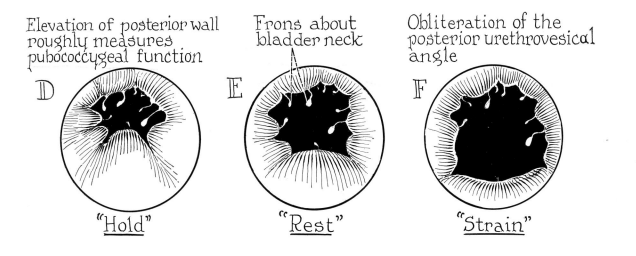

Elevation of posterior wall roughly measures pubococcygeal function

D "Hold"

Frons about bladder neck

E "Rest"

Obliteration of the posterior urethrovesical angle

F "Strain"

tion anterior to Mercier's bar. Continent patients may have a deep bas-fond with no defect of the trigone.

Trigone Tests

Some of the anatomic defects accessory to the incompetent bladder neck and the probable end results of operation can be studied by what we have come to call trigone tests. The bladder neck is studied during manipulation by an Allis clamp placed on the anterior vaginal wall in the region of the interureteric ridge. To evaluate the role that descensus and anterior wall relaxation may play, the anterior lip of the cervix may also be manipulated with a tenaculum. After the bladder has been filled with 250 ml. of saline solution, the patient is taught to cough with sufficient violence to allow a trickle of water to escape if such can be demonstrated. In all subsequent tests she is told to cough with approximately the same stress. Stress must be differentiated from simple urination or precipitancy. With stress there is an increase in intravesical pressure directly proportional to the increase in intra-abdominal pressure caused by coughing. With a conscious effort to urinate, there is relaxation of the perineum and less increase in intra-abdominal pressure. We are not interested in the latter at the moment.

A speculum is placed in the vagina and turned sideways to visualize the urethra and bladder neck. With a long needle and small-bore syringe, a wheal of 1 per cent procaine is raised in the vaginal wall at the level of the interureteric ridge. This wheal is then grasped with an Allis clamp inserted posteriorly between both blades of the speculum so that the latter may be removed and the clamp left in place. By the same approach a tenaculum is made to grasp the anterior lip of the cervix and the speculum is removed.

The patient gives one or two coughs with each maneuver and the degree of incontinence is roughly estimated. The cervix is first pulled down and then replaced. The bladder neck is depressed and pulled toward the introitus. Next it is placed approximately in the position one might expect to achieve by an anterior colporrhaphy with plication of the bladder neck. Then it is placed far up behind the symphysis where one would suspend it with some type of sling operation or cervicocystopexy. Traction is then made on the cervix while the bladder neck is replaced and vice versa, and the effects are studied. The perineal body is depressed and spread while making traction on the Allis clamp and the result noted. With the patient in the standing position, over a towel, various maneuvers are done. It is necessary to hold the handle of the Allis clamp from behind to manipulate the bladder neck properly in the standing position. Finally, the trigone is depressed by traction while the patient walks in a circle. Some patients demonstrate incontinence in this way without the added factor of stress. It must be pointed out that in cases where one or more operations have been performed for this condition, the circumstances under which the patient is incontinent are often variable. It is seldom necessary to perform all these tests in detail to diagnose the common case. But there is the unusual patient who insists she is wet under the most bizarre circumstances who requires the most careful consideration in locating the mechanism of her stress incontinence. This is particularly true of the patient with incontinence on walking, where a complicated group of muscular motions forces open the weakened bladder neck. The mechanics of the pelvic floor still require much study in the living anatomy.

Roentgenographic methods are utilized to confirm or exclude occult spina bifida and bladder diverticula. Where it is possible to take some type of cystourethrogram, this should be done in patients having a history of operative failures. The course of the urethra, its mobility, and the position of the bladder neck are determined. These facts are valuable in planning the surgical procedure as well.

Classification of Stress Incontinence

The principal objectives in classifying this condition are to emphasize the underlying pathologic physiology and to directly suggest adequate operations for its cure. A classification is needed since some surgeons commonly apply the same operation to a variety of patients with different anatomic defects and associated factors. The only common denominator among many of these patients is the symptom of stress incontinence. Another objective is to establish a basis for comparison of results since our studies to date have little meaning when series of cases contain all types of patients. Some further objectives are the emphasizing of accuracy in description of the symptoms and findings, the need of the well-trained gynecologist to master the diagnostic devices used in female urology, the contribution a classification can make to a more accurate prognosis and to students' understanding of this condition, as well as the physiology of the pelvic floor. Finally, it is desired to emphasize the advantages of gynecologic surgery from the space of Retzius, particularly in the management of incontinence.

Charts V and VI show a simple method of classifying a patient with stress incontinence. Thus, complex urethroscopic, cystometric, and urethrographic procedures, which would result in the same staging of a given patient, are not necessary. However, it is not to be inferred that these procedures are not useful adjuncts which contribute detail to the study and refinement to the surgery. The first step is to determine by history and examination the frequency and degree of incontinence. This may be further clarified during the examination by filling the bladder with 250 ml. of water or saline solution and having the patient cough in the lithotomy and standing positions. A patient continuously and grossly incontinent almost always has aggravating factors, but in the rare instance where such severe incontinence exists without demonstrable aggravation, a patient may be placed in Stage II on this basis alone. Second, the presence of aggravating medical factors is determined. Some of the common factors have been listed. Third, the state of the pubococcygeal function is determined by the following test: The index finger

is passed a few centimeters within the introitus along each lateral sulcus of the vagina. With the finger tip flexed, the anterior thickened edge of the pubococcygeus is identified by having the patient alternately hold back the urine and strain down. The patient is directed to hold, relax, or strain down several times until an estimate of the strength of the action is appraised. In the same way the finger palpates the length of the urethra while the patient holds or relaxes to determine the degree of mobility or fixation. Scarring and distortion are observed. Dysfunction infers the presence of pubococcygeal action but of a degree insufficient to elevate the bladder neck and maintain continence. Malfunction is present when scarring and distortion do not permit the remains of the pubococcygeus to act normally. Not infrequently muscle action is felt, but it will be well posterior to the bladder neck in the ileococcygeus and not where it can affect bladder control.

By such a classification, attention is focused on the selection of a primary operation that is adequate for the patient instead of a trial-and-error procedure. This requires a more extensive primary procedure but should reduce the number of failures. By a more extensive operation is inferred a procedure which attacks the problem not only from the vaginal side, but also from an abdominal approach through the space of Retzius. Depending on the training and preference of the surgeon, the procedure selected may be a sling-type operation, such as the Goebell-Stoeckel, the Millin-Read, the Aldridge and Studdiford types, or other modifications. The simple suprapubic suspension of Marshall and Marchetti recently stimulated interest and gave new promise in the relief of this condition. I have had excellent results with the introduction of a dual plication of the bladder neck of the vaginal and then the abdominal aspect of the bladder neck, followed by a cystopexy to the rectus tendons. In any event the operation should correct the funneling of the bladder neck and the forward and downward descent of the urethra by something more than a simple vaginal plication. It should restore the posterior urethrovesical angle.

Recurrent incontinence constitutes the most common indication at present for a combined type of operation. We feel there are many patients with recurrent incontinence who would have been cured by the first procedure if the operation selected were of the combined type. Barring some specific contraindication, an operation can often be planned to take care of stress incontinence at the time of another procedure. It is our practice to do a combined operation after one failure. It is our goal to be selective enough to pick out the prospective failures and do more adequate surgery from the start.

The short, squat, heavy-boned, overweight female sent to our incontinence clinic for study is so frequently an operative failure that she should be studied thoroughly before the first operation. I feel that the obese individual with severe stress incontinence should have a combined type of operation as a primary procedure. While the addition of an abdominal approach to the bladder neck increases the morbidity, the increased percentage of successful operations is justified by this. The heavy abdominal panniculus and fat-laden intra-abdominal contents put an unusual strain on the entire levator sling. This is impressive when the degree of incontinence is compared in the lithotomy and standing positions. It is almost invariably more severe in the latter position.

Radium causes changes in the vagina and bladder base, which, when combined with previous displacement of the bladder neck by parturition, create very unfavorable conditions for vaginal surgery. The vagina is shortened, is decreased in caliber, and shows loss of pliability. The cardinal and uterosacral thickenings retract and tend to pull the bladder base downward. Endarteritis and fibrosis result in a poor blood supply. The bladder neck and base may be adherent to the vaginal wall due to irradiation which contributes to a displacement of the bladder neck to a position unfavorable for proper function. Patients are seen with gross incontinence where the retrac-

tion caused by intracavitary radium for benign disease leaves a contracted vagina with no obvious urethrocele or cystocele to correct by surgery. This is because the vaginal aspect of the bladder neck does not indicate the degree of funneling of the bladder neck as seen intravesically. It is especially important to free the urethra and bladder neck from the vaginal wall and then depend on the abdominal phase to effect reposition and plication. The effects of intracavitary radium on the anterior bladder wall are minimal, so why not utilize this healthy aspect of the bladder to correct incontinence. Late radiation cystitis with stress incontinence requires a combined operation as the initial procedure.

Coughing is the most common form of stress that causes incontinence when the bladder neck is incompetent to withstand increased intravesical pressure. Patients with chronic coughs from bronchitis, bronchiectasis, excessive smoking, or other causes not only wet themselves more often, but also put a great deal of strain on the bladder neck after any surgery for correction. This is true for many years as well as for the immediate postoperative period. They virtually cough everything down when the support of the pelvic floor alone is depended upon in the operation designed for cure. While existence of a chronic cough provides a handy excuse for operative failures when the postoperative patient returns still incontinent, it does not provide any satisfaction to the surgeon who performed an inadequate simple colporrhaphy and plication under these adverse circumstances. The vaginal aspect of the bladder neck is subjected to every intra-abdominal stress which tends to displace its attachments laterally. This can only result in the displacement of the bladder neck downward and forward, which has been shown to result in funneling and incompetency. Knowing that the patient will probably cough just as much after the operation as before, the surgeon should select a combined operation that promises the utmost support.

Patients are seen with stress incontinence (and their genital tracts confirm the fact) who

CHART V

BASIS OF THE CLASSIFICATION OF STRESS INCONTINENCE

1. Frequency and degree of incontinence

2. Presence of aggravating medical factors such as:

    a. Obesity

    b. Chronic coughs

    c. Bronchial asthma

    d. Hay fever

    e. Bronchiectasis

    f. Diabetes mellitus

    g. Neurologic complications

    h. Radiation changes in vagina and bladder base

    i. Other similar medical factors

3. Function of the pubococcygeus

CLASSIFICATION

	INCONTINENCE	MEDICAL FACTORS	PUBOCOCCYGEUS
STAGE 0	None	Variable	Normal or attenuated
STAGE I	Mild to moderate	None	Dysfunctional
STAGE II	Moderate to severe	Yes	Dysfunctional
STAGE III	Moderate to severe	Variable	Malfunctional

CHART VI

CLASSIFICATION OF STRESS INCONTINENCE

STAGE 0—POTENTIAL INCONTINENCE

   a. No incontinence

   b. Bladder neck susceptible to *unintentional derangement during pelvic surgery*

   c. May have aggravating medical factors

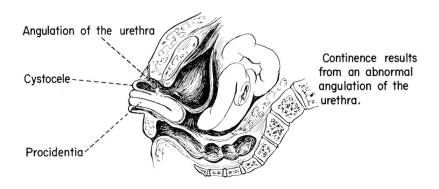

Angulation of the urethra

Cystocele

Procidentia

Continence results from an abnormal angulation of the urethra.

STAGE I—DYSFUNCTIONAL INCONTINENCE

   a. Moderate loss of urine on occasions with stress

   b. No aggravating medical factors

   c. Pubococcygeal function present but inadequate; abnormal forward mobility and funneling of the urethra without fixation

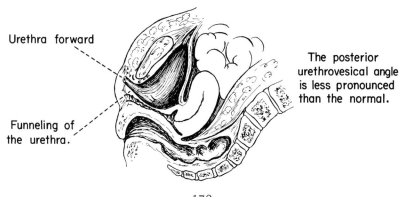

Urethra forward

Funneling of the urethra.

The posterior urethrovesical angle is less pronounced than the normal.

CHART VI (Concluded)

CLASSIFICATION OF STRESS INCONTINENCE

STAGE II—AGGRAVATED DYSFUNCTIONAL INCONTINENCE

    a. Frequent considerable loss of urine with stress

    b. *Aggravating medical factors compound the degree of incontinence*

    c. Pubococcygeal function present but inadequate; abnormal forward mobility and functioning of urethra often more marked but without fixation

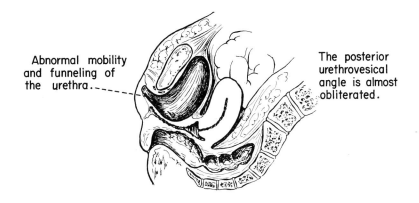

STAGE III—MALFUNCTIONAL INCONTINENCE

    a. Variable degrees of severity; sometimes grossly incontinent even in recumbent position

    b. May have aggravating medical factors.

    c. *Malfunction of the pubococcygeus;* abnormal forward fixation, distortion, and funneling of urethra; frequently seen following operative failures

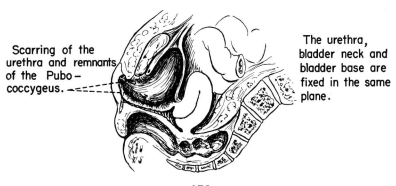

have not borne children and, indeed, some who have not had sexual relations. Whether these patients should be distinguished from those with neurologic defects associated with incontinence is conjectural. Not infrequently they have a history of enuresis or weak bladder in childhood or puberty and volunteer this information. When examined, however, I am impressed with the number of these patients in whom the entire pelvic sling seems to be lower and more attenuated and in whom the ability to elevate the pelvic floor or compress the examining fingers is limited. The muscular action of the puborectalis division of the levator ani is not impressive. It would appear that this muscle is thinner than usual, exemplifying the weakness of the pelvic floor. While difficult to demonstrate, it is my impression that the line of insertion of the entire levator system is more caudad in these patients than is normally seen. This makes for poor support of the bladder neck, which must be reposed up and behind the symphysis in order to remain small in diameter and efficient. In the literature there are statements that anterior wall relaxation, even given the distinction of being cystoceles, can result from vigorous intercourse and produce conditions causing incontinence. Just how sexual intercourse in any frequency, position, or known anatomic variation can duplicate the passage of and cause relaxation the same as a bony, albeit malleable, fetal head, about 9.5 cm. in biparietal diameter is difficult to imagine. The clinical impression in these patients is that some developmental variation in the muscle rather than a neurologic defect is present. When the history elicits such a story and complete examination confirms a patient with congenital stress incontinence, the operative procedure should include an abdominal approach of some type in order to give permanent support.

Surgical Anatomy of the Female Bladder

The bladder is a distensible vesicle situated dorsal to the symphysis and ventral to the uterus. Its relations as well as its shape change with the degree of filling so that what may be true of the empty bladder is not applicable to the full one. The lateral aspect of a distended bladder extends to the obliterated umbilical artery as it passes forward on the sidewall of the pelvis. It is also closely related to the obturator vessels and nerve. The shape of this ever-changing organ must be appreciated from every anatomic view to appreciate the distortions that may occur after multiple operations. The bladder neck is that portion of the bladder that joins the urethra and forms a funnel with the upper portion of the latter. Extending upward, a definite triangle, the trigone, may be observed on the internal surface. The base is that portion of the posterior wall above the trigone that extends upward to the level of the vesicouterine reflection of the peritoneum. The superior surface extends from the peritoneal reflection to the anterior abdominal wall and attachment of the urachus. The portion of the bladder to which the urachus is attached is called the vertex. The anterior or inferolateral surfaces of the bladder extend from the vertex to the bladder neck and rest upon the pelvic diaphragm. Those portions between the vertex and the base are termed the body. The anterior border of the inferolateral aspect looks downward and forward toward the symphysis pubis, from which it is separated by the space of Retzius. The inferolateral surface on each side is separated from the levator ani and obturator internus by subperitoneal connective tissue and ensheathes the bladder vessels and nerves. The vertex is at the level of the upper border of the symphysis when the bladder is empty but may rise almost to the umbilicus when it is full. The superior surface is pointed upward into the abdominal cavity. The base of the bladder rests on the upper part of the anterior wall of the vagina and cervix. The trigonal area rests on the lower part of the anterior wall of the vagina. The adult bladder when moderately distended measures about 12.5 cm. in its long axis and about 7.5 cm. in its transverse and has an average capacity of about 500 ml. The measurements vary with the age and habits of the individual.

The bladder is surrounded by a covering of

loose connective tissue except over the trigone and base, where this areolar layer is thicker and stronger. The latter is continuous with the fascia covering the inside of the levator ani, and this extension of the parietal connective tissue along the inferolateral border of the bladder becomes further condensed with the inferior vesical arteries, veins, nerves, and lymphatics. The middle pubovesical ligament (triangular ligament) is a condensation of the connective tissue which extends from the lower part of the anterior wall of the bladder and upper urethra through the space of Retzius to the posterior surface of the pubic bones at the sides of the symphysis. This condensation of areolar tissue is constantly seen in the space of Retzius during gynecologic surgery. At first it appears to be an artifact due to the tissue being more adherent to the interpubic fibrocartilage than to the adjacent bone. However, we still observe it in the elderly patients in whom bony union of the symphysis has occurred. How this tissue—that can be dissected from the symphysis by the weight of the surgeon's hand—can be called a "ligament" and contribute to the support of the bladder neck is incredible. The middle umbilical ligament is formed by the urachus, which is the obliterated portion of the allantoic stalk extending from the vertex of the bladder to the umbilicus. The false ligaments are formed by folds of peritoneum. The two posterior false ligaments are called the uterovesical ligaments and contain the obliterated hypogastric arteries, the ureters, the vessels, and the nerves passing to the bladder. The lateral false ligaments are peritoneal folds extending between the sides of the bladder and the lateral walls of the pelvic cavity. The superior false ligament is the fold of peritoneum which passes from the summit of the bladder to the abdominal wall and covers the urachus and obliterated hypogastric arteries.

The detrusor muscle comprises all of the bladder musculature except the trigone. It is composed of thin outer and inner longitudinal layers with a thicker circular layer between. The thickness varies greatly in different sub-

jects and also with the degree of distention. When moderately stretched, it is about 3 mm. thick, but when contracted it may be as thick as 12 mm. The thickest portion is the base. The inner muscular layer is somewhat retiform, and with the bladder wall distended, the layer becomes so thin that open meshes are left between the muscle bundles. These bundles may become hypertrophied and form ridges with saccules in between. The bladder is lined by a layer of transitional epithelium, and in the empty state the mucosa is thrown into numerous irregular folds. When the bladder is distended, the mucosa appears as a pearly white membrane, through which the larger blood vessels in the submucosa can be seen. The submucosa is quite loose throughout, except in the trigone, and permits folding and stretching of the mucosa.

The trigone is a separate structure which merits individual description. Its base is formed by a line drawn between the ureteral orifices, and its apex is the internal urethral orifice. In the trigone the inner longitudinal layer is more fully developed by reinforcements from the longitudinal coats of the ureters. The lateral ridges of the trigonal muscles are known as Bell's muscles. The thickened edge between the ureteral orifices is called the interureteric ridge or Mercier's bar. Other fibers spread out over the trigone and decussate with those from the opposite side, and some of them extend through the vesical orifice into the upper part of the urethra. The submucosa is absent in the trigone, and the mucosa is closely attached to the muscularis, for which reason it always remains smooth. The relative immobility of the trigone as compared with the remainder of the bladder base is important in bladder surgery, radiation, and the repair of fistulas.

The female urethra is a tubular structure 3 to 5.5 cm. in length and 7 to 10 mm. in diameter. The internal orifice lies about 2 cm. behind and about 0.5 cm. above the inferior border of the symphysis in the nulliparous woman but is lower and farther forward in parous females. From here the urethra passes downward and slightly forward to the external meatus, which opens in the vestibule of the vagina 2.0 cm. in front of and 1.5 cm. below the inferior borders of the symphysis in nulliparous subjects. The urethra may be divided into three portions: the pelvic, between the bladder and the triangular ligament; the membranous, between the layers of the triangular ligament; the vaginal, between the triangular ligament and the meatus. The muscular coats are continuous with those of the bladder and consist of inner and outer longitudinal layers with a circular layer between them. There is a mucosa of transitional epithelium which merges anteriorly into stratified squamous epithelium at variable distances from the meatus. The urethra contains branched, tubular glands emptying into paraurethral ducts.

The duct openings are most common in the anterior third of the urethra and diminish toward the bladder neck. In the posterior third they are represented by crypts and lacunae. The arterial supply is derived from the inferior vesical and pudic arteries. Veins drain into the vesicovaginal and pubic plexuses, while the lymphatics drain into the hypogastric and inguinal nodes in association with lymphatics about the neck of the bladder. The urethra has a cavernous layer due to the numerous veins in the loose areolar tissue of the submucous coat. The nerve supply is intimately related to that of the bladder. Muscle fibers of the trigone pass over the bladder neck into the upper part of the urethra, creating the most prominent fold in the canal, known as the crista urethrae. Distal to the bladder neck some fibers of the pubococcygeus pass along the lateral wall to be inserted into the vaginal cuff surrounding the urethra. The urethra then passes through the superior and inferior layers of the urogenital diaphragm, with the fibers of the deep transverse perineal muscles between. Beyond this, fibers of the ischiocavernosi, fasciculi from the bulbocavernosi, and the superficial transverse perineal muscles pass intimately associated with the outer muscular fibers of the urethra to their places of insertion. Kennedy describes an arrangement of muscle bundles in the wall of the urethra which he calls the muscle of micturition. His studies show fibers passing between the circular and external longitudinal coats from the anteromedial facies of the pubic rami obliquely back and around the urethra and acting as a purse string. This muscle of micturition, observed on histologic sections, is difficult to visualize as a functional unit closing the bladder neck. The part played by the levator ani in urinary control cannot be dismissed. It is probable that muscular control of urination is achieved by a combination of the actions of the intrinsic muscles of the bladder neck and proximal urethra and the puborectalis division of the levator ani.

Three pairs of vessels provide the main blood supply to the bladder: the superior, middle, and inferior vesical arteries. The two former arise from the hypogastric arteries proximal to their points of obliteration and supply the body of the bladder. The inferior vesical arteries often arise in common with the middle hemorrhoidal arteries from the anterior trunks of the hypogastric arteries. The inferior vesical arteries supply the base, trigone, vesical neck, and proximal urethra and give off vaginal branches. The veins form a fine anastomosis in the connective tissue surrounding the bladder and drain into veins along the course of the arteries. The mucosa has only lymph spaces, but a definite network is visible in the submucosa. Small lymphatics then run in staircase fashion through the adjacent muscularis and join larger collectors in the connective tissue surrounding the organ. There is very little anastomosis from side to side on the anterolateral surfaces, and the larger collectors from here pass laterally and downward to the uterovesical angle and the groove between the ureter and obliterated hypogastric artery. Occasional intercalated nodes are found in the connective tissue between the obliterated hypogastric artery, ureter, and bladder wall. The collectors then pass to the internal and middle chains of the external iliac chains, but with anastomoses to nodes along the course of the ureter and along the obliterated hypogastric artery to hypogastric nodes and to the obturator nodes. Over the superior surface anastomoses are more common from side to side. Some of the collectors pass directly to the middle and internal group of the external iliac chain of nodes, while the remainder pass down to run in the uterovesical angle and thence to nodes, as do the anterior channels. Between channels of the bladder neck, trigone, and base and the anterior vaginal wall and cervix there is free anastomosis. The collectors here drain into the external iliac chains and also follow the course of the ureter to hypogastric nodes and may go up to a common iliac node.

The autonomic innervation of the bladder consists of sympathetic fibers originating from the first and second lumbar segments of the spinal cord and parasympathetic fibers that arise from the second, third, and possibly fourth sacral segments. Efferent sympathetic fibers pass by way of the presacral nerve, dividing into the hypogastric nerves and passing through the hypogastric ganglia to reach the bladder near the sites of entrance of the ureters. Sympathetic fibers innervate the muscular layers of blood vessels, ureters, and the trigonal musculature with its extension into the crista urethralis. The parasympathetic fibers pass through the hypogastric plexuses and innervate the detrusor and urethra. Afferent fibers from stretch receptors in the bladder muscle run with the parasympathetic fibers to the sacral roots. Sensory fibers running with the sympathetic trunks and blood vessels innervate the mucosa; a few fibers ending in the mucosa join the parasympathetic nerves. The striated muscle about the urethra is innervated by branches of the pudendal nerves arising from the third and fourth sacral segments.

Surgical Principles in Operations for Stress Incontinence

The proper operation for the cure of stress incontinence must be selected for each patient. The surgery for correction of stress incontinence has been so replete with failures and partial failures that patients now have heard that "bladder operations don't turn out well."

The technique of an anterior colporrhaphy cannot be changed very much, but the method of plication of the bladder neck has been the object of so many techniques of placing the sutures as to be a source of confusion. Whether placed horizontally, vertically, singly or in layers, mattressed or otherwise, the results are about the same when appraised critically. The obvious answer is that a different surgical approach is needed. You cannot apply the same operation to a relatively young woman with minimal stress incontinence and also to a patient in the fifth or sixth decade, with one or more previous vaginal plastic operations, diabetes, and a history of insertion of radium for benign disease. Yet this is exactly what has been done in the past with the anticipated high percentage of failures or partial cures. This is a plea for more extensive primary surgery in selected patients.

Vaginal plastic surgery requires careful preoperative planning just as does plastic surgery in other locations. If this is not done, vaginal constrictions, painful scars, recurrent incontinence, and a persistence of the same symptoms of bearing down will persist. Certainly if one vaginal plastic operation has failed to cure the patient, this patient should now be given the benefit of all of the diagnostic and prognostic facilities at our disposal. We feel it is possible to select from the start those patients who constitute the majority of the operative failures. This being so, such patients should have a different operation as a primary procedure. Surgery should be definitive and conclusive. There is no place in modern gynecology for the attitude that "if this doesn't work, we can then try a sling operation or something else." The preoperative study of the patient can be, in most instances, conclusive as to the type of procedure that should be employed. The final decision can even be delayed until the vaginal plastic operation is done. If urethroscopy does not show an adequate reduction in caliber of the bladder neck and an increase in the effective length of the proximal urethra at the operating table, one should go further and do the abdominal stage.

Indications for Operation in the Various Stages

Relief of stress incontinence should be offered any patient who is able to tolerate surgery and who can be assured that the chances of failure are minimal. The indications for the type of operation to be performed are the important considerations. For clarity, these will be grouped under the stages of the condition advocated by the author.

Indications for Stage O Patients

A common example of potential incontinence is seen in the patient with procidentia who is continent because of urethral angulation at the urogenital diaphragm and incontinent after reposition with a pessary. Unless this is appreciated, a vaginal hysterectomy may repose the internal meatus and proximal urethra in suitable alignment for gross incontinence. The pubococcygeus is elongated and attenuated, and there may or may not be associated aggravating medical factors. A prophylactic plication should be done to prevent postoperative incontinence. In the presence of aggravating factors, such as severe asthma with procidentia, the outlook for good postoperative urinary control is discouraging. The wisdom of considering such a patient in the category of Stage II must be considered. After a Fothergill-Hunter procedure or even simple anterior colporrhaphy, the urethrovesical angles and relationships may be so disturbed as to create an incompetent bladder neck. After successful closure of a vesicovaginal fistula one may find the patient with severe stress incontinence. An incidental procedure to correct stress incontinence can often be done during these other procedures. Patients subjected to laparotomy for pelvic disease or other lower abdominal conditions with medical factors known to aggravate bladder control, but whose bladder necks have not as yet decompensated, may be spared surgery later by a simple prophylactic plication from the abdominal route. The anterior aspect of the bladder neck is identified in the space of Retzius and plicated, followed by a ventrofixation of the anterolateral walls of the bladder just above the neck to the rectus sheaths. This effectively tightens the bladder neck and adds only a few minutes to the operation during the closure of the abdomen and can be done through most of the common lower abdominal incisions. The suspension and plication are done before the peritoneum is closed and before the bowel and omentum, packed into the upper abdomen, is replaced in the pelvis. This permits excellent exposure of the space of Retzius especially in short, obese patients (see Steps of the Operation described under Abdominal Phase, page 193).

Indications for Stage I Patients

Characteristically there is minimal anterior wall relaxation with intact pubococcygeal function. The latter is inadequate, but in the absence of aggravating factors the frequency and degree of incontinence are not marked. If the bladder neck is visualized urethroscopically, the funneling is not marked and the action noted when the patient attempts to restrain urination is prompt and without distortion. A lateral urethrogram taken in a standing position will confirm the funneling and obliteration of the posterior urethrovesical angle. It will also show the abnormal mobility on straining. By exposures, with the patient attempting to hold her urine, the strength of the pubococcygeus can be studied, but these procedures are not necessary to use this classification. The operation indicated here is a partial vaginal vesico-urethrolysis and plication.

In this operation the mobilization of the urethra is extensive but does not include detachment from its normal relationship to the pelvic diaphragm. The usefulness of the pubococcygeus is to be preserved and aided in its function. A full-length plication of the urethra, bladder neck, and base is done, followed by additional plication with on-end mattress sutures at the bladder neck to restore the posterior vesicourethral angle (see Steps of the Operation described under Anterior and Posterior Repair, page 118, Plate 14, *E* to *M*).

Indications for Stage II Patients

The characteristic finding in Stage II patients is the presence of one or more aggravating medical factors. The physical findings are basically the same as in Stage I patients. The frequency and degree of incontinence are generally exaggerated by these medical conditions. During the levator test or urethroscopy, the patient is not infrequently able to demonstrate rather forceful levator action since she has been unconsciously exercising these muscles in a vain attempt to keep dry despite her anatomic derangement and aggravated stress. The urethrogram will confirm these findings and often shows greater abnormal mobility and loss of the normal urethrovesical contour. A combined operation is indicated to ensure permanent results. These patients constitute the bulk of the operative failures seen after a simple bladder neck plication. I cannot concur in the concept that a simple plication should be tried first and combined operations reserved for failures. Such thinking is not progressive gynecology when one operation may only set the stage for a second. Some of the individual reasons for a primary combined vaginal and abdominal operation will be discussed in detail later.

The suggested combined operation consists of a vaginal stage as suggested for Stage I patients and an abdominal stage of the type suggested as a prophylactic procedure during laparotomies. When these procedures are combined, a very effective reduction in the caliber of the bladder neck is achieved. The advantages of surgery from the space of Retzius will be readily apparent to the surgeon. The walls are thin and pliable, the intra-abdominal forces and pressure will not tend to disrupt the procedure or put strains on it in the future, and the area is free of scarring from parturition or other surgery. Having once approached the surgical correction of stress incontinence from the space of Retzius, one will become increasingly conscious of its potentialities in the cure of this and other gynecologic conditions.

Indications for Stage III Patients

Distinctive of Stage III patients is the forward fixation, distortion, and adhesions of the urethra and bladder neck so that the pubococcygeal function is abnormal and impotent in so far as helping to maintain a competent bladder neck. The usual patient has had previous surgery and represents an operative failure. Radium for benign disease with secondary contraction and fibrosis may be superimposed upon existing anatomic displacements to give the same picture. Occasionally a patient who has had a particularly traumatic delivery with paraurethral lacerations presents the same findings. On performing the levator test or urethroscopy, it is noted that the bladder neck is sluggish, almost fixed, and widely funneled and barely flickers when the patient attempts to hold urination. A lateral urethrogram shows the same forward fixation and immobility on exposures with the patient attempting to hold urination. The operation indicated is a complete lysis of the urethra, vaginally and abdominally, plication from both aspects, and a ventral cystopexy.

The procedure requires the disruption of the pelvic diaphragm to mobilize the urethra and bladder neck completely. Plication from both aspects decreases the caliber and increases the functional length of the urethra and bladder neck. The anterior plication is more extensive than necessary for Stage II patients. Several weeks postoperatively one can observe the unscarred portions of the iliococcygeus exert their influence on the bladder neck. The levator test shows action several centimeters posterior to the usual edge of the pubococcygeus. In addition, one notes that the direction of pull is more posterior and less back and up than before disruption of the portions of the pelvic diaphragm adjacent to the urethra and bladder neck. It is impressive, however, how this mechanism is now a functional one, substituting good muscle tissue for the scarred.

Stage III may include patients with a secondarily contracted bladder. There frequently has been long-standing incontinence and disease with a hypertonic detrusor. On urethroscopy, with the bladder distended, a contraction may occur which will force urine or saline solution about the instrument. Trabeculation is frequently observed, and cystometric studies indicate a low capacity. The condition of the tissues is evident at the time of operation. One gets the impression that the bladder wall, especially the bladder neck and proximal urethra, is thinner than usual. To meet the resistance of the hypertonic detrusor and added stress, the operation must, in effect, create a long and resistant channel. A full-length plication can be done abdominally and additional sutures placed at the bladder neck to create a long and resistant channel. A full-length plication can be done abdominally and additional sutures placed at the bladder neck to create an artificially long bladder neck and urethra. If it is felt that anything can be added by a vaginal stage, this is also done. In many patients with a secondarily contracted bladder one should not expect a perfect result, although enough control may be anticipated to make the situation tolerable.

COMPOSITE INCONTINENCE OPERATION
Steps of the Operation

1. Allis clamps are placed on either side of the urethra on the folds that indicate the remnants of the urogenital diaphragm. A third Allis clamp may be placed on the posterior lip of the external meatus, or this may be held by a smooth forceps as the incision is made. The anterior vaginal wall is opened retrograde from the urethra to the bladder base just beyond the bladder neck. The scarring of the vaginal wall usually present in the recurrent cases makes blunt dissection difficult so this is best done by knife and knife handle. Not infrequently the normal plane of cleavage between the bladder and vaginal wall was not entered during the previous surgery or disturbed by obstetric trauma, and if this cleavage plane can be located, the dissection proceeds with ease.

2. The alternate method is to start near the cervix, or the vaginal vault if the cervix has been removed, and dissect toward the urethra with a curved scissors. In any event the full thickness of the vaginal wall is separated from the bladder.

3. The index finger of the right hand is now introduced astride the urethra and close against the posterior surface of the descending ramus of the pubic bone (Plate 22, A). Scars, in addition to the remains of the origin of the puborectalis, will be felt, and the puborectalis will have defects in its anterior border, all of which contribute to the

distortion and fixation of the urethra. With a rolling motion toward the midline, the urethra is freed from all adhesions and the finger then enters the lateral recess of the space of Retzius. Some sharp dissection is needed for the more dense scars, and this is done by knife or scissors, whichever is easier. When the urethra is completely free on this side, the anterior part of the puborectalis and some fibers of the pubococcygeus will have been detached from their origins, and the extensions of the parietal connective tissue (endopelvic fascia, obturator fascia) toward the urethra and bladder neck will have been lysed. This step of the operation is much less traumatic than it would appear and is essential to the success of the operation, especially where the urethra and bladder neck are solidly bound down by connective and scar tissue.

4. Using the left index finger, the same maneuver is repeated on the left side. The scarring subsequent to parturition is likely to be greater on the left than on the right side. The exact reason for this in the mechanism of labor is not clear, but it has been reported by many observers. The mobilization, however, should be just as complete as on the right side.

5. In some patients fracture of the veins in the plexus of Santorini may give rise to considerable bleeding. It is not practical to attempt to control this type of bleeding by ligature from the vaginal aspect. Hot, wet, gauze sponges are packed into the lateral recesses to minimize blood loss, and they are removed from above (Plate 22, B). Usually these sponges will stop the bleeding by the time the second stage of the operation from above proceeds to the region of the space of Retzius. If not, the bleeding points can be readily seen from this aspect and clamped and ligated. The surgical nurse properly accounts for any sponges left in order to keep her sponge count correct.

6. A complete full-length plication of the urethra, bladder neck, and bladder base is performed (Plate 22, B). Additional on-end mattress sutures are placed in the bladder neck (Plate 22, B), and as in a simple anterior repair the full thickness of the vaginal wall is closed with interrupted sutures. It is seldom necessary or advisable to trim the anterior wall to a great extent. It is usually quite straight from previous surgery and one should attempt to restore some semblance of a normal urethrovesical angle. Also, if the wall is scarred and stretches between the descending rami of the pubic bone, there is scarcely enough vaginal wall to bridge the gap without any trimming.

186

7. Further surgery on the posterior vaginal wall, if indicated, is then done. A two-inch plain vaginal pack is placed in the vagina. With a free mobilization of the urethra such as has been done, the pack elevates the bladder neck, urethra, and bladder base up behind the symphysis and facilitates the second stage of the operation. A small caliber catheter, No. 12 or 14 Fr., is left in the bladder. A Foley catheter can also be used to identify the bladder neck as it is seen from the space of Retzius. However, the complete mobilization of the urethra outlines the anatomy so clearly that the use of bulb catheters is seldom necessary to recognize the anatomic landmarks of the bladder.

Modification of the Vaginal Stage to Perform a Partial Urethrolysis for Stage II Stress Incontinence

1. Stage II patients that have sufficient, useful, levator function to preserve have a partial urethrolysis in the first stage. Steps 1 and 2 of the operation are the same except that some operators may select the technique of opening the bladder from the cervix or vault forward rather than using the retrograde method. The mobilization of the urethra is almost as complete but does not entail detachment of the puborectalis or rupture of the extensions of the obturator (parietal, endopelvic) fascia and connective tissue extensions. The lysis of the urethra and bladder neck is carried up behind the symphysis to the point where the origin of the puborectalis division of the levator ani is palpated, and here the dissection stops. Since it has been ascertained that some useful function still exists, this muscle is left intact.

2. The remainder of the vaginal phase is continued as in a complete urethrolysis until the trimming of the full thickness of the vaginal wall is undertaken. Since many patients in this stage have had no previous anterior wall surgery, a more liberal correction of the cystocele is done. Again the posterior urethrovesical angle must be preserved.

Abdominal Stage of the Operation

1. A low Pfannenstiel incision is preferable unless a previous incision exists in the lower abdomen that requires excision for cosmetic reasons. The rectus muscles are separated in the midline from the symphysis to the dome of the bladder (Plate 22, C). The muscles are then retracted laterally to expose the dome and anterolateral surfaces of the bladder. The friable areolar tissue about the bladder contains some easily ruptured vessels that are ligated as encountered.

2. A self-retaining retractor or individual lateral retractors are used to hold the rectus muscles out of the field of operation. The right hand of the operator is used to detach the bladder from the back of the symphysis. The fragile areolar tissue in the space of Retzius, often described as the lateral and medial pubovesical ligaments, actually allows the organ to be mobilized by the weight of the hand. The index and middle fingers straddle the urethra in the dissection (Plate 22, D). The landmarks are now clear. Should it have been necessary to leave sponges in the space of Retzius during the vaginal phase of the operation, these are removed and accounted for by the surgical nurse.

3. The areolar thickening (medial pubovesical ligament) contains some small blood vessels, which is the reason for its slight condensation, and these vessels are clamped, cut, and tied. The landmarks deeper in the space of Retzius are now evident (Plate 22, E).

4. A tagged 4 by 4 gauze sponge is now packed in each lateral recess of the space of Retzius (Plate 22, F). This controls any annoying bleeding, which is minimal in any event since it is not necessary to disturb tissue in this region. The areolar sheath enclosing the bladder is now dissected off the upper half of the urethra, the bladder neck, and lower few centimeters of the anterolateral walls of the bladder (Plate 22, F). This is to expose the muscular wall of the bladder for the anterior plication of the bladder neck and subsequent cystopexy to the rectus tendons.

5. In Plate 22, F, is shown a vessel labeled the "pilot vein." This vein I have observed frequently running from the right to the left in an oblique downward course immediately at the bladder neck. A small artery is seen to accompany it. This pilot vein provides an excellent landmark for the anterior plication of the bladder neck.

6. Using the pilot vein as a guide, an on-end mattress suture is placed at the bladder neck (No. 1 as shown in Plate 22, G). A second suture is placed distal to this (No. 2) and another proximal (No. 3). The reduction in the caliber of the bladder neck is impressive when these sutures are tied. These sutures also restore the anterior urethrovesical angle. For the plication, 0 chromic catgut is used. Nonabsorbable suture material is not used, for the bladder mucosa is frequently penetrated and it might form the nidus of a bladder stone. If the bladder is filled with dilute methylene blue at this point, leakage about the

Text continued on p. 193.

Plate 22

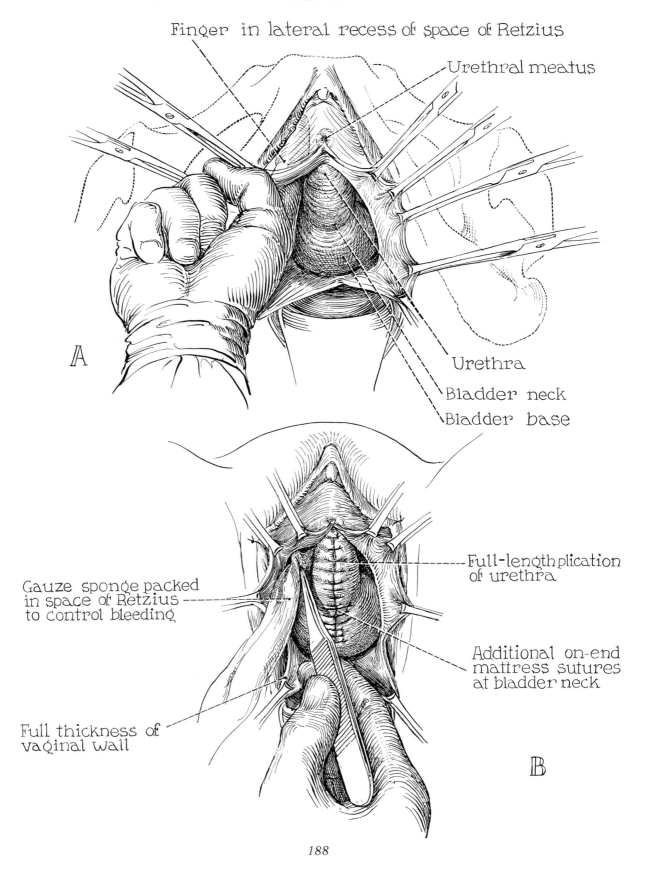

Finger in lateral recess of space of Retzius

Urethral meatus

Urethra

Bladder neck

Bladder base

A

Gauze sponge packed
in space of Retzius
to control bleeding

Full-length plication
of urethra

Additional on-end
mattress sutures
at bladder neck

Full thickness of
vaginal wall

B

Plate 22 (Continued)

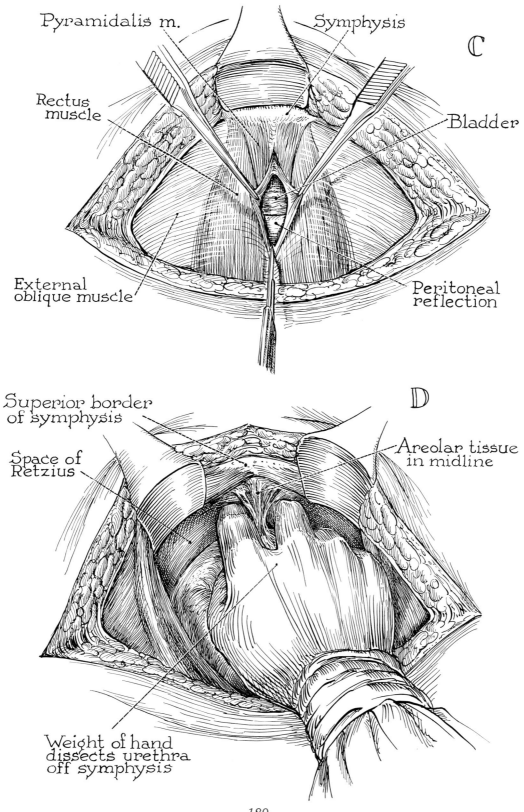

Pyramidalis m. — — — Symphysis

C

Rectus muscle

Bladder

External oblique muscle

Peritoneal reflection

D

Superior border of symphysis — — —

Areolar tissue in midline

Space of Retzius

Weight of hand dissects urethra off symphysis

Plate 22 (Continued)

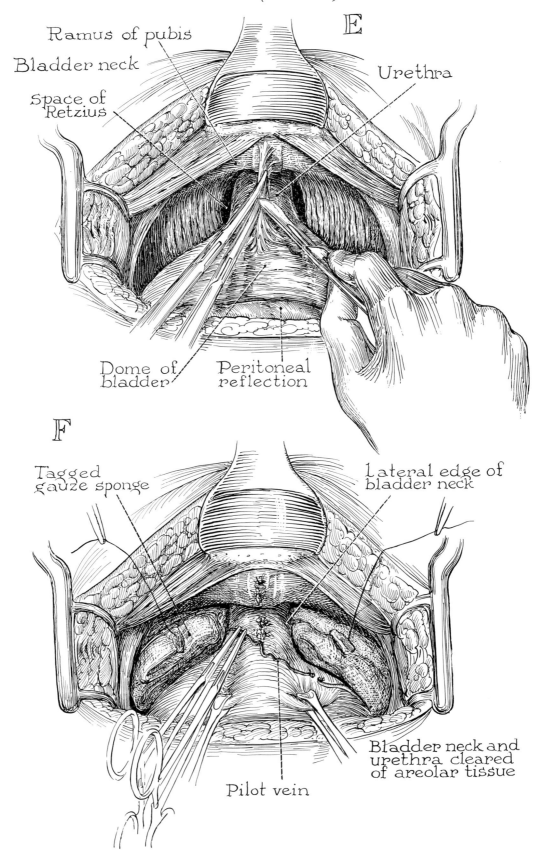

E

Ramus of pubis

Bladder neck

Space of
Retzius

Urethra

Dome of
bladder

Peritoneal
reflection

F

Tagged
gauze sponge

Lateral edge of
bladder neck

Bladder neck and
urethra cleared
of areolar tissue

Pilot vein

Plate 22 (Continued)

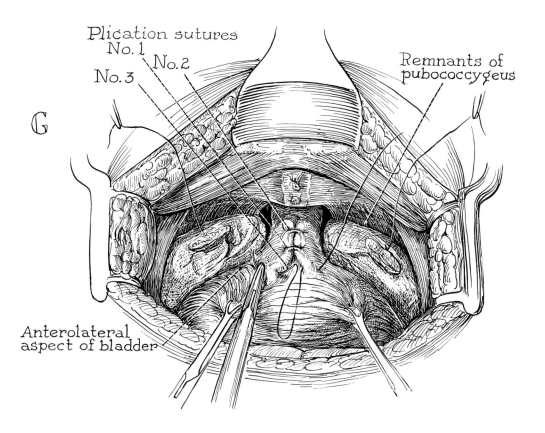

G

Plication sutures
No. 1
No. 2
No. 3

Remnants of
pubococcygeus

Anterolateral
aspect of bladder

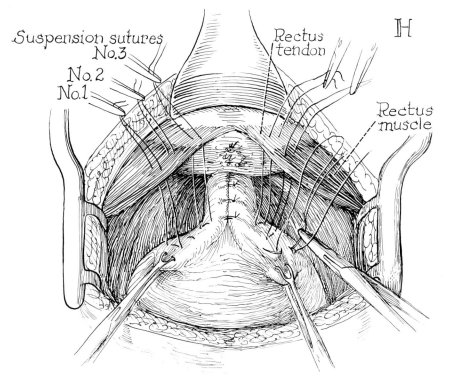

H

Suspension sutures
No. 3
No. 2
No. 1

Rectus
tendon

Rectus
muscle

Plate 22 (Concluded)

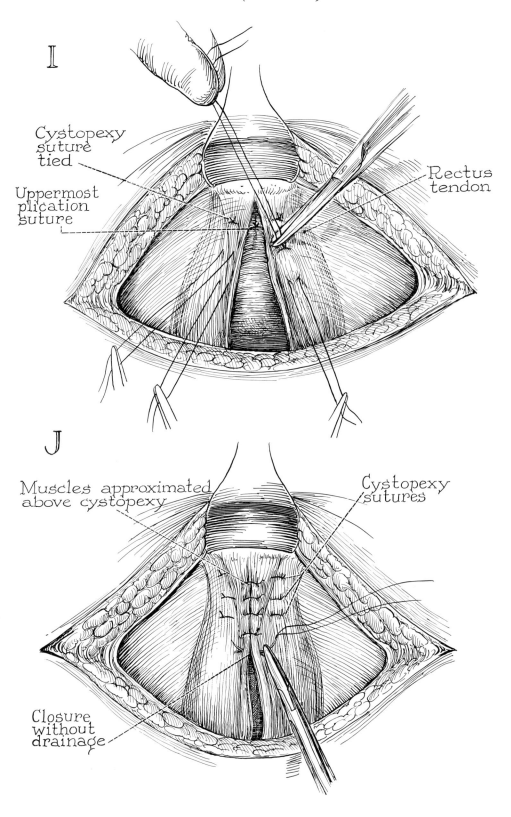

I

Cystopexy
suture
tied

Rectus
tendon

Uppermost
plication
suture

J

Muscles approximated
above cystopexy

Cystopexy
sutures

Closure
without
drainage

sutures is often seen despite the surgeon's care in placing the plication sutures. The penetration of the bladder mucosa by absorbable catgut sutures does no more harm than similar sutures used to close a cystostomy.

7. The anterior walls of the bladder, bladder neck, and urethra are thinner than the posterior walls. Further, they have not been scarred by parturition or by previous vaginal surgery. The use of this tissue to reduce the funneling of the bladder neck is logical and the surgeon will be impressed with the effectiveness of the plication from this aspect as contrasted with the vaginal route. When the bladder neck has first been mobilized from below, the ease of working in the space of Retzius is surprising. Babcock clamps can be placed above the bladder neck to bring the structures closer to the operator (Plate 22, *G*). It is seldom necessary to place a Foley bulb in the bladder or to distend it with colored fluid to do this operation, although some surgeons may find this convenient while demonstrating the procedure to colleagues. The self-retaining retractor, if used, is now removed to allow the cystopexy sutures to be placed. It can be loosened and moved cephalad with adequate exposure of the operative field.

8. Two or three paired suspension sutures are now placed in the anterolateral wall of the bladder, beginning proximal to the bladder neck. This is a change from the original technique in which the suspension sutures were placed more distal and also in the paraurethral tissues. In the evolution of the operation it was found that the suspension of the bladder was much less important than the plication in creating an effective anterior urethrovesical angle. Gradually the sutures were placed more and more proximal to the bladder neck with just as good results and a simplification of the technique. By angulating the mobile anterolateral walls of the bladder forward, an acute urethrovesical angle is formed (Plate 22, *H*). The sutures take two bites in the bladder wall for hemostasis, and the ends, untied, are passed up through the rectus tendon or muscle on the same side. The degree of mobility of the bladder and the configuration of the symphysis and rectus muscles govern the exact placing of the cystopexy or suspension sutures. This can be decided by placing a Badcock clamp at various points on the anterolateral wall of the bladder and drawing it toward the under surface of the rectus tendon and muscle of that side. Self-retaining or other retractors should be relaxed during this maneuver to simulate the normal position of the recti muscles. The sutures should be placed and adjusted to avoid tension or abnormal stretching of the

bladder. The bladder, distal to the sutures, becomes adherent to the posterior aspect of the symphysis and adjacent descending rami of the pubis in a position conducive to easy and effective closure of the bladder neck.

9. The tagged sponges in the lateral recesses, as well as the retractors, are now removed. The rectus muscles fall together in the midline. Rarely one encounters a general ooze in one or other of the recesses of the space of Retzius, and if it is not possible to locate the bleeding points specifically, a drain may have to be left. The cystopexy sutures are now tied in pairs, beginning at the symphysis (Plate 22, *I*). With the rectus muscles falling together in the midline, the bladder is easily drawn up without tension. The most distal sutures from the symphysis may have to be placed in the muscle itself, depending on the development of the tendinous insertion (Plate 22, *I*).

10. The rectus muscles from the symphysis, medial to the cystopexy sutures and up to the peritoneal reflection, are approximated with interrupted sutures of fine silk, and the fascia, subcutaneous tissue, and skin are closed in routine fashion (Plate 22, *J*).

Abdominal Phase of the Operation With Peritoneal Cavity Open

The principle difficulty in the abdominal phase of this operation is the exposure of the field of operation. Many of the patients are obese with a deep funnel pelvis. Without the peritoneal cavity open and the bowel packed into the upper abdomen, the sigmoid colon and loops of terminal ileum and the omentum fill the pelvis and indirectly crowd the upper reaches of the operative field.

When the peritoneal cavity is opened and the bowel and omentum systematically packed into the abdomen above the pelvic brim, the space of Retzius can be exposed with more than adequate room to operate. The dome and anterolateral walls of the bladder fall into the hollow of the sacrum when detached from the symphysis and pelvic sidewalls. The bladder neck and proximal urethra can be readily mobilized if there has been no other surgery in the space of Retzius. Traction on the dome of the bladder toward the sacrococcygeal junction makes all the landmarks stand out. This cannot be done without the peritoneum opened and the mobile contents of the pelvis displaced into the abdomen.

Two situations exist in which this approach to the space of Retzius is utilized. First, the abdominal phase of the operation may follow intra-abdominal surgery. The plication and suspension are then done before the packed-off bowel is replaced and the peritoneal cavity closed. Second, an extremely obese, short patient with a deep symphysis and funnel pelvis may make adequate exposure impossible. Here, it is worth the slightly added risk of opening the peritoneal cavity, packing off the bowel and omentum, to provide a well-exposed adequate field of operation.

Postoperative Care

If drains were placed in the space of Retzius, they are withdrawn about two inches the first postoperative day and a few inches farther the second day and are removed on the third day. The postoperative care otherwise follows that previously described under Anterior and Posterior Repair (page 120).

RECURRENT INCONTINENCE
THE FROZEN BLADDER SYNDROME AND SPECIAL SITUATIONS
Introduction

The normal bladder is a distensible, pliable organ that changes position with the degree of filling. Furthermore, the presence of a fetal head or breech, large fibroid tumors of the uterus, bilateral ovarian tumors, malignancies with general carcinomatosis of the abdomen, and many other purported insults to its proper functioning find the bladder adapting to its compromised position with remarkable agility. One marvels at the lack of symptoms from large masses encroaching on this organ. Bladder complaints, ascribed to pressure from such things as benign ovarian cysts and fibroid tumors of the uterus, seldom parallel the physical findings of tumor masses impinging on the bladder. The presence of extrinsic sources of pressure on the bladder should be noted, and then the urologically oriented gynecologist should start searching for the true cause.

Etiology

The iatrogenic causes of bladder discomfort often do not permit the organ to adjust to its changed position. The development of scar tissue hinders its mobility. The new alignment of the urethra with the bladder neck may make voluntary and involuntary musculature control impossible in so far as closure of the internal meatus and continence are involved. Further, suture of the urethra, bladder neck, and adjacent anterior wall of the bladder to the cartilage of the symphysis and the adjacent periosteum of the descending rami of the pubis permanently fixes the anterior wall of an organ that normally rides freely over these skeletal structures. Whether the fixation is from the urethra and bladder or, in modifications of the Marshall Marchetti procedure, from the adjacent vaginal wall, these operations attach a mobile organ to a fixed bony structure.

Reconstructive surgery, with due allowance for the situations in which this is impossible, should attempt to restore normal function. Operations for urinary incontinence that create scar tissue by slings, periosteal suspensions, use of foreign bodies, and other distortions are complicated and inconsistent with many simple principles compatible with the physiologic function of the female bladder. Why should not trauma from sutures, dug into the fibrocartilage of the symphysis and adjacent periosteum of the descending rami of the pubis, be just as painful as that caused by trauma to the periosteum and cartilage by fractures and severe contusions to bone in other parts of the body? The periosteal suspension may have been done with such enthusiasm that the sutures about the bladder neck may sharply angulate the terminal ureter. One case report deals with the accidental ligation of the intraumural ureter by a suture passing to the periosteum.

With such extensive dissections in the space of Retzius the amount of scar tissue is proportionately increased. The sutures are frequently passed with large caliber Mayo needles. In many patients the persistence of discomfort for many years is the price paid, whether the result is a successful or unsuccessful procedure. The ideal operation would restore the anatomy and physiology to normal. This is not possible. What is possible is this: Restore the anatomy without bizarre procedures that further hinder function and permit this organ, with a remarkable capacity for regeneration, to function again approaching its normal manner.

In summary, operations upon the bladder for benign conditions such as urinary incontinence should be done by a method that corrects the anatomic and physiologic defects without compromising its normal distensibility and mobility. Pain, urgency, precipitancy, and other symptoms that detract from the patient's evaluation of the success of the operation should not be created by the operative technique. Elemental principles of plastic surgery, such as restoring the structure or organ as nearly as possible to its anatomic and physiologic basic structure, avoiding bizarre innovations not compatible with the physiology of the organ, and not engaging in perchance operations with the attitude that if these do not succeed something else may be tried, should be the surgeon's objective. There should be sufficient study of the individual patient to pattern the operation to her particular anatomy and complicating factors so that a procedure is arrived upon that is adequate, or more than adequate, to give her urinary control.

Few, if any, sufferers from chronic illness face both the symptoms of their disease and social ostracism as does the patient with urinary or fecal incontinence. Colostomies are, for the most part, successful in diverting the fecal stream with reasonable control. Diversion of the urinary tract for benign disease carries hazards many patients will not risk, even in preference to their miserable existence. Most urinary diversions are done as last resort procedures in malignant disease or other obstructive uropathies that threaten the life of the patient. This leaves a large group of patients, both female and male, whose lives are not jeoparidzed by their chronic illness of the lower urinary tract but who live an intolerable existence not only for themselves but also for those about them who may have to limit their social life because of the incontinent parent or relative in the family circle.

It is to this group that much sincere but unrewarding research has been devoted by urologists, physiologists, and urologically-oriented gynecologists over the past few decades. Drugs to control the spastic, hypertonic bladder, local therapy with various chemicals to reduce irritation, and countless mechanical devices to keep the patient dry fail for the most part. Although there were earlier advocates of splanchnic nerve resection for the hypertonic bladder syndrome, regardless of etiology, the researches of A. M. Meirowsky by the abdominal route and those of A. Axel Ingelman-Sundberg in Sweden via the vaginal route have stimulated other workers to expand the scope of surgery with the advantages of improved anesthesia and blood replacement in an area unfamiliar to most surgeons.

Hypertonicity of the bladder with overflow incontinence, the "tormented bladder syndrome," is increasing as a gynecologic problem. This condition is never fatal to its long-suffering victims, occasionally it is so relentless in its persistent physical and social manifestations that patients will accept any chance of relief, but it has defied every approach to a definitive cure. Why is this so? A discussion of the etiologic factors, some iatrogenic, some the result of more aggressive cancer surgery, some just the result of survival into the later decades, will point up the problem.

Physiology of Micturition

Although the exact mechanisms for pain, urge to void, and the initiation and interruption of micturition in the female has not been determined, research in bladder physiology has demonstrated the following observations.

Efferent Pathways

Stimulation of the anterior roots of S3 and S4 stimulate the detrusor. In paraplegics damage to these sacral cord segments results in a hypotonic bladder with waves in the cystometer curve of low amplitude inadequate for complete voiding. A complete motor paralysis of the musculature of the pelvic floor accompanies the cord damage. Stimulation of the sympathetic (presacral and inferior hypogastric nerves) contracts the ureteral orifices, trigone, and vesical neck. Presacral neurectomy results in some relaxation of the bladder neck.

Stimulation of the pudendal nerves causes contraction of the striated cloacal muscles (ischiocavernosus, bulbocavernosus, and transverse perinei). Also stimulated are the muscles of the pelvic floor, the levator ani, and coccygeus. Contraction of the bladder neck can be observed cystoscopically when the peripheral stump of the pudendal nerve is stimulated, indicating that the insertion of striated muscle fibers of the puborectalis portion of the levator ani and their intermingling with the smooth muscle elements plays an important role in female urinary incontinence.

Afferent Pathways

The desire to void is mediated by parasympathetic fibers. This is demonstrated since presacral neurectomy and pudendal nerve section or anesthesia leaves this function intact. Not only is pain perceived as long as the sympathetic afferent pathways are intact, but it also travels in the parasympathetic afferent fibers, indicating that both are mixed nerves. The sympathetic pathways enter the cord at or above T9 so that cord injuries must be above this level to abolish all of the pain reflex arcs.

Pathologic Anatomy

Any extensive procedure performed on the bladder in the space of Retzius disrupts the flimsy areolar tissue between the bladder and the adjacent symphyseal fibrocartilage and posterior aspect of the descending rami of the pubic bone. If the operation requires further dissection along the anterolateral walls of the bladder, the areolar tissue between the bladder and obturator fascia is disturbed. While some slight condensations of this areolar tissue are evident, nothing is found to merit the textbook descriptions of anterior and paired lateral pubovesical ligaments. Postoperatively, scar tissue forms in the operative area, particularly along the course of drains and suture lines that is more dense than the original adventitia surrounding the bladder.

In failures of the periosteal suspension opera-

tions it is postulated that the bladder comes away from the symphysis. Some surgeons have even reoperated with the intention of resuspending the urethra and bladder neck because it had broken down. Nothing could be further from the actual findings. The bladder and urethra are still firmly attached and are dissected free only with the greatest difficulty. In fact, it is seldom possible to revise the procedure without entering the bladder unintentionally.

What actually happens when the Marshall-Marchetti operation and sling-type procedures fail is this: The anterior and anterolateral walls of the bladder remain adherent where they were sutured or became adherent during healing. The posterior wall of the bladder neck descends, causing a straightening of the posterior urethrovesical angle. At the same time the anterior and anterolateral walls of the bladder, scarred and functionless from the surgery, become stretched and attenuated. A segment of the bladder, normally attached to the surrounding structures by a tenuous connective tissue, is now an adherent, functionless part of an organ that should have the utmost pliability and distensibility. It is this adherent segment of the bladder that is responsible for the annoying side effects of an operative failure, such as suprapubic pressure or pain, urgency and precipitancy, and the low capacity, hypertonic bladder syndrome. Operation invariably confirms these findings. The degree of scarring, thinning of the bladder wall in the operative area, and the difficulty in revising the previous operation is directly related to the extent of the original surgery, postoperative infection, number and length of time drains were employed, hematomas in the space of Retzius, size and number of sutures used, and any factors contributing to poor wound healing. But the anterior wall of the bladder does not come away from the symphysis and adjacent structures; it is, in fact, abnormally adherent from the previous procedure.

There are other than iatrogenic causes of the frozen bladder syndrome. They are rare. Crushing injuries to the pelvis could cause the same limitations to bladder mobility as surgery in the space of Retzius. Radiation therapy could cause changes in the pliability of the bladder wall with a succession of symptoms such as these patients experience. A particularly traumatic delivery might be followed by infection that would immobilize the bladder. We are dealing with an iatrogenic disease.

SPECIAL HISTORY, PHYSICAL EXAMINATION, AND TEST FOR THE FROZEN BLADDER SYNDROME AND OTHER CONDITIONS WITH A HYPERTONIC BLADDER AND OVERFLOW INCONTINENCE

History

I. Postoperative failure or multiple failures
 A. Time relationship, the immediate recurrence
  1. Patients seen within three months of operation; wound infection of anterior vaginal wall, inadequate correction during surgery, creation of mechanical conditions for stress incontinence in formerly continent female, hematomas of operative site, poor choice of vaginal plastic operation selected, and inadequate preoperative study of entire problem involved in patient's urinary control provide immediate failures seen during convalescent period
 B. Time relationship, the late recurrence
  1. Patients seen several years after operation may report other factors contributing to recurrence; some may have been in childbearing period and permitted to deliver vaginally after successful operation for urinary stress incontinence, an inexcusable clinical judgment; age decreases the resiliency and distensibility of tissues about urethra while atrophy takes its toll of musculature of pelvic floor; patient may have become obese, developed chronic cough, diabetes, hay fever, bronchiectasis, or myriad of other aggravating accomplices that exaggerate urinary incontinence; frequently, combination of overflow incontinence and stress incontinence misdiagnosed at original surgery and hypertonic, secondarily contracted, low-capacity bladder was present and obviously could not be corrected by simple, standard operations employed
 C. Details of previous operations from patient, abstracts, examinations by other surgeons
  1. Febrile postoperative course suggestive of infected wound
  2. Postoperative sanguineous drainage suggestive of hematoma in anterior vaginal wall
  3. Wound breakdown or postoperative bleeding requiring resuture of operative area
  4. Wound healing as observed four to six weeks after operation with regard to delayed closure
  5. Prolonged suprapubic drainage after periosteal suspension
  6. Duration of suprapubic drainage and position of drains against periosteum associated with febrile course
  7. Suture material used or unusual complications of operation
II. Study to determine whether previous surgery was done in presence of interstitial cystitis or other primary cause of hypertonic, secondarily contracted, low-capacity bladder
 A. Details of suprapubic pain with particular regard to onset after surgery
 B. Hematuria, spontaneous or after bladder distention* as diagnostic test; records of previous tests
 C. Specific details of overflow incontinence and aggravating factors
III. Secondarily contracted bladder in geriatric patient
 A. Age and age at onset of symptoms of overflow incontinence
 B. Examination for evidence of atrophy of lower genital tract
IV. Special situations
 A. Late radiation bladder with secondary contracture
 B. Bladder neoplasms with bladder resection
 C. Bladder neoplasms treated with interstitial radium or other radioactive sources
 D. Ill-advised transurethral resections of female bladder neck for retention, so-called bar deformity, and other indications for this questionable procedure
 E. Over-zealous fulguration of bladder neck for chronic posterior urethritis and trigonitis
 V. After multiple attempts and eventually successful fistula closure and secondary contracture of the bladder

---

Bladder distention test for interstitial cystitis. Many observers have noted hematuria following over-distention of the bladder in the presence of interstitial cystitis. When this disease is suspected the bladder is distended until the patient experiences pain. This may vary from 100 ml. to 500 ml., depending on the severity of the disease and its effect on the pliability of the bladder wall. Although it is difficult to prove by actual biopsy of the bleeding areas when they are demonstrated, rupture of small vessels about the areas of muscular infiltration cause the hemorrhage. When fresh bleeding occurs without any other explanation, the test is valuable. The absence of hematuria does not exclude interstitial cystitis as the primary cause of the patients' complaints.

A. Fistulas associated with previous roentgen or radium therapy
B. Fistulas not associated with radiation reaction
VI. Bladder injuries
    A. Incontinence after bladder injuries with or without fracture of pubis or symphysis
    B. Straddle wounds to bladder base with or without traumatic fistula formation

Physical Examination

The findings on abdominal and vaginal examination of many of these operative failures become less shocking as one becomes more inured to seeing what can happen from either a minor error or an unavoidable complication of vaginal plastic surgery. Indeed, a virginal girl may start with the unthinkable, but unsinkable, operation of uterine suspension done to correct a normal variation of the usual position of the uterus. I have seen several who ended their surgical excursions with almost total urinary incontinence, and these were not surgical addicts.

The object now is to determine what you have to undo before it is possible to plan the revision. The studies outlined for simple urinary incontinence are done or already may be a matter of record, page 166. The revision of the patient's anatomy in the last resort surgical procedure, short of diversion of the urinary stream, should be undertaken only after a detailed study indicates a reasonable chance of success. The following observations will guide the surgeon in so far as the distortion of the normal anatomic features he may be expected to encounter. They may be appalling. Reintegration is seldom possible, but the restoration of near normal function may be possible.

1. The symphysis and adjacent pubic rami are palpated for areas of tenderness that may have resulted from a periosteitis.

2. The immediate suprapubic area and abdominal scar are palpated for pliability, particularly at the sites of drainage of the spaces of Retzius. This gives some information concerning the difficulties that may be encountered during the approach to the abdominal revision.

3. The outlet is observed for scarring and contracture, with specific attention paid to the amount of exposure the operator will have

during the vaginal urethrolysis and whether an episiotomy will be necessary.

4. Palpation of the periurethral areas with the patient instructed first to "hold" or attempt to restrain urination and then to "strain" as if to initiate urination suggests the degree of fixation of the urethra.

5. Any deviation of the urethra from the midline is noted since technical difficulties from scar tissue are more often noted on the side to which the urethra is retracted. This is usually the left side of the patient if the previous operator was right-handed. Presumably a deeper bite of tissue into or about the periosteum of the decending ramus of the pubis causes more reaction on this side among operative failures.

6. The usual tests of levator function by grasping the anterior edge of the levators between the thumb and index finger are done to determine what if any, function still exists. The trigone tests described in the work-up of the less complicated cases (page 174) are repeated.

7. The anterior vaginal wall is carefully palpated for specific areas of dense scar tissue with reference to reproduction of any pain the patient may have, particularly if she complains of "bladder spasms."

8. Lateral traction tests* are performed. Lysis of the urethra in the revision of operative failures is essential to success. Several areas of dense scar tissue are commonly encountered. First, the region of the urogenital diaphragm, at or near the junction of the middle and outer thirds of the urethra, is frequently badly

---

Lateral Traction Tests. Lateral traction tests are performed in the following manner. A No. 24 French sound, straight or curved, a No. 8 Hegar dilator, or the equivalent of these instruments is introduced into the urethra with the tip past the internal meatus. The index finger of the left hand then palpates the periurethral tissues on the patient's right side while the sound is used to retract the urethra to the patient's left. Bands of scar tissue and the general mobility of the urethra, bladder neck, and lower anterolateral wall of the bladder are studied. Reversing hands, the difficulties to be encountered are studied on the patient's left side. The patient is now placed in the knee-chest position, and the same maneuvers repeated. This is a more satisfactory method of observation. Retraction of the posterior wall of the vagina and the perineal body by the nurse assistant permits the tests to be done with maximum exposure, providing, at times, direct visualization of the densely scarred areas or specific firm bands of scar tissue. These may stand out sharply when firm traction is made to the opposite side.

scarred. Proximal to this and extending up behind the symphysis and posterior wall of the descending ramus of the pubis, dense bands of scar tissue may be encountered, part of which may be lysed vaginally with the remainder to be freed from the abdominal approach. Third, the anterolateral wall of the bladder and the bladder neck may be firmly adherent to the periosteum of the descending ramus of the pubis and the extensions of the obturator fascia over the obturator foramen. Some of the difficulties in store for the surgeon may be anticipated by lateral traction tests.

Special Tests for the Hypertonic Bladder Syndrome Complicating Stress Incontinence or Operative Failures After the Standard Operations for Urinary Incontinence

The history is frequently sufficient to establish the existence of overflow incontinence together with a simple mechanical stress incontinence. Both may have specific etiologies, both be iatrogenic, or one or the other causes be either specific or the result of previous surgery. Symptoms of pain, tenesmus, frequency, urgency, voiding in small amounts, and bladder spasms with overflow incontinence will establish the diagnosis before examination. Nevertheless, confirmation of the hypertonic bladder syndrome requires special tests. More important than diagnosis, which may be already obvious, is the prediction as to whether a combined superior hypogastric and pelvic splanchnic sympathectomy may afford relief and is a necessary adjunct to the operation or revision contemplated.

1. Parasympatheticolytic drug response tests are informative.* Drugs that block nerve impulses at postganglionic sites have been isolated principally for the management of peptic ulcer. Their direct effects on another smooth muscle, hollow viscus, the bladder, have been used in the management of the hypertonic, irritable, bladder. After the classic drug used for this purpose, atropine, many drugs having the same or even more potent anticholinergic action without severe side reactions have been discovered. Some of these are: methantheline bromide (Banthine); a more potent analogue by ten times, proantheline bromide (Probanthine); methscopolamine bromide (Pamine); oxyphencyclimine hydrochloride (Daricon); isopropamide iodide (Darbid); and diphemanil methylsulfate (Prantal). These and others in combination with other drugs are purported to soothe the bladder mucosa. Each new drug of this type comes under clinical study by researchers in this field, and none has provided a solution without a review of all the pharmacologic properties of each and clinical observations of patients treated with these drugs. Dosages reported to effect a reduction of gastric secretion and motility provide the bladder cripple with little or no relief. A controlled clinical study with the development of a more sensitive method of cystometrics would have to replace our clinical impressions before one drug could be designated as a superior agent. However, in this confused and difficult area of bladder physiology, any small tidbit of information is welcome. The response of the patient to drug therapy adds a little to the knowledge of the problem. Typical of the studies is the following quotation from an investigator's summary of one of the newer compounds.

"Intravenous Daricon in doses of 0.01 to 10 mg./kg. produced inconsistent degrees of blockade of the pelvic nerve-urinary bladder response, i.e., 15 to 43 per cent reduction in bladder contraction for 30 to 90 minutes. As with the nictitating membrane, the dogs were apparently refractory to successive and increased doses of the compound. However, in one dog that received a second dose of 10 mg./kg. 3 hours following the first, the blockade was reproduced. Atropine was similar to Daricon in that it never produced complete blockade (75 per cent) in doses up to 10 mg./kg.; but it did obviously evoke a greater degree of depression of bladder response to electrical stimuli. Pro-Banthine produced a 50 to 100 per cent blockade, with recovery in 30 to 60 minutes, following doses of 1 mg./kg."*

---

*Parasympatheticolytic Drug Response Tests. One or other of the anticholinergic drugs is given in doses sufficient to cause dryness of the mouth, gastric distention or feeling of epigastric fullness, blurring of vision, urinary hesitancy or retention, or constipation. The patient's bladder symptoms, particularly pain or suprapubic discomfort, are evaluated. Alternate periods of therapy and withdrawal are studied in a sort of personal double-blind study of a drug, but only one patient is involved. Patients who report symptomatic relief with these drugs are those most likely to benefit by a sympathectomy of the bladder in so far as this is possible without further knowledge of the bladder innervation both from sympathetic and parasympathetic nerves.

---

*Investigators Summary of Information, Pfizer Laboratories Medical Department, The Chas. Pfizer Company, New York, N. Y.

2. Cystometric studies of the bladder have been handicapped by the insufficiencies of the method, but even the most crude estimation of the bladder capacity and irritability provide some information and guidance. A tracing is made and compared with the normal capacity of the female bladder for retention, urgency to void, pain, leakage about the catheter, or other abnormalities. One learns that many iatrogenic symptoms may be created by surgery and, with a normal cystometric examination by our present methods, still have an irritable bladder. The instruments used vary from hospital to hospital and may be home-made or purchased from a surgical supply house. None give much useful information about the irritability of the female bladder, particularly those bladders previously attacked by many surgical procedures. Minor abnormalities in the tracing are often associated with incapacitating symptoms as far as the patient is concerned. Since the patient has to live with her bladder, the clinician must use his judgment as to whether his operation should be extended to interrupt the sensory supply of the bladder.

3. In the event of an abnormal cystogram or even minor changes in the tracing accompanied by complaints of pain or unusual discomfort, a "bladder block test"* is done to determine whether the tracing is modified by interruption of the nerve supply of the bladder in so far as this can be done by local infiltration. The operator is encouraged to proceed with a combined hypogastric and inferior splanchnic sympathectomy when the test shows a significant change. The patient's temporary

relief after the injection, if any, must be tempered by any suggestive therapy that is inherent in any test for which a patient must sign permission for an injection to block nerves. These patients have had, almost without exception, enough doctors and hospitals to make them rather astute if not hypercritical in evaluating results. Patients who have discomfort, suprapubic pressure, tenesmus, pain, and drawing sensations associated with urination or change of position and who have ordinary mechanical stress incontinence are not going to be happy about any surgery that relieves the stress incontinence without relief of the overflow incontinence and its usual symptoms as enumerated. To stop their shuttling back and forth between gynecologist and general urologist, one complete study to determine the part played by mechanical stress incontinence and that caused by a hypertonic bladder is done before embarking on any of the many surgical procedures devised for female urinary incontinence.

WEDGE RESECTION OF THE BLADDER IN REVISION OF FAILED RETROPUBIC OPERATIONS FOR STRESS INCONTINENCE
Introduction

A select group of patients may have recurrent incontinence without secondary contraction of the bladder and overflow. Their periosteal suspensions or sling operations may have failed, but they have a normal bladder capacity without hypertonicity. These patients require a revision of the previous operation with a correction of the iatrogenic source of their symptoms. It is not easy. Surgeons who have re-invaded the space of Retzius after the Marshall-Marchetti or other operations will testify as to the distortion of the bladder anatomy. Those patients whose previous operations did not result in a limitation of their bladder capacity are fortunate. A revision of their previous operation will usually relieve their incontinence.

The author has devised and utilized an operation for recurrent incontinence after peri-

---

*Bladder Block Test. Wheals of 1 per cent Novacaine, Xylocaine, or any suitable local anesthetic solution are raised in the anterior fourchette at seven and five o'clock in relation to and about 2 cm. from the external urinary meatus. A long spinal needle, No. 22 or smaller, is introduced into the paraurethral tissues posterolateral to the urethra. Local anesthetic solution (10 ml.) is then injected as the needle is guided by a finger in the vagina and underneath the ureter into the paravesical tissues of the bladder base. The needle is directed posterolaterally as it proceeds so as to remain retroperitoneal, and the final few milliliters of solution are aimed toward the iliac spine. This should block a substantial number of fibers of the pelvic plexus both near the bladder and some distance away. The injection is repeated on the opposite side. A finger or sponge stick is used to massage the solution into the tissues lateral to the bladder.

osteal suspensions and other retropubic operations of the sling-type that, in an adequate number of patients with a normal bladder capacity for clinical evaluation, has been successful enough to warrant inclusion in this text. This operation is designed to restore as nearly as possible the normal anatomic and physiologic function of the female bladder. Perhaps the need to devise new operations for the correction of the original procedure will stimulate thought as to the proper selection of the first operation.

Surgical Principles and Refinements in Technique

The previous operation or operations leave the surgeon dealing with an operative failure with the original complaint of incontinence in addition to any new symptoms subsequent to the surgery. Since the simplest procedure results in a certain amount of scarring and distortion, it follows that any subsequent operations should be adequate to cure the condition but be as uncomplicated as possible. A technique that recreates the normal anterior and posterior urethrovesical angles, that replaces the bladder neck at or near its normal topographic relationship with the symphysis, and that does not unnecessarily cause scar tissue or further limit the mobility and distensibility of this organ is the ideal operation.

Except to suggest another try at surgery, little study has been forthcoming for an answer to the total failure after periosteal suspensions and sling procedures. This method of revision of the failed operations is based upon the premise that complicated, bizarre, unanatomic, grotesque operations must be first undone. Then, an attempt is made to give the bladder a chance to resume something approximating its normal function. How is this done? First, the firm, often stony-hard adhesions of the urethra, bladder neck, and trigone to the descending rami of the pubis must be lysed vaginally. If a retropubic and intravaginal infection complicated the primary procedure, dense scar tissue will have fixed the normally mobile bladder to the surrounding bony structures. This must

first be revised before the scarred, functionless segment of the bladder in the space of Retzius is approached. Organs that have a great ability to regenerate do this from their normal components. The revision aims at the resection of all scar tissue so that the normal musculature, newly approximated, may expand and proliferate to form a bladder of normal capacity within the limitations of plastic surgery of this type.

The proximal third of the urethra and the adjacent anterior and anterolateral bladder walls are scarred, attenuated, and useless. This segment of the bladder must be excised, and pliable, normal, distensible bladder wall approximated. This can and will subsequently proliferate new musculature, for which the bladder has an unusual capacity, after the patient's incontinence is cured. The distribution of scar tissue will determine the mode of excision. Commonly, a diamond-shaped wedge, with the transverse diameter of the diamond at the bladder neck, lends itself to complete excision of the nonfunctioning bladder wall and proximal urethra. In the closure of such a wedge of tissue, this method of resection permits a narrowing of the bladder neck, which, with the subsequent plication of the bladder over this primary closure, creates an excellent anterior urethrovesical angle.

Often the degree of scarring and contraction does not permit a subsequent suspension of the anterior bladder wall to the rectus tendons, except that, as these sutures tend to accentuate the anterior urethrovesical angle, they have become less and less important in the management of recurrent incontinence. Should it appear that they might limit the expansion of the bladder by fixing the anterior wall where decreased capacity, secondary contraction, and overflow incontinence are part of the physical findings they are frequently omitted. This operation is designed to free the "frozen bladder." It does nothing that would further compromise its normal mobility. The latter characteristic of the bladder, after one failure, is never restored.

While the occasional patient will present

the symptom of stress incontinence without urgency, frequency, precipitancy, suprapubic pain or discomfort, initial or terminal tenesmus, or acute pain with what they describe as "bladder spasms," the majority will require more extensive study to determine whether the bladder should be partially denervated. However, the release of the scar tissue, both vaginally and in the space of Retzius, and the removal of the scarred nonfunctioning segment of proximal urethra and bladder are mandatory.

Preoperative Care and Anesthesia

Urinary incontinence does not threaten the patient's life. It does inflict upon her a social punishment that is often intolerable. The preoperative study, with its attention to every detail, does much to give her assurance. This support of the patient must be carried out to the moment of induction of anesthesia since her disillusionment with previous operative failures can only be counteracted by an honest appraisal of the chances of success. Since the immediate postoperative period is much the same as in any major surgery, all efforts on the part of the surgeon and the anesthetist who sees her before surgery may well determine the patient's determination to get well and cooperate in all the complexities of the postoperative management of these operations. A general anesthetic is usually employed. Spinal anesthesia could be used, but the length of the procedure would require a continuous type. Urinary antiseptics known to be tolerated from past history or sensitivity tests are given in the usual dosage forty-eight hours before surgery to ensure an adequate blood level at the time of operation.

Steps of the Operation
Vaginal Phase

1. Allis clamps are placed at the external urinary meatus and on each side at the fold of mucosa marking the posterior border of the remnants of the urogenital diaphragm. This dissection is essentially the same as that described for the combined incontinence operation described on page 186 and illustrated in Plate 22, A and B. Since these patients may have considerably more scar

tissue in the bladder base than those patients with operative failures not demonstrating a secondary contraction of the bladder, the mobilization of the bladder and the excision of nonfunctional scar tissue are more extensive.

2. An incision is made in the midline from the external meatus for a distance of 4 to 5 cm. This is through the full thickness of the vaginal wall. The operator will not find a natural line of cleavage in this section of the anterior vaginal wall. Scar tissue will be trimmed from the normal musculature of the urethra later in the operation. If plaques of scar tissue are removed at this time, a general ooze of blood may be expected that obscures the subsequent dissection.

3. By alternately incising the mucosa and retracting with clamps, the incision is extended to the vaginal vault or anterior fornix if cervix, uterus, or amputated cervix are still present.

4. Here the operator may have the good fortune to find a natural line of cleavage not entered during the previous operative procedures. This plane, or the best possible line of cleavage, is further developed until the medial edge of the descending ramus of the pubis is felt. At this time the dense scar tissue resected by sharp dissection will be replaced by adherent anterolateral bladder wall that usually can be lysed by blunt dissection. A complete urethrolysis into the space of Retzius is done on both sides, freeing the bladder neck, adjacent bladder base, and urethra from all adhesions created by the previous surgery.

5. Plaques of scar tissue may be seen adherent to the bladder wall and urethra. These are dissected off until normal musculature is encountered so that they are not incorporated into the line of sutures when the bladder is plicated. The surgeon should not be disturbed if the bladder is entered in this dissection. Densely scarred areas are a source of pain and bladder irritability. Since they must be removed and this should result in the bladder being entered, the edges are freed of scar tissue and pliable healthy bladder musculature and mucosa are reapproximated. A rent in the bladder is closed with a layer of 000 plain catgut, and interrupted sutures are placed through the full thickness of the bladder wall except the mucosa if this can be done technically. A second layer of interrupted sutures of 00 chromic catgut inverts the primary layer.

6. A full-length plication of the urethra is done with careful attention to the relationship of urethra and bladder so that overcorrection of the cystocele or advancement of the bladder base

prevents the establishment of a satisfactory, functional, posterior urethrovesical angle. The suture material used throughout is 00 chromic catgut.

7. On-end mattress sutures are placed at the bladder neck, to create a posterior urethrovesical angle approaching the normal relationship.

8. The full thickness of the bladder mucosa is rarely trimmed to any extent. Since there must be enough tissue to bridge the subpubic arch without retracting across and downward in the healing process, frequently no tissue is removed. Dense scar tissue in the midline is removed from the vaginal wall in order to approximate pliable tissues.

9. The mucosa is approximated with interrupted sutures of 00 chromic catgut.

10. A No. 18 French indwelling catheter is placed in the bladder, and a light pack is inserted in the vagina.

Retropubic Phase

1. The preferred incision for this operation is a high Pfannenstiel incision that permits delineation of the dome of the bladder to start the revision. Since many of the patients have had multiple surgical procedures, some through abdominal approaches, excision of the old scar can still be done with adequate exposure. Occasionally drains may have to be placed straddling the cystostomy tube. Whether the incision is in the midline or transverse, the short-lived drains are placed near the midline and removed as early as any sizable quantity of serosanguineous fluid drains, regardless of the direction of the skin incision. Although drainage is a part of the end of the procedure, its necessity is thought of during the planning of the original incision.

2. After the skin incision or excision of abdominal scar, the dissection is carried down to the rectus fascia and external oblique sheath and aponeurosis laterally. A midline or paramedian incision would not be carried so wide. Either an incision of the fascia in the midline or transverse incision of the fascia and external oblique aponeurosis is carried out, depending on the skin incision.

3. Seldom can the normal anatomy of the abdominal wall be recognized. But if the recti muscles can be identified in the midline, they are separated from the underlying transversalis fascia near the dome of the bladder, and the muscles are spread laterally by a self-retaining retractor. Each patient will differ, but, if the dissection is started high on the anterolateral wall of the bladder, some semblance of the normal

planes of dissection may be entered before the more distorted areas are encountered.

4. Plate 23, *A*, shows the artist's concept of one such dissection. The underlying bladder is densely adherent to the under surface of the recti muscles. Sharp dissection is necessary to free the dome of the bladder and anterolateral walls. Areas in which drains were left at prior operations may be extremely difficult. The recti muscles may be attenuated and hardly recognizable in some patients. Alternate use of Metzenbaum scissors and knife, and patience, eventually permits the surgeon to discern some of the normal landmarks.

5. Frequently it will be apparent that the previous suspension has caused such firm adhesions to bone and obturator fascia that multiple rents are inevitable. Then, it is best to perform a cystotomy so that the bladder wall can be observed both from within and without during the dissection and in this way avoid unnecessary tears into adjacent normal bladder musculature. If the dissection proceeds with reasonable ease, and there is seldom an easy dissection, the cystotomy is done later in the operation (Plate 23, *C*).

6. As the vicinity of the lateral recesses of the space of Retzius, that formerly contained the plexuses of Santorini, are reached, many new vessels in the scar tissue and adhesions that must be lysed will cause annoying bleeding. Where specific bleeding points cannot be tied off, it is best to control the general oozing with hot packs in one area while diverting the dissection to another portion of the bladder (Plate 23, *B*).

7. The areas on the posterior border of the symphysis where the periosteal suspension sutures were placed at the previous surgery may be particularly difficult to lyse. The scarred urethra is detached from the symphysis until the inferior border of the interpubic fibrocartilage can be palpated. Although the distal one-half of the urethra is not resected as part of the anterior wedge resection, it must be lysed to permit the surgeon sufficient mobility and room between symphysis and urethra to close without tension the proximal one-third of the anterior wall of the urethra that will subsequently be resected (Plate 23, *B*).

8. The completely lysed anterior and anterolateral walls of the bladder are now surveyed to determine the extent of nonfunctional, scarred bladder wall that must be removed (Plate 23, *C*). Generally the removal of a diamond-shaped wedge of tissue with the transverse diameter of the diamond at the bladder neck will eliminate the scar tissue and narrow the bladder neck during the closure.

Text continued on p. 208.

Plate 23

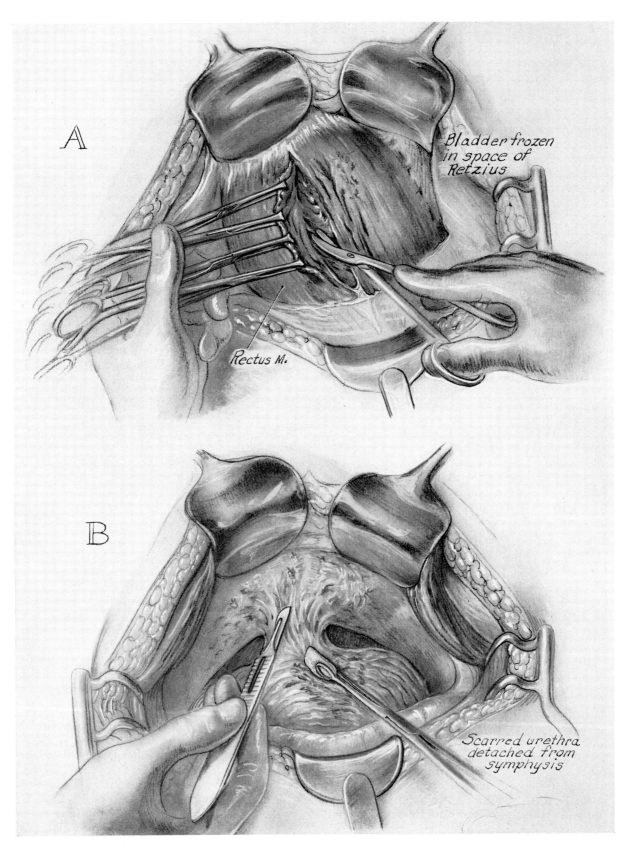

A — Bladder frozen in space of Retzius

Rectus M.

B — Scarred urethra detached from symphysis

Plate 23 (Continued)

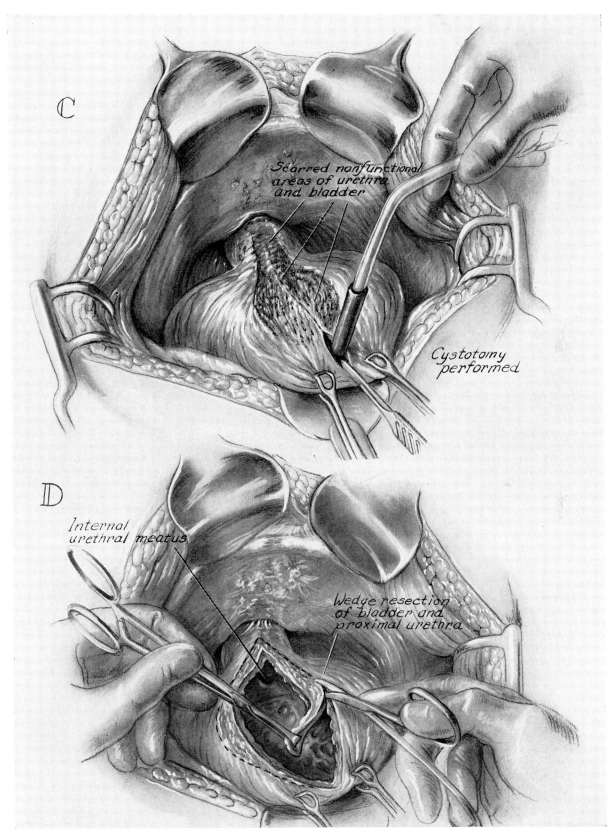

Plate 23 (Continued)

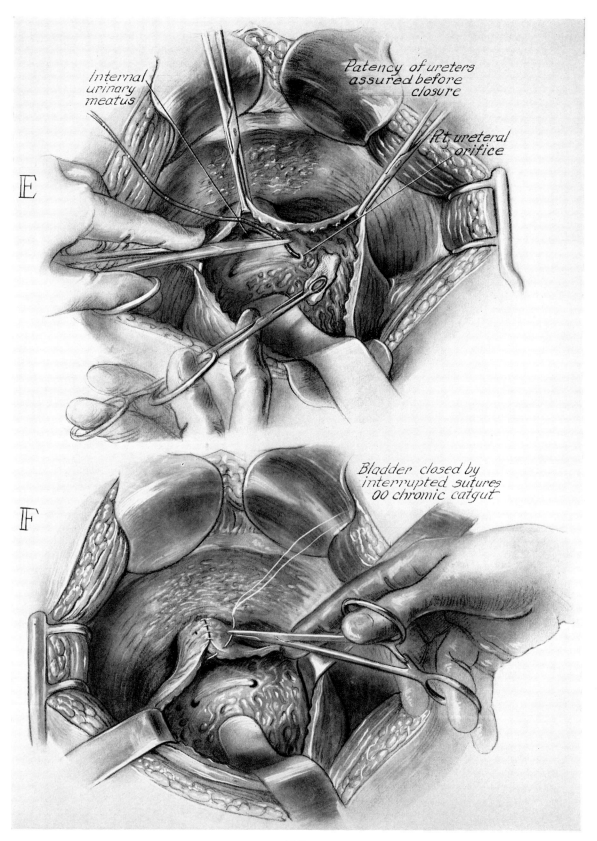

Plate 23 (Concluded)

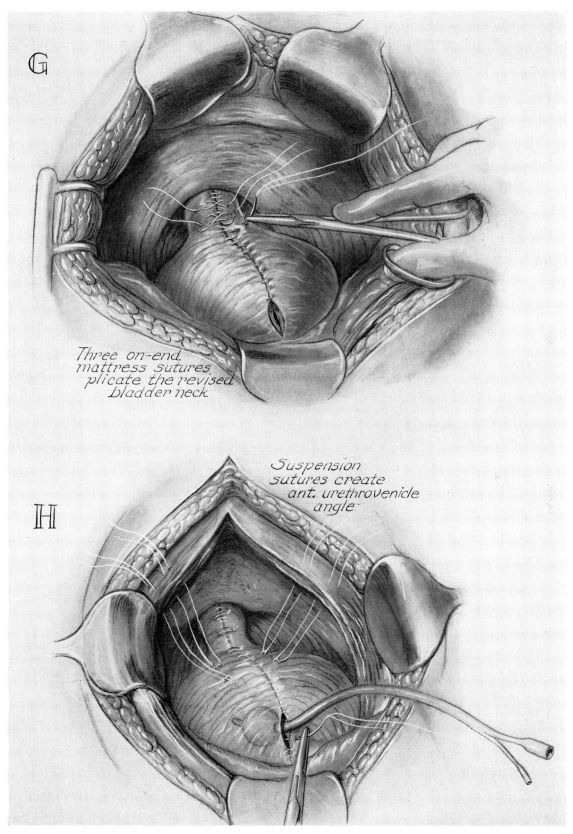

G

*Three on-end
mattress sutures
plicate the revised
bladder neck*

H

*Suspension
sutures create
ant. urethrovenicle
angle*

9. A cystotomy is now performed unless is was done earlier in the operation to aid in the dissection (Plate 23, C). This is extended distally to open up the bladder, bladder neck, and proximal third of the urethra in the midline. The interior of the bladder can now be surveyed to determine the extent of scarring and the areas that must be removed to permit the approximation of functional bladder musculature in the closure.

10. Metzenbaum scissors are used to resect the wedge of tissue and trim the edges until pliable bladder musculature is recognized (Plate 23, D). This may require a wider resection of scar tissue on one side than on the other. This is unimportant in so far as distortion is concerned since the primary objective is the approximation of healthy bladder musculature (Plate 23, D).

11. The revision of the previous operation may require lysis of scar tissue far laterally in the spaces of Retzius, both from below and from the abdominal approach. Since the ureters may have been distorted during the previous operations, their courses and continuity are determined before closure of the cystotomy. Ureteral catheters are passed up both ureters under direct vision (Plate 23, E). They are also observed for a clear efflux of urine. Should they be compromised, this is the time to correct any distortion, angulation, or constriction. The field of operation is well exposed, and the sutures or ties causing the obstruction to the passage of the catheter are released. In practice this is seldom observed in any of the operations performed in the space of Retzius, but the possibility of such a complication must be eliminated.

12. The bladder wall is then closed with interrupted sutures of 00 chromic catgut on fine Ferguson needles. The sutures should pass through the full thickness of the musculature and into the submucosa. Rarely will all sutures avoid penetrating the mucosa, but this does not cause any complications, and some urologists use a through-and-through type of closure with good approximation and healing. However, since we wish to avoid scar tissue in the suture line, continuous sutures are avoided, and the minimum amount of catgut is left in the bladder wall (Plate 23, F).

13. An on-end mattress suture of 00 chromic catgut is then placed at the new bladder neck, inverting the primary layer of closure. Similar sutures are placed about 2 cm. distal and proximal to the bladder neck to complete the plication. This should recreate an anterior urethrovesical angle, although more sutures may be necessary in some cases. This plication must be individualized by the surgeon (Plate 23, G).

14. A cystopexy is done by a few sutures well up on the bladder wall. This may be omitted entirely if it would appear that the suspension will limit the mobility of the bladder. The purpose of the sutures is to exaggerate the anterior urethrovesical angle and obliterate dead space. If the suspension does not add this relatively unimportant step to the operation because of some peculiarities of the individual patient such as a high symphysis with much scarring and contraction of the bladder, it is omitted (Plate 23, H).

15. Where suspension will contribute to restoring the anterior angle, one or two 0 chromic sutures are passed into the bladder wall in figure-of-eight fashion for hemostasis and brought out through the rectus tendons. The first pair of sutures are placed about 3 cm. above and 2 cm. lateral to the proximal plication suture. The second suspension sutures are placed about 2 cm. above the first and more lateral, depending on the configuration of the anterolateral bladder wall. They are brought out through the rectus tendons on each side at a level where they can be tied without tension (Plate 23, H).

16. Transurethral drainage is preferred to a suprapubic cystostomy in order to eliminate another source of postoperative scarring. Drains are placed only if absolutely necessary for the same reason. If drainage cannot be avoided, the drains are placed in each lateral recess and brought out near the midline a few centimeters from the symphysis. They are brought out through whatever incision has been used and not through stab wounds. In the event drains are used, a suprapubic cystostomy can be utilized for drainage (Plate 23, H).

17. The closure of the abdominal incision must be modified, depending on the findings at operation. If the medial edges of the recti muscles have been largely replaced by scar tissue and atrophic muscle fibers, it is best not to approximate this layer since it might limit the postoperative expansion of the bladder by forming a layer of firm, nonpliable connective tissue deep to the external oblique and rectus fascia which must of necessity be approximated. If the recti have escaped and are normal, a few sutures can be used to bring them together in the midline.

18. The fascia is closed with interrupted medium silk sutures. Drains and cystostomy tubes are anchored to the skin rather than the fascia. The skin is closed with interrupted fine silk sutures.

Postoperative Care

Urinary antiseptics are continued in the infusion during the operation and ordered parenterally and orally during the first few days after surgery. I dislike not being specific about the agents used, dosage, and route of administration, but the profusion of drugs and individualization of urinary tract therapy defy outlining a standard regime. Fluid and electrolyte replacement is seldom a problem but is carried out as outlined in Chapter 30.

If drains were used, these are advanced about 6 cm. the first postoperative day and removed the second day unless the drainage of serum is unusually profuse, when they are left longer. The sooner drains can be removed from contact with bone exposed in this operation the less they are likely to be a cause of morbidity. If a cystostomy tube was left as the means of bladder drainage, this is irrigated daily with warm saline to ensure prompt drainage of urine. An indwelling catheter is left five days. A cystostomy tube is removed in eight days.

An intake and output chart is kept by the nurse or patient. An order for catheterization every four hours as necessary is left, and residual urine is noted at least once daily. Difficulty in initiating urination is not uncommon. The measures outlined in Chapter 9 may be tried. Frequency of urination for several weeks after operation reflects the preoperative lack of normal bladder capacity. If the patient has frequent voidings of small quantity, she is instructed to practice spacing urination further and further apart. To do this she must voluntarily restrain herself from voiding until further waiting would result in precipitancy of urine. Several weeks may be necessary to re-train the bladder and attain a capacity approaching normal.

Combined Superior Hypogastric and Pelvic Splanchnic Sympathectomy
Surgical Anatomy

The presacral plexus (prelumbar, superior hypogastric) has several variations (see also page 359). Whatever its formation the plexus divides below the level of the sacral promontory that forms the base of the interiliac trian-gle (the triangle formed by the sacral promontory at its base, the common iliac arteries as the sides, and the bifurcation of the aorta as the apex). As I have pointed out before, the designation of this plexus as being presacral in location is erroneous and a source of error and confusion in teaching pelvic surgery. Although the bulk of the fibers are the result of the joining of the paired aortic plexuses, some communications join the plexus from the lower part of the lumbar chain, and these must come from behind and between the common iliac vessels rather than lie over them. Retraction of the ureters and complete mobilization of the plexus between the right common iliac artery and left common iliac vein will usually cut these twigs and result in a complete neurectomy (Plate 24, A and B).

Since this plexus is resected in the course of operations for the relief of overflow incontinence accompanied by pain, its variations become significant. The most common type is an obvious plexus of nerves that have to be gathered together from the edges and under the common iliac artery on the right and the left common iliac vein. This is found in about three out of four dissections. The next common formation is a single nerve as found by anatomists who have studied this plexus. It can also be represented by parallel strands or form an arch-shaped plexus just at the promontory, the dome of which is directed cephalad. My own experience at the operating table has been bizarre since I have had to dissect the plexus from the anterior surface of a pelvic kidney on two occasions. An obvious plexus is the usual finding. A thorough dissection is done only if the terminal branches of the inferior mesenteric artery (superior hemorrhoidal or this plus the lowermost sigmoidal artery) are mobilized on the left side. The plexus frequently lies more to the left of the midline. These vessels to the sigmoid and more particularly the terminal sigmoidal branch have been regarded as essential to the blood supply of the sigmoid colon and this area of the sigmoid mesocolon called the critical angle. With recent advances in pelvic surgery and many radical operations

Plate 24

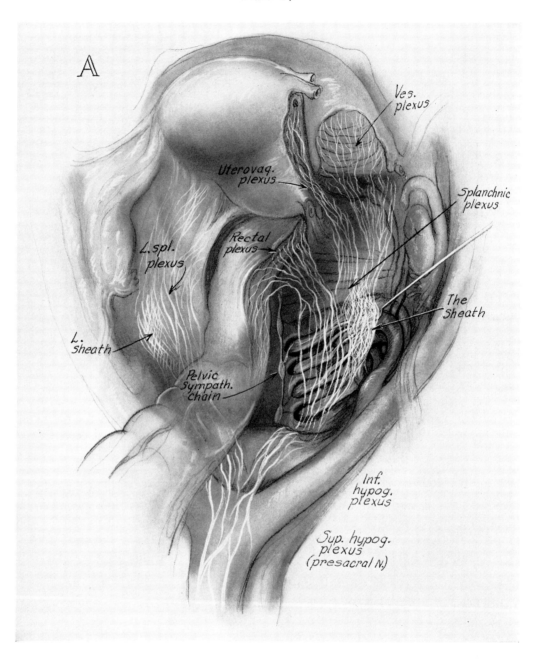

A

Ves.
plexus

Uterovag.
plexus

Splanchnic
plexus

Rectal
plexus

L. spl.
plexus

The
Sheath

L.
sheath

Pelvic
Sympath.
chain

Inf.
hypog.
plexus

Sup. hypog.
plexus
(presacral N.)

Plate 24 (Concluded)

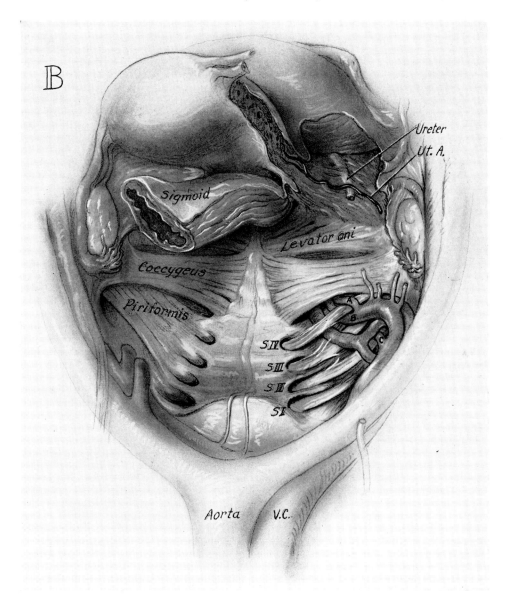

in the fields of abdominal, gynecologic, and urologic surgery, the sigmoid colon has been found to survive the interruption of its terminal sigmoidal artery, and the rectum has been found to do without its superior hemorrhoidal artery. Thus, if these vessels must be ligated because of some variation in the prelumbar plexus, the bowel can be observed for ischemia, and, if this should happen, resection can be carried out. However, it is quite improbable that this would ever be necessary. After the lowermost sigmoidal artery and superior hemorrhoidal artery are lifted up and displaced laterally, the medial edge of the left common iliac vein is encountered before the left common iliac artery. When pain and suprapubic pressure are the chief complaints of these bladder cripples, it is imperative that any afferent pain fibers be interrupted. The variations of the plexus must be recognized at the operation, and the dissection done to interrupt the maximum number of fibers.

The middle sacral artery and vein lie behind the plexus. These must frequently be ligated for a thorough dissection. They may originate or drain into the bifurcation of the abdominal aorta or the inferior vena cava. They may originate or drain into the left common iliac artery and vein. Whatever the formation, they must frequently be ligated to complete the dissection.

The inferior hypogastric plexuses are the paired divisions of the presacral (prelumbar, superior hypogastric) nerves. When these nerves are joined by sacral parasympathetic components from S3 and S4, they are designated as the pelvic plexuses. The paired inferior hypogastric plexuses pass downward and laterally on the pelvic wall, firmly embedded in the connective tissue of the pelvis. At the level of the fifth sacral vertebra the pelvic splanchnic nerves (parasympathetic fibers) join in forming the pelvic plexuses. The picture is further complicated by the fact that some branches from the pelvic sympathetic chain also join the plexus. In the male the pelvic splanchnic nerves from S3 and S4 are called the nervi erigentes. In the female they are called the

pelvic splanchnic nerves or just pelvic nerves (Plate 24, *A* and *B*).

The splanchnic nerves arise from the anterior primary rami just after they have emerged from the anterior sacral foramina. In dissections at the operating table twitching of legs is sometimes seen when the motor fibers of the lumbosacral plexus are accidentally stimulated. The fibers from S3 are invariably larger than the contributions from S4. If any fibers arise from S2 or S5, they are relatively small.

The pelvic splanchnic nerves contain both efferent and afferent fibers. Observations after section of these nerves indicate that they are a more important pathway for the conduction of pain from the pelvic viscera than afferent fibers (sympathetic) carried in the inferior hypogastric plexus. Thus in a small, contracted bladder, subject to painful spasms, the resection of both the parasympathetic and sympathetic afferent fibers is necessary to provide relief.

The sacral sympathetic chains typically present three or four more ganglia on each side. They enter the pelvis behind or deep to the common iliac vessels and extend downward on the front of the sacrum gradually converging toward and frequently fusing together over the coccyx to form the ganglion impar. In contrast to the thoracic and lumbar chains, the sacral chains are connected to the spinal nerves by gray rami communicantes (postganglionic fibers) only. The lowest limit of origin of preganglionic fibers (white rami communicans) is the second or possibly the third lumbar nerve. They supply some slender fibers to the pelvic plexuses, the functional importance of which is not known but could be a pathway by which sympathetic fibers reach the pelvic organs without transversing the superior hypogastric plexus. Their fibers go to the limbs, but their resection is unnecessary for denervation of the extremities since all the functional or preganglionic denervation is obtained by lumbar sympathectomy.

The pelvic splanchnic nerves course downward and laterally ventral to the piriformis muscle and hypogastric vessels and join the inferior hypogastric plexus to form the pelvic plexus on each side. When the pelvic plexus is retracted medially, these nerves can frequently be seen in their short course. If the largest contribution comes from S3, as is the usual finding, these nerves will pass between the inferior gluteal artery and vein and the lateral sacral artery and vein. Some observers report that some pelvic splanchnic fibers pass directly to the bladder without joining the pelvic plexuses so that total denervation of the bladder would necessitate a most thorough dissection fraught with technical difficulties (Plate 24, *A* and *B*).

Several muscles and bony landmarks are in the immediate operative field. The piriformis muscle originates on the pelvic surface of the second, third, and fourth sacral vertebrae just lateral to the anterior sacral foramina. The sacral portion of the lumbosacral plexus lies on its surface as well as the gluteal arteries and veins. The coccygeus is a small muscle forming the most posterior portion of the pelvic floor. It arises from the ischial spine and inserts on the lateral borders of the lower two sacral vertebrae and upper two coccygeal vertebrae. It is a fan-shaped muscle diverging to its point of insertion. Between the piriformis and coccygeus, the major branches of the sacral plexus leave the pelvis, passing through the greater sciatic notch. The internal pudendal artery and vein and the inferior gluteal artery and vein pass down the anterior surface of the sacral plexus to exit through the lower part of the greater sciatic foramen. The internal pudendal artery is the smaller of the two and is typically situated anterior or lateral to the inferior gluteal. The internal pudendal artery curves forward around the sacrospinous ligament, while the inferior gluteal artery passes through the branches of the sacral plexus to enter the gluteus maximus muscle. Control of bleeding from these vessels, should they be severed and subsequently retract behind the sacral plexus and between the piriformis and coccygeus muscles, is exceedingly difficult.

Besides the hazards of bleeding from the hypogastric artery and vein with its variable distribution, the operator must preserve the lumbosacral plexus which lies directly underneath and upon the piriformis and coccygeus muscles. During the operation, irritation of some of the motor nerves of the lumbosacral plexus are noticed as muscle groups in the leg contract. A review of the common formation of the plexus will clarify some refinements in technique in the operation.

The lumbosacral trunk, composed of a portion of the anterior primary ramus of the fourth lumbar nerve and all of the primary ramus of the fifth lumbar nerve descends into the pelvis usually as a single trunk but occasionally as two closely parallel trunks. This trunk emerges from the inferomedial surface of the psoas major muscle and lies deep in the angle between the muscle edge and the sacral promontory. In one common formation of the plexus, the lumbosacral trunk is then joined by the anterior primary divisions of the first three sacral nerves to form the sciatic nerve, together with smaller branches to various muscles. The components of the lumbosacral plexus are directed laterally and somewhat downward on the anterior surface of the piriformis muscle, after giving off the superior gluteal nerve which passes out of the pelvis above the upper edge of the piriformis and through the lowest part of the greater sciatic foramen. These branches are: the sciatic, inferior gluteal, posterior femoral cutaneous, and pudendal, together with small muscular branches to the gemelli, obturator internus, and quadratus femoris. The pudendal nerve or plexus is the most medial as it leaves the pelvis.

Those branches of the hypogastric artery and veins that exit from the pelvis must pass through the lumbosacral plexus of nerves. Variations exist, but commonly the superior gluteal artery passes between the lumbosacral trunk and first sacral nerve. The inferior gluteal artery and vein or veins leave the pelvis below the piriformis muscle and on the upper edge of the coccygeus muscle. It may emerge in the buttock between the sciatic and pudendal nerves or may pass through the origin of the sciatic nerve. The internal pudendal artery lies medial to the sacral plexus, passing between the third sacral nerve and its branches. It also passes through the greater sciatic foramen but is more anteriorly placed and passes over the sacrospinous ligament close to the ischial spine and enters Alcock's (pudendal) canal in its course through the ischiorectal fossa. Should any of these vessels be injured during the operation, blind clamping should be avoided or nerves of the sacral plexus may be crushed. For the same reasons the excision of a retroperitoneal tumor in this area may present insurmountable technical difficulties.

With the preceding landmarks as a background, further description of the position and gross appearance of the pelvic plexus is possible. After the inferior hypogastric plexus is dissected off the pelvic wall below the level of the third sacral foramina and drawn medially, a closely meshed, almost solid sheet of fibers can be gently elevated off the inferior gluteal and pudendal vessels as they exit from the pelvis. The cephalic or superior edge of this is usually at the level of the superior edge of the greater sciatic notch and slightly caudad (inferior) to the second sacral foramina. This will be seen to be about 2.5 cm. in height and 3 to 5 cm. in length and appear more like a fascial sheath than connective tissue containing many nerve bundles. The pelvic splanchnic nerves join the lateral or deep surface (Plate 24, *A* and *B*).

Slightly firmer traction on the inferior hypogastric plexus medially and toward the symphysis pubis puts the splanchnic nerves and sheath of parasympathetic fibers on the stretch to further expose the vessels behind and somewhat laterally. The pudendal nerve, occasionally referred to as a plexus, is lateral to the pelvic splanchnic nerves and somewhat lateral to the pudendal vessels since the pudendal nerve like the splanchnic nerves is derived from the anterior divisions of S2, S3, and S4.

The subsidiary plexuses to rectum, uterus, and bladder emerge from the pelvic plexuses on their medial, their anterior, and finally the lower borders. The rectal (hemorrhoidal) plexus is seen as a series of nerves arising from the posteroinferior border of the pelvic plexus. It passes downward on the anterolateral aspect of the rectum together with the middle hemorrhoidal artery to terminate in the rectal wall. The uterovaginal plexus courses forward and anteriorly on the anterolateral wall of the rectum and then turns medially with the uterosacral thickenings (ligaments) and finally with the uterine vessels to enter the uterus near the internal os and with some fibers continuing into the vaginal wall. The remainder of the pelvic plexus becomes the vesical plexus and passes under the cardinal thickenings (ligaments) and then anteriorly with the true lateral ligaments of the bladder to mingle with the connective tissue of the inferior vesical artery and the ureter to a final distribution in the bladder wall, trigone, vesical neck, and urethra.

Surgically, the interruption of the sympathetic nerve supply to the bladder should be best done by section of the pelvic splanchnic plexus immediately after its formation. Because of the variations in the anatomy of the plexus, the operation must be extended further to interrupt nerve fibers in the vesical plexus itself. This permits a more complete denervation of an organ that anatomically almost defies complete interruption of its nerve supply. The ureter is dissected out as it approaches its intramural segment in the same manner as one does with an extended radical hysterectomy. Since the patient does not have cancer and since she usually will not have had extensive radiotherapy, or a combination of both when dealing with malignant disease, the problem of fistula formation does not present a contraindication to the technique of this operation that I have described.

Interruption of the rectal plexus results in some discomfort from the distention of the rectosigmoid. A feeling of fullness in the descending colon and sigmoid results from this procedure. Patients adjust to this slight discomfort within a period of several weeks but must be advised to avoid constipation or dry stools due to an inadequate fluid intake.

Preoperative Care and Anesthesia

The urinary tract should be free of infection before this operation is undertaken. Had there been previous episodes of urinary tract infections and the bacteria responsible cultured and subjected to sensitivity tests, the urinary antiseptic known to control this organism is started forty-eight hours before the surgery. This permits an adequate blood and urinary level of the urinary antiseptics to be built up and avoid postoperative complications. Without any previous sensitivity tests a combination of a sulfonamide and a wide-spectrum antibiotic is given these patients, since almost without exception they have had many courses of therapy with urinary antiseptics.

A general anesthetic is satisfactory. Unless the surgeon is accustomed to controlling small bleeding points by fulguration, cyclopropane may be administered. A spinal anesthetic can be used when inhalation anesthesia is contraindicated. The operation does present the possibility of the sudden loss of blood from the tearing of a major vessel in a field where large arteries and veins are so abundant. There should be 2,000 ml. of blood on call, and this demand on the blood bank can be cancelled after the hazardous areas of the dissection are completed without incident.

Steps of the Operation

1. The incision selected should permit a complete exposure of the pelvis and lower abdomen well above the bifurcation of the aorta. Since most patients will have had previous pelvic surgery, the revision of previous incisions may be a consideration. If the patient is short, obese, with a deep funnel pelvis (as is frequently the problem in the multiple operative failures), an interiliac incision with section of the recti muscles ensures maximum exposure of the pelvis and lower abdomen. See Chapter 33 for technique of this incision.

2. Any adhesions from previous surgery are lysed so that the bowel can be packed into the upper abdomen and the sigmoid colon outlined in its course in the pelvis. This also delineates the sigmoid mesocolon through which the left inferior hypogastric plexus must be traced during the resection of the nerves entering the left side of the bladder.

3. The parietal peritoneum over the fifth lumbar vertebra is identified. Vasopressin solution, two

units diluted up to 20 ml., is used to infiltrate the retroperitoneal connective tissue and prevent minor areas of bleeding along the course of the incision shown in Plate 25, *A*. Sixty ml. of 1 per cent solution of procaine can be used for the same purpose. The equivalent of 0.06 ml. of epinephrine solution 1:1000 per 5 ml. of procaine may be added to prolong the effect unless contraindicated.

4. The parietal peritoneum is incised longitudinally and carried cephalad up to the bifurcation of the aorta. The incision is then carried downward and laterally from the promontory of the sacrum along the lateral pelvic wall to end just lateral to the right uterosacral ligament (Plate 25, *A*).

5. The peritoneum over the fifth lumbar vertebra is tagged with sutures on each side for lateral traction. The right side is gently lifted up to expose the right ureter. This is retracted with a vein retractor and lifted anteriorly. The right common iliac artery is thus exposed in order to dissect all of the fibers of the superior hypogastric plexus (prelumbar or presacral plexus) from the common iliac artery and underlying common iliac vein (Plate 25, *B*).

6. On the left side, depending on the length and configuration of the sigmoid mesocolon, the inferior mesenteric or the superior hemorrhoidal artery is retracted laterally to expose the left common iliac artery and underlying vein. The left ureter is lateral to these structures and displaced laterally with them during the dissection of the nerve bundles from the iliac vessels.

7. The superior hypogastric plexus is then mobilized by gently dissecting all of the fibers from the vessels toward the midline and off the periosteum of the body of the fifth lumbar vertebra. Ties of medium silk are passed under the plexus with an angle clamp or Kelly hemostat, the ligatures are tied distally and proximally as far as possible depending on the configuration of the plexus, and the nerve bundles between are resected (Plate 25, *B*).

8. The distal end of the resected plexus is used as traction, and the plexus is further dissected beyond the promontory until its division into right and left inferior hypogastric plexuses is evident. The middle sacral artery and vein will usually have to be ligated in the course of this dissection. The left inferior hypogastric plexus is mobilized and divided just as it passes under the sigmoid mesentery and superior hemorrhoidal artery (Plate 25, *C*).

9. The right inferior hypogastric plexus is now drawn toward the left anterolateral quadrant of

Text continued on p. 220.

Plate 25

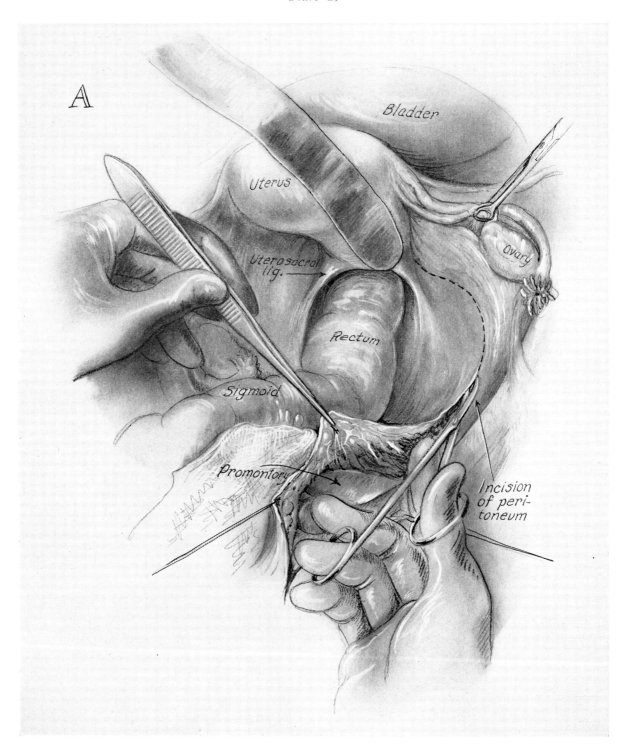

A

Bladder

Uterus

Ovary

Uterosacral lig.

Rectum

Sigmoid

Promontory

Incision of peritoneum

Plate 25 (Continued)

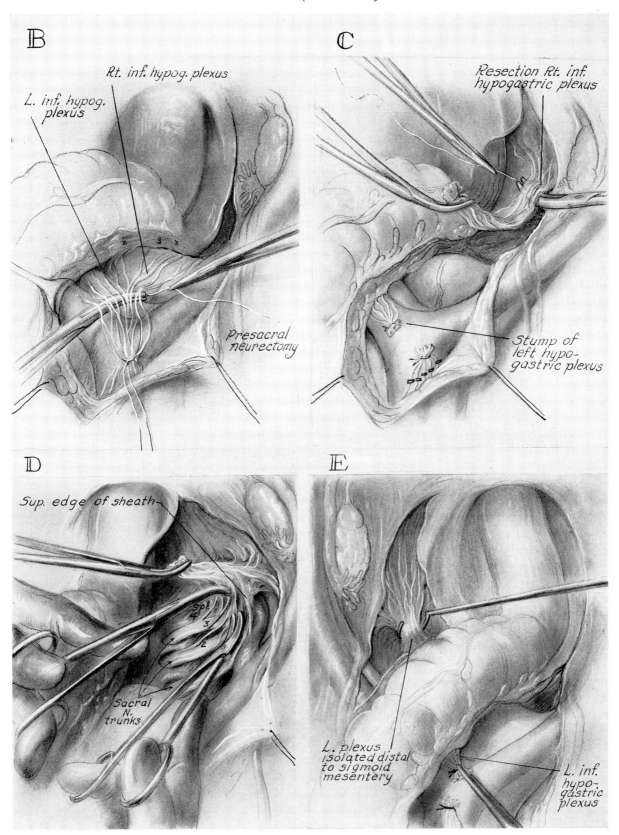

B

L. inf. hypog. plexus

Rt. inf. hypog. plexus

Presacral neurectomy

C

Resection Rt. inf. hypogastric plexus

Stump of left hypogastric plexus

D

Sup. edge of sheath

Sacral N. trunks

E

L. plexus isolated distal to sigmoid mesentery

L. inf. hypogastric plexus

Plate 25 (Continued)

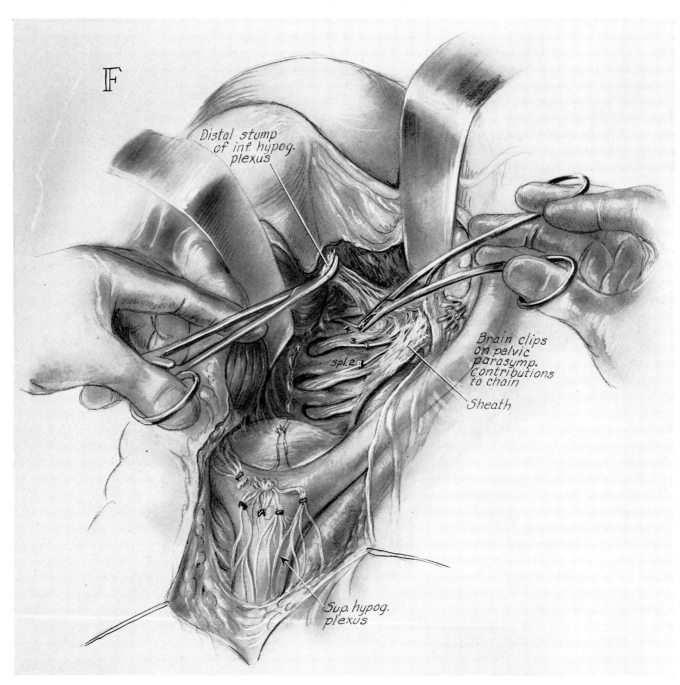

Plate 25 (Concluded)

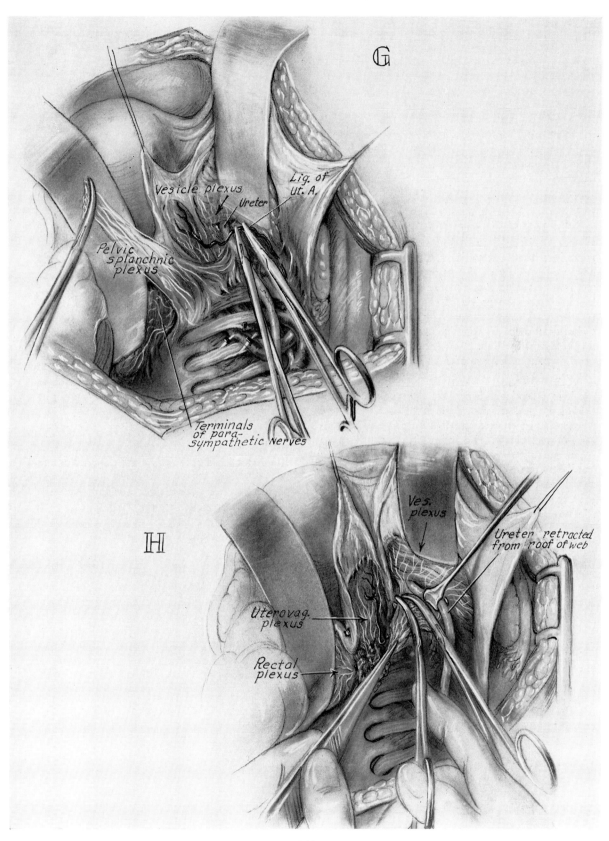

G

Vesicle plexus

Lig. of
Ut. A.

Ureter

Pelvic
splanchnic
plexus

Terminals
of para-
sympathetic Nerves

H

Ves.
plexus

Ureter retracted
from roof of web

Uterovag.
plexus

Rectal
plexus

the pelvis (Plate 25, *C*). This places the nerve bundles lying over the hypogastric artery and medial aspect of the pelvic ureter under tension and more readily identifiable. The ureter is drawn laterally with a vein retractor while the plexus is dissected from the lateral pelvic sidewall down to about the level of the second sacral foramina. The nerve bundles, lymphatics, and areolar tissue from the retracted ureter to the pelvic mesocolon are mobilized by alternate dissection with scissors, angle clamps, or small (peanut) sponges. A ligature of medium silk is tied around the plexus distally, and the plexus resected (Plate 25, *C*).

10. Each of the plexuses are individually labelled and sectioned to observe the number of nerve bundles in the specimen. This indicates the completeness of the denervation and guides the surgeon in subsequent patients. Brain clips can also be placed on any of the stumps, should it be desired to retain an x-ray record based on the bony landmarks of the pelvis of the level of resection of the various plexuses. Any of the approved techniques of x-ray pelvimetry will permit this mensuration. In Plate 25, *C*, brain clips are shown on the proximal stump of the superior hypogastric plexus.

11. The lateral pelvic wall is then palpated with the distal end of the right inferior hypogastric plexus drawn toward the left anterolateral quadrant of the pelvis. The index finger slides down over the piriformis muscle until the inferior border of the ala of the sacrum is felt. A slightly softer area which is the superior border of the greater sciatic notch is identified. The pulsation of the superior gluteal artery is felt, and its course carefully noted. The palpating finger gently explores the area of pelvic sidewall a few centimeters beyond the superior gluteal artery where contact will be made with the superior edge of the splanchnic nerve sheath. The proximal part of this broad, tough, fibrous band can be teased off the vessels by the exploring finger, but beyond this the dissection should proceed by direct vision (Plate 25, *D*).

12. The distal stump of the inferior hypogastric plexus is then drawn toward the left anterolateral wall of the true pelvis (Plate 25, *D*). This tenses the sheath and exposes the small parasympathetic contributions to the plexus from the anterior primary divisions of S-2, S-3, and S-4.

13. By sharp and blunt dissection the parasympathetic nerves and the sheath are further delineated and raised off the branches of the hypogastric artery and veins. This is a delicate dissection, and the operator should try to work in a

field with excellent hemostasis since accidental fracture or laceration of the major vessels in the area due to blood in the field will result in severe hemorrhage that is difficult to control. Plate 25, *D*, shows the artist's drawing of one such dissection. Many variations of the plexus occur, but, as one performs more operations, the consistency with which the sheath is found as described and its general dimensions proves to be a reliable landmark.

14. The surgeon must now decide whether to complete the operation on the right side or start the dissection on the left side. If there is minor oozing of blood at this point, I prefer to place a hot pack in the area and proceed with the dissection on the left side.

15. Two choices are possible in the dissection of the left inferior hypogastric plexus. The plexus can be traced under the sigmoid mesentery, or the length of the plexus under the sigmoid can be left intact and the plexus identified to the left of the colon. Unless the peritoneum over the plexus has been distorted by previous surgery, pelvic inflammatory disease, or some other condition, it is simpler to make traction on the proximal stump of the plexus to the right of the colon. This makes the distal portion to the left of the sigmoid stand out where it can be isolated (Plate 25, *E*).

16. An aneurysm needle or angle clamp is used to pick up the nerve fibers as they are isolated to the left of the colon. The superior hemorrhoidal artery is avoided in the dissection although its ligation, if necessary, does not impair the blood supply to the pelvic sigmoid colon (Plate 25, *E*). The dissection is then carried on in the same manner as on the right side of the pelvis.

17. Plate 25, *F*, shows the further dissection of right side. At or near the exit point of the superior gluteal vessels the parasympathetic (pelvic splanchnic) contribution from the anterior division of the second sacral nerve is observed. A brain clip is placed on the nerve filament flush with the pelvic sidewall, and it is resected. The brain clip serves to control minor oozing from vessels about the nerve.

18. The sheath is then teased from the pelvic sidewall and retracted toward the midline, along with the distal stump of the inferior hypogastric plexus (Plate 25, *F*).

19. By sharp and blunt dissection, the band is removed from the underlying vessels and nerves. The parasympathetic contributions from the third sacral nerve, anterior division, are clamped and cut. These usually number two or more filaments.

The inferior gluteal artery and veins and the pudendal artery and veins now come into view as the dissection proceeds. Finally, some small filaments may be observed coming from the anterior division of the fourth sacral nerve. Any fibers coming from the pelvic sympathetic chain to contribute to the pelvic splanchnic plexus are so small that individual identification is impractical. This stage of the nerve resection is shown in Plate 25, *F*.

20. The surgeon should be sure that the contributions of the third sacral nerve, anterior division, the largest and most consistent, have been specifically identified to ensure their interruption. I have seen at the operating table and in the anatomy laboratory two types of formations of the parasympathetic contributions to the splanchnic plexus from the third sacral nerve. More frequently than not, in a limited number of dissections, two nerve filaments are seen. They probably arise as a single branch and diverge before entering the sheath. In several cases one rather large filament is seen to enter the sheath.

21. The fibers from the anterior division of the fourth sacral nerve join the plexus in the depths of the pelvis, deep to the level of the cul-de-sac, and medial to the inferior gluteal vessels and nerves. The surgeon should not be concerned if these fibers are not specifically identified since some anatomists consider these contributions as inconsequential. The internal pudendal artery and veins are less likely to be injured since they exit from the pelvis more lateral and just posterior to the ischial spine before entering Alcock's canal.

22. The more lateral of the sympathetic fibers, lymphatics, and the accompanying connective tissue, together with the lateral edge of the sheath, is still intact. Laterally these are the terminal branches of the now fully formed splanchnic plexus as they proceed to the bladder. Medially, branches pass to the rectum (rectal plexus), to the uterus (Frankenhäuser's uterine plexus), and probably to the bladder by other than the routes that can be traced during this operation. Although not unlike a thorough lymphadenectomy, the objective here is the identification and resection of nerve fibers and bundles. This should be done with exact anatomic identification at each anatomic level to ensure interruption of the nerve supply to the bladder rather than the all-inclusive gleaning of the pelvis for lymphatic extensions of a malignant tumor as one does for an extended radical hysterectomy.

23. As the dissection continues deeper in the pelvis, the rectal plexus is resected as well as the uterovaginal nerve bundles. This is done since it is not possible to single out a distinct vesical plexus, and, if fibers cross over within the splanchnic plexus, they will be interrupted by sectioning all the nerve bundles adjacent to those going to the bladder.

24. The uterine artery is ligated as it passes over the ureter (Plate 25, *G*). The dissection has now proceeded almost to the point of entry of the nerve bundles into the pelvic organs. To ensure interruption of the maximum number of nerve fibers to the bladder, the terminal ureter is mobilized just before becoming intramural in position. The ligation of the uterine artery is necessary to accomplish this.

25. To completely mobilize and excise the vesical plexus, the rectal and uterovaginal plexuses are clamped, cut, and tied close to their respective organs. Then, with the distal ends of these nerves retracted to the left (for the dissection on the right side of the patient), the terminal bundle of fibers of the vesical plexus stands out as it passes beneath the ureter and into the wall of the bladder (Plate 25, *H*).

26. The ureter is carefully retracted with a vein retractor, and the plexus clamped, cut, and tied. Since the ureter is not detached from any small arteries supplied from the uterine artery in this technique, the terminal ureter is not compromised. Many patients will have had a hysterectomy so that the uterine artery, if still patent lateral to the ureter, would amount to a direct branch to the terminal ureter from the hypogastric artery (Plate 25, *H*).

27. Meticulous hemostasis is secured in the field of operation, the color of the ureter noted, and a hot, wet, tagged sponge left in the field.

28. The dissection on the left side is then begun. In my own experience the "sheath" is encountered a few centimeters cephalad of its counterpart on the right side. I cannot support this by any series of cadaver dissections, but it is possible that the course of the sigmoid mesentery could alter the anatomy of the formation of the splanchnic plexus to this extent if this is found to be a consistent finding.

29. The surgeon should appreciate the difference in the arterial supply to the left of the rectosigmoid. Here the unpaired superior hemorrhoidal artery freely anastomoses with the middle hemorrhoidal artery to create a slight change in the dissection.

30. The dissection is completed on the left side in the same manner as on the right side of the patient

except for the minor variations in the anatomy. Where the peritoneum can be reapproximated without distorting the course of the ureter, this is done. Some areas may have to be left devoid of peritoneum especially in those patients who have had one or more pelvic operations. Hemostasis should be so complete as to make drains unnecessary.

Postoperative Care

A vaginal pack and indwelling catheter are inserted. The vaginal pack is removed the first postoperative day. Some patients may require a suprapubic cystostomy, in which event this is left for nine or more days. When a urethral catheter is used for bladder drainage, this is removed on the fifth postoperative day. Urinary antiseptics that preoperative studies have shown to be effective against any of the bacteria cultured from the patient's urine in the past are given in adequate dosage. When the previous organisms are unknown, knowing that many drugs have been used, I order one sulfonamide in combination with one wide-spectrum urinary antiseptic. This can be left to the judgment of the surgeon and the limitations or selections of his own hospital's formulary.

After the indwelling catheter is removed, the patient should be instructed to voluntarily increase the time between voidings to permit the bladder to regain its normal capacity. It should be explained that she will have a period during which urinary frequency is to be expected and that she should resist voiding until the urge is strong. This requires a few weeks of training. Cystoscopy, an intravenous pyelogram, and cystometrics are repeated four to six weeks after operation to assess the operative result by these means as well as the more important evaluation provided by the patient's report of symptomatic relief.

References

Aldridge, A.: Transplantation of Fascia for Relief of Urinary Stress Incontinence, Am. J. Obst. & Gynec. 44: 398, 1942.

Amreich, G.: Incontinence of Urine in Women, Chirurg 4: 234, 1932.

Arnold, J. H.: The Vesical Adaptometer: A New Concept in Cystometry, J. Urol. 82: 651, 1959.

Baker, W. J., and Callahan, D. H.: Interstitial Cystitis, J. Urol. 81: 112, 1959.

Balfour, J., and Ankenman, G. J.: Atonic Neurogenic Bladder as a Manifestation of Diabetic Neuropathy, J. Urol. 76: 746, 1956.

Ball, T. L.: Topographic Urethrography, Part I, Am. J. Obst. & Gynec. 59: 1243, 1950.

Ball, T. L.: Combined Vaginal and Abdominal Plication of the Bladder Neck and Cystopexy, Am. J. Obst. & Gynec. 63: 1245, 1952.

Ball, T. L., Douglas, R. Gordon, and Fulkerson, L.: Topographic Urethrography, Part II, Am. J. Obst. & Gynec. 59: 1252, 1950.

Ball, T. L., and Douglas, R. Gordon: Topographic Urethrography in "Continent" and "Incontinent" Women, Part III, Tr. New England Obst. & Gynec. Soc. 4: 65, 1950.

Ball, T. L., and Fulkerson, L.: Female Urinary Incontinence, Urol. & Cutan. Rev. 55: 591, 1951.

Beneventi, F.: A Study of the Posterior Urethra in the Newborn Female, Surg., Gynec. & Obst. 76: 64, 1943.

Berkow, S.: Paraurethral Fixation: a New Operation for the Cure of Relative Incontinence of Urine in Women, Am. J. Obst. & Gynec. 41: 1051, 1941.

Berkow, S.: The Corpus Spongiosum of the Urethra: Its Possible Role in Urinary Control and Stress Incontinence in Women, Am. J. Obst. & Gynec. 65: 346, 1953.

Berkow, S.: Paraurethral Fixation for Stress Incontinence, Obst. & Gynec. 5: 74, 1955.

Berry, J. L.: A New Procedure for Correction of Urinary Incontinence: Preliminary Report, J. Urol. 85: 771, 1961.

Blundon, K. E., and Lane, J. W.: Diagnostic Difficulties in Ureteral Ectopia, J. Urol. 84: 463, 1960.

Bors, E.: Segmental and Peripheral Innervation of the Urinary Bladder, J. Nerv. & Ment. Dis. 116: 572, 1952.

Bors, E.: Topical Anesthesia of the Vesical Mucosa as a Tool for the Management of the Neurogenic Bladder, J. Urol. 79: 431, 1958.

Bourque, J. P.: Surgical Management of the Painful Bladder, J. Urol. 65: 25, 1951.

Brandstetter, J., and Haschek, H.: The Irritable Female Bladder, (Die Reizblase der Frau), Zschr. Urol. 53: 295, 1960.

Burch, J. C.: Urethrovaginal Fixation to Cooper's Ligament for Correction of Stress Incontinence, Cystocele, and Prolapse, Am. J. Obst. & Gynec. 81: 281, 1961.

Burford, E. H., and Burford, C. E.: Hunner Ulcer of the Bladder: A Report of 187 Cases, J. Urol. 79: 952, 1958.

Carpenter, F. G., and Root, W. S.: Effect of Parasympathetic Denervation on Feline Bladder Function, Am. J. Physiol. 166: 686, 1951.

Carson, R.: Retropubic Vesicourethral Suspension, J. Urol. 79: 844, 1958.

Chait, A., Pons, T., and Roland, V. A.: Neurogenic Bladder Caused by Sacral Echinococcus Cyst, J. Urol. 80: 183, 1958.

Chavigny, C. L.: Specialized Retractor for Use in the Marshall-Marchetti Operation, Obst. & Gynec. 8: 371, 1956.

Comarr, A. E.: Present Day Treatment of the Traumatic Cord Neurogenic Bladder, J. Urol. 83: 34, 1960.

Comarr, A. E.: Transurethral Vesical Neck Resection: An Adjunct in the Management of the Neurogenic Bladder, J. Urol. 72: 849, 1954.

Comarr, E.: Further Observations on Excretory Cystometry, J. Urol. 79: 714, 1958.

Counseller, V., and Symmonds, R.: Vesicourethral Suspension for Urinary Stress Incontinence; a Study of the Results Obtained in 82 Patients, Am. J. Obst. & Gynec. 75: 525, 1958.

Cowley, R. A., and Yeager, G. H.: Anatomic Observations on the Lumbar Sympathetic Nervous System, Surgery 25: 880, 1949.

Crabtree, E. G., Brodney, M. L., Kontoff, H. A., and Muellner, S. R.: Roentgenological Diagnosis of Urological and Gynecological Diseases of the Female Bladder, J. Urol. **35:** 52, 1936.

Denny-Brown, D.: Nervous Disturbances of the Vesical Sphincter, New England J. Med. **215:** 647, 1936.

deSousa, Meleiro, e Gomes, Kirio: Incontinência de urina ao esforco na mulher. Separata da: Rev. clin. d. inst. maternal, Lisboa **4:** 23, 1952.

Engelking, R. L., and Alcaine, T. P.: Female Epispadias: Treatment of Incontinence by the Marshall-Marchetti Technique, J. Urol. **84:** 555, 1960.

Francis, W.: The Onset of Stress Incontinence, J. Obst. & Gynaec. Brit. Emp. **67:** 899, 1960.

Frank, R.: Operation for the Cure of Incontinence of Urine in the Female, Am. J. Obst. & Gynec. **53:** 618, 1947.

Frankel, D. S.: Full-Thickness Anterior Colporrhaphy for Correction of Urinary Stress Incontinence, Am. J. Obst. & Gynec. **76:** 1185, 1958.

Fulkerson, L.: Incontinence of Urine in Women. Urethrocele; Relaxed Vesical Sphincter; Urethral Dilatation, Urol. & Cutan. Rev. **43:** 569, 1939.

Fulkerson, L.: Incontinence of Urine in Women: Evaluation of Recent Studies, New Operations and New Methods for Diagnosis and Cure of Stress Incontinence, Urol. & Cutan. Rev. **56:** 72, 1952.

Gaker, L. B., Smith, K. M., and Helfman, H.: Preliminary Report on Modified Vesicourethropexy, J. Urol. **85:** 781, 1961.

Goff, B. H.: An Histological Study of the Perivaginal Fascia in a Nullipara, Surg., Gynec. & Obst. **52:** 32, 1931.

Greco, P. A., and Anllo, V.: Urethrocystopexy for Stress Incontinence in the Female; Experience With the Marshall-Marchetti Procedure, J. Urol. **85:** 776, 1961.

Harper, J., and Russell, J.: A Clinical Evaluation of Urethrovesical Lysis for the Cure of Urinary Stress Incontinence in the Female, Am. J. Obst. & Gynec. **74:** 1322, 1957.

Hepburn, T. N.: Prolapse of the Female Urethra, Surg., Gynec. & Obst. **31:** 83, 1920.

Hepburn, T. N.: Prolapse of the Urethra in Female Children, Surg., Gynec. & Obst. **44:** 400, 1927.

Hodgkinson, C. P., and Kelly, W. T.: Urethrovesicopubic Relationships and Urinary Stress Incontinence, IV. The Uterine Suspension Syndrome, Am. J. Obst. & Gynec. **76:** 1114, 1958.

Huffman, J. W.: The Detailed Anatomy of the Paraurethral Ducts in the Adult Human Female, Am. J. Obst. & Gynec. **55:** 86, 1948.

Hutch, J. A.: Sacral Rhizotomy for Treatment of Paraplegics With Hydronephrosis, J. Urol. **77:** 123, 1957.

Ingelman-Sundberg, A.: Plastic Repair of the Pelvic Floor, Acta obst. et gynec. scandinav. **30** (supp. 7): 318, 1950.

Ingelman-Sundberg, A.: Vaginal Slingoperation, Nordisk forening for obstetrikk og gynekologi, Kongress I, Oslo, 1957.

Ingelmann-Sundberg, A.: Parametriografi, Nordisk forening for obstetrikk og gynekologi, Kongress I, Oslo, 1957.

Ingelman-Sundberg, A.: Partial Denervation of the Bladder; a New Operation for the Treatment of Urge Incontinence and Similar Conditions in Women, Acta obst. et gynec. scandinav. **38:** 487, 1959.

James, T.: Incontinence of Urine and the Neurogenic Bladder in Childhood, With Illustrative Case, Arch. Pediat. **69:** 253, 1952.

Jeffcoate, T. N. A., and Roberts, H.: Observations on Stress Incontinence of Urine, Am. J. Obst. & Gynec. **64:** 721, 1952.

Jeffcoate, T. N. A.: Stress Incontinence of Urine, J. Obst. & Gynaec. Brit. Emp. **59:** 685, 1952.

Kasdon, S.: Interposition of Uterine Ligaments Following Vaginal Hysterectomy in 100 Patients With Urinary Stress Incontinence, Am. J. Obst. & Gynec. **75:** 1048, 1958.

Kaufman, J. J.: A New Recording Uroflometer: A Simple Automatic Device for Measuring Voiding Velocity, J. Urol. **78:** 97, 1957.

Kegel, A. H.: The Nonsurgical Treatment of Genital Relaxation; Use of Perineometer as Aid in Restoring Anatomic and Functional Structure, Ann. West. Med. & Surg. **2:** 213, 1948.

Kennedy, W. T.: Incontinence of Urine in the Female; Some Functional Observations of Urethra Illustrated by Roentgenograms, Am. J. Obst. & Gynec. **33:** 19, 1937.

Kennedy, W. T.: Muscle of Micturition; Its Role in Sphincter Mechanism, With Reference to Incontinence in the Female, Am. J. Obst. & Gynec. **52:** 206, 1946.

Kennedy, W. T.: Incontinence of Urine in the Female: Effective Restoration and Maintenance of Sphincter Control, Am. J. Obst. & Gynec. **69:** 338, 1955.

Kuntz, A., and Farnsworth, D. I.: Distribution of Afferent Fibers Via the Sympathetic Trunks and Gray Communicating Rami to the Brachial and Lumbosacral Plexuses, J. Comp. Neurol. **53:** 389, 1931.

Langley, L. I., and Kimura, K.: The Afferent Pathway of the Vesicorenal Reflex, J. Urol. **82:** 476, 1959.

Langworthy, O. R., Drew, J. E., and Vest, S. A.: Urethral Resistance in Relation to Vesical Activity, J. Urol. **43:** 123, 1940.

Langworthy, O. R., Kolb, L. C., and Lewis, L. G.: Physiology of Micturition, Baltimore, 1940, Williams & Wilkins Co.

Langworthy, O. R., and Murphy, E. L.: Nerve Endings in the Urinary Bladder, J. Comp. Neurol. **71:** 487, 1939.

Lapides, J., and others: Further Observations on the Kinetics of the Urethrovesical Sphincter, J. Urol. **84:** 86, 1960.

Lapides, J., and others: Physiopathology of Stress Incontinence, Surg., Gynec. & Obst. **111:** 224, 1960.

Leadbetter, W. F., and Shaffer, F. G.: Ileal Loop Diversion, Its Application to the Treatment of Neurogenic Bladder Dysfunction, J. Urol. **75:** 470, 1956.

Learmonth, J. R.: Neurosurgery in the Treatment of Disease of the Urinary Bladder. I. Anatomic and Surgical Considerations, J. Urol. **25:** 531, 1931.

Learmonth, J. R.: Neurosurgery in the Treatment of Disease of the Urinary Bladder. II. Treatment of Vesical Pain. J. Urol **26:** 13, 1931.

Learmonth, J. R.: A Contribution to the Neurophysiology of the Urinary Bladder in Man, Brain **54:** 147, 1931.

Learmonth, J. R.: Neurosurgery in Diseases of the Urinary Bladder, Am. J. Surg. **16:** 270, 1932.

Learmonth, J. R.: Operations on Nerves of the Urinary Bladder, Edinburgh M. J. **39:** 43, 1932.

Leger, L.: La cervico-cystopexie par lambeau aponevrotique dans le traitement de l'incontinence orthostatique des urines chez la femme, J. urol., Paris **56:** 78, 1950.

Lepage, F., and DeTourris, H.: Present Concepts on Micturition in Women. Incidences on the Orthostatic Incontinence of Urine (Conceptions actuelles sur la miction de la femme; incidences sur l'incontinence orthostatique d'urine), Gynéc et obst. **59:** 57, 1960.

Long, D. M., and Bernstein, W. C.: Sexual Dysfunction as a Complication of Abdominoperineal Resection of the Rectum in the Male: An Anatomic and Physiologic Study, Dis. Colon & Rectum **2:** 540, 1959.

Lowenberg, R. I., and Morton, D. E.: The Anatomic and Surgical Significance of the Lumbar Sympathetic Nervous System, Ann. Surg. **133:** 525, 1951.

Lund, C. J., Fullerton, R. E., and Tristan, T. A.: Cinefluorographic Studies of the Bladder and Urethra in Women; II. Stress Incontinence, Am. J. Obst. & Gynec. **78:** 706, 1959.

McCrea, L. E.: Interstitial Cystitis, J. Urol. **84:** 311, 1960.

McCrea, L. E., and Kimmel, D. L.: A New Concept of Vesical Innervation and Its Relationship to Bladder Management Following Abdominoperineal Proctosigmoidectomy, Am. J. Surg. **84:** 518, 1952.

Macleod, D.: Trigonal Muscle With Special Reference to Its Composition and Urinary Function, Brit. J. Urol. **13:** 135, 1941.

Marchetti, A. A., Marshall, V. F., and Shultis, L. D.: Simple Vesicourethral Suspension for Stress Incontinence of Urine, Am. J. Obst. & Gynec. 74: 57, 1957.

Marshall, V. F., and others: Osteitis Pubis Treated With Adrenocorticotrophic Hormone, J. Urol. 67: 364, 1952.

Melick, W. F., Naryka, J. J., and Schmidt, J. H.: Experimental Studies of Ureteral Peristaltic Patterns in the Pig: I. Similarity of Pig and Human Ureter and Bladder Physiology, J. Urol. 85: 145, 1961.

Meredith, J. M.: The Importance of Anatomic Precision in Differential Sacral Neurotomy for "Cord Bladder," Am. J. Surg. 87: 819, 1954.

Miller, N. F.: Construction of a Vulvar Urethra for Selected Problem Cases of Urinary Incontinence, Obst. & Gynec. 2: 107, 1953.

Milner, W. A., and Garlick, W. B.: Selective Sacral Neurectomy in Interstitial Cystitis, J. Urol. 78: 600, 1957.

Moulder, M. K., and Meirowsky, A. M.: The Management of Hunner's Ulcer by Differential Sacral Neurotomy: Preliminary Report, J. Urol. 75: 261, 1956.

Muellner, S. R.: Lack of a Specific Urethral Lesion in Exertional Urinary Incontinence, New England J. Med. 234: 400, 1946.

Muellner, S. R.: The Voluntary Control of Micturition in Man, J. Urol. 80: 473, 1958.

Muellner, S. R., and Fleischner, F. G.: Normal and Abnormal Micturition: A Study of Bladder Behavior by Means of the Fluoroscope, J. Urol. 61: 233, 1949.

Mulvany, J.: Stress Incontinence in Women: Its Mechanism and Treatment, J. Obst. & Gynaec. Brit. Emp. 64: 531, 1957.

Mulvaney, J.: Vesicourethrolysis for Urinary Incontinence in Women, Surg., Gynec. & Obst. 107: 511, 1958.

Murphy, J. J., and Schoenberg, H. W.: Observations on Intravesical Pressure Changes During Micturition, J. Urol. 84: 106, 1960.

Nathan, P. W.: Sensations Associated With Micturition, Brit. J. Urol. 28: 126, 1956.

Natvig, H.: Incontinence of Urine in Women, Norsk mag. laegevidensk. 92: 325, 1931.

Nesbit, R. M., and Lapides, J.: The Physiology of Micturition, J. Michigan Med. Soc. 58: 384, 1959.

Ney, C., Tausend, M. E., and Friedenberg, R. M.: Deviation of the Bladder in Neurogenic Lesions, J. Urol. 81: 659, 1959.

Nunes de Barcelos, O.: Urinary Stress Incontinence in the Female; Report on 135 Cases (Incontinecia urinaria de esforco na mulher; relatorio sobre 135 casos a consideracoes gerais), Rev. Brasil. Cirurg. 32: 521, 1956.

Parrott, M.: Adequate Anterior Colporrhaphy; a New Surgical Approach for the Relief of Stress Incontinence in Women, Am. J. Obst. & Gynec. 80: 381, 1960.

Paxon, N. F., Campbell, E. W., and Kannapel, A. R.: Urinary Stress Incontinence: a Comparison of the Treatments Used, Obst. & Gynec. 2: 112, 1953.

Pick, J.: The Identification of Sympathetic Segments, Ann. Surg. 145: 355, 1957.

Plum, F.: Autonomous Urinary Bladder Activity in Normal Man, A. M. A. Arch. Neurol. 2: 497, 1960.

Plum, F., and Colfelt, R. H.: The Genesis of Vesical Rhythmicity, A. M. A. Arch. Neurol. 2: 487, 1960.

Prochorow, M.: A New Operation for Stress Incontinence, Ginek, Pol. 29: 157, 1958.

Raia, A., and Haddad, J.: Sexual Function and Fecal Continence Following Abdominoperineal Resection of Rectosigmoid for Acquired Megacolon, Surg., Gynec. & Obst. 111: 357, 1960.

Rattner, W. H., Fink, S., and Murphy, J. J.: Pressure Studies in the Human Ureter and Renal Pelvis, J. Urol. 78: 359, 1957.

Reynolds, C. L., and Smith, R.: Practical Approach to the Male Chronic Neurogenic Bladder, J. Urol. 84: 710, 1960.

Riba, L. W.: The Role of the Lymphatics in Interstitial Cystitis (Hunner's Ulcer), J. Urol. 79: 942, 1958.

Richer, V.: Traitement des cystites tuberculeuses rebelles et des cystalgier néoplasique par la section des nerfs erecteurs, J. d'urol. 39: 60, 1935.

Ritter, J. S., and Sporer, A.: Physiological Principles Governing Therapy of the Neurogenic Bladder, J. Urol. 61: 528, 1949.

Roedling, H. A., and others: Paravertebral Alcohol Block of Lumbar Sympathetic Nerves: Evaluation by Sweating Tests in 351 Patients, J. A. M. A. 165: 799, 1957.

Rose, D. K.: Physiology of the Bladder, J. Urol. 43: 190, 1940.

Rose, D. K.: Urethroceles in Urology, J. Urol. 58: 349, 1947.

Scott, J. E.: The Anatomy of the Pelvic Autonomic Nervous System in Cases of High Imperforate Anus, Surgery 45: 1013, 1959.

Shaw, Wilfred: An Operation for the Treatment of Stress Incontinence, Brit. M. J. 1: 1070, 1949.

Shev, E. E., and Finkle, A. L.: Reversible Neurogenic Bladder Following Cerebral and/or Spinal Cord Concussion, J. Urol. 81: 653, 1959.

Simmons, J. L.: Interstitial Cystitis: An Explanation for the Beneficial Effect of an Antihistamine, J. Urol. 85: 149, 1961.

Studdiford, W.: The Problem of Stress Incontinence and Its Surgical Relief, Surg., Gynec. & Obst. 83: 742, 1946.

Talbot, H. S.: The Management of the Spastic Bladder in Paraplegia, J. Urol. 79: 759, 1958.

Taussig, F.: A New Operation for Urinary Incontinence in Women by Transposing Levator Ani Muscles, Am. J. Obst. & Gynec. 77: 881, 1918.

Taverner, D., and Smiddy, F. G.: An Electromyographic Study of the Normal Function of the External Anal Sphincter and Pelvic Diaphragm, Dis. Colon & Rectum 2: 153, 1959.

Teinturier, M. J.: Une technique de suspension du col dans l'incontinence orthostatique chez la femme, J. urol., Paris 57: 847, 1951.

Thackston, L. P., Price, N. C., and Richardson, A. G.: Use of Antispasmodics in Treatment of Spastic Ureteritis, J. Urol. 73: 487, 1955.

Thompson, I. M., and Jackson, I. J.: Urologic Evaluation as a Neurologic Adjunct, South. M. J. 51: 428, 1958.

Todd, T. Wingate: Age Changes in the Pubic Bone. I. The Male White Pubis, Am. J. Phys. Anthropol. 3: 285, 1920.

Todd, T. Wingate: Age Changes in the Pubic Bone. II. The Pubis of the Male Negro-White Hybrid; III. The Pubis of the White Female; IV. The Pubis of the Female Negro-White Hybrid, Am. J. Phys. Anthropol. 4: 1, 1921.

Todd, T. Wingate: Age Changes in the Pubic Symphysis. VII. The Anthropoid Strain in Human Pubic Symphyses of the Third Decade, J. Anat. 57: 274, 1922-23.

Twombly, G. H., and Landers, D.: The Innervation of the Bladder With Reference to Radical Hysterectomy, Am. J. Obst. & Gynec. 71: 1291, 1956.

Ullery, J. C.: Stress Incontinence in the Female, New York, 1953, Grune & Stratton, Inc.

Van Duzen, R. E., and Looney, W. W.: Further Studies on the Trigone Muscle; the Anatomy and Practical Considerations, J. Urol. 27: 129, 1932.

Webber, R. H.: An Analysis of the Sympathetic Trunk, Communicating Rami, Sympathetic Roots and Visceral Rami in the Lumbar Region in Man, Ann. Surg. 141: 398, 1955.

Weyrauch, H. M., and Melody, G. F.: Marshall-Marchetti Operation for Prolapse of Vesical Neck, Surg., Gynec. & Obst. 92: 115, 1960.

Wharton, L. R.: Innervation of the Ureter, With Respect to Denervation, J. Urol. 28: 639, 1932.

Wharton, L. R.: The Nonoperative Treatment of Stress Incontinence in Women, Am. J. Obst. & Gynec. 66: 1121, 1953.

Youssef, A. F.: Cystometric Studies in Gynecology and Obstetrics, Obst. & Gynec. 8: 181, 1956.

11 · Urinary Tract Fistulas

General Considerations

Several factors have resulted in an increase in the number of urinary tract fistulas from gynecologic surgery. At the same time there has been a decrease in these complications from obstetric causes. The increasing popularity of the total abdominal hysterectomy rather than the subtotal operation has resulted in more injuries to the ureter and bladder. This does not mean that the total operation should not be done as the procedure of choice in all but rare instances. The recent employment of radical pelvic surgery in the management of pelvic cancer has increased the number of fistulas. When surgery is employed after radiation, the incidence of urologic complications is exceedingly high. Fistulas as a result of prolonged labor and difficult forceps operations have decreased in number with the better recognition of cephalopelvic disproportion, a better selection of patients requiring cesarean section, and the avoidance of prolonged, ineffectual labors by the use of intravenous Pitocin. Fistulas may result from the use of radium and x-ray without surgery. Better screening techniques and higher voltage x-ray deliver larger tumor doses without severe radiation effects on the adjacent vital structures.

Etiology and Pathologic Anatomy

Plate 26, A, shows some of the types of fistulas that may be encountered. Vesicoabdominal and vesicoperitoneal fistulas are rare but tend to occur after damage to the bladder during abdominal surgery. They may be the result of penetrating wounds in this area. Urethrovaginal, bladder neck, and vesicovaginal fistulas occur after damage to the anterior vaginal wall and bladder base by surgery, radia-tion, or parturition. A combination of fistulas is possible, and the tracts may course through several structures. Vesicouterine, vesicocervico-vaginal, and vesicorectovaginal fistulas are indicated on Plate 26, A. One or more fistulas may exist at the same time. Plate 26, B, shows an additional group of fistulas, some of which involve the pelvic ureter. A fistula may exist after accidental injury between the ureter, peritoneal cavity, and abdominal wall. A uretero-peritoneal fistula that subsequently drains into the vaginal vault is often the result of trauma during a difficult hysterectomy. Injury to the ureter nearer the ureterovesical junction results in the more common ureterovaginal fistula. The ureter may be damaged from vaginal as well as abdominal surgery in this location. Fistulas may go from the bladder into the peritoneum and then to the vagina, and such a vesicoperitoneovaginal fistula may result from a difficult dissection in which the bladder base is strongly adherent to the lower uterine segment and cervix. A fistula may be in a midline location in the immediate retrotrigonal area. Birth trauma usually is the cause of the fistula. Fistulas from the bladder to the small and large bowel or to walled-off areas within the pelvic cavity are possible. The variety of fistulas is almost endless, and the path of each fistula must be individually studied and determined.

Symptoms and Diagnosis

The symptoms and diagnosis of fistulas suspected in the immediate postoperative period or within several weeks after operation or delivery are discussed under Bladder Injuries (page 536) and Ureteral Injuries (page 537). The innumerable variety of fistulas do not lend

PLATE 26

URINARY TRACT FISTULAS

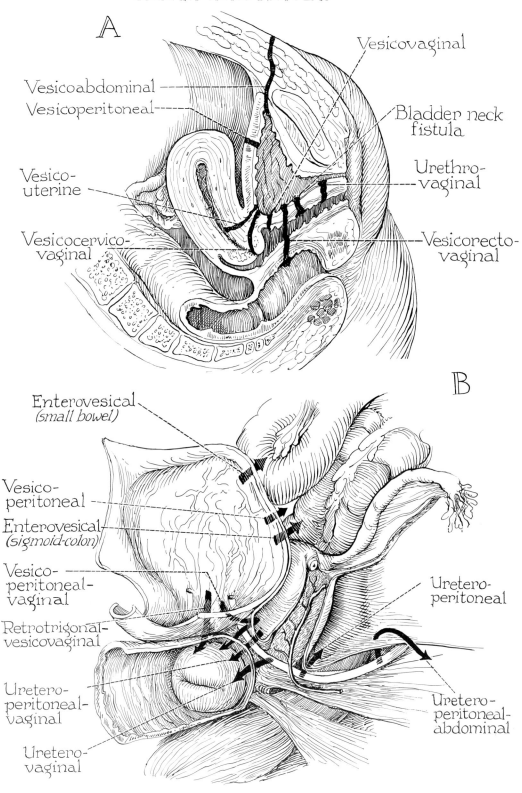

A

Vesicovaginal

Vesicoabdominal

Vesicoperitoneal

Bladder neck fistula

Vesico-uterine

Urethro-vaginal

Vesicocervico-vaginal

Vesicorecto-vaginal

B

Enterovesical (small bowel)

Vesico-peritoneal

Enterovesical (sigmoid-colon)

Vesico-peritoneal-vaginal

Retrotrigonal-vesicovaginal

Uretero-peritoneal-vaginal

Uretero-vaginal

Uretero-peritoneal

Uretero-peritoneal-abdominal

themselves to a characteristic description of the signs and symptoms of each.

Twenty-Five Surgical Principles in Bladder Fistula Surgery

The surgical principles concerned with modern fistula surgery of the bladder and adjacent structures may be divided into the following general categories: (1) Those principles concerned with the preoperative preparation of the fistulous tract and adjacent structures and with the general condition of the patient regarding nutrition, electrolytes, and other factors concerned with the primary union of a surgical incision. (2) Consideration of the accessibility of the site of operation, the best approach or combined approach, and incidental means of improving exposure of the area. (3) Those principles concerned with the cause of the fistula, the direction, density, and degree of retraction of the fibrous tissue about its tract, and the painstaking study needed to avoid a hasty dissection when time spent analyzing the ultimate strain on the suture line is more important. (4) The methods of obtaining a closure that approximates without tension or strangulation and approximates mucosa to mucosa within the bladder. (5) The postoperative care and methods of bladder drainage that are so important in the success of the operative closure.

1. Surfaces are to be opposed that will require all the factors concerned with the union of tissues to be as near normal as possible. Evaluate the patient's general health and nutrition. Postpone operation until any nutritional deficiencies are corrected by diet and supplementary therapy. Investigate the patient's blood chemistry with attention to the plasma proteins, blood sugar, and electrolytes. Latent diabetes should be suspected and a sugar tolerance test performed in patients who have experienced multiple failures. The most skillful closure may fail when the essential conditions for proper wound healing are neglected.

2. Infection and the deposition of urinary salts about the edges of the fistula compromise healing. Upper urinary tract disease should be eliminated by appropriate study and treatment and the bladder freed of infection by urinary anti-septics. An intravenous pyelogram, cystoscopy, and retrograde studies as indicated should precede the operation. Urine cultures and sensitivity tests—so you know you have one or more agents effective against any organism identified—guide your choice of antibiotics and other urinary antiseptics. The importance of confirming the presence of healthy edges by cystoscopic observation will be apparent to those who attempt a closure only to find themselves inverting tissue into an encrusted bladder mucosa. The preoperative preparation of the fistulous tract requires attention to bladder irrigations and vaginal douches. The solutions should be mildly acid since the deposition of urinary encrustations is most frequent in an alkaline urine. Water intake should be forced despite the discomfort attendant upon the increased output.

3. Study the accessibility of a fistula and the means by which the position on the operating table (lithotomy, Sims, knee-chest) may help to bring it into the field. As Kelly said regarding accessibility, "Either the operator must go up to the fistula or the fistula must be brought down to the operator; or a combination of both may be necessary for success."

4. Regardless of how distant the tract may seem from the vaginal aspect, it is not, with few exceptions, so far away as it is through a large abdominal panniculus, deep pelvis, and across the bladder through a suprapubic cystotomy. In short, everything favors the vaginal approach to all but a few fistulas. *From the abdomen you operate in the dark so far as the vaginal wall is concerned and at the bottom of a chasm on the bladder wall; from the vagina you see the vaginal wall directly, and the mucosa of the bladder can be visualized as frequently as necessary by the simplest of endoscopes!*

5. Remember that fistulas in the lateral sulci are accessible only with some risk of damage to the ureter unless this structure is positively identified. Place a catheter in the ureter, if possible, on the side of the fistula, and remove it only when all sutures in the fistula closure have been placed and tied. A small catheter can be left in place as a splint if the particular fistula involves the intramural ureter. If the catheter is removed, the ureteral orifice should be visualized with a simple observation endoscope to note the efflux of urine and whether it contains blood.

6. Schuchardt's incision, correctly performed, makes a high fistula readily accessible. This is true even in fistulas following a hysterectomy and

wound infection in the vault with dense scar tissue and retraction. *This operation is not a paravaginal incision but a means of displacing the rectum out of the field (for right-handed surgeons) and should be called a rectal displacement incision.*

7. Vesicovaginal fistulas recognized on the delivery table are closed immediately only if the edges of the tear are clean, not edematous or necrotic, and the patient's condition is good. The frantic closure of a fistula after a long labor, edema and ischemia of the edges, and contamination of the field by repeated examinations and instrumentation will most surely result in complete breakdown of the wound and complicate future closure. Exercise restraint since the fistula may close spontaneously or be a simple procedure in a few months.

8. Develop the patience to study before and during a fistula repair the direction, density, and firmness of the scar tissue adjacent to the fistula, not only in all directions, but also along its course directly to the bladder or through other structures. Master gynecologic surgeons—renowned for dexterity and speed—have the wisdom to proceed painstakenly and deliberately in performing a fistula repair. Remember that you can observe the pliability of the bladder wall through a cystoscope while manipulating the vaginal aspect of the fistulous tract and add to your information regarding the direction of forces that may disrupt your repair.

9. Midline vesicovaginal fistulas are best approached by a vertical (in axis of vagina) incision that circumscribes the vaginal orifice of the fistula. After the separation and mobilization of the vaginal and bladder walls, the bladder is closed transversely and the vaginal wall vertically. By this method the ultimate strain on the suture lines is minimized and the blood supply left intact to both layers.

10. Lateral sulcus fistulas of small dimensions are best approached with a transverse vaginal incision since the blood supply to the vagina originates from that direction. A long vertical incision in the lateral vaginal wall, while leaving the lateral vaginal flap of the closure with an intact blood supply, may compromise the medial flap since it would have to receive vessels from above or across the midline.

11. Adequate mobilization of the bladder frequently requires a total hysterectomy, either vaginal or abdominal. This is necessary to remove a uterus to which the bladder is adherent by dense

scar tissue that would cause retraction of the edges of the fistula closure if left behind.

12. Fistulas not infrequently course through a cervical stump when they are the result of an emergency Porro section or other surgery to stem bleeding. Elimination of the entire fistula is best accomplished by excision of the cervical stump, which effects an adequate mobilization of the bladder at the same time.

13. *Study the cause of a fistula and you will learn where to expect its edges to be scarred and retracted!* An example of this is a vault fistula following a total abdominal hysterectomy. The posterior edge of such a fistula is farthest from the introitus and coincides with the transverse scar of the vaginal vault. *This, then, is the segment of the opening that must be carefully mobilized!* In an obliteration type of procedure (Latzko) this must be appreciated so that an adequate denudation is done posteriorly to cover the opening that anatomically lies in the anterior vaginal wall just as it is reflected anteriorly from the scar of the closed vaginal vault.

14. Recognize a situation in which the blood supply adjacent to the fistula is so impaired as to require some type of transplant as an artificial means of providing nourishment to the flaps used in the closure. The gracilis muscle or a Martius graft (bulbocavernosus and vestibular bulb) is a source of providing a new blood supply.

15. Will the patient have gross urinary stress incontinence from an incompetent bladder neck after a successful fistula closure and thus be little better off than before? Studies of the position of the bladder neck before surgery by urethroscopy and urethrography may anticipate this complication, permitting the surgeon to incorporate some type of bladder neck plication for restoration of the posterior urethrovesical angle and a competent bladder neck in his fistula repair.

16. The principles of bladder fistula surgery that permit approximation of the edges without strangulation or tension are put into effect the moment tissue is touched. Use traction sutures to gain exposure or fix tissues for dissection wherever this is possible.

17. Crushing instruments must not be used, and *all tissues are delicately handled and as little as possible!*

18. Aim for the approximation of broad, raw, healthy surfaces.

19. When a suture has to be tied under tension, the dissection has been inadequate, and this suture

should be removed. It will only cause a sloughing of the immediate area and may doom the entire procedure to failure.

20. The availability of strong, small caliber, and atraumatic suture material has outmoded nonabsorbable material such as silkworm gut and silver or steel wire. Use small, round-body, atraumatic needles and interrupted sutures throughout. Purse-string, figure-of-eight, and other fancy variations are tissue stranglers and have no place in fistula surgery.

21. Characteristic of the anastomosis in most hollow structures (bowel, ureterovesical and ureterointestinal transplants, vascular surgery), the success of the closure depends, to a great extent, upon the approximation of the internal lining of the structure. Strive to approximate mucosa to mucosa, with your sutures passing in the submucosa in the closure of a bladder fistula.

22. Close the bladder and vaginal walls in different planes so that as little as possible of one suture line is superimposed on the other. The exception to this principle is a situation where such a closure would cause undue tension. The direction of retraction of the edges of the fistula may necessitate closure in the same plane to avoid tension, and this is more important than superimposition of the suture lines.

23. Do not neglect the use of the cystourethroscope during the course of an operation. It is invaluable in determining the proper eversion of healthy tissue and mucosa-to-mucosa approximation within the bladder.

24. A vaginal cystotomy through healthy tissue will close spontaneously after the catheter is removed and is the ideal type of dependent drainage. This is true for most fistulas except those involving the posterior part of the bladder base. A urethral catheter is satisfactory for fistulas in the base, provided it does not lay on the suture line. A suprapubic cystotomy is used after an abdominal approach to some fistulas or a combined approach.

25. Postoperatively the urinary tract is kept free of infection by the use of an effective urinary antiseptic or a combination of drugs. The patient's nutrition is important, and appropriate electrolyte studies are done as indicated. Patients should be mobilized immediately and careful attention paid to the avoidance of straining at stool, coughing, or sneezing. Complete immobilization of the patient would seem to add little to the chance of successful closure since the patients still have to strain to evacuate their bowels.

Treatment of Urinary Tract Fistulas

The following techniques are applicable to the late repair of urinary tract fistulas and emphasize the vaginal approach. Each fistula is different and requires careful preoperative planning. Some of the more common fistulas and the methods of repair are described in detail.

Preoperative Care and Anesthesia

A complete urologic study is done in the presence of any urinary tract fistula. The patient's general nutrition is carefully managed so that the best possible circumstances for primary wound healing are provided. If possible, the urinary tract should be free of infection, and prophylactic urinary antiseptics are routinely given prior to surgery. A general or spinal anesthetic is used. Fistula surgery may require considerable time, and this should be considered in the selection of the anesthetic.

OPERATIONS IN THE CLOSURE OF FISTULAS
MULTIPLE-LAYER CLOSURE OF VESICOVAGINAL FISTULA
Steps of the Operation

1. Plate 27, *A,* shows a vesicovaginal fistula in the bladder base that is readily accessible. The ureters are catheterized to identify them in the event that the dissection is extended near the intramural ureter. Four traction sutures are placed about the fistulous tract, and the tissue is grasped by instruments only when absolutely necessary. The scar tissue about the fistulous tract is studied, and the direction of any retraction caused by this tissue is noted (Plate 27, *A*).

2. The scar tissue about the fistula is completely excised (Plate 27, *B*), including that which has formed in the bladder musculature as well as the vaginal wall.

3. By sharp dissection the plane of cleavage between the bladder and vaginal wall is located. Flaps, free of scar tissue, are mobilized for some distance from the fistula (Plate 27, *C*). The mobilization of healthy tissue extends far enough away from the fistulous tract to ensure approximation without tension.

4. The bladder mucosa is inverted toward the interior of the bladder by interrupted sutures of

PLATE 27

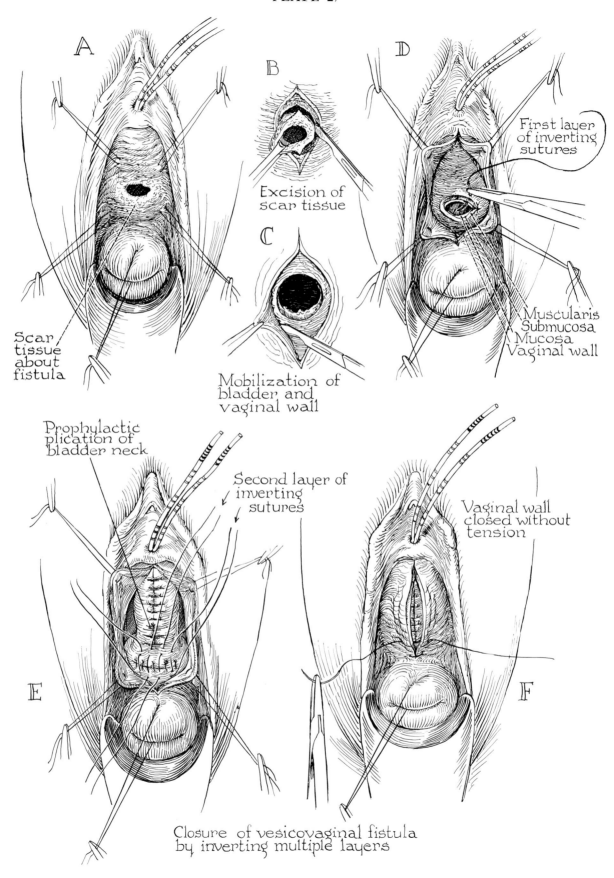

A

B

Excision of scar tissue

C

Mobilization of bladder and vaginal wall

D

First layer of inverting sutures

Muscularis
Submucosa
Mucosa
Vaginal wall

Scar tissue about fistula

Prophylactic plication of bladder neck

Second layer of inverting sutures

Vaginal wall closed without tension

E

F

Closure of vesicovaginal fistula by inverting multiple layers

0000 chromic catgut on atraumatic needles (Plate 27, D). This suture passes through the muscularis of the bladder down to, but not including, the mucosa (Plate 27, D).

5. In Plate 27, E, a second layer of inverting sutures has been placed in the bladder, and when the sutures are tied, the bladder mucosa in the area of the former fistula will be precisely inverted toward the interior.

6. If the fistula is in the bladder base and pre-operative studies have indicated that the patient, after successful closure of the fistula, would have ordinary stress incontinence, a prophylactic plication of the bladder neck is done (Plate 27, E).

7. The vaginal wall is closed with interrupted sutures in the opposite (longitudinal) direction to the closure of the bladder wall (Plate 27, F).

Postoperative Care

The postoperative care as outlined for plastic vaginal surgery applies here. Catheters, regardless of the route of drainage, are left for eight to ten days or longer. Antibiotic therapy is continued for two weeks or more, with substitution of sulfonamides or other antimicrobial agents should resistance appear and a bacteriuria persist. Strict attention is paid to the patient's nutritional requirements for sound wound healing. Immobilization of the patient is advised by some surgeons, but it would seem the resulting debility from this would impair healing and offset any advantages gained by bed rest. Except under unusual circumstances, the patient is mobilized early.

PARAVAGINORECTAL DISPLACEMENT INCISION (SCHUCHARDT)
Indications and Surgical Principles

This technique of making the upper vagina accessible for fistula closure or radical surgery has been poorly understood. Many surgeons make a superficial cut in the perineum to permit the introduction of a larger retractor and describe this as the operation originally described by Schuchardt. Correctly performed, a paravaginorectal incision displaces the vagina and rectum to the left (for right-handed operators) and changes the vagina from a tubular structure to a wide-open field of operation.

This incision provides wide exposure of the operative field from the introitus to a point a few centimeters distal to the fistula. It extends posteriorly and laterally along the extensions of the obturator fascia on the levator ani. It is impossible not to cut some of the fibers of the levator muscles that pass posteriorly.

Steps of the Operation

1. Make an incision in the left lateral sulcus of the vagina about 6 cm. above the introitus and carry it down through the full thickness of the vaginal wall. Continue this to the vulva, curving more laterally after the edge of the puborectalis is passed.

2. At the mucocutaneous junction the incision is continued in a half circle about the anus to the midline posteriorly. It should clear the anus by at least 3 cm. in order to avoid any fibers of the external sphincter ani muscle (Plate 28, A).

3. The incision is now carried deeper along the lateral wall of the rectum. Bleeding points from the inferior and middle hemorrhoidal vessels will be numerous and require ligation. The extension of the incision to the deeper layers in the perineum will cut the superficial and deep layers of the urogenital diaphragm, and the anal, deep and superficial transverse perineal branches of the pudendal artery, vein, and nerve.

4. Deaver retractors are placed on either side to further expose the vaginal vault. The rectum and vagina tend to fall caudad from loss of support and in this way bring the vaginal vault closer to the operator (Plate 28, C).

5. The incision (after completion of the fistula repair) is closed in layers, using 00 chromic catgut (Plate 28, F). Dead space is avoided particularly where the incision has opened up the ischiorectal fossa.

Postoperative Care

The postoperative care is the same as that described under Anterior and Posterior Repair (page 120).

VAULT OBLITERATION OPERATION (LATZKO)
Steps of the Operation

1. A paravaginal rectal displacement incision is performed as previously described.

231

PLATE 28

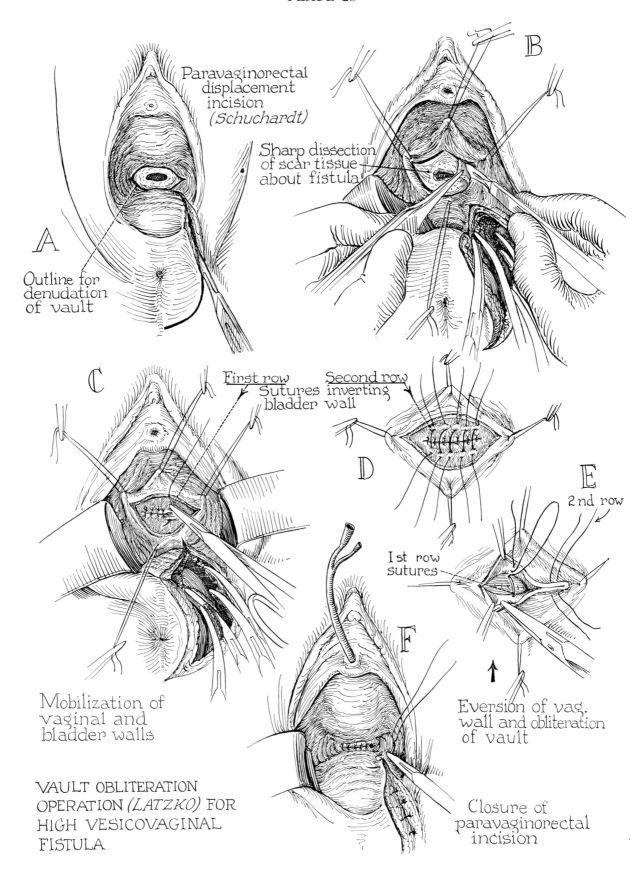

Paravaginorectal
displacement
incision
(Schuchardt)

Sharp dissection
of scar tissue
about fistula

A

Outline for
denudation
of vault

B

C

First row
Sutures inverting
bladder wall

Second row

D

E

2nd row

1st row
sutures

Mobilization of
vaginal and
bladder walls

F

Eversion of vag.
wall and obliteration
of vault

VAULT OBLITERATION
OPERATION *(LATZKO)* FOR
HIGH VESICOVAGINAL
FISTULA

Closure of
paravaginorectal
incision

2. Plate 28, *A*, shows the outline for denudation of the vault about the area of the fistula.

3. The scar tissue about the fistula is completely excised from both the vaginal and bladder walls. This excision should be carried a sufficient distance from the edges of the fistula to ensure removal of all the scar tissue even though it is anticipated that the vault will be shortened (Plate 28, *B*).

4. The vaginal and bladder walls are mobilized for some distance from the fistula. The bladder wall is then inverted toward the interior of the bladder by two rows of sutures of 0000 chromic catgut on atraumatic needles (Plate 28, *C* and *D*).

5. The vaginal vault is partially obliterated by eversion of the vaginal wall toward the vaginal aspect. This is accomplished by two rows of sutures as shown in Plate 28, *E*. These sutures are placed so that broad, healthy surfaces oppose each other as the incision heals.

6. The paravaginorectal incision is closed in layers (Plate 28, *F*).

Postoperative Care

The postoperative care is the same as that described under Multiple-Layer Closure of Vesicovaginal Fistula (page 231).

TRANSVESICAL CLOSURE OF VESICOVAGINAL FISTULA
Indications and Surgical Principles

Vesicovaginal fistulas are closed transvesically when it is necessary to explore carefully the interior of the bladder or, in some instances, the peritoneal cavity. The bladder has a remarkable capacity for healing even after a segmental resection of a large part of the organ. The difficulties of exposing the field of operation by this method, particularly in an obese individual, can be partially overcome by bisecting the bladder in the midline in order to operate on the bladder base. If the bladder wall is healthy, other than at the site of the fistula, the extent to which the bladder is opened has relatively little effect upon healing.

Steps of the Operation

1. A suprapubic cystotomy is performed, amounting to a bisection of the dome of the bladder, part of its anterior wall, and part of the bladder base. Retractors are placed within the bladder and the ureteral orifices identified. Catheters are threaded retrograde for a distance of 8 to 10 cm. above the ureteral orifices (Plate 29, *A*).

2. The scar tissue about the fistulous tract is removed, exposing the full thickness of the vaginal wall and bladder base. The bladder wall is separated from the vaginal wall throughout the circumference of the fistula to permit eversion of the vaginal wall into the vagina (Plate 29, *A*).

3. If possible, the vaginal wall is closed in a longitudinal direction, although this is technically difficult from this aspect. When the vaginal wall can only be closed transversely, as shown in Plate 29, *A*, the bladder wall is closed so the two lines of sutures are in a different transverse plane.

4. The vaginal wall is everted in two layers which permits approximation of wide areas of healthy muscularis of the vagina.

5. The bladder wall is closed in two layers. The second row of sutures further inverts the bladder wall and mucosa toward the interior of the bladder (Plate 29, *B*).

6. The ureteral catheters are removed and the orifices observed for a clear efflux of urine. The cystotomy is closed in two layers with interrupted sutures leaving a cystostomy tube in place.

Postoperative Care

Suprapubic drainage is usual after this type of closure. The postoperative care is otherwise the same as that described under Multiple-Layer Closure of Vesicovaginal Fistula (page 231).

TRANSPERITONEAL APPROACH TO VESICOVAGINAL FISTULAS
Indications and Surgical Principles

An exploratory laparotomy may be indicated in the presence of a high vesicovaginal fistula. A fistula may exist when the surgeon must do other surgery within the pelvis, particularly if there is a malignancy. Such a situation could arise from cancer in any part of the genital tract. The fistula may be closed after the pelvic exploration. In the absence of any indication to explore the abdomen, the transperitoneal approach represents a rather extensive procedure to close a vault fistula that can

PLATE 29

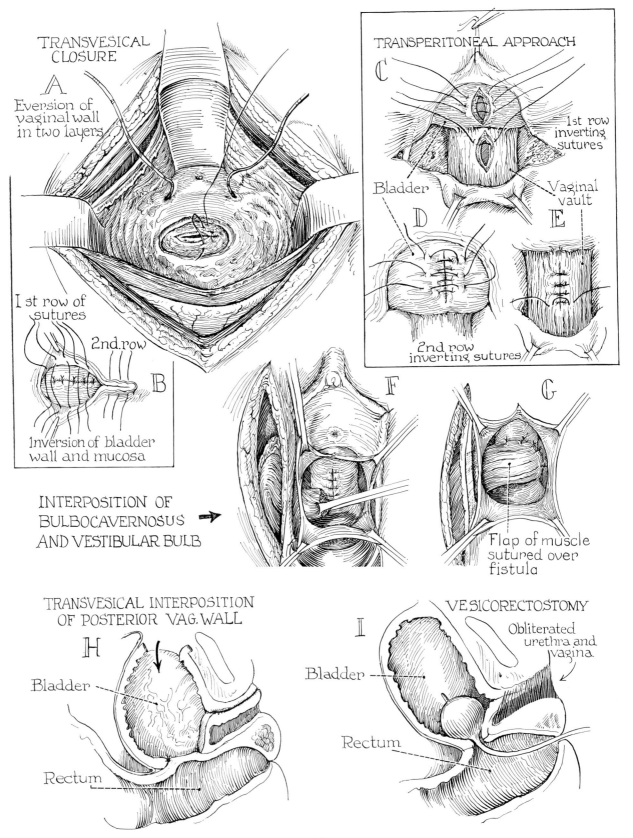

TRANSVESICAL
CLOSURE

A

Eversion of
vaginal wall
in two layers

1st row of
sutures

2nd.row

B

Inversion of bladder
wall and mucosa

TRANSPERITONEAL APPROACH

C

Bladder

1st row
inverting
sutures

Vaginal
vault

D

E

2nd row
inverting sutures

INTERPOSITION OF
BULBOCAVERNOSUS
AND VESTIBULAR BULB

F

G

Flap of muscle
sutured over
fistula

TRANSVESICAL INTERPOSITION
OF POSTERIOR VAG. WALL

H

Bladder

Rectum

VESICORECTOSTOMY

I

Bladder

Rectum

Obliterated
urethra and
vagina

almost always be closed by a rather simple vaginal vault obliteration from below.

Steps of the Operation

1. The vaginal vault and the adjacent, adherent bladder are separated after the fistulous tract has been identified. This dissection in the vesicovaginal septum should continue far enough down so that healthy tissue well beyond the site of the fistula is mobilized (Plate 29, C).

2. Two rows of inverting sutures of fine chromic catgut invert the bladder side of the fistula into the interior of the bladder (Plate 29, C and D).

3. Two rows of sutures are likewise used to invert the muscularis and mucosa of the vagina into the vaginal vault (Plate 29, C and E).

4. Flaps of peritoneum are mobilized both from the bladder and from the adjacent vaginal vault, and these are closed together to form a new vesicovaginal reflection of peritoneum well below the site of the old fistulous tract.

Postoperative Care

The postoperative care is the same as that described under Multiple-Layer Closure of Vesicovaginal Fistula (page 231).

INTERPOSITION OF BULBOCAVERNOSUS IN A FISTULA REPAIR
Indications and Surgical Principles

The interposition of the bulbocavernosus and part of the vestibular bulb can be utilized to improve the blood supply in the area of a fistula closure. The muscle itself has been interposed between the bladder and vaginal wall to actually form a bridge of tissue across the fistula when sufficient healthy tissue cannot be mobilized to close the tract. The interposition of the bulbocavernosus has also been used to elevate the bladder neck and increase the posterior urethrovesical angle for the cure of urinary stress incontinence.

Steps of the Operation

1. The scar tissue about the fistula is completely excised, and flaps of the full thickness of the vaginal wall are mobilized from the bladder.

2. If the fistula is not too large, it is possible to close the fistula in at least one layer. Should the area of closure appear ischemic and devitalized, the bulbocavernosus may be sutured over the closure in an effort to improve the blood supply (Plate 29, F).

3. A lateral incision over the labia majora is made, and the bulbocavernosus and part of the vestibular bulb are mobilized, with care being exercised not to disturb the blood supply of the bulbocavernosus, which comes from the deep perineal branch of the external pudendal artery. This approaches the muscle near its point of origin, so care should be exercised not to disturb the major vessels. The vaginal wall is mobilized further on the lateral edge of the incision, and finally the anterolateral wall is dissected free along the upper portion of the descending pubic rami. A canal is formed behind the labia majora and vaginal wall, through which the bulbocavernosus can be drawn (Plate 29, F).

4. The bulbocavernosus is detached anteriorly and the free edge observed for viability. The muscle is sutured across the area of the fistula or to the periosteum of the opposite pubic ramus (Plate 29, G).

5. The full thickness of the vaginal wall is closed by interrupted sutures. The incision in the labia majora is likewise closed, and the skin edges are everted by interrupted sutures.

Postoperative Care

The postoperative care is the same as that described under Multiple-Layer Closure of Vesicovaginal Fistula (page 231).

TRANSVESICAL INTERPOSITION OF POSTERIOR VAGINAL WALL
Indications and Surgical Principles

This operation, which amounts to a partial vaginal obliteration, may be done from the abdominal aspect as a palliative procedure when it is necessary to explore the interior of the bladder or the pelvis. The patients encountered in a gynecologic practice who would require such a procedure would have had some type of radical surgery, and usually the cervix and fundus of the uterus are absent. The principle of the operation is to obliterate a portion of the vagina, bringing the posterior vaginal wall up to form a new bladder base.

Steps of the Operation

1. A suprapubic cystotomy is performed and the base of the bladder widely exposed (Plate 29, H).

2. The edges of the fistula are dissected of scar tissue in so far as possible and are mobilized sufficiently to permit the placing of sutures throughout the circumference of the defect.

3. An area on the posterior vaginal wall as seen transvesically is outlined and then denuded of vaginal epithelium. It may be possible to leave a small center of vaginal mucous membrane in the area that is to be utilized as a new bladder base. In Plate 29, *H,* is diagrammed the method of suturing the edges of the fistulous tract to the area outlined in the posterior vaginal wall. Care is exercised not to have the sutures pass into the rectum during the closure.

Postoperative Care

The postoperative care is the same as that described under Multiple-Layer Closure of Vesicovaginal Fistula (page 231).

VESICORECTOSTOMY FOR URINARY CONTROL
Indications and Surgical Principles

Vesicorectostomy for urinary incontinence not amenable to correction by any other means short of urinary tract diversion is not applicable to the female with the uterus and cervix present. A cloaca can be created by performing a colpocleisis or complete obliteration of the vaginal opening and then creating a fistula from the bladder, through the vaginal wall, into the rectum. Gynecologists have resorted to this, on rare occasions, for many years. The operation would also be possible by performing a hysterectomy and then approximating the bladder base to the rectum and creating a fistula. General urologists recommend this procedure in the male for complete incontinence due to inadequacy of the bladder neck, urethral carcinoma, severe stricture, exstrophy of the bladder, intractable Hunner's ulcer, tuberculous cystitis, and after radical prostatectomy with total urinary incontinence.

Steps of the Operation

1. A Kelly clamp or similar instrument is inserted through the anus and made to impinge on the posterior vaginal wall opposite the bladder base. An incision about 2 cm. long is made through the full thickness of the posterior vaginal and rectal walls.

2. If, as is usually the situation, the major part of the bladder base is destroyed, a retention catheter is introduced through the rectum into the bladder (Plate 29, *I*). Should the fistula be in the trigone or farther forward, a new opening is created in the bladder base to shunt the urine into the rectal ampulla.

3. A total colpocleisis is performed. The terminal urethra is excised and the resected end closed with several sutures. The labia minora and mucous membrane of the vestibule are denuded and approximated with interrupted sutures to complete the obliteration.

Postoperative Care

Measures previously described for postoperative care in Multiple-Layer Closure of Vesicovaginal Fistula (page 231) are instituted. The retention catheter is left in position for ten days until the colpocleisis is healed and the fistulous tract into the rectum well established. Careful attention is directed to fluid and electrolyte balance as with any operation that diverts urine into the bowel.

GRACILIS INTERPOSITION OPERATION
Surgical Anatomy of the Gracilis Muscle

The gracilis is a long, flat muscle that is the most medial of the adductors of the thigh. The fact that its upper portion is wide and flat, with an abundant blood supply, together with its proximity to the vagina, make it ideal for inclusion in plastic procedures for the cure of fistulas. It arises from the medial margin of the body and ramus of the pubis by a thin, broad tendon about 6 cm. in width. It becomes more round in the lower thigh and terminates in a round tendon, which passes behind the medial condyle of the femur, over the internal lateral ligament of the knee joint, and between the tendons of the semitendinosus and sartorius, to be inserted into the proximal part of the medial aspect of the shaft of the tibia below the medial tuberosity. The long saphenous nerve passes between the tendons of the gracilis and sartorius. Loss of the gracilis as an adductor of the thigh and flexor of the knee is of no importance, since the remaining muscles of the adductor group are more than adequate. (Plate 30, *B.*)

The gracilis receives its blood supply from the anterior branch of the obturator artery. The obturator artery enters the thigh through the upper part of the obturator foramen beneath the obturator nerve. It divides into two branches, an anterior and posterior, that encircle the foramen under cover of the obturator externus. The obturator artery has a liberal anastomosis with the medial circumflex and inferior gluteal arteries. (Plate 30, *B*.)

The obturator nerve supplies the gracilis, and its fibers are from the second, third, and fourth lumbar nerves. It leaves the pelvis, in company with the obturator vessels but lying above them, through the obturator foramen. Like the artery, it divides into anterior and posterior branches. The anterior branch descends in front of the obturator externus and adductor brevis and beneath the pectineus and adductor longus. It communicates with the medial cutaneous and long saphenous nerves to form the subsartorial plexus. Fibers from the anterior branch supply the gracilis.

Indications and Surgical Principles

When the leg is abducted in the lithotomy position, it renders the gracilis tense and easier of dissection. The nerve and blood supply of the muscle must be kept intact, or the interposed muscle will slough and the purpose of the operation fail. The difference in retractility of various structures must therefore be kept in mind. Muscles unattached to the shaft of a long bone, such as the gracilis, will retract strongly. Nerves retract very little and may swell into bulbous and sensitive ends. Arteries are highly retractile, but their accompanying veins are less so.

The adductor longus is a good landmark in locating the gracilis as well as being used in differentiating a femoral from an inguinal hernia. The adductor longus is superficial and arises from the front of the body of the pubis below the crest. When the leg is abducted strongly in the lithotomy position, the tendon of origin of the adductor longus can be distinctly felt. It orients the surgeon to the pubic tubercle and the bulge of a hernia. An in-guinal hernia will be to the medial side of the muscle and a femoral hernia to the lateral side of the tendon of the adductor longus, while the tendon of origin of the gracilis is medial and just adjacent to the origin of the adductor longus. (Plate 30, *E*.) The adductor longus could be used in this operation if technical difficulties arose in which the nerve and blood supply of the gracilis were compromised. Between the adductor longus and the sartorius and superficial to the fascia lata is the great saphenous vein. Deeper in the same plane, in Hunter's canal, are the femoral artery, vein, and nerve.

The most important point in this operation is the location of the anterior branches of the obturator artery, vein, and nerve. If these are compromised, the adductor longus or another substitute must be used to complete the procedure. The surgeon should review the cross-sectional anatomy of the leg from the head of the femur beyond Hunter's canal. The anterior branches of the obturator artery, vein, and nerve pass medial to the pectineus at a level just below the lesser trochanter. They then emerge between the adductor longus and brevis and communicate with the internal (medial) cutaneous and long saphenous (saphenous) vessels and nerves. About 10 cm. distal to the tendon of origin of the gracilis the belly of this muscle should be retracted medially and the belly of the adductor longus retracted laterally, both with utmost care. The anterior branches of the obturator artery, vein, and nerve will emerge between the muscles and pass obliquely to the gracilis. The transplantation of muscle tissue without its original nerve and blood supply ends in necrosis and replacement of the transplant with fibrous tissue. In the repair of fistulas, as everyone knows, we have enough of this to deal with at the start of the operation. However, if the blood and nerve supply of a muscle is intact, it is a most useful structure to provide blood supply, restore contour, reinforce other muscles, check bleeding, and, in the case of the gracilis, give contour to the bladder neck. A muscle flap must be treated very carefully, but it has a wide field of usefulness in all types of reconstructive surgery.

Few appreciate that the orifice of the obturator canal can be palpated through the vagina. Were a rare obturator hernia to be found, it would present beneath the pectineus muscle, to the inner side of the capsule of the hip, behind and to the inner side of the femoral vessels, and to the outer side of the adductor longus tendon. To do the gracilis interposition operation, an obturator hernia must be created, although in the lower or caudad part of the membrane near the ischial tuberosity. It has to be made large enough to permit the passage of the belly of the gracilis without constricting the muscle. The surgeon, obviously, must not compromise the obturator artery, vein, and nerve during the preparation of the tract for the muscle transplant. Despite the descriptions of the membrane as a thin, interlacing complex of fibers, it is difficult to rupture with the finger to perform this operation. (Plate 30, C to E.)

From the point of deflection of the gracilis with its nerve and blood supply to the implantation of its substance in the anterior vaginal wall between vagina and bladder is some distance. The route is as follows, and the vital structures to be preserved are noted: The caudad segment of the obturator membrane is to be perforated to allow the passage of the belly of the gracilis. To do this, the exploring finger dissects on the medial side of the gracilis and between the adductor brevis and magnus. When the obturator membrane is reached, the belly of the obturator externus may be palpated and the dissecting finger should go below this. It may be difficult to avoid rupturing some vessels of the posterior division of the obturators and some branches from the internal circumflex vessels in the blunt dissection, but the gracilis will be drawn through the area, and a muscle transplant is the hemostatic par excellence. Part of the obturator internus arises from the inner surface of the obturator membrane but not many fibers from the posterior part that forms the canal to admit the obturator membrane. Most of its fibers originating on the obturator membrane arise from the tendinous arch that comprises the obturator canal. The pudendal artery crosses the spine of the ischium under the sacrospinous ligament and re-enters the pelvis on the outside of the ischiorectal fossa and on the surface of the obturator internus. The muscular branches to the levator ani, obturator internus, piriformis, and coccygeus may be fractured in opening the obturator membrane. This, as well as rupture of the inferior hemorrhoidal, is unavoidable. The main vessels, in Alcock's canal, are quite well protected by these extensions of the obturator fascia making up this canal and usually escape damage. Since the pudendal artery contributes to the blood supply of the vagina and urethra, its preservation is desirable. There now remains to avoid the origins of the levator ani (specifically the puborectalis) that also arise from the pubis and obturator membrane. This is seldom a problem since they have usually been sclerosed, scarred, or otherwise rendered useless by the process that necessitates the surgery.

When the route of the muscle flap has been determined, it remains for the surgeon to pass the viable muscle through the above structures. A large aneurysm needle, with a suture in the distal tendon of the gracilis, is quite useful in drawing the muscle between bladder and vagina. The surgeon will frequently improvise his own method and selection of instruments for lysing the obturator membrane through which the gracilis muscle is drawn. A double-curved kidney clamp is a useful instrument to have available. A finger knife would facilitate enlargement of the rent through the obturator membrane which must be opened widely so that the muscle is not constricted. It should not be forcefully positioned, placed with any constrictions, or sutured where the stitches cut through viable muscle. The angle at which the muscle is reversed in direction to enter the vagina should not be acute and constrict the blood supply and nerve. This is regulated by a piece of rubber dam at this critical point so the muscle is not inadvertently traumatized or stretched at the source of its blood supply. (Plate 30, C).

The general principles of fistula surgery—viable, fresh edges for approximation, liberal dissection to avoid tension of the suture lines, and the use of fine, atraumatic, catgut—apply here in every particular. Since the interposition of the muscle is done to supply blood to tissue with an inadequate supply, it is important to excise every fragment of scar tissue from the edges of the fistulous tract. Excision of scar tissue may enlarge the opening, but, if it removes scarred edges, the size of the fistula is unimportant.

Frequently, the decision to use a new source of blood supply at the site of the fistula will be determined at the time of operation. The operator will have excised the fistulous tract. He then begins to mobilize layers to approximate viable tissue to viable tissue but finds that he is cutting through avascular scar tissue that cuts like plaster board and bleeds little. The patient should have signed an informed operative permit since the leg incision to mobilize the gracilis is the length of the thigh. This should have been explained in detail. The patient should also be told that, if in the judgment of the surgeon the closure shows a good chance for success without a transplant, the muscle will not be used.

Steps of the Operation

1. The medial aspect of either the right or left leg is prepared and draped from the genitocrural fold to the region of the medial epicondyle of the knee. The vagina and vulva are prepared and draped. The preparation of the vaginal flaps about the fistula may be done in the knee-chest position and the patient turned around for the gracilis transplant. It is awkward to attempt to mobilize the gracilis in the knee-chest position. If exposure is adequate, the entire procedure is better done in the dorsal lithotomy position. The sketches accompanying this description were drawn in the dorsal lithotomy position, and the right gracilis was transplanted.

2. The edges of the fistula are denuded of all scar tissue, and the natural line of cleavage between the bladder and anterior vaginal wall is entered when reasonably normal tissue is found some distance from the fistula. Continue the dissection farther until the bladder is freely mobilized and until the edges of the fistula will come together without tension. With large fistulas this may not be possible, and the transplanted muscle will be used to fill the gap. If the edges will come together, they are loosely approximated with interrupted sutures of 0000 atraumatic, chromic catgut. No attempt should be made to close the fistula in several layers, which adds a lot of suture material in the wound. The area of the fistula is then avoided and protected from trauma and pressure during the rest of the operation. (Plate 30, A.)

3. If the fistula is at the bladder neck, trigone, or adjacent bladder base, the patient should be drained by a vaginal cystotomy as illustrated in Plate 30, A. A fistula in the bladder base may be drained by an indwelling catheter as long as it does not cause pressure on the edges of the wound or muscle transplant. A suprapubic cystotomy is preferable to an indwelling urethral catheter and can be done as a preliminary operation or at the time of the gracilis transplant procedure.

4. The medial epicondyle of the femur is then palpated and an incision made through the skin and subcutaneous tela from here to a point on the descending ramus of the pubis and 2 cm. below the inferior border of the symphysis (Plate 30, B). The fascia lata is then split along the course of the incision to within a few centimeters of the knee, where it thickens and sends fibers into the joint capsule. The fascia lata is then dissected laterally and medially, exposing the gracilis, adductor longus, and, medial to the gracilis, the edge of the adductor magnus.

5. The success of the transplant depends on the next maneuver. Retract the fascia lata laterally about 12 cm. distal from the origin of the gracilis muscle. Gently lift up its lateral edge and look for the anterior branch of the obturator artery, vein, and nerve. It will be seen entering the lateral edge of the muscle together with some connective tissue extensions of the muscle sheath. In some patients the vessels are located by retracting the lateral edge of the gracilis medially. This is best done with a vein retractor, and once the bundle of vessels and nerve are located, the area must be carefully protected.

6. To protect the blood and nerve supply, a rubber dam is sutured across the point of entrance of the vessels and attached to skin or adjacent muscle. During the ensuing phase of the operation, the blood and nerve supply can be compromised as the surgeon draws the muscle through the obturator foramen and under the bladder. The rubber dam serves as a landmark and prevents traction on the vessels (Plate 30, C).

PLATE 30

Gracilis

Adductor longus

B

Adductor brevis

A

Adductor magnus

Artery and vein

Br. of obturator n.

C

Rubber dam to protect a.,v.,and n.

PLATE 30 (Concluded)

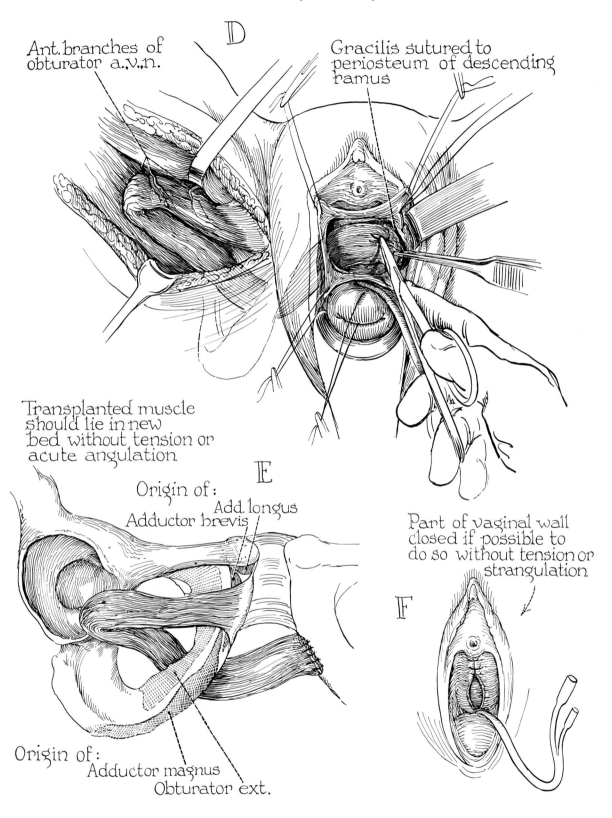

D

Ant. branches of
obturator a.,v.,n.

Gracilis sutured to
periosteum of descending
ramus

Transplanted muscle
should lie in new
bed without tension or
acute angulation

E

Origin of:
Add. longus
Adductor brevis

Origin of:
Adductor magnus
Obturator ext.

Part of vaginal wall
closed if possible to
do so without tension or
strangulation

F

7. The gracilis is now dissected free from the other muscles of the adductor group to a point where its tendon is overlapped by the tendon of the sartorius. This portion of tendon is useful in passing the muscle through the obturator space but is later resected almost down to the belly of the muscle since the latter is the part that has an abundant blood supply. The distal portion of the muscle is bathed in wet gauze while the path for its transplantation between bladder and vaginal wall is being prepared.

8. The index finger is now inserted between the medial edge of the gracilis and the medial edge of the adductor magnus that lies behind and at a deeper level. Direct the dissecting finger posteriorly between the adductor magnus and the adductor brevis, which is anterior to the adductor magnus. This may avoid injuring the posterior branches of the obturator artery, vein, and nerve. The index finger of the other hand is then inserted between the bladder and vaginal wall and directed laterally until the most caudad edge of the obturator membrane is felt. The finger dissecting from the thigh then separates some of the fibers of the obturator externus to meet the vaginal finger, with the obturator membrane interposed between them. The finger in the vagina will rupture some of the fibers of the levator ani and obturator internus in this dissection.

9. A long, curved Kelly clamp is then passed along the index finger, dissecting from the thigh until the tip reaches the most caudad part of the obturator membrane. The clamp is then forced through the membrane and opened to make a passageway of sufficient size to admit the belly of the gracilis. It is important to make the opening adequate so the edges do not necrose the muscle or constrict its blood supply.

10. A silk traction suture is then inserted in the tendon of the gracilis. A large curved clamp or large aneurysm needle is passed from the vaginal aspect, through the rent in the obturator membrane, and between the muscles, to emerge medial to the gracilis and a few centimeters from its origin. The traction suture is then drawn through this pathway and out the vagina. A clamp then grasps the tendon of the gracilis, and by a combination of pushing with the clamp and traction on the suture, the muscle is inserted through the obturator fossa and between the bladder and vaginal wall to the opposite descending ramus of the pubis (Plate 30, D). This must be accomplished without tension or angulation of the blood and nerve supply of the muscle (Plate 30, E). Since the detached distal end of the muscle retracts, it frequently seems that there is not enough muscle to reach across the vagina. This is not the case, and one finds ample length to span even the widest pubic arch.

11. The viable ends of the muscle or tendon that have not been disturbed by traction suture or clamp are then sutured to the inner aspect of the opposite descending ramus of the pubis. These sutures pass through the remains of the attachment of the levator ani and the extensions of the obturator fascia that once formed the inferior layer of the urogenital diaphragm that in these patients has long since lost its identity. The muscle should now lie between the bladder and vaginal wall without tension and should cover the fistula. With large fistulas the muscle will present into the interior of the bladder and with a successful transplant soon become covered with bladder mucosa (Plate 30, F).

12. If the vaginal wall can be closed without tension, this is done with interrupted sutures of 00 chromic catgut, tied to provide approximation without strangulation. Should the anterior vaginal wall be so deficient that approximation is not feasible without tension, the edges should be sutured to the muscle graft in a few places to eliminate dead space, but again the sutures should be few and far between and not tied tightly (Plate 30, F). The vagina should not be packed, nor should petroleum jelly gauze or other foreign bodies be placed against the suture lines to impede vascularization and healing.

13. The leg incision is closed in layers with fine and medium silk sutures.

Postoperative Care

Measures previously described for postoperative care in Multiple-Layer Closure of Vesicovaginal Fistula (page 231) are instituted. Regardless of the site of bladder drainage, the indwelling catheter is left in position for ten days or longer, depending on the appearance of the vaginal wound. Sutures are removed from the leg incision on the seventh postoperative day. There is no contraindication to early mobilization of the patient.

References

Babcock, W.: The Operative Treatment of Vesicovaginal and Related Fistulas, South. Surgeon 8: 34, 1939.
Benson, R., and Hinman, F.: Urinary Tract Injuries in Obstetrics and Gynecology, Am. J. Obst. & Gynec. 70: 467, 1955.
Collins, C. G., Pent, D., and Jones, F. B.: Results of Early

Repair of Vesicovaginal Fistula With Preliminary Cortisone Treatment, Am. J. Obst. & Gynec. 80: 1005, 1960.

Counseller, V.: Surgical and Postoperative Treatment of Vesicovaginal and Rectovaginal Fistulas, Surg., Gynec. & Obst. 74: 738, 1942.

Counseller, V.: Etiology, Prevention and Treatment of Vesicovaginal Fistula, South. Surgeon 13: 752, 1947.

Deming, C. L.: Transplantation of the Gracilis Muscle for Incontinence of Urine, J. A. M. A. 86: 822, 1926.

Emmett, T.: Vesico-vaginal Fistula From Parturition and Other Causes; With Cases of Recto-vaginal Fistula, New York, 1868, W. Wood & Co.

Everett, H. S., and Mattingly, R. F.: Vesicovaginal Fistula, Am. J. Obst. & Gynec. 72: 712, 1956.

Falk, H. C.: Inoperable Vesicovaginal Fistula, Obst. & Gynec. 15: 646, 1960.

Falk, H. C.: Vesical Fistula After Cesarean Section, Obst. & Gynec. 15: 492, 1960.

Falk, H. C., and Tancer, M. L.: Loss of the Urethra, Obst. & Gynec. 9: 458, 1957.

Foda, M. S.: Evaluation of Methods of Treatment of Urinary Fistulae in Women; a Report of 220 Cases, J. Obst. & Gynaec. Brit. Emp. 66: 372, 1959.

Frith, K.: Diverticulum of the Female Urethra; Report of Two Cases With Review of the Literature, J. Obst. & Gynaec. Brit. Emp. 67: 314, 1960.

Goodwin, W. E., Turner, R. D., and Winter, C. C.: Rectourinary Fistula: Principles of Management and a Technique of Surgical Closure, J. Urol. 80: 246, 1958.

Goodwin, W. E., Winter, C. C., and Turner, R. D.: Fistula Between Bowel and Urinary Tract, J. Urol. 84: 95, 1960.

Hewett, A. L., and Headstream, J. W.: Pericystitis Plastica, J. Urol. 83: 103, 1960.

Ingelman-Sundberg, A.: The Treatment of Uterine or Vaginal Recurrence of Cancer of the Cervix. Repair of Vesicovaginal and Rectovaginal Fistulas Following Fulguration of Recurrent Cancer of the Cervix After Radiation. In Meigs, J. V.: Surgical Treatment of Cancer of the Cervix, New York, 1954, Grune & Stratton, Inc.

Kelly, H.: The History of Vesico-vaginal Fistula, Tr. Am. Gynec. Soc. 31: 225, 1906.

McClausland, A. M., and others: A Comparative Study of Vesicovaginal Fistulas Following Delivery, Am. J. Obst. & Gynec. 79: 1110, 1960.

Mackenrodt, A.: Die operative Heilung grosser Blasenscheidenfisteln, Zentralbl. Gynäk. 18: 180, 1904.

Mahfouz, N.: Urinary Fistulas in Women, J. Obst. & Gynaec. Brit. Emp. 64: 23, 1957.

Martius, H.: Operation of Urinary Fistula, Deutsche med. Wchnschr. 64: 269, 1938.

Milbert, A.: Urovaginal Fistula; a New Device for Effective Control of Urinary Incontinence, Obst. & Gynec. 16: 743, 1960.

Moir, J.: Vesicovaginal Fistulas, Lancet 1: 57, 1954.

Noszkay, A.: Experience With the Surgical Treatment of Vesicovaginal Fistula (Erfahrungen mit der Operation der Blasenscheidenfistel) Ztschr. urol. 51: 206, 1958.

Pec, J.: The Treatment of Vesicovaginal Fistula (Beitrag zur Behandlung der Blasenscheidenfistel), Ztschr. urol. 51: 236, 1958.

Phaneuf, L., and Graves, R.: Vesicovaginal Fistula and Its Management, Surg., Gynec. & Obst. 88: 155, 1949.

Roen, P. R.: Combined Vaginal and Transvesical Approach in Successful Repair of Vesicovaginal Fistula, A. M. A. Arch. Surg. 80: 628, 1960.

Russell, C. S.: Urinary Fistulas and Their Management, J. Obst. & Gynaec. Brit. Emp. 63: 481, 1956.

Schuchardt, K.: Weitere Erfahrungen über die paravaginale Operation, Arch. klin. Chir. 53: 473, 1896.

Shaw, W.: The Martius Bulbo-cavernosus Interposition Operation, Brit. M. J. 2: 1251, 1949.

Sims, J.: On the Treatment of Vesicovaginal Fistula, Am. J. M. Sc. 23: 59, 1852.

Ward, G.: The Operative Treatment of Inaccessible Vesicovaginal Fistulae, Surg., Gynec. & Obst. 11: 22, 1910.

Ward, G.: The Repair of Inaccessible Vesico-vaginal Fistulae Following Hysterectomy, Surg., Gynec. & Obst. 11: 22, 1910.

Ward, G.: The Operative Technique Employed in the Closure of an Extensive Vesico-vaginal Fistula, Surg., Gynec. & Obst. 33: 150, 1921.

Ward, G.: Reconstruction of Urethra After Complete Loss, Complicating an Extensive Vesico-vaginal Fistula, Surg., Gynec. & Obst. 37: 678, 1923.

Ward, G.: Experiences in the Treatment of Some Difficult Urinary Fistulae, Urol. & Cutan. Rev. 48: 66, 1944.

Zimmerman, I. J., Precourt, W. E., and Thompson, C. C.: Direct Uretero-cysto-neostomy With the Short Ureter in the Cure of Ureterovaginal Fistula, J. Urol. 83: 113, 1960.

12 · Regional Bladder and Ureteral Surgery in Gynecology

MINOR SURGICAL CONDITIONS OF THE URETHRA
CHRONIC ANTERIOR URETHRITIS AND SKENEITIS

The anterior urethra contains several large glands commonly known as Skene's glands. In addition, there are many small glands that are involved in the inflammatory diseases of the urethra. Either occlusion of the ducts of the larger glands or pinching off of the intra-urethral ducts may result in a chronic urethritis. While relatively innocuous, minor pathology gives rise to a disproportionate volume of symptoms. Since the anterior structures of the female introitus, the clitoris and urethra, are exceedingly sensitive in the healthy state, minimal abnormalities may give rise to distressing symptoms. A simple anterior urethritis may cause nocturia, urgency-frequency, hesitancy, dysuria, overflow incontinence, a bearing-down sensation in the lower abdomen, and suprapubic pain—all this despite the insignificance of the lesion. Palpation of the urethra reveals pain on pressure, especially when it is compressed against the inferior border of the symphysis. Purulent material is expressed from the infected glands and cultured. Urethroscopy is done to determine the extent of the inflammation. The orifices of infected glands are probed and the number and depth of the lesions determined. Specific therapy is started prior to fulguration or excision. Rarely a gonococcus will turn up in the cultures of patients with a chronic condition and surgery is deferred. Under Pentothal sodium anesthesia the glands are individually destroyed with a needle and cutting current. An alternative procedure is the excision of the terminal urethra and infected tissue.

URETHRAL CARUNCLE

Urethral caruncles result from retraction of the mucous membranes of the vestibule and eversion of the mucous membrane of the urethra about the posterior lip of the meatus. This is a normal occurrence coincident with atrophic changes about the external genitalia after the menopause. The majority of the caruncles are asymptomatic and do not require treatment. Some become sessile or pedunculated and cause painful micturition or dyspareunia. They may be very vascular and bleed profusely if traumatized. Many of these can be cured by several applications of silver nitrate, 10 per cent, at two-week intervals. The patient applies an estogenic cream to the meatus and intravaginally twice daily between office visits. An occasional pedunculated caruncle has to be excised by cautery of knife.

PROLAPSE OF THE URETHRAL MUCOUS MEMBRANE

Prolapse of the urethral mucous membrane occurs in elderly women with chronic coughs or other conditions which cause increased intra-abdominal pressure. It is seen in children following severe episodes of coughing. The mucous membrane prolapses throughout the entire circumference of the external meatus and becomes edematous and congested, resembling a raspberry. Segments may become infarcted and cause severe pain. Urinary reten-

244

tion is not uncommon if the condition is neglected. The condition requires immediate attention and surgery. A small catheter is passed to relieve the distention. A circular incision is made proximal to the lesion, preserving as much healthy mucous membrane of the vestibule as possible. The distal one third of the urethra can be amputated, if necessary, without disturbing urinary control. The lesion is amputated in guillotine fashion. Fine, atraumatic, on-end mattress sutures are used to close the edges. The sutures invert the squamous epithelium of the vestibule toward the lumen of the urethra and decrease the caliber of the external meatus so as to prevent recurrence.

THE URGENCY-FREQUENCY SYNDROME

The urgency-frequency syndrome represents a female urologic condition in which, more than in any other problem, the degree of disturbance of function is grossly out of proportion to the demonstrable pathology. Pages have been written on the psychosomatic etiology of ulcers, colitis, eczema, and seborrhea, but the psychosomatic aspects of the urgency-frequency syndrome of the female bladder have had scant study. The sequence of events in urination suggests the psychic influences to which the bladder is subjected. The impulse to urinate, after initiation by contraction of the abdominal muscles and an indirect increase in intravesical pressure, is followed by a contraction of the detrusor (or bladder as a whole), which is under sympathetic and parasympathetic innervation. Certainly any organ that is so sensitive in its reaction must also be the site of subjective symptoms of psychic influences. The blood vessels about the proximal one third of the urethra probably react to psychic stimuli, and their role in continence and incontinence is yet to be determined. Frequency of urination and dribbling are common accompaniments of anxiety. It is most revealing to observe the number of women seeking relief for the urgency-frequency syndrome in a female urology clinic in whom little or nothing is seen on cystoscopy. But, in the same clinic, patients with cervical malignancies who have

had a course of radiation (with its inevitable bladder effects) are so preoccupied with their known or suspected malignant disease that they seldom complain of minor urinary symptoms. What happens to the close relation between sexuality and micturition in a patient afflicted with a disease that intimately involves the bladder? The importance of micturition in infantile sex behavior, if carried into adult life, certainly seems to disappear when the patient is threatened with a fatal disease.

Certain characteristics are seen in patients with urgency incontinence. There is a tendency to hypochondria and preoccupation with health that centers on the bladder. These patients may be depressed, are easily fatigued, and appear to hold the unconscious belief that they have some secret malady for which magic medicine is required. Observing these patients over a period of years, one becomes impressed with how often the severity of their symptoms parallels traumatic events in their lives.

The organic lesion associated with the urgency-frequency syndrome is chronic nonspecific urethrotrigonitis. The diagnosis is made from the patient's medical history since cystoscopy rarely reveals any lesions not seen in many patients who have no symptoms. Medical treatment is at best a form of nonspecific psychotherapy. The urethra is dilated to admit a No. 28 Fr. or No. 8 Hegar dilator. Two per cent Xylocaine jelly may be used as a lubricant for the dilators. Silver nitrate up to 1:500 dilution is instilled, starting with 30 ml. of a 1:5,000 solution and increasing the strength at weekly treatments. Drugs such as Pro-Banthine, 15 mg. every six hours, or Daricon, 10 mg. at the same intervals, may have some effect in relaxing the bladder musculature. Fulguration of the trigone and posterior one third of the urethra is successful in helping some patients.

Patients with the mild urgency-frequency syndrome who do not have organic disease that limits the bladder capacity should be sharply distinguished from those with a secondarily contracted bladder and overflow incontinence of a severe degree. The latter are crippled by their disease whether caused by specific, nonspecific, or iatrogenic factors. These patients require extensive urologic study, may require extensive surgery, may require diversion of the urinary stream, or may be distined to live with their almost intolerable affliction. These patients and their management are discussed in Chapter 10.

CHRONIC INTERSTITIAL CYSTITIS (HUNNER'S ULCER)

Interstitial cystitis consists of an inflammatory reaction in the muscularis of the bladder. Small areas are infiltrated with round cells and later sclerose and contract, causing superficial ulcers in the mucous membrane that may bleed when the bladder is distended. The etiology is unknown. The disease has become so extensive in rare instances that diversion of the urinary stream is necessary. The symptoms are marked urgency and frequency, suprapubic pain, and marked burning at the end of urination. The diagnosis is made on cystoscopy by noting the small contracted areas and limited bladder capacity. In the mild cases treatment consists of dilatations and instillations together with the administration of drugs to relax the bladder musculature. Pro-Banthine, 15 mg. every six hours, is used for this purpose. Cortisone has been used with some improvement in the severe cases. Surgical treatment consists of fulguration of the ulcerated areas. One per cent procaine and hyaluronidase can be injected into the bladder wall of the involved areas. Treatment is generally unsatisfactory.

OTHER RARE LESIONS OF THE URETHRA

Several rare lesions of the urethra may be encountered if urethroscopy is routinely done for recurrent urethritis or cystitis. These include congenital valves, minute urethral diverticula, polyps, and dense strictures. The latter may form in the wake of a long-standing granular urethritis. Valves, polyps, and strictures should be resected by using a fulgurating wire with the bipolar coagulating current. If resection is not possible by this means in the case of diverticula, surgical excision is done. The use of the resectoscope in the region of

the female bladder neck is fraught with danger because of the high incidence of fistulas and stress incontinence following resections. In patients with strictures that almost close the urethra, the urethra is dilated with filiforms and followers for temporary relief, but eventually more definitive surgical therapy is required.

SUBURETHRAL DIVERTICULUM
Etiology and Pathologic Anatomy

Suburethral diverticula are stages or complications of suburethral abscesses. The original process starts as an inflammation of one or more of the urethral glands that subsequently enlarge with recurrent infections. While the possibility exists that some cases may be on a congenital basis, this has been difficult to prove from study of the tissue removed at operation. The opening of the diverticulum is usually in the midline in the posterior urethral wall. It can, however, originate from the lateral walls or from the anterior wall of the urethra. The diverticulum may originate anywhere along the course of the urethra but must be distinguished from small infected glands at the external urethral meatus. Not infrequently a suburethral diverticulum is a multiloculated structure, and the possibility that it contains one or more calculi should not be overlooked.

Symptoms and Diagnosis

Patients with a suburethral diverticulum complain of dysuria of long-standing duration. They have urgency and frequency, and these symptoms are afforded only temporary relief from most types of therapy. Infection of the diverticulum with formation of a suburethral abscess is attendant upon acute, severe, suprapubic pain, pyuria, and other signs of an acute infection. Patients are aware of a tender mass just underneath the urethra. They complain of a sense of fullness or pressure and, though they have just voided, they feel the urge to urinate again. The diverticulum may contain a few cubic centimeters of urine, and the patients notice posturinary dribbling when they assume the erect posture. One patient was able to identify the location of her diverticulum by pressing on a specific spot underneath the right descending ramus of the pubis and ejecting a small stream of urine. The steps of the operation illustrated in Plate 31, that shows some of the principles of surgery for this condition, were sketched during this patient's operation.

The diagnosis is completed by employing a direct vision cystourethroscope or panendoscope to identify the internal urethral opening. The urethra is observed through the endoscope and the wall of the urethra, or the bulge suggesting the sac of the diverticulum is massaged and the escape of either urine or purulent material observed. A catheter may be passed into the pocket and palpated through the urethra. A malleable sound serves the same purpose. The surgeon should be aware that the diverticulum may have multiple openings into the urethra or that the diverticulum itself may be multiloculated. Anteroposterior, oblique, and lateral films taken after the injection of x-ray opaque material into the sac will reveal the ramifications of the diverticulum. Operative failures result from the incomplete removal of a diverticulum, particularly when multiple openings into the urethra or multiple loculations are present. Several devices can be arranged to x-ray the urethra in the female. The opening of the main channel of a Foley catheter is closed by a ligature and an opening proximal to the bulb is made. The catheter is introduced into the bladder and the bulb distended with water and seated in the bladder neck. Opaque material is injected and pressure is exerted around the external meatus to prevent leakage. The urethra, as well as the various pockets of the diverticulum, is distended. Differential diagnosis necessitates distinguishing suburethral diverticulum from the presence of an ectopic ureter that opens into the urethra. Excision of the former would result in serious complications. The operator should be alert to the possibility of metastatic disease extending along the submucosa of the vagina and into the urethra which may be mistaken for a benign lesion. Suburethral varicosities of large size

may simulate a urethral diverticulum, but the external appearance and the failure of urethroscopy to demonstrate any opening into the urethra should make the differential diagnosis clear. Abscesses of Skene's glands near the external meatus are smaller. Since they are not subjected to the full force of the urinary stream, they do not give the common symptoms of suburethral diverticula. Gartner's duct cysts are more lateral in location than the urethra. Unless they are large and cause a displacement or compression of the urethra, they do not cause any bladder symptoms.

Indications and Surgical Principles

Diverticula of any size are symptomatic since they are sources of inflammation with subsequent complications. Diverticula that distort the urinary stream or cause retention must be removed. Annoying symptoms of urgency, frequency, and dysuria require relief by surgery. Excision of a suburethral diverticulum ideally lends itself to the combined endoscopic-external dissection technique. In this method the line of suture is observed with a panendoscope or urethroscope, with special attention to the inversion of the mucosal layer. At the same time the external layers of the urethral musculature are approximated along a large surface area. Following a closure on this principle, the vaginal wall and vaginal mucosa are everted toward the vaginal aspect of the urethra. This effects a multiple-layer closure, with the mucous membrane of the urethra and vagina being sutured so as to present in opposite directions. Postoperative drainage of the bladder in this operation is best accomplished by a vaginal cystostomy. An indwelling urethral catheter rests on the line of closure of the wound and its use is inadvisable on this account.

Preoperative Care and Anesthesia

The urine is rendered bacteria free by the administration of appropriate urinary antiseptics for several days prior to surgery. If there is a stone in the suburethral diverticulum, it is impossible to clear up the infection, and

PLATE 31

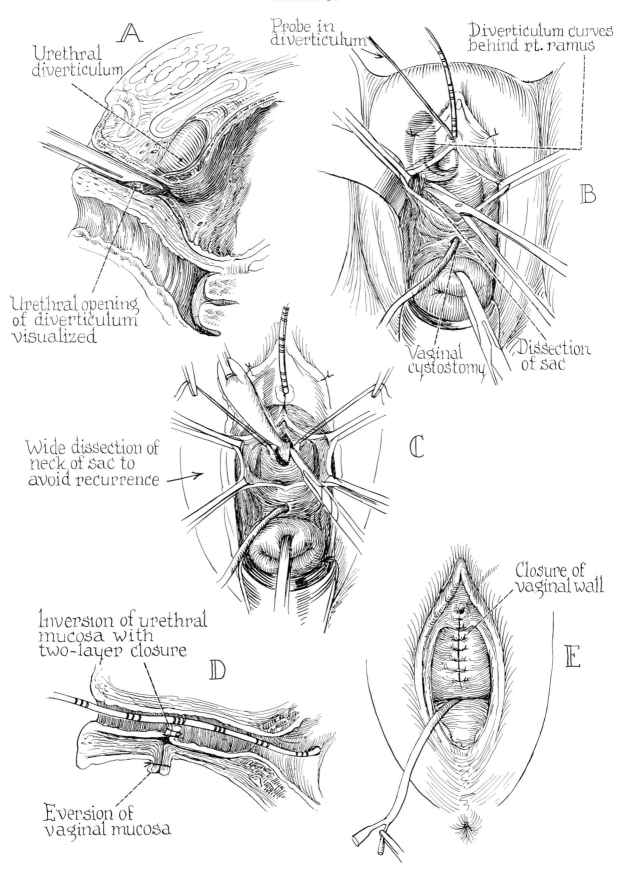

A

Urethral diverticulum

Probe in diverticulum

Diverticulum curves behind rt. ramus

Urethral opening of diverticulum visualized

B

Vaginal cystostomy

Dissection of sac

Wide dissection of neck of sac to avoid recurrence

C

Inversion of urethral mucosa with two-layer closure

D

Eversion of vaginal mucosa

Closure of vaginal wall

E

attempts should be made to remove the impacted stone before the actual obliteration of the suburethral pocket or pockets is undertaken. A general anesthetic is preferred, and if the surgeon prefers the knee-chest position for the operation, the patient should be intubated before being placed in this position. Spinal or saddle block types of anesthesia can be used, but, again, if the patient is operated upon in the knee-chest position, the anesthetic level must be carefully controlled.

Steps of the Operation

1. The position of the internal opening of the diverticulum is again visualized with either a panendoscope or direct-vision cystourethroscope (Plate 31, *A*). The point opposite this opening on the vaginal aspect of the urethra is noted. In the operation shown, the diverticulum that had been overlooked during two previous operations had an opening in the midline of the urethra at approximately the junction of the middle and posterior thirds. The major portion of the sac extended up behind the right ramus of the pubis and was of considerable size (Plate 31, *A* and *B*).

2. If the diverticulum curves posteriorly along the anterolateral aspect of the urethrovesical junction, a catheter is placed in the ureter on this side, since it is exposed during the dissection. A vaginal cystostomy is done prior to the dissection of the sac (Plate 31, *B*). This is the simplest method of draining the bladder and avoids a suprapubic cystostomy. A probe is passed into the diverticulum to aid the surgeon in the dissection (Plate 31, *B*). The complete sac is dissected free. All locules of a loculated diverticulum are excised. It is unimportant if the sac is inadvertently opened, since the dissection of the neck of the sac and its opening into the urethra will be widely excised under direct vision in the next step.

3. In Plate 31, *C*, the sac has been completely freed and the neck of the sac, together with the adjacent urethral wall and mucosa, is being excised. It is not necessary to perform this part of the operation by having a large catheter in the urethra, since the operator should excise the neck of this sac under direct vision. What is more important, he should be prepared to pass an endoscope at any time and to visualize the interior of the urethra to be sure that all of the edges of the urethral opening are adequately excised. Fresh edges are subsequently approximated (Plate 31, *C*).

4. Plate 31, *D*, shows a lateral view of the closure of the incision. The first line of sutures encompassed the submucosa of the urethra and inverted the mucosa toward the interior. The second layer closed the musculature of the urethra, permitting an adequate approximation of wide areas of the muscular layer. The preferred suture material is 0000 chromic catgut on atraumatic needles.

5. The vaginal wall is closed by interrupted sutures after it has been adequately mobilized. This allows closure with eversion of the vaginal mucosa toward the vaginal aspect of the urethra (Plate 31, *E*).

Postoperative Care

The cystostomy tube is connected to a bedside drainage tube and receptacle. The patient is mobilized as soon as she has reacted from the anesthetic. Urinary antiseptics are continued and urine cultures taken frequently during the postoperative course. Sensitivity tests on the organisms isolated are done as indicated. The cystostomy tube is usually removed on the seventh or eighth day. The opening closes spontaneously within twenty-four to thirty-six hours, and the patient may be expected to void spontaneously after removal of the catheter. She should be warned that a certain amount of urgency, frequency, and dysuria may persist for some time. She is seen at frequent intervals postoperatively and the urethra sounded to a No. 28 Fr. dilator to prevent the development of a soft stricture.

RECONSTRUCTION OF THE URETHRA
Indications and Surgical Principles

The posterior and posterolateral walls of the urethra are sloughed away as the result of plastic surgery on the anterior vaginal wall with the use of large caliber, ineptly placed, strangulating sutures. The surgeon frequently has utilized a "favorite stitch" that passes though the full thickness of the vaginal wall in the region of the bladder neck and into the musculature of the bladder wall to "anchor it." This duplicates in every particular the method used for the experimental creation of a fistula, except that the closure is more difficult and the gynecologic operating room is not a

PLATE 32

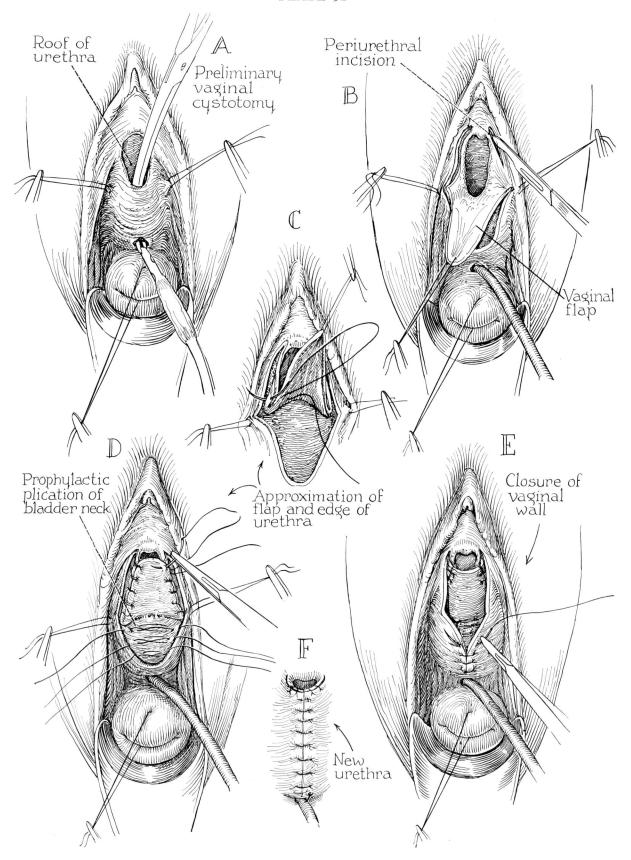

A — Preliminary vaginal cystotomy

Roof of urethra

B — Periurethral incision

Vaginal flap

C

D — Prophylactic plication of bladder neck

Approximation of flap and edge of urethra

E — Closure of vaginal wall

F — New urethra

laboratory. An injury of this type as the result of a neglected labor could occur under unusual circumstances.

Steps of the Operation

1. A preliminary vaginal cystotomy is performed (Plate 32, *A*). A Kelly hemostat is inserted into the bladder until it impinges on the bladder wall in the anterior fornix. The tips of the instrument are spread, and an incision is made through the full thickness of the vaginal and bladder walls. The Kelly hemostat is inserted through this small incision and the catheter drawn inside. The bag of the Foley catheter is inflated and seated in the bladder base. The roof of the urethra is all that remains, and a new floor for the urethra is to be reconstructed (Plate 32, *A*).

2. A vaginal flap is developed that is roughly triangular in shape with the base at the bladder neck (Plate 32, *B*). The full thickness of the vaginal wall is separated from the bladder base and a traction suture placed in the edge of the flap to avoid instrumentation; other fine sutures are used for traction as shown in Plate 32, *B*.

3. A second periurethral incision along the lateral edges of the remains of the roof of the urethra is made (Plate 32, *B*) and carried down until it joins the vaginal flap in the region of the bladder neck. The angle at which these incisions join on each side is the critical point of the operation because it is from the base of these two flaps that the blood supply for the new urethra must originate.

4. The lower flap is brought anteriorly and sutured so that the muscular coat of the vaginal wall approximates the same layer of tissue along the sides of the remaining roof of the urethra. In Plate 32, *C*, is shown the method of placing the sutures, which has the effect of rolling the edges together and approximating the open edges of the flaps. In this method the mucosal surface of the vaginal flap now becomes the interior surface of the posterior urethral wall. The tip of the flap will form the posterior circumference of the new external urethral meatus (Plate 32, *C*).

5. Many patients who have lost the urethra through surgical or obstetric trauma will be incontinent on stress following a successful urethral reconstruction. A prophylactic plication of the bladder neck can be done before the closure of the vaginal wall. The sutures used in the plication should be 00 chromic catgut or smaller and should be placed in such a manner as not to impair the blood supply at the critical angle of the vaginal flap (Plate 32, *D*).

6. The vaginal wall is further mobilized to allow closure without tension. The vaginal wall is closed with interrupted sutures of fine chromic catgut (Plate 32, *E*).

7. At the conclusion of the procedure the new urethra will have the appearance shown in Plate 32, *F*. Sutures placed about the new external meatus should be tied so as just to approximate the edges without strangulation. This is the terminal portion and least viable part of the vaginal flap.

Postoperative Care

The postoperative care is the same as that described under Suburethral Diverticulum (page 249).

SUPRAPUBIC CYSTOTOMY AND CYSTOSTOMY
Indications and Surgical Principles

A suprapubic cystotomy with subsequent retention of a catheter (cystostomy) is frequently indicated in gynecologic surgery for accidental injury to the bladder. The bladder may be opened to visualize the closure of the perforation and to effect drainage subsequently by means of a suprapubic catheter. Certain situations encountered by the gynecologist lend themselves to bladder injury. A hysterectomy, after a previous myomectomy, is a frequent cause. The bladder may have been advanced over the line of incision or incisions used to remove the fibroids. A strong scar exists between the bladder base and the wall of the uterus, and in separating these organs the bladder may be entered. Excision of a cervical stump, either by the vaginal or abdominal route, may cause bladder injury. After a subtotal hysterectomy, the bladder normally falls over the top of the stump, to which it becomes firmly adherent. Bladder injuries are not uncommon in the course of radical pelvic surgery, and these are more likely to occur at or near the ureterovesical junction. Ovarian cancer with metastatic deposits over the bladder and in the vesicouterine reflection of peritoneum may result in bladder injury as the operator attempts to remove the primary tumors and the larger metastatic masses. Pelvic surgery in a

PLATE 33

SUPRAPUBIC CYSTOTOMY
AND CYSTOSTOMY

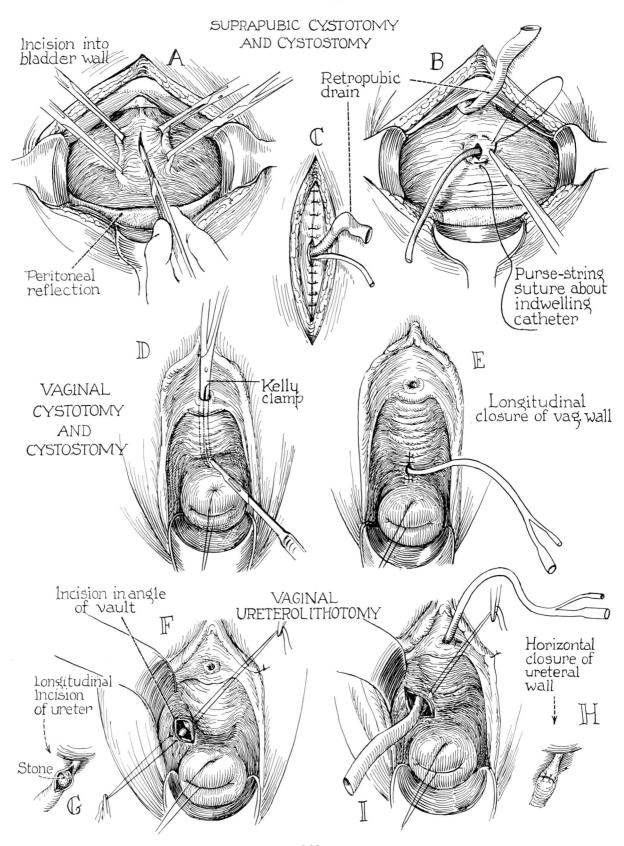

Incision into
bladder wall

A

Peritoneal
reflection

B

Retropubic
drain

C

Purse-string
suture about
indwelling
catheter

VAGINAL
CYSTOTOMY
AND
CYSTOSTOMY

D

Kelly
clamp

E

Longitudinal
closure of vag. wall

Incision in angle
of vault

F

VAGINAL
URETEROLITHOTOMY

Longitudinal
Incision
of ureter

Stone

G

Horizontal
closure of
ureteral
wall

H

I

patient who has had previous intracavitary radium or external irradiation results in some injuries to the bladder, which has become secondarily contracted and fibrotic from the radiation. The bladder is also injured during vaginal plastic surgery, particularly during repeat operations for recurrent relaxation.

Steps of the Operation

1. The bladder is mobilized anteriorly for a short distance by dissecting it from the posterior border of the symphysis pubis. Four Allis clamps are used to grasp the dome of the bladder prior to making the incision. The bladder may be distended with 250 to 300 ml. of normal saline solution at this time. This is a particularly useful measure if the normal outline of the bladder has been distorted by other pelvic disease. If a long incision into the bladder is contemplated to utilize this approach for intravesical procedures, such as visualizing the site for a ureteroneocystostomy, for fistula repair, or removal of a stone, the peritoneal reflection is identified and the bladder further mobilized by dissecting the peritoneum from the dome and part of the bladder base (Plate 33, A).

2. A simple cystostomy is performed as shown in Plate 33, B. A purse-string suture is placed about the opening into the bladder and a Foley or other type indwelling catheter inserted. The purse-string suture is lightly tied about the catheter and a drain placed in the retropubic space (Plate 33, B).

3. The wound is closed in layers, bringing the retropubic drain out just anterior to the catheter (Plate 33, C).

Postoperative Care

Urinary antiseptics are routinely given as is the case with any indwelling catheter in the bladder. The retropubic drain is withdrawn halfway the day after operation and is removed on the following day, unless drainage continues to be profuse. Other measures in the postoperative care of the patient will depend on the indication for the cystostomy.

VAGINAL CYSTOTOMY AND CYSTOSTOMY
Indications and Surgical Principles

A vaginal cystostomy is the preferred method of drainage after many fistula repairs. This is particularly true of the repair of retrotrigonal,

bladder neck, and urethrovaginal fistulas. Fistulas should not be drained by a catheter lying across the line of closure of the bladder or urethra, and a vaginal cystostomy, at the bladder base, provides excellent drainage. It is the ideal type of drainage for the successful healing of the fistula repair. A vaginal cystotomy or cystostomy may be performed in the event of injury to the bladder and frequently provides the best site for continuous drainage.

Steps of the Operation

1. A long Kelly clamp is introduced through the urethra and the tip advanced to the bladder base (Plate 33, D). The tip of the clamp is spread so that it impinges on and can be felt at the anterior fornix of the vagina. An incision is made through the full thickness of the vaginal wall and the clamp passed into the vagina (Plate 33, D).

2. The tip of a Foley or other type of retention catheter is grasped with the open Kelly clamp and the catheter drawn into the bladder. One or two sutures are placed through the full thickness of the vaginal wall above and below the catheter (Plate 33, E).

Postoperative Care

Urinary antiseptics are administered, and the catheter is connected to a bedside drainage tube and receptacle. If the vaginal cystostomy was performed as a method of bladder drainage for a fistula, the catheter is usually removed on or about the tenth postoperative day. The success or failure of the fistula closure will have been decided. Since the cystostomy site was made in normal bladder and vaginal wall, the fistula created by the cystostomy tube promptly closes. If the patient is able to void spontaneously, she frequently does not notice any drainage from the vagina after thirty-six to forty-eight hours. The time of the removal of the indwelling catheter varies with the reason for which the cystostomy was performed. Other postoperative measures are instituted, depending on the reason for the primary operation.

VAGINAL URETEROLITHOTOMY
Indications and Surgical Principles

A stone in the terminal ureter or impacted at the ureterovesical junction may be felt vaginally. Vaginal ureterolithotomy should be considered when the stone is readily located because of the simplicity of this operative approach to the terminal ureter. A stone impacted for a considerable length of time may be adherent to the ureteral wall, with the ureteral mucosa actually growing over and surrounding the stone. In a parous woman, and particularly if there is some degree of prolapse, the terminal ureter is readily exposed through the vagina and frequently presents an approach technically more simple than the accepted retroperitoneal approach to the terminal ureter from an incision in the flank. Should a resection of the terminal ureter and a ureteroneocystostomy be necessary, this can be done vaginally, although one has to look to the pelvic and urologic surgeons—on the continent and several generations back—to find anyone who has had an appreciable experience with this method. Should the removal of a stone in the terminal ureter necessitate resection and transplantation, and if removal has first been approached by the vaginal route, there is no reason why the vaginal wound cannot be closed and the more conventional route, in this country, used to transplant the ureter.

Steps of the Operation

1. The stone is palpated through the vaginal wall, and traction sutures are placed in the subjacent vaginal wall on either side of the stone. An incision is made through the full thickness of the vaginal wall over the ureter, which is exposed above and below the stone (Plate 33, *F*).

2. A longitudinal incision is made in the ureter over the stone (Plate 33, *G*), and the stone is extracted with a minimal amount of trauma to the terminal ureter. Care is exercised in those cases of long duration where the reaction about the foreign body has been considerable.

3. The ureter is closed transversely, using 0000 chromic catgut on atraumatic needles (Plate 33, *H*). The color of the ureter above and below the point of closure is observed for several minutes to determine the adequacy of its blood supply.

4. A small drain is placed in the vaginal wall, if there is oozing, although if the field is dry, it is preferable to close the full thickness of the vaginal wall, everting the edges toward the vagina

in the same manner as a fistula closure (Plate 33, *I*).

Postoperative Care

The use of a small, splinting ureteral catheter has no precedent with which we may be guided. If the ureter has an adequate lumen above and below the transverse line of closure, it is reasonable to omit both a splinting catheter and any type of drain. Even with the present urinary antiseptics available, and provided that the inevitable urinary tract infection present under these circumstances can be brought under control, there is no assurance that an indwelling ureteral catheter will add much to the successful healing of the wound and prevention of contracture of the ureter about the suture line. An indwelling urethral catheter is left in place for several days to irrigate the bladder and remove any blood clots that may accumulate. Other forms of treatment, postoperatively, will depend on the condition of the urinary tract on the involved side and on observations of its function. The usual follow-up of such urologic procedures, such as cultures and intravenous and retrograde pyelograms and other intravesical observations by cystoscopy, is done.

PARTIAL CYSTECTOMY AND URETERECTOMY
Indications and Surgical Principles

A partial cystectomy and ureterectomy is usually indicated in gynecologic surgery for recurrent pelvic malignancies involving the bladder base and terminal ureter. It is often a palliative procedure in that the patient may refuse a complete pelvic exenteration or such an operation may not be feasible. Plate 34 was sketched during an operation on a patient who had had a complete course of pelvic irradiation and vaginal cone therapy for cancer of the cervix, followed by a recurrence of the tumor that involved the terminal portion of the right ureter and adjacent bladder base. In such a patient, the fibrosis, contraction, and endarteritis subsequent to the radiation and radical surgery make it unlikely that a ureteroneocystostomy would be successful. In order to preserve the function of the right kidney, the

PLATE 34

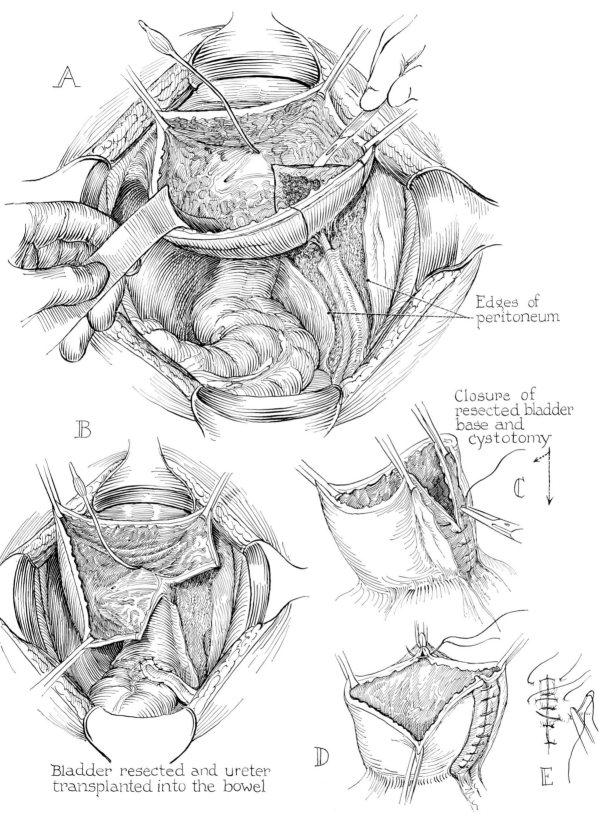

A

Edges of peritoneum

B

Bladder resected and ureter transplanted into the bowel

Closure of resected bladder base and cystotomy

C

D

E

ureter may be transplanted either to the skin or into the bowel. The method of diversion of the urinary stream on the involved side is individualized for each patient and is sometimes governed by what the patient, herself, will accept.

Steps of the Operation

1. No attempt is made to perform this operation as an extraperitoneal procedure. The necessity of examining the pelvis plus lymphatic stations along the course of the aorta for prognostic reasons requires that the peritoneum be opened. The operation could conceivably be done if the ureter were brought to the skin as an extraperitoneal procedure; however, if the ureter is to be placed in the bowel, the abdomen is opened.

2. A cystotomy is performed by bisecting the dome of the bladder in order to expose its interior completely (Plate 34, A).

3. The ureter is mobilized from the brim of the pelvis to a point well above the involved area. A flap of peritoneum for nourishment is permitted to remain on the uninvolved upper segment of the ureter (Plate 34, A).

4. A wedge-shaped incision is made to include an adequate segment of uninvolved bladder adjacent to the tumor (Plate 34, A). The intramural ureter and terminal portion of the ureter involved in the tumor will be removed in one block. Active bleeding points are clamped and ligated as encountered. In a postradiation bladder and ureter, the amount of bleeding is rarely alarming.

5. The ureter is transplanted into the bowel by one of the several techniques described. The site selected for transplantation of the ureter is usually at or near the pelvic brim to utilize ureter that is well away from the site of recurrent cancer. In Plate 34, B, the segmental resection of the bladder and terminal ureter has been completed. A catheter is seen in the urethra which indicates the normal landmarks.

6. The area of resection is closed by interrupted sutures of 00 chromic catgut. This first layer of sutures passes through the deeper layer of musculature of the bladder, and, if possible, just beneath the bladder mucosa (Plate 34, C).

7. The cystotomy is closed with interrupted sutures placed in the same manner (Plate 34, D), leaving an area for insertion of a cystostomy tube.

8. The line of incision for the cystotomy plus the line of incision of the segmental resection of the bladder are closed by a second layer of interrupted sutures as shown in Plate 34, E.

Postoperative Care

The cystostomy tube is connected to dependent drainage and is irrigated at intervals to prevent obstruction from clots of blood that follow surgery in the bladder. Urinary antiseptics are administered in adequate doses, and the patient is observed for signs of a developing pyelonephritis or obstruction in the ureterointestinal or ureterocutaneous transplant, as the case may be. Electrolyte studies are done daily during the first few postoperative days, with particular reference to the avoidance of hyperchloremic acidosis in the event that the ureter was transplanted to bowel. The function of the kidneys and other details concerning the success or failure of the transplanted ureter are determined by intravenous pyelograms and renal function tests. If a ureter is transplanted to the skin, retrograde studies are done simply by the insertion of a catheter and the injection of dye by gravity. Since this operation is usually indicated as a palliative procedure for recurrent cancer, where a complete exenteration is either impossible or refused, the general nutritional, supportive, and comprehensive care for the patient is individualized for each situation.

URETEROINTESTINAL ANASTOMOSIS
Indications and Surgical Principles

Transplantation of the ureters either into the bowel or skin is commonly indicated in gynecologic surgery because of ureteral obstruction after radical surgery or radiation. Cancer of the cervix, cancer of the fundus, and cancer of the vagina are the common malignancies that may extend to involve the pelvic ureter. Intracavitary radium and external radiation cause ureteral injuries in addition to radiation changes in the bladder that may compromise the continuity of the excretory system and require transplantation of the ureters. Among the benign conditions requiring transplantation, the most common gynecologic lesion is a large vesicovaginal fistula that has resisted every method of closure, as a result of which the patient is completely incontinent. Ureteral injuries at the level of the pelvic brim during surgery for benign disease may require ureterointestinal anastomosis. Sufficient length of ureter may not be available for ureteroneocystostomy or for one of the other methods of ureteroureterostomy. After studying the possibility of the utilization of bladder flaps, the seriousness of the situation may necessitate transplantation of the ureters into the bowel as an emergency measure. Patients with advanced interstitial cystitis have been known to have such severe pain, together with an overflow incontinence, as to be incapacitated. In these rare cases transplantation of the ureters into the bowel may establish a useful existence to the patient. The general urologic indications are bladder or other malignancies involving the lower urinary tract and pelvic ureter.

The surgical principles involved in ureterointestinal anastomosis are concerned with the prevention of stricture and the prevention of reflux of feces and gas. Many techniques have been designed over the years, and seldom is one anastomosis done in an identical manner to another. Techniques that utilize an elaborate tunnel at the point of anastomosis possibly result in more strictures. Techniques that do not employ tunnels and approximate mucosa to mucosa are perhaps guilty of more reflux of gas and fecal contents into the ureter. Combinations of these two principles in one technique frequently look good in retrospect in those patients in whom the anastomosis functions well. There is no technique that invariably ensures a good result. The ureter may be transplanted into small or large bowel, into the cecum, or into an isolated ileal segment. There is an endless variety of sites that may be selected, and each one has its own individual problems insofar as anchoring the bowel near the site of anastomosis and bringing the ureter to this site without angulation or tension. When a colostomy must be performed, the site of the colostomy will modify the site selected for the ureterointestinal anastomosis. The gynecologist transplants the ureters into the bowel above a permanent colostomy after a total pelvic evisceration. Less commonly, the ureters may be transplanted into the bowel after an anterior evisceration, in which event the rectal ampulla is converted into a cloaca.

Preoperative Preparation and Anesthesia

In addition to the usual general medical study of the patient prior to this major procedure, the urinary tract is completely studied in regard to its function and any possible congenital or acquired deformities that may complicate the procedure. Urine cultures and sensitivity tests are done on urine specimens from both kidneys during the course of retrograde studies. Prior to surgery, appropriate urinary antiseptics, to which any organisms cultured from the urine is sensitive, are administered in adequate dosage. The bowel is prepared for the anastomosis by the administration of a saline cathartic each night for three or four nights prior to surgery. The following morning a tap water enema is given. The patient may be kept on a regular diet if necessary for nutritional reasons, and this may be modified to include clear liquids on the day prior to surgery. Forty-eight hours before operation, neomycin, 1 Gm. every four hours, is begun. This effectively cuts down the bacterial flora of the large bowel by the day of surgery. A general or spinal anesthetic is used, and if an extensive procedure such as a pelvic exenteration is to be done at the same time, a hypotensive anesthetic reduces the blood loss. An anesthetist trained in this type of anesthesia is necessary.

Steps of the Operation

1. The position of the bowel is studied, together with the ureters that have been mobilized. The taenia may be selected as a site of anastomosis, but this is not necessary, and other areas of the bowel can be used. The bowel is studied with the ureter from each side to determine how the flaps of the peritoneum or serosa of the bowel can be mobilized to subsequently anchor the site of anastomosis. The flaps are used to cover and splint the area during the final steps of the operation.

PLATE 35

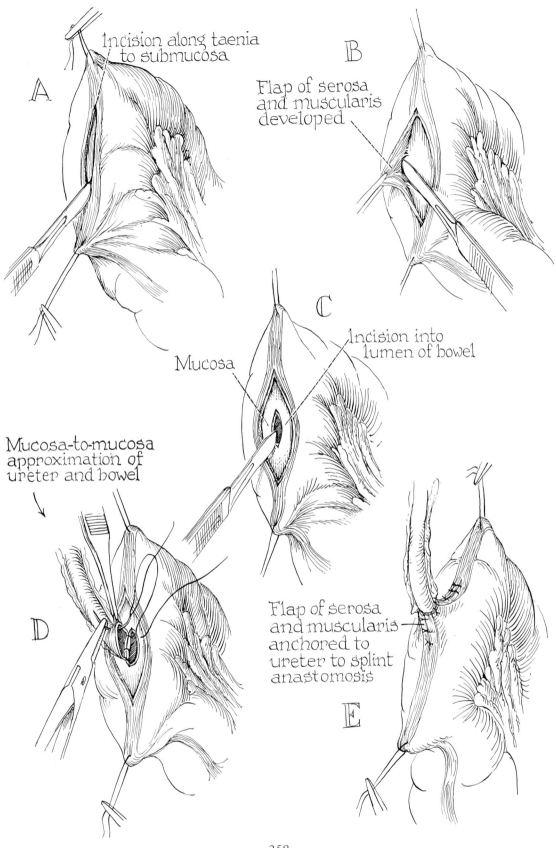

A — Incision along taenia to submucosa

B — Flap of serosa and muscularis developed

C — Mucosa — Incision into lumen of bowel

Mucosa-to-mucosa approximation of ureter and bowel

D

E — Flap of serosa and muscularis anchored to ureter to splint anastomosis

2. An incision is made along the taenia down to the submucosa (Plate 35, *A*) for a distance depending on the size of the lumen of the ureter to be transplanted. Traction sutures are placed above and below the incision to mobilize the area during this delicate procedure (Plate 35, *A*).

3. A flap of serosa and muscularis is developed (Plate 35, *B*) and mobilized laterally for a centimeter or two from the site of the original incision.

4. An incision is made into the lumen of the bowel and the mucosa allowed to evert (Plate 35, *C*).

5. Interrupted sutures of 0000 chromic catgut on atraumatic needles are used to approximate mucosa to mucosa between the ureter and the bowel (Plate 35, *D*).

6. The flap of serosa and muscularis that was undermined as shown in Plate 35, *C*, is brought up a centimeter or so along the course of the terminal ureter and is anchored by several interrupted sutures so as to splint the actual site of anastomosis (Plate 35, *E*). The sutures should be few in number and be placed in such a way as not to cause a stricture.

7. A flap of peritoneum, mobilized either from the side of the bowel wall or from the mesentery, may be sutured over the terminal ureter and site of anastomosis. The source of this flap or the method of preparing it must be individualized for each patient, depending on the site of anastomosis and the position and length of the bowel segment where the anastomosis has been done.

Postoperative Care

The patient is started on adequate urinary antiseptics given intravenously until fluids are tolerated by mouth. The usual postoperative enemas are omitted, and the return of normal peristalsis in the abdomen is encouraged by the early administration of a full diet. A rectal tube can be used at intervals and may add to the patient's comfort. The management of the patient's fluid intake and nourishment will depend on the indication and extent of the original operation and on whether or not the anastomosis was part of another major procedure (see Management of Electrolyte Abnormalities in Gynecologic Surgery, page 543). The patient should be observed for the development of a pyelonephritis. This is the most serious complication that develops from this operation. Intravenous pyelograms are taken at any time during the postoperative course if there are signs of impaired kidney function or other complications. An intravenous pyelogram should be done on or about the tenth postoperative day in the average patient to determine kidney function and the development of a hydroureter and hydronephrosis. This will be repeated at intervals to confirm the success or failure of the anastomosis.

ISOLATED BOWEL SEGMENT OPERATION
Indications and Surgical Principles

Ureterointestinal anastomosis using an isolated bowel segment has the following advantages: (1) Hyperchloremia and acidosis are minimized by the presence of less bowel mucosa for absorption of electrolytes; (2) there is less back pressure on the excretory channels of the kidney; and (3) the segment is free of the fecal stream that causes ascending infections. The exact mechanism of hyperchloremic acidosis subsequent to ureterointestinal transplants is not known. Two mechanisms, or a combination of both, are possible: (1) The process may be compared to intoxication by ammonium chloride such as occurs with an overdose of this drug; (2) the cause of the syndrome may be a renal tubular insufficiency. Biochemists and biophysicists have made important observations. The bowel resorbs chloride, sodium, and ammonia. This resorption is greatest in the upper small bowel, and becomes less and less in the lower small bowel and large intestine. The area of contact is important—so transplants into the upper tract provide a correspondingly greater length of bowel and surface. The rate of evacuation of the urine is important, since the length of contact of the urine with the bowel mucosa affects the total quantity of ammonia and chlorides retained. Diversion of the urinary stream into an isolated segment minimizes these factors. A nephrosis or lower nephron syndrome may be at fault or a consequence of the above chemical changes. Enough studies have not been accumulated on the histology of kidneys after ureterointestinal anastomosis in patients in whom the kidney is functioning well. Most of the kidneys are examined after the patient has died. On the basis of autopsy material it is safe to presume that a normal kidney does not exist after ureterointestinal anastomosis. Those patients in whom chlorides are very readily absorbed from the lower bowel can be determined by a simple preoperative test. The rectum is distended with a pint of hypertonic sodium chloride solution, and blood studies for sodium, chloride, and carbon dioxide combining power are done within a few hours. While this test has not been widely used and studied, an occasional patient may be found who resorbs chlorides from the lower bowel with significant changes in the serum electrolytes. Such a patient should have an isolated segment operation or cutaneous transplant. One or both ureters may be transplanted to the isolated ileal segment. This can be done by an end-to-end or an end-to-side anastomosis. If there is only one ureter, it can be put into the end opposite that brought out on the skin for the permanent stoma.

Preoperative Care and Anesthesia

A modified bowel preparation is prescribed to reduce the bacterial content of the lower ileum. This is adapted to the individual patient, since the usual cathartics, enemas, and reduction of food intake for preparing the bowel must not upset the patient's electrolyte balance preoperatively. Forty-eight hours prior to surgery the patient receives 1 Gm. of neomycin every four hours. A light diet is ordered two days before surgery, and liquids are ordered the day before operation. The patient's intake of electrolytes and proteins is regulated as near to normal as the patient's disease permits. A general anesthetic or a continuous spinal anesthetic is used, for several hours are required for the anastomoses between bowel, ureters, and skin.

Steps of the Operation

1. An extended right rectus incision is preferred unless the abdomen has been entered by some other approach for the primary surgery. Exploration of the pelvis and abdomen should reveal that the patient's disease is confined at the time. The procedure is not indicated if there will be only a short-term survival.

2. An appendectomy is performed.

3. A segment of the terminal ileum, 14 to 16 cm. in length, located 8 to 10 cm. from the ileocecal junction, is selected for isolation. The mesentery is incised so that one or more primary arcades remain intact to the isolated loop (Plate 36, A). The incision in the mesentery is continued to the origin of the primary arcades from the intestinal artery. Bleeding points in the incised mesentery are clamped and tied.

4. Straight Kocher clamps are placed across the bowel at the distal and proximal ends of the isolated loop (Plate 36, A), and the segment is resected.

5. The continuity of the small bowel is restored by anastomosing the distal end of the ileum to the end of the segment of terminal ileum entering the cecum (Plate 36, B). The mesentery of the newly anastomosed ileum is closed without constricting or impairing the vessels supplying the isolated segment (Plate 36, B). Defects are closed through which small bowel may herniate and become obstructed.

6. The ureters are mobilized with a flap of peritoneum for nutrition and are resected deep in the pelvis clear of any suspected area of tumor (Plate 36, B).

7. The right ureter is mobilized several centimeters above the pelvic brim so that it can be brought posterior to the isolated loop and gently curved toward the antimesenteric border of the ileum for implantation (Plate 36, B). The left ureter is mobilized 4 or 5 cm. above the pelvic brim and underneath the superior hemorrhoidal and sigmoidal vessels (Plate 36, B). The bridge of peritoneum over the promontory between the flaps created for the ureters is lifted from the bodies of the fifth lumbar and first sacral vertebrae, and the left ureter is brought retroperitoneally to the right of the midline (Plate 36, B). The superior hemorrhoidal and lower sigmoidal arteries are not ligated. They are prevented from angulating the ureter, as it sweeps in a gentle curve from left to right, by carefully closing and anchoring the parietal peritoneum. The mobilization of the left ureter will vary if the sigmoid and rectum have been removed in the course of the primary surgery or if a left permanent inguinal colostomy was performed.

PLATE 36

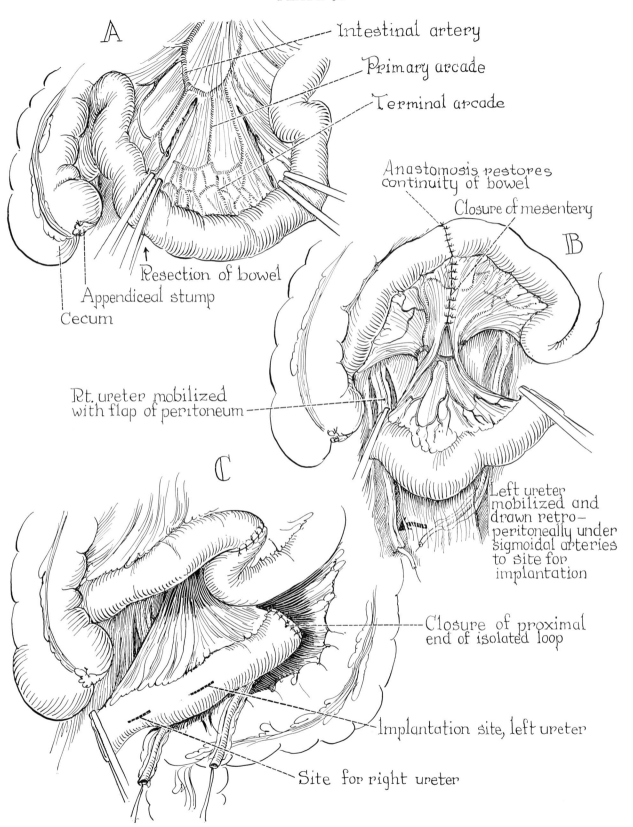

A

Intestinal artery

Primary arcade

Terminal arcade

Resection of bowel

Appendiceal stump

Cecum

Anastomosis restores
continuity of bowel

Closure of mesentery

B

Rt. ureter mobilized
with flap of peritoneum

C

Left ureter
mobilized and
drawn retro-
peritoneally under
sigmoidal arteries
to site for
implantation

Closure of proximal
end of isolated loop

Implantation site, left ureter

Site for right ureter

261

PLATE 36 (Concluded)

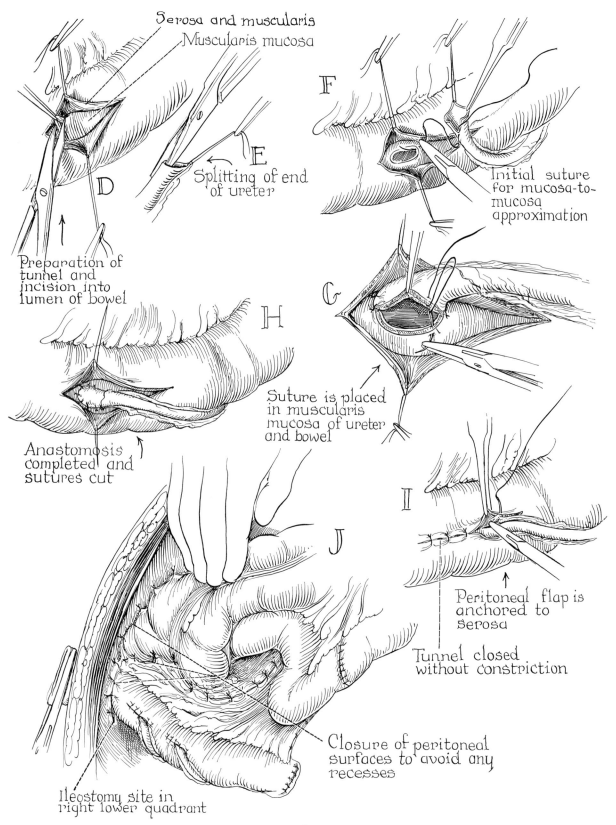

Serosa and muscularis

Muscularis mucosa

D

Preparation of
tunnel and
incision into
lumen of bowel

E

Splitting of end
of ureter

F

Initial suture
for mucosa-to-
mucosa
approximation

G

Suture is placed
in muscularis
mucosa of ureter
and bowel

H

Anastomosis
completed and
sutures cut

I

Peritoneal flap is
anchored to
serosa

Tunnel closed
without constriction

J

Closure of peritoneal
surfaces to avoid any
recesses

Ileostomy site in
right lower quadrant

262

8. The proximal end of the isolated loop is closed by interrupted sutures of fine silk (Plate 36, C). The isolated loop and the ureters are studied to decide the site for transplantation. The location for the ileostomy in the right lower quadrant is decided (Plate 36, C).

9. Both ureters are transplanted by an end-to-side technique as in the operation illustrated. Plate 36, D, shows the preparation of a tunnel down to the muscularis mucosa and a small incision made into the bowel.

10. The end of the ureter is split in preparation for a combined mucosa-to-mucosa anastomosis, with a small tunnel to anchor the site of anastomosis (Plate 36, E). The mucosa of the ureter and mucosa of the ileum are approximated by fine interrupted sutures of 0000 chromic catgut (Plate 36, F). The details of this closure are shown enlarged in Plate 36, G. If possible, the sutures pass in the muscularis mucosa of the ureter and bowel.

11. Plate 36, H, shows the anatomosis complete, with the flaps of serosa and muscularis retracted. The tunnel of serosa and muscularis is closed with interrupted sutures of 0000 chromic catgut without constricting the ureter. The peritoneal flap left on the ureter is anchored to the serosa of the bowel by several interrupted sutures (Plate 36, I).

12. A muscle-splitting incision is made in the right lower quadrant at the site selected for the ileostomy (Plate 36, J). The bowel is drawn to the outside and the mesentery of the isolated loop and the ureters observed for any signs of tension.

13. The isolated loop is sutured to the parietal peritoneum and the adjacent cecum to avoid any recesses in the peritoneal flaps (Plate 36, J).

Alternate Method of Treatment of Ileostomy Stoma

Even exteriorized serosa of the bowel does not tolerate digestive secretions well. If the stoma is simply brought out and anchored, the serosa is bathed in secretions and becomes inflamed just as the peritoneum in a bowel perforation. This, in turn, causes an inflammation of the skin, with prolonged healing and poor adaptation to the collecting device.

Sufficient length of bowel is brought out so that the exteriorized portion can be turned back on itself to form a cuff. This approximates serosa to serosa and protects its from the secretions of the small bowel. It also prevents stric-

ture of the stoma that results from infection and scarring, more common when other techniques are used.

Postoperative Care

The following shows the loss of fluid from exteriorized segments of bowel at various levels:

Duodenum and jejunum	8,000-12,000 ml./24 hr.
Mid-ileum	12,000 ml./24 hr.
Terminal ileum	480 ml./24 hr.
Anus	200-300 ml./24 hr.

Thus, when the fecal stream is diverted, the amount of fluid lost is dependent on how high in the gastrointestinal tract the diversion is done. Effort is made to save the terminal ileum whenever possible because of the enormous absorption in this segment.

Postoperative care involves the special problems after bowel resection and after ureterointestinal anastomosis. (See Intestinal Surgery Incident to Gynecologic Procedures, page 586, and Management of Electrolyte Abnormalities in Gynecologic Surgery, page 543.)

CUTANEOUS URETEROSTOMY: TREATMENT OF THE TERMINAL URETER
Indications and Surgical Principles

The ideal cutaneous ureterostomy is one that remains viable without stricture, does not retract beneath the skin surface, and lends itself adequately to a collecting device. The site of the ureterostomy is placed away from any bony prominences, previous scars, and the colostomy stoma, if one is present. A number of methods of treating the terminal ureter are used, varying from simply anchoring it to the skin to complicated skin flaps and pedicles. Regardless of the method used, successes and failures are unpredictable. The following method utilizes a simple skin flap to provide blood supply and to prevent retraction of the cutaneous ureterostomy.

Steps of the Operation

1. A site is selected in the abdomen, usually opposite the anterior superior spine. The selection

263

PLATE 37

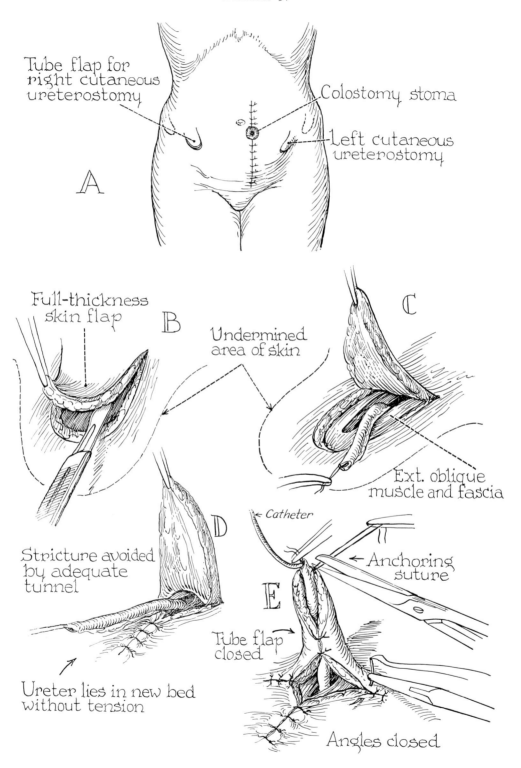

Tube flap for right cutaneous ureterostomy

Colostomy stoma

Left cutaneous ureterostomy

A

Full-thickness skin flap

B

Undermined area of skin

C

Ext. oblique muscle and fascia

Stricture avoided by adequate tunnel

D

Ureter lies in new bed without tension

Catheter

Anchoring suture

E

Tube flap closed

Angles closed

of the site is individualized for each patient, depending on the existence of previous scars, other stomas, or the condition of the skin from radiation (Plate 37, *A*).

2. A full-thickness skin flap is then cut at the area selected for the cutaneous ureterostomy (Plate 37, *B*). This should point downward and somewhat medially so as to better adapt itself to a collection device. The receptacle may be carried between the legs. An area of the skin adjacent to the flap is undermined for 2 to 3 cm. to aid in the subsequent closure (Plate 37, *B*).

3. The ureter is brought out to the skin retroperitoneally and through the transversalis and internal and external oblique muscles. An adequate canal is created by splitting the muscles and the aponeurosis of the external oblique, so that they do not contract about the ureter as it passes through the abdominal wall (Plate 37, *C* and *D*).

4. The area of skin that was undermined beyond the distal end of the flap is closed by interrupted sutures (Plate 37, *D*).

5. The ureter is anchored to the tip of the skin flap and the flap closed about the ureter without tension (Plate 37, *E*). Several sutures are placed at the angle of the base of the flap, but care is exercised not to constrict the ureter at any point. A small area is left open to granulate and also to drain any blood or serum that may emerge from the canal created for the transplanted ureter (Plate 37, *E*).

Postoperative Care

A small, soft rubber catheter is placed in the ureter and connected to a tube and bedside drainage bottle. Multiple, open, 4 by 4 sponges are placed around the cutaneous ureterostomy and flap. A small rubber catheter or polyethylene tubing is inserted among the open sponges in order to inject saline solution from time to time to keep the area moist. The transplanted ureter and flap are inspected for viability on the third postoperative day, and if healing is progressing well, the wound is lightly dressed and protected from pressure or other trauma. Since the skin about the transplant may become excoriated from urine that leaks about the catheter, it is kept clean and is painted with tincture of benzoin every other day. The catheter is replaced and irrigated from time to time, but excessive manipulation of the catheter

and operative area is to be avoided. Urinary antiseptics are given, and the usual postoperative care and electrolyte studies incidental to major pelvic and urologic surgery are carried out. By the tenth postoperative day or sooner the wound may be adequately healed, and the adaptation of a collecting device is started. The sooner the patient accepts and undertakes the care of the transplant, the better it is for her emotionally. The psychologic preparation of the patient preoperatively for this type of surgery will pay handsome dividends at this time.

References

Abbott, A. C., Macdougall, J. T., and Goodhand, T. K.: Hydronephrosis in a Solitary Kidney: Its Treatment by Nephro-ileo-neocystostomy (Calyco-ileo-neocystostomy), J. Urol. 84: 505, 1960.

Abeshouse, B. S., and others: Intestinovesical Fistulas, Report of 7 Cases and Review of the Literature, J. A. M. A. 164: 251, 1957.

Amar, A. D.: Clinical Importance of Ureteral Duplication and Ectopia, J. A. M. A. 168: 881, 1958.

Anson, B. J., and Daseler, E. H.: Common Variations in Renal Anatomy, Affecting Blood Supply, Form, and Topography, Surg., Gynec. & Obst. 112: 439, 1961.

Arconti, J. S.: The Isolated Ileal Segment in Urinary Surgery, J. Urol. 77: 182, 1957.

Arduino, L. J., and Miller, E. V.: Bladder Pouch for Tubeless Cystostomy, J. Urol. 84: 615, 1960.

Ashworth, A.: Papillomatosis of the Urethra, Brit. J. Urol. 28: 3, 1956.

Azoury, B. S., and Williamson, S. W.: Anastomosis of Stenosed Uterine Cervix to Urinary Bladder, Obst. & Gynec. 12: 113, 1958.

Baker, R., and others: Subtotal Cystectomy and Total Bladder Regeneration in Treatment of Bladder Cancer, J. A. M. A. 168: 1178, 1958.

Baker, W. J., and Graf, E. C.: Transplantation of the Ureters to an Isolated Ileostomy, J. Urol. 76: 557, 1956.

Ball, T.: Management of the Urological Complications of Pregnancy, M. Clin. North America 35: 3, 1951.

Bivens, M. D.: Postirradiation Vesicocervicovaginal Fistula, Obst. & Gynec. 9: 89, 1957.

Bohne, A. W., and Urwiller, K. L.: Experience With Urinary Bladder Regeneration, J. Urol. 77: 725, 1957.

Bourque, J.: Colocystoplasty for Enlargement and Substitution of Bladder: Preliminary Report of 25 Cases, J. Urol. 84: 527, 1960.

Boyd, M. L.: Transplantation of the Ureter Into the Bladder, J. A. M. A. 164: 651, 1957.

Butcher, H. R.: The Utility of Ureteroleal Urinary Diversion the Treatment of Irreparable Ureteral Obstructions, Surg., Gynec. & Obst. 109: 521, 1959.

Byron, R. L., and others: Ureterostomy in situ for Temporary Control of Ureteral Obstruction, Am. J. Obst. & Gynec. 81: 814, 1961.

Cesare, F., and Parsons, L.: Bilateral Sigmoid Transplantation of Duplicate Ureters, a Report of Two Cases, Obst. & Gynec. 14: 200, 1959.

Charnock, D. A., Riddell, H. I., and Lombardo, L. J.: Retroperitoneal Fibrosis Producing Ureteral Obstruction, J. Urol. 85: 251, 1961.

Chavigny, C. L.: Beaded Chain and Catheter for Cystograms, Obst. & Gynec. 10: 296, 1957.

Chovnick, S. D., Boyarsky, S., and Newman, H. R.: Clinical Value of Indirect Methods for the Determination of Residual Urine Volume, New York J. Med. **60:** 259, 1960.

Cibert, J., Durand, L., and Soler, A.: Urinary Complications Following Radical Treatment of Uterine Cancer, J. Urol. Med. **62:** 305, 1956.

Cohen, D.: The Ectopic Ureter, M. J. Australia **2:** 857, 1954.

Collins, C. G., and Jones, F. B.: Preoperative Cortisone for Vaginal Fistulas, Obst. & Gynec. **9:** 533, 1957.

Comarr, A. E.: Excretory Cystometry: A More Physiologic Method, J. Urol. **77:** 622, 1957.

Compere, D., and others: Ureteral Polyps, J. Urol. **79:** 209, 1958.

Cordonnier, J. J.: Ileal Bladder Substitution: An Analysis of 78 Cases, J. Urol. **77:** 714, 1957.

Crowell, J.: Ureteral Injury in Pelvic Surgery: Report of a Case, Am. J. Obst. & Gynec. **74:** 1266, 1957.

Davis, D.: The Process of Ureteral Repair: A Recapitulation of the Splinting Question, J. Urol. **79:** 215, 1958.

Davis, H. J., and TeLinde, R. W.: Urethral Diverticula: An Assay of 121 Cases, J. Urol. **80:** 34, 1958.

Davis, J. F., and Biel, L.: The Action of Pipenzolate Methylbromide on the Bladder as Determined by Cystometric Study, J. Urol. **82:** 596, 1959.

Douglas, R., Ball, T., and Davis, I.: Terramycin in Urinary Tract Infections, California Med. **73:** 463, 1950.

Douglas, R., McLellan, M., and Ball, T.: Aureomycin in the Treatment of Urinary Tract Infections in Obstetrics and Gynecology, M. Rec. & Ann. **45:** 4, 1951.

Drake, W. M., Jr.: The Uroflometer: An Aid to the Study of the Lower Urinary Tract, J. Urol. **59:** 650, 1948.

Drake, W. M., Jr.: The Uroflometer in the Study of Bladder Neck Obstructions, J. A. M. A. **156:** 1079, 1954.

Draper, J. W., Sierp, M., and Karam, O.: Simultaneous Studies of the Effect of Various Cholinergic and Anticholinergic Drugs on End Organs of the Autonomic Nervous System: Stomach, Colon, and Urinary Bladder, J. Urol. **77:** 214, 1957.

Dreyfuss, W., and Goodsitt, E.: Acute Regional Ureteritis, J. Urol. **79:** 202, 1958.

Eberhart, C.: Avulsion Therapy for Female Urethritis, J. Urolg. **79:** 293, 1958.

Eberhart, C.: The Etiology and Treatment of Urethritis in Female Patients, J. Urol. **79:** 293, 1958.

Edwards, E., and Beebe, R.: Diverticula of the Female Urethra, Obst. & Gynec. **5:** 729, 1955.

Ehrlich, H.: A Method of Artificial Closure of an Inoperable Vesicovaginal Fistula (Ueber einen kuenstlichen Verschluss inoperabler Blasenscheidenfisteln), Geburtsh. u. Frauenh. **88:** 1137, 1956.

Ellik, M.: Diverticulum of the Female Urethra: A New Method of Ablation, J. Urol. **77:** 243, 1957.

Everett, H., and Brack, C.: Unusual Lesions of the Female Urethra, Obst. & Gynec. **1:** 571, 1953.

Everett, H., and Long, J.: The Treatment of Urinary Infections, Am. J. Obst. & Gynec. **67:** 916, 1954.

Everett, H. S.: Diseases of the Female Urethra, J. A. M. A. **166:** 206, 1958.

Falk, H., and Bunkin, I.: Ureteral Injuries, Obst. & Gynec. **4:** 4, 1954.

Falk, H. C., and Tancer, M. L.: Vaginal Cystostomy, Obst. & Gynec. **9:** 86, 1957.

Felton, L. M., and Read, P. M.: An Evaluation of Bladder Flap and Skin Flap Cystostomies, J. Urol. **84:** 619, 1960.

Ferris, D. O.: Enlargement of the Urinary Bladder With a Segment of Ileum, J. Urol. **77:** 826, 1957.

Fretz, H. Z.: Granular Urethritis in Women, J. A. M. A. **169:** 933, 1959.

Furniss, H.: Ureterovesical Anastomosis, Surg., Gynec. & Obst. **27:** 339, 1918.

Furniss, H.: Sub-Urethral Abscesses and Diverticula in the Female Urethra, J. Urol. **33:** 498, 1935.

Garrett, R. A., and Vaughn, W. R.: Regeneration of Bladder, J. Urol. **77:** 718, 1957.

Gentil. F.: Bilateral Ureteroileal Anastomosis With Ileorectosigmoidostomy, Following Cystectomy for Cancer of Bladder: Preliminary Report, J. Urol. **80:** 20, 1956.

Gentil, F., and Shahbender, S.: The Use of Segments of Small Intestine in Surgery, Internat. Abstr. Surg. **109:** 417, 1959.

Gil Vernet, J. M.: Technique for the Construction of a Functioning Artificial Bladder, J. Urol. **83:** 39, 1960.

Goldman, H. J., and others: Monilial Cystitis—Effective Treatment With Instillations of Amphotericin B, J. A. M. A. **174:** 359, 1960.

Goodwin, W. E., and Winter, C. C.: Technique of Sigmoidocystoplasty, Surg., Gynec. & Obst. **96:** 370, 1959.

Goodwin, W. E., Winter, C. C., and Barker, W. F.: "Cup-Patch" Technique of Ileo-cystoplasty for Bladder Enlargement or Partial Substitution, Surg., Gynec. & Obst. **96:** 240, 1959.

Goodwin, W. E., Winter, C. C., and Turner, R. D.: Replacement of the Ureter by Small Intestine: Clinical Application and Results of the "Ileal Ureter," J. Urol. **81:** 406, 1959.

Graham, S. D.: The Use of Clorpactin WCS-90 for Routine Bladder Irrigations, J. Urol. **82:** 322, 1959.

Greenfield, M.: Eversion Stripping in the Production of a Nonsecretory, Nonabsorptive Urethral Emptying Ileal Bladder, J. Urol. **81:** 543, 1959.

Grey, D. N., Flynn, P., and Goodwin, W. E.: Experimental Methods of Ureteroneocystostomy: Experiences With the Ureteral Intussusception to Produce a Nipple or Valve, J. Urol. **77:** 154, 1957.

Hazard, J. B., McCormack, L. L., and Belovich, D.: Exfoliative Cytology of the Urine With Special Reference to Neoplasms of the Urinary Tract: Preliminary Report, J. Urol. **78:** 182, 1957.

Hinman, F.: Ureteral Repair and the Splint. J. Urol. **78:** 376, 1957.

Hinman, F., and Oppenheimer, R.: Functional Characteristics of the Ileal Segment as a Valve, J. Urol. **80:** 448, 1958.

Hinman, F., Jr., and Oppenheimer, R.: Ureteral Regeneration: VI. Delayed Urinary Flow in the Healing of Unsplinted Ureteral Defects, J. Urol. **78:** 138, 1957.

Hodgkinson, C. P.: Direct Urethrocystometry, Am. J. Obst. & Gynec. **79:** 648, 1960.

Hodgkinson, C. P.: Urethrovesicopubic Relationships in the Female, Am. J. Obst. & Gynec. **73:** 518, 1957.

Hodgkinson, C. P., and Kelly, W. T.: Urinary Stress Incontinence in the Female. III. Round-Ligament Technic for Retropubic Suspension of the Urethra, Obst. & Gynec. **10:** 493, 1957.

Hoffman, W. W., and Grayhack, J. T.: The Limitations of the Intravenous Pyelogram as a Test of Renal Function, Surg., Gynec. & Obst. **110:** 503, 1960.

Hudson, P. B., and Fox, H: Ureteroileosigmoidostomy, a Preliminary Report, Am. J. Obst. & Gynec. **74:** 368, 1957.

Ingelman-Sundberg, A.: An Operation for the Relief of Urinary Retention Caused by Paralysis of the Detrusor Muscle, Urol. internat. **4:** 249, 1957.

Ingelman-Sundberg, A.: Urinary Fistulae and Disturbances of the Bladder Function in Women, Gaz. Egypt. Soc. Gynec. & Obst. **6:** 6, 1957.

Ingelman-Sundberg, A.: Vaginal Slingoperation, Nordisk forening for obstetrikk og gynekologi, Kongress 1, Oslo, 1957.

Jude, J. R., Harris, A. H., and Smith, R. R.: The Physiological Response to the Ileal Bladder, Surg., Gynec. & Obst. **109:** 173, 1959.

Jude, J. R., Lusted, L. B., and Smith, R. R.: Radiographic Evaluation of the Urinary Tract Following Urinary Diversion to an Ileal Bladder, Cancer **12:** 1134, 1959.

Kane, J. T.: Stones in Urethral Diverticulum, New York J. Med. **57:** 3989, 1957.

Karcher, G.: The Indications for Permanent and Temporary Renal Fistulas in Obstructions of the Ureter and Renal Pelvis; Report of 75 Cases (Die Indikationen der permanenten und temporaren Nierenfistel bei Harnleiter-und Nierenbeckenverschluessen) Arch. klin. chir. **282:** 967, 1955.

Katzen, P., and Twatchman, B.: Diagnosis of Vaginal Ectopic Ureter, J. Urol. 72: 808, 1954.

Kickham, C. J. E., and Colpoys, F. L., Jr.: Periureteral Fascitis, J A. M. A. 171: 2202, 1959.

Kimura, C., Harada, N., and Tatsumi, W.: Antepubic Vesico-ileal-neourethrostomy, J. Urol. 77: 227, 1957.

Kittredge, W. E., and Brannan, W.: Cystitis Glandularis, J. Urol. 81: 419, 1959.

Kotzschke, G. H., and Sieber, E.: Studies Concerning the Hyperchloremic Acidosis Following Ureterosigmoidostomy (Untersuchungen ueber die hyperchloraemische Azidose nach Ureterosigmoidostomie) Ztschr. Urol. 49: 213, 1956.

Lapides, J., Ajemian, E. P., and Lichtwardt, J. R.: Cutaneous Vesicostomy, J. Urol. 84: 609, 1960.

Leadbetter, G., and Leadbetter, W.: Ureteral Re-implantation and Bladder Neck Reconstruction; Four and One-Half Years' Experience, J. A. M. A. 175: 349, 1961.

Leader, A. J.: A Useful Tool for Subpubic Repair of Vesicovaginal Fistula, J. Urol. 81: 494, 1959.

Levin, H. A.: Simplification of Ureteral Catheter Drainage, J. Urol. 84: 685, 1960.

Levin, J., Sneider, S., and Andrews, J.: An Appraisal of Renal Function and Infection in Advanced Bladder Cancer Treated With Ileal Bladder Construction and Irradiation, Surg., Gynec. & Obst. 112: 53, 1961.

McCormack, J. L., and Kretz, A. W.: Some Principles in the Care of Urinary Tract Injuries, J. A. M. A. 164: 1180, 1957.

McDonald, H. P., Upchurch, W. E., and Artime, M.: Urethritis-Cystitis Syndrome in the Female, J. A. M. A. 171: 2291, 1959.

McDonald, J. H., and Heckel, N. J.: Uretercutaneous Anastomosis Without the Use of Catheters, J. A. M. A. 163: 911, 1957.

MacDonald, S. A., and Kataria, P. N.: Ureteral Substitution by Isolated Ileal Loop: Ileoureteroplasty and Ileopyeloplasty, J. Urol. 77: 437, 1957.

McInnes, G. F., and Engler, H. S.: Experiences With the Ileal Bladder in Radical Pelvic Surgery, Cancer 9: 1219, 1956.

McNamara, R. J., Farber, E. M., and Roland, S. I.: Problems and Treatment of the Circumileostomy Skin, J. A. M. A. 171: 1066, 1959.

Malcolm, D. C.: Experiences With Ureterointestinal Anastomosis, J. Urol. 77: 173, 1957.

Marchetti, A. A., Marshall, V. F., and Shultis, L. D.: Simple Vesicourethral Suspension, Am. J. Obst. & Gynec. 74: 57, 1957.

Marshall, F. C., Uson, A. C., and Melicow, M. M.: Neoplasms and Caruncles of the Female Urethra, Surg., Gynec. & Obst. 110: 723, 1960.

Martin, L. S. J.: Uroepithelial Lined Ileal Segment as a Bladder Replacement: Experimental Observations and a Brief Review of Literature, J. Urol. 82: 633, 1959.

Martin, L. S. J., Duxbury, J. H., and Leadbetter, W. F.: Uroepithelial Lined Small Bowel as a Ureteral Substitute, Surg., Gynec. & Obst. 108: 439, 1959.

Masterson, J. G.: An Experimental Study of Ureteral Injuries in Radical Pelvic Surgery, Am. J. Obst. & Gynec. 73: 359, 1957.

Mathison, W., and others: Renal Function in Dogs Following Transplantation of the Ureters to an Isolated Sigmoid Pouch, J. Urol. 77: 27, 1957.

Mellinger, G. T., and Suder, G. T.: Ileal Reservoir (Ureteroileourethral Anastomosis), Method of Urinary Diversion, J. A. M. A. 167: 2183, 1958.

Mendel, E. B., and Bone, F. W.: Suprapubic Vesicourethral Suspension: Its Use as a Primary Procedure; a Preliminary Report of 52 Cases, Obst. & Gynec. 10: 493, 1957.

Merricks, J. W., and others: Surgical Treatment of Urethral Diverticulum (Female), J. A. M. A. 163: 386, 1957.

Morales, P., Askari, S., and Hotchkiss, R. S.: Ileal Replacement of the Ureter, J. Urol. 82: 304, 1959.

Morales, P. A., and others: Sigmoidocystoplasty for the Contracted Bladder, J. Urol. 80: 455, 1958.

Morris, J. McL., and Keggi, K. J.: Clinical and Cineradiographic Evaluation of the Mathisen Ureterosigmoidostomy, Surg., Gynec. & Obst. 112: 481, 1961.

Muellner, S. R.: The Anatomies of the Female Urethra, Obst. & Gynec. 14: 429, 1959.

Mulvany, J. H.: Stress Incontinence in Women: Its Mechanism and Treatment, J. Obst. & Gynaec. Brit. Emp. 64: 531, 1957.

Murphy, J., and Schoenberg, H.: Diagnosis of Bladder Outlet Obstruction, J. A. M. A. 175: 354, 1961.

Murphy, J. J., and Mikuta, J. J.: Urinary Diversion in Pelvic Exenteration, Surg., Gynec. & Obst. 112: 743, 1961.

Nelson, N. M., and others: Transurethral Resection of the Bladder Neck in the Female, J. Urol. 77: 198, 1957.

O'Conor, V. J., Jr., and Dawson-Edwards, P.: Role of the Ureter in Renal Transplantation: 1. Studies of Denervated Ureter With Particular Reference to Ureteroureteral Anastomosis, J. Urol. 82: 566, 1959.

Ormond, J. K.: Idiopathic Retroperitoneal Fibrosis; an Established Clinical Entity, J. A. M. A. 174: 1561, 1960.

Paquin, A. J., Jr.: Ureterovesical Anastomosis: The Description and Evaluation of a Technique, J. Urol. 82: 573, 1959.

Pasquier, C. M., Jr., and Campbell, J. H.: Further Observations on the Problems of Vesicoureteral Reflux, South. M. J. 52: 967, 1959.

Pereyra, A. J.: A Simplified Surgical Procedure for the Correction of Stress Incontinence in Women, West. J. Surg. 67: 223, 1959.

Pool, T. L.: Irradiation Cystitis, J. A. M. A. 168: 854, 1958.

Pool, T. L., Mackinnon, M., and Pratt, J. H.: Diverticulum of the Female Urethra, S. Clin. North America 39: 953, 1959.

Powell, E.: Effect of Hydrocortisone on Urethritis, J. Urol. 84: 340, 1960.

Powell, N. B., and Powell, E. B.: Transurethral Bladder Neck Resection in the Female, J. Urol. 80: 479, 1958.

Prentiss, R. J., Mullenix, R. B., and Feeney, M. J.: Ureteral Implantation: Clinical Experiences, J. Urol. 77: 600, 1957.

Rattner, W. H., Moran, J. J., and Murphy, J. J.: The Histological Appearance of Small Bowel Segments Used as Urinary Conduits, J. Urol. 82: 236, 1959.

Reed, D. C., and Dodson, A. I.: Ureteral Injury, J. Kansas M. Soc. 58: 505, 1957.

Richardson, E. J.: Ileal Loop Substitute in Ureteral Injuries, J. Urol. 80: 17, 1958.

Robbins, J. J.: Vesicorectostomy, J. Urol. 77: 34, 1957.

Shackman, R.: Urinary Deviation in Gynaecological Surgery, J. Obst. & Gynaec. Brit. Emp. 65: 548, 1959.

Shoemaker, W. C., and Long, D. M.: Functional Studies on Transplanted Intestinal Smooth Muscle Grafts Used to Reconstruct the Denervated Canine Bladder, Surg., Gynec. & Obst. 108: 523, 1959.

Shram, M., and Silverstein, L. M.: Female Suburethral Diverticulum, New York J. Med. 59: 634, 1959.

Simon, H. B., and Nygaard, K. K.: Ureteral Obstruction Due to Idiopathic Retroperitoneal Fibrosis; Report of One Case and Collective Review of Thirty-four Additional Cases, J. A. M. A. 174: 1569, 1960.

Sinatra, T. J.: Use of Y-Plasty for Obstruction of Vesical Neck, J. Urol. 77: 614, 1957.

Sinatra, T. J., and Weinverg, S. R.: Functional Analysis of the Bladder After Ileocystoplasty, J. Urol. 80: 180, 1958.

Smith, R. A.: Clorpactin XCB: Its Use in Urology in the Sugical Treatment of Malignant Neoplasms, J. Urol. 81: 554, 1959.

Symmonds, R. E.: Present Concepts and Management of Urinary Stress Incontinence, S. Clin. North America 39: 933, 1959.

Tauber, A. S., and Maluf, N. S. R.: Anterior Approach to the Upper Ureter, J. Urol. 80: 13, 1958.

TeLinde, R.: Urological Aspects of Gynecology, Am. J. Obst. & Gynec. 74: 1305, 1957.

Ulm, A. H.: An Incision for the Removal of Stones Impacted in the Lower Ureter, Surg., Gynec. & Obst. 94: 637, 1957.

VanDuzen, R., and Duncan, C.: Anatomy and Nerve Supply of Urinary Bladder, J. A. M. A. 153: 1345, 1953.

Wade, W. H., Stephenson, H. E., and Todd, C.: Use of the Real Conduit in Traumatic Paraplegia, A. M. A. Arch. Surg. 80: 162, 1960.

Wallingford, A. J., and Gabriels, A. G.: Ectopic Ureter: A Cause of Female Urinary Incontinence; Reports of Four Cases, Obst. & Gynec. 10: 95, 1957.

Walsh, A.: Hazards of Bladder Surgery Following Irradiation, J. Urol. 84: 627, 1960.

Weaver, R. G.: Basic Surgical Principles of Ureteral Repair, Surg., Gynec. & Obst. 110: 594, 1960.

Weinberg, S., and Maletta, T.: Measurement of Peristalsis of the Ureter and its Relation to Drugs, J. A. M. A. 175: 15, 1961.

Weinberg, S. R., and Waterhouse, K.: Function of the Bladder After Ileocystoplasty, J. Urol. 82: 80, 1959.

Wharton, L. R., and Creecy, A. A., and Bealzie, F. S.: Regeneration of the Female Urethra Following Severe Injury and Observation on the Localization of Urinary Control, J. Urol. 82: 105, 1959.

Wilkins, S. A.: Experience With Uremic Complications After Ureterointestinal Transplantation, With Comment on the Use of the Rectal Bladder, Cancer 11: 40, 1958.

Wilkins, S. A., and Wills, S. A.: The Rectal Bladder for Urinary Diversion, Surg., Gynec. & Obst. 109: 1, 1959.

Winter, C. C.: A Clinical Study of a New Renal Function Test: The Radioactive Diodrast Renogram, J. Urol. 76: 182, 1956.

Winter, C. C., and Goodwin, W. E.: Results of Sigmoidocystoplasty, J. Urol. 80: 467, 1958.

Wishard, W. N., Nourse, M. H., and Mertz, J. H. O.: Diverticulum of the Female Urethra, With Special Reference to Diverticular Carcinoma, South. M. J. 52: 890, 1959.

Wishard, W. N., Jr., Nourse, M. H., and Mertz, J. H. O.: Use of Clorpactin WCS 90 for Relief of Symptoms Due to Interstitial Cystitis, J. Urol. 77: 420, 1957.

Woodburne, R. T.: Structure and Function of the Urinary Bladder, J. Urol. 84: 79, 1960.

Youngblood, V., and others: Exfoliative Cytology of the Senile Female Urethra, J. Urol. 79: 110, 1958.

Youngblood, V. H., Tomlin, E. M., and Davis, J. B.: Senile Urethritis in Women, J. Urol. 78: 150, 1957.

Youssef, A. F.: Cystometric Studies in Gynecology and Obstetrics, Obst. & Gynec. 8: 181, 1956.

Section VI · PROCTOLOGY ASSOCIATED with GYNECOLOGIC SURGERY

13 · General Considerations and Surgical Principles in Proctology Encountered by the Gynecologist

General Considerations

The gynecologist can no more remove himself from the diseases of the anorectum in the practice of his specialty than he can dissociate himself from the female bladder. Many anorectal lesions are corrected at the time of gynecologic surgery, and the experienced vaginal plastic surgeon will correct these with equal skill. Should he be trained in radical pelvic surgery, the gynecologist is able to combine the most formidable procedures on the rectosigmoid with the removal of other organ systems in the pelvis.

Symptoms and Diagnosis in Anorectal Disease

The two most common complaints in benign anorectal disease are bleeding and pain. Bright red blood comes from lesions near the anus, while dark blood is indicative of some disease higher in the bowel. Pain suggests an anal ulcer, a foreign body, or a thrombosed hemorrhoid. This symptom is generally out of proportion to the seriousness of the lesion except in advanced malignancies. Pruritus is so common that it adds nothing to the differential diagnosis as a symptom of anorectal disease. Protrusion of hemorrhoids and polyps is common, with the differential diagnosis being evident on inspection. A discharge of mucus or pus suggests an inflammatory process, the origin of which is usually evident on examination. Constipation and diarrhea are not significant symptoms in themselves unless there is a change of bowel habits.

On rectal examination the thickened, roll-like feel of the contracted external sphincter is first felt. The thinner, broader internal sphincter extends up from this about 2 cm., and just above this the medial edge of the puborectalis can be felt on each side. The finger then passes into the more or less dilated ampulla of the rectum proper. By palpating laterally, the condition of the ischiorectal fossa is determined and the extent—above or below the levator sling—of a perirectal abscess can be noted. The mobility of the coccyx and the presence of pain on movement (coccygodynia) are observed. Of particular interest to the gynecologist is the palpation of the rectovaginal septum and the cervix through the rectal wall. Thickening and induration are noted so that they can be compared with the observations on proctosigmoidoscopy. The palpation of the paracolpium, the uterosacral thickenings, and the cardinal thickenings through the rectal wall is generally more informative than anything learned by vaginal palpation.

Nothing can take the place of a proctosigmoidoscopic examination since it reveals lesions not large enough (in the rectosigmoid area) to be seen on x-ray or fluoroscopic examination and those too far above the examining finger to be felt or seen by simple anoscopy. A proctosigmoidoscopic examination should precede any rectal surgery, however minor, undertaken in the course of gynecologic surgery. In the rectum, ulcerations, papillomas, tumors, and other suspicious lesions are biopsied. In the region of the pectinate (anorectal, dentate) line, cryptitis, papillitis, fistulas, and ulcers and, above the line, the presence and extent of internal hemorrhoids are diagnosed.

Surgical Principles in Proctology Encountered by the Gynecologist

1. Pelvic surgeons need not feel awkward in performing anorectal surgery in the lithotomy position. The impaction of the fecal stream against the perineal body results in most of the simple lesions of the anal canal being located in the posterior half. The gynecologist, therefore, works in the most comfortable position. Think of how we work on the anterior vaginal wall! While the lithotomy position causes considerable orthopedic strain on the patient, the operative field for anorectal surgery is well exposed. Gynecologists learn to perform vaginal surgery with the hands flexed toward the radius and extended dorsally. This is the exact opposite to the position of the hands used by all craftsmen, in every trade, to perform delicate pieces of work! In fact, it is in an opposite direction to all the precision movements men have learned since birth. We have adapted ourselves to work so as not to shift the position of the patient because of the resultant anesthetic complications. Anorectal surgery can be done from the lithotomy position with ease.

2. Although high rectal pain in the female is most frequently the result of gynecologic disease and menstruation rather than of intrinsic rectal disease, the indications for proctosigmoidoscopic study are just as imperative. Endometriosis is a skilled imitator of cancer in the rectum and sigmoid colon!

3. Proctologic surgery is postponed during pregnancy. Especially in the third trimester, only imperative operations are undertaken, since the congestion and swelling of the tissues make hemostasis difficult. The susceptibility of the pregnant patient to thrombosis contraindicates any but the most urgent procedures.

4. External thrombotic hemorrhoids—common but not exclusive in pregnancy—are not really clots in a hemorrhoid. They result from the rupture of small veins near the skin surface, with the collection of several pockets of coagulated blood. This is evident to anyone who has evacuated such a mass. Thrombotic hemorrhoids should be excised, not incised, in the early months of pregnancy. More conservative measures are indicated for palliation later in pregnancy when such hemorrhoids may have to be treated by applications to relieve pain or by incision of the larger pockets.

5. Hemorrhoids may be caused by invasion of the rectum from genital tract malignancies as well as from intrinsic disease.

6. Fulguration of lesions on the vaginal side of the rectum causes more reaction and must be done with greater care than does fulguration of lesions on the lateral or posterior walls. This is because of the better blood supply to the posterolateral aspect of the rectum.

7. The height of lesions in the rectum is important. Those above the peritoneal reflection are much more dangerous and the complications more serious. No surgeon is more competent than the gynecologist, who knows the level of the cul-de-sac peritoneum in the various degrees of prolapse, to decide on the extension of a rectal lesion in the female.

8. If the external rectal sphincter is markedly hypertrophied and is contributing to the recurrence of fissures or causing rectal tenesmus, a posterior proctotomy is indicated. Vaginal surgeons, skilled in the approximation of the tissues of the perineal body, compensate for this with an effectual and functional perineorrhaphy.

Preoperative Care and Anesthesia

Patients prepared for gynecologic surgery need have only a few more cleansing enemas and they are ready for rectal surgery. This does not apply to operations for malignancy, where a major procedure is to be done. Many surgeons have noted that patients experience prolonged urinary retention after combined gynecologic and proctologic operations. The reason for this is not clear, but preoperative and postoperative use of antimicrobial therapy protects the urinary tract from serious infection until normal bladder function returns.

The bulk of gynecologic surgery is done

under general anesthesia, and this is quite satisfactory for the additional anorectal operation. Many minor proctologic operations are preferably done under local anesthesia. Either procaine, 1 per cent, or Xylocaine, 0.5 to 2.0 per cent, with or without the addition of epinephrine, is satisfactory, as are several other preparations. Many preparations are available that contain hyaluronidase. One common preparation contains 300 TR (turbidity-reducing) units of hyaluronidase in 50 ml. of 1 per cent procaine, with 0.5 ml. of epinephrine solution, 1:1,000, added. The diffusion of the procaine because of the hyaluronidase effect has its enthusiastic supporters. Much more important than the choice of drugs or combinations is the skill of the operator in infiltrating this highly sensitive area. The surgeon must be fast and meticulous in his technique. Long, angled or curved, special rectal needles are used to spare the patient multiple primary introductions of the needle into the skin.

Surgical Anatomy of the Rectum and Anus

The rectum begins where the pelvic mesocolon ceases, and it is divided into two parts. The first part is 10 to 12 cm. long and is concave forward, following the curve of the sacrum and coccyx. The second part (anal canal) begins on the pelvic floor and curves downward and backward to the anus. The lower portion of the first part presents a dilation (ampulla) due to the accumulation of feces. This part is sometimes described as the infraperitoneal portion of the rectum proper. The anal canal (second part) is from 2.5 to 3.5 cm. in length, passes through the pelvic floor, and ends at the anus. It is entirely surrounded by two sphincter muscles.

The structure of the rectum differs from the colon in that its walls are smoother, there are no epiploic appendages, and it derives a well-developed longitudinal muscle layer from the taeniae found on the colon. The taeniae spread out on the rectum to form a longitudinal muscle layer that is better developed anteriorly and posteriorly than it is laterally. This is referred to in some texts as O'Beirne's

sphincter. Its function in defecation and rectal symptomatology is not understood. Three constant transverse folds (valves of Houston) project into the lumen of the rectum. One, on the right side, is at the level of the reflection of the peritoneum from the bowel to the uterus and upper vagina (cul-de-sac of Douglas). Two are on the left side, one above and one below the fold on the right side. All the folds contain smooth muscle and project for varying distances into the lumen of the rectum. The upper fold is near the junction of the rectum with the colon, where the bowel is often constricted. The fold on the right side is the largest and is located about 7.5 cm. above the anus. The lowermost fold is on the left side a few centimeters below the larger middle fold on the right.

The structure of the anal canal creates many landmarks useful in the practice of proctology. Rectal columns (columns of Morgagni) are a series of longitudinal folds of mucous membrane containing some smooth muscle fibers. They become more prominent as they extend downward. Just above the anus, each two adjoining columns unite by an archlike fold of mucous membrane. These folds are called anal valves, while the small fossae behind them are known as anal crypts. On the anal surface of some of the folds, small, papillary, fibrous structures called the anal papillae arise. They are subject to much trauma and inflammation in addition to considerable apprehension when their enlargement suggests a malignant change. The crypts and papillae in the posterior half of the anorectal (pectinate, dentate) line are especially prone to infection since the fecal mass impinges upon this part of the line almost at right angles to the long axis of the rectum. Cryptitis is the first stage of an anal fistula, and one should search for the internal opening of the lesion just distal to the anorectal line, where the floor of the rectovaginal wall starts to incline anteriorly into the body of the perineum. The mucous membrane of the anal canal is more firmly attached to the muscularis than it is in the rectum. First or second degree rectal prolapse starts with the mucous membrane of the lower portion of the ampulla being extruded because of this firm attachment. The area below the valves and extending to the anus is variously divided by a number of anatomic lines that are equally significant in anorectal pathology. The anorectal line is the same as the dentate line or the pectinate line. All three terms are variously used among anatomists and clinicians writing about the rectum and anus. This line is the upper end of the anal canal and represents the union of modified anal skin (anoderm) with the rectal mucosa above. Above this line the blood supply is from the superior hemorrhoidal artery and middle hemorrhoidal artery. The contribution of the latter and its anastomoses is not clearly understood. The venous drainage above the anorectal line from a clinical standpoint is into the portal circulation. Below the anorectal line the inferior hemorrhoidal branch of the internal pudendal artery provides the blood supply. Above the dentate line the innervation is sympathetic in origin, while below this line the anoderm is supplied by the cerebrospinal system. This line (anorectal, dentate, pectinate) also divides internal from external hemorrhoids that are reportable as separate conditions to most surgical insurance carriers, although it has ever been a mystery to most surgeons as to how you could operate for one type to the total exclusion of the other. Duty compels me to continue to clarify the nomenclature of this area. Many of the anatomic landmarks have several names and, used interchangeably, confuse the descriptions of the anorectal anatomy. The white line of Hilton is at the junction of the middle and lower thirds of the anal canal, where the internal sphincter overlaps the external sphincter. Between this and the anorectal line (dentate, pectinate) is the pecten (pecten line), because underneath the anoderm is a fibroelastic band (pecten band) that immediately overlies the intermuscular septum between the internal and external sphincters. This band is regarded by many proctologists as pathologic, since it causes contracture in response to chronic inflammation. The constriction of

this band due to inflammatory reaction (pectenosis) does not yield under anesthesia. An hypertrophied and spastic sphincter would dilate under the same circumstances according to those who advocate the pecten band as a distinct entity. Obstetricians and gynecologists accustomed to dilatations permitting the passage of a fetal head 10 cm. or more in diameter may take a dim view of this theory.

The anus is the aperture by which the intestine opens externally. Due to the sphincters that surround the terminal part of the anal canal, the skin is wrinkled. The internal sphincter is a thickening of the circular fibers of the rectum, is about 2 to 3 mm. thick, is composed of smooth muscles, and surrounds the lower part of the anal canal. The voluntary muscles of the rectum are the external sphincter, levator ani, and rectococcygeal. The external sphincter ani is a thin, flat plate of muscle, elliptical in shape and adherent to the skin around the margin of the anus. It is 2 to 3 cm. broad and from 8 to 10 cm. from its anterior to its posterior extremity. Three parts, not always distinct, are recognizable. A small subcutaneous division surrounds the anus just under the skin. A superficial division, the main portion of the muscle, arises from a narrow tendinous band, the anococcygeal raphe, which stretches from the tip of the coccyx to the posterior margin of the anus. The muscle then encircles the anus to insert into the central point of the perineum. The anterior fiber bundles interdigitate with one another and also with the transverse perineal muscles and bulbocavernosi. The deep division surrounds the canal and is intimately connected with the internal sphincter. It is separated from fibers of the puborectalis division of the levator ani by connective tissue accompanying the inferior hemorrhoidal vessels. The nerve supply is from the fourth sacral nerve and a twig from the inferior hemorrhoidal branch of the internal pudic nerve.

The blood supply of the rectum and anus, from above downward, arises from the superior hemorrhoidal branch of the inferior mesenteric artery, the middle hemorrhoidal branch of the hypogastric artery, and the inferior hemorrhoidal branch of the internal pudic artery. The superior hemorrhoidal artery divides into two branches which pass down on either side to within about 12 cm. of the anus. Here they split into about six branches which pierce the muscular coats of the rectum and also anastomose with branches of the middle hemorrhoidal artery. The middle hemorrhoidal artery usually has a common origin with the internal pudendal artery. It passes to the rectum several centimeters below the middle of the rectum and anastomoses with the branches of the superior and inferior hemorrhoidal arteries. The inferior hemorrhoidal artery rises from the internal pudendal as it passes above the tuberosity of the ischium. Crossing the ischiorectal fossa, it is distributed to muscles and walls of the anal region and adjacent skin. The connective tissues surrounding these vessels and also the nerves, together with the levator ani, help support the rectum and have been called collectively the suspensory ligament of the rectum. A rent in the bowel, whether sigmoid or rectum, rarely develops into a fistula, even after radiation and the most radical surgery. The blood supply of the rectum precludes this. For some reason, when the urinary stream has been diverted to the bowel, and subsequent injury occurs to the segment containing both feces and urine, fistulas are more likely to occur. Since the use of vaginal cone radiotherapy by any of the various techniques, the rectovaginal wall, just in front of the posterior fornix, has been subjected to intense dosages of deep therapy. This is especially true when a relaxed outlet permits a high rectocele to bulge in the path of the vaginal cone. Some fistulas have resulted from a necrotizing dose in this area.

About 2.5 cm. above the levator ani two fibrous bands insert into the rectum. They are known as the rectococcygeal muscles or rectal stalks. They arise from the area of the second and third coccygeal vertebrae and, together with fibers surrounding the middle hemorrhoidal vessels, pass to either side of the rectum. The main support of the rectum, the levator

ani, is described completely under The Statics of the Female Pelvic Viscera (page 103). This muscle divides the perineum from the pelvis. Above it and its connective tissue extensions from the obturator fascia is the pelvirectal or supralevator fossa and below it is the ischiorectal fossa. Fibers of the puborectalis portion of the levator ani converge toward the anorectal (dentate, pectinate) line.

The lymphatics of the anus and rectum arise from two networks. The lymphatics of the skin at the anal margin pass to the superficial inguinal nodes. Some lymphatics from the skin drain deeper to join the lymphatics from the submucous plexus of the rectum. The regional lymph vessels of the rectum pass to the pararectal nodes, to the nodes along the middle hemorrhoidal artery, and to nodes along the inferior hemorrhoidal artery. A node near the origin of the internal pudic artery is quite constant. The efferents from these nodes terminate in the inferior mesenteric nodes. Since the rectal lymphatics accompany the blood vessels, a complete resection of the vessels and attached mesentery and visceral extensions of the parietal connective tissue will remove the greatest number of nodes in anorectal surgery for malignant disease.

The nerve supply of the rectum and anus is derived from the inferior mesenteric plexus and paired hypogastric plexuses. The inferior mesenteric plexus is derived from the left side of the aortic plexus and sends fibers which surround the inferior mesenteric artery. Left colic and sigmoid plexuses are formed, as well as a superior hemorrhoidal plexus, which supply their respective organs. The hypogastric plexuses supply the viscera of the pelvic cavity. They are derived from the presacral plexus and accompany branches of the hypogastric artery in innervating the pelvic viscera.

The ischiorectal fossa is situated between the end of the rectum and the ischial tuberosity. It is triangular in shape, with its base directed toward the skin. Its apex corresponds to the point of division of the obturator fascia and the thin membrane given off from it that covers the outer surface of the levator ani. Its dimensions are about an inch in breadth at the base and about two inches deep. It is bound, internally, by the anal sphincter, the levator ani, and the coccygeus. Externally it is bounded by the tuberosity of the ischium and the obturator fascia. Behind, it is limited by the margin of the gluteus maximus and the great sacrosciatic ligament. In front it is bounded by the line of junction of the deep layer of the superficial fascia with the base of the triangular ligament. It is filled with fatty tissue, an important factor in dealing with infections about the rectum.

Medical Treatment of Anal Pruritus

The patient with anal pruritus should be reassured by carefully explaining the physical findings responsible for the itching. The psychogenic factors that aggravate this and other similar complaints about the body are best enumerated after medical treatment has been initiated and the patient experiences some relief. The scratch-itch cycle must be interrupted by local treatment known to relieve the majority of mild cases and to make the severe problems more bearable. Woolen or nylon underwear or close-fitting garments keep the area moist and aggravate the symptom. Tight girdles press the buttocks together and prevent proper ventilation, which results in chafing and irritation.

Local treatment in females necessitates the correction of any vaginal discharge that may bathe the perineum and anus and thus add to the irritation in the area. Douches normally used to produce an acid medium in the vagina should be generally favored if they do not contain any ingredients to which the patient appears sensitive. In many instances the anal pruritus is only a part of a general irritation of the area, and a concurrent vulvovaginitis is frequently found. Treatment must then be focused on the whole problem and not just the anus.

Anal hygiene is clearly and simply explained to the patient. No coarse tissue, which amounts to scratching the area, should be used. Wet tissue or cotton is used after defecation, and then the anus is blotted dry with soft tissue. Soap should not be used directly on the anal skin, and if an ointment is prescribed, this is applied before bathing to prevent contact of the anal area with soap.

Diet is important and should be prescribed so as to produce an acid-ash residue. Studies of the pH of the anal secretions and ampulla of the rectum reveal a pH of 7.5 or less as a normal value. In many patients with severe pruritus the pH of the ampulla is from 7.5 to 9, and this favors the growth of many fungi and pathogenic bacteria not common to the area. A diet that produces lactic acid on fermentation in the intestinal tract includes dairy products of all types and cultured buttermilk. Beta-lactose can be added to the milk for greater production of lactic acid. Carbohydrates and fruits such as prunes, plums, and cranberries produce an acid-ash. Proteins are de-emphasized during the acute phase, since they encourage the growth of putrefactive bacteria although producing an acid medium in their metabolism.

Viable *Lactobacillus acidophilus* can be given in several ways, and several products containing the organism in tablet form are available. This organism is especially useful in the management of pruritus following the use of the wide-spectrum antibiotics that sterilize the intestinal tract to some degree and reduce its normal acidophilic flora. Alcohol and spices are avoided in the acute phase. Anything that produces a loose stool, such as beer or ale, is contraindicated, although a dry, firm stool is likewise to be avoided. Mineral oil, which may leak through the anus and take irritating substances with it, has caused more rectal symptoms than it has ever alleviated.

A vigorous attack upon the alkalinity of the rectal ampulla by the use of rectal irrigations is most effective in getting at the basis of the problem and affording prompt relief. The rectal irrigation is made up by adding 1 teaspoonful of 20 per cent lactic acid solution to a pint of warm water and is administered as a low enema. This can be repeated up to three times daily. The pH of the rectal ampulla is roughly determined with nitrazine paper prior to the above treatment. Rectal irrigations of this type also remove residual feces, mucus, and other irritating substances.

Local applications such as Burow's solution, 1:10, and potassium permanganate, 1:4,000, are both useful. An ice collar can often afford dramatic relief. Local anesthetics in an oily base are not recommended for long-term relief. A mild paste that will protect the perianal skin from the irritating secretions is desirable. Unna's soft zinc paste can be used for long periods without inducing local symptoms from its own contents. Zinc oxide and castor oil in equal parts, frequently used about colostomies, has a protective, soothing, emollient action. When a fungicidal preparation is indicated, mild preparations of gentian violet, malachite green, Castellani's paint, and other dyes may be applied. In the very acute cases they should be diluted three or more times with some mild ointment.

The use of hydrocortisone ointment, 2.5 per cent, in the management of anal pruritus produces dramatic results in relieving the symptoms but should be used in conjunction with specific therapy of the underlying cause. It affords relief within a few days, but the results are not permanent if the anal skin continues to be bathed in irritating secretions. Frykman advises the addition of neomycin to the hydrocortisone ointment when the presence of secondary infection is evidenced by scattered excoriations in the area. The very chronic cases with lichenification of the skin frequently respond to x-ray therapy. The hyperexcitability of the skin is decreased and the scratch-itch cycle interrupted. The usual precautions against a radiodermatitis are taken, and the skin must be observed with each treatment to single out those patients who do not tolerate the therapy well.

Indications and Surgical Principles in the Treatment of Anal Pruritus

Surgical therapy consists of the injection of long-lasting anesthetics, sclerosing solutions, and undercutting operations. An aqueous preparation of Diothane and benzyl alcohol is very good for local injection and is safer than the anesthetics in oil. Redundancy of the mucous membrane may sometimes be corrected by the injection of a sclerosing solution into the submucosa, causing it to become adherent to the underlying muscularis. Five per cent phenol in olive oil is one of several good agents. Primary, extensive undercutting operations are reserved for intractable, incapacitating cases. The perianal skin should be routinely undercut during the course of surgery for other rectal conditions. This is true in practically all minor rectal and anal surgery, for itching is usually present, even if it is not the primary symptom that brings the patient to her physician. This interruption of the sensory nerves will last for several months, during which time the skin of the anus can be restored to normal. (See Surgical Management of Anovulval Pruritus, page 95.)

References

Abel, A. L.: The Pecten; the Pecten Band; Pectenosis and Pectenotomy, Lancet 1: 714, 1932.
Abramson, D. J.: An Improved and Rotatable Anoscope, J. A. M. A. 160: 874, 1956.
Adriani, J.: Anesthesia for Anorectal and Colonic Surgery, New York J. Med. 59: 1066, 1959.
Alexander, R. M., and Manheim, S. D.: Preliminary and Short Reports. The Effect of Hydrocortisone Acetate Ointment on Pruritus Ani, J. Invest. Dermat. 21: 223, 1953.
Anderson, M. J.: Perianal Hidradenitis Suppurativa; a Clinical and Pathological Study, Dis. Colon & Rectum 2: 23, 1959.
Bockus, H. L., and others: Early Clinical Manifestations of Cancer of the Colon and Rectum, Dis. Colon & Rectum 2: 58, 1959.
Bowman, F. B.: Proctosigmoidoscopy for the Family Physician, Canad. M. A. J. 68: 244, 1953.
Buckwalter, J. A., and Jurayj, M.: Relationship of Chronic Anorectal Disease to Carcinoma, A. M. A. Arch. Surg. 75: 352, 1957.
Fansler, W. A.: Proctoscopy and Proctologic Office Procedures, G. P. 15: 101, 1957.
Finney, J. M. T., Jr., and Stone, D. H.: The Fallibility of Roentgenograms in Diagnosing Lesions of the Colon, Ann. Surg. 137: 682, 1953.
Foote, R. F., De La Cruz, T., and Hill, M.: Muscle Rehabilitation in Anorectal Surgery, Dis. Colon & Rectum 4: 135, 1961.
Frykman, H. M.: Anal Pruritus, Minnesota Med. 38: 19, 1955.
Gianturco, C., and Miller, G. A.: Program for the Detection of Colonic and Rectal Polyps, J. A. M. A. 153: 1429, 1953.
Hellwig, C. A., and Barbosa, E.: How Reliable is Biopsy of Rectal Polyps? A Clinical and Morphological Study of 107 Cases, Cancer 12: 620, 1959.
Jackman, R. J.: The Importance and Technic of Proctoscopy, Dis. Colon & Rectum 2: 139, 1959.
Jackman, R. J., and Swartzlander, F. C.: Source of Bleeding From the Lower Bowel, New York J. Med. 56: 397, 1956.
Judd, E. S., Jr.: Progress in the Surgical Management of

Diverticulitis of the Colon, J. Iowa M. Soc. 46: 577, 1956.

Lucas, M. A., and Bowling, E. C.: Incidence of Lesions in 6,000 Consecutive Proctoscopic Examinations, J. Kentucky Med. A. 55: 431, 1957.

Manheim, S. D., and Alexander, R. M.: Further Observations on Anorectal Complications Following Aureomycin, Terramycin, and Chloromycetin Therapy, New York J. Med. 54: 231, 1954.

Mayo, C. W., and Cullen, P. K.: Diverticulosis and Diverticulitis of the Colon, New York J. Med. 59: 2391, 1959.

Moon, L. E.: Proctologic Help for the General Practitioner and the Diagnostician, J. A. M. A. 154: 138, 1954.

Necheles, H., Jefferson, N. C., and Sporn, J.: New Gastrointestinal and Urinary Spasmolytic Drugs, Am. J. Gastroenterol. 26: 464, 1956.

Osborne, E. D., and Stoll, H. L.: Pruritis Ani et Vulvae, J. A. M. A. 169: 124, 1959.

Paine, J. R.: Early Diagnosis of Carcinoma of the Gastrointestinal Tract, J. Indiana M. A. 46: 737, 1953.

Pope, C. E.: An Anorectal Plastic Operation for Fissure and Stenosis and its Surgical Principles, Surg., Gynec. & Obst. 108: 249, 1959.

Portes, C., and Majarakis, J. D.: Proctosigmoidoscopy—Incidence of Polyps in 50,000 Examinations, J. A. M. A. 163: 411, 1957.

Raskin, H. F., Palmer, W. L., and Kirsner, J. B.: Exfoliative Cytology in Diagnosis of Cancer of the Colon, Dis. Colon & Rectum 2: 46, 1959.

Rauch, R. F.: Coexisting Diverticulitis and Carcinoma of the Colon, A. M. A. Arch. Surg. 73: 823, 1956.

Rosenberg, I.: The Use of Corticosteroid Ointments in the Management of Postoperative Anorectal Wounds, Dis. Colon & Rectum 3: 50, 1960.

Sauntry, J. P., and Knudtson, K. P.: A Technique for Marking the Mucosa of the Gastrointestinal Tract After Polypectomy, Cancer 11: 607, 1958.

Shackelford, R. T., and McGeehan, J. S.: Improved Technique of Coloscopy, J. A. M. A. 167: 280, 1958.

Shatz, B. A., and Freitas, E. L.: Area of Colon Visualized Through the Sigmoidoscope, J. A. M. A. 156: 717, 1954.

Turell, R.: Adenomas and Hemorrhoids. Problems of Rectal Bleeding, Wisconsin M. J. 54: 413, 1955.

Turell, R.: Modern Treatment of Pruritus Ani, Surg., Gynec. & Obst. 104: 233, 1957.

Turell, R.: Colonic and Anorectal Function and Disease, Internat. Abstr. Surg. 107: 417, 1958.

Turell, R., and others: The Healing of Anorectal Wounds With Reference to "Rectal Medication," A. M. A. Arch. Surg. 73: 870, 1956.

Turell, R., and Garson, B. J.: Sigmoidoscopy and Biopsy, New York J. Med. 50: 89, 1950.

Turnbull, R. B.: The Value of Sigmoidoscopic Examination, Dis. Colon & Rectum 2: 33, 1959.

Wasserman, I. F.: New Suction-Lavage Sigmoidoscope, J. A. M. A. 172: 1036, 1960.

Waugh, J. M., and Walt, A. J.: Changing Concepts in the Treatment of Diverticulitis of the Sigmoid, Journal-Lancet 76: 373, 1956.

Wilkins, B. D.: Gastrointestinal Bleeding as Seen by a Proctologist, J. A. M. A. 163: 1214, 1957.

14 · Minor Anorectal Operations and Conditions Complicating Gynecologic Surgery

CRYPTECTOMY
Indications

An isolated, infected crypt is excised when it is responsible for subjective symptoms. Mild degrees of cryptitis exist in a large group of patients who do not require surgery. Many infected crypts are removed in the course of other anorectal operations, especially during a complete hemorrhoidectomy. The removal of one or more infected crypts, as an isolated procedure, is done in the office.

Steps of the Operation

1. After local preparation with pHisoderm, followed by Zephiran, 1:1,000 solution, 1.0 ml. or less of a 1 per cent solution of procaine or other suitable local anesthetic is injected into the base of the crypt (Plate 38, *A*).

2. A crypt hook or other suitable instrument is introduced into the diseased crypt, which is drawn upward by traction (Plate 38, *B*).

3. A small curved Kelly clamp is used to crush the base of the inflamed crypt. It is excised with a curved scissors (Plate 38, *C*).

4. Crushing the base usually provides sufficient hemostasis. However, should there be active bleeding, the vessels are ligated with suture ligatures of 0000 chromic catgut on atraumatic needles.

Postoperative Care

The following orders are suitable for most patients having had a cryptectomy or other surgery for benign anorectal conditions. They are modified as indicated for the individual patient:

1. Continuous hot dressing of 2 per cent boric acid, normal saline, or witch hazel are ordered to begin as soon as the patient reacts from anesthesia or when sensation returns after spinal anesthesia.

2. Morphine sulfate, 15 mg., or its equivalent of other opiate derivatives is ordered every four hours p.r.n.

3. The patient is placed on a progressive diet.

4. Orders are left for catheterization every four hours p.r.n.

5. The patient is mobilized as soon as possible—on the day of operation if the operation has taken place early in the morning.

6. On the first postoperative day, a blunt glass rod or metal rod is dipped in an aqueous solution of 1 per cent gentian violet, an aqueous solution of 4 per cent Mercurochrome, an aqueous solution of Zephiran, 1:1,000, or an aqueous solution of Merthiolate, 1:1,000, and the rod is inserted into the rectum. This prevents the development of adhesions in addition to informing the patient indirectly that the best way to prevent a postoperative stricture is to return the anal canal to normal function as soon as possible. It should be explained to the patient that the sooner she can pass a normal stool, the better the postoperative result will be.

7. On the second postoperative day a warm mineral or olive oil enema, 240 ml., is given with a No. 14 soft rubber catheter. This will initiate peristalsis and the expulsion of gas. On the night of the second postoperative day the patient is given an ounce of milk of magnesia.

8. On the third postoperative day the patient is started on sitz baths in six inches of warm

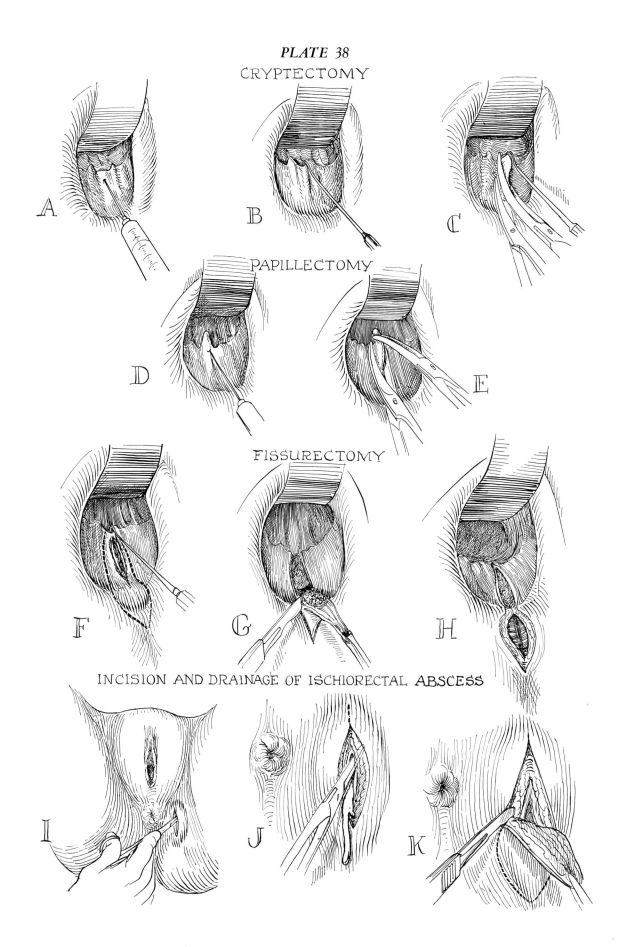

PLATE 38

CRYPTECTOMY

PAPILLECTOMY

FISSURECTOMY

INCISION AND DRAINAGE OF ISCHIORECTAL ABSCESS

water. By this time they will be taking a regular diet and may have a spontaneous bowel movement.

9. The following day sitz baths can be given two or three times a day and the duration of each bath continued up to fifteen minutes. At this time the surgeon inserts a well-lubricated finger into the rectum to break up any adhesions and to determine whether the incisions within the anorectum are healing properly.

10. If the patient did not have a bowel movement following the oil instillation, a tap water enema is given on the fourth postoperative day. The patient can be discharged the following day with instructions to continue the sitz baths at home plus mild catharsis with milk of magnesia as indicated. It is important to examine the patient within a week after discharge from the hospital to take measures against postoperative adhesions, contracture, or failure of adequate wound healing.

PAPILLECTOMY
Indications

Infected and hypertrophic papillae are removed when they are causing pain and tenderness. Usually they are seen with other anorectal lesions, and a complete operation is best done in the hospital. However, one or more isolated infected papillae can be removed as an office procedure.

Steps of the Operation

1. The base of the infected papilla is injected with a suitable local anesthetic (Plate 38, *D*).

2. The papilla is grasped with a curved hemostat (Plate 38, *E*) and gentle traction is made. The entire papilla is excised with a curved scissors. One or more hemostatic sutures of 0000 chromic catgut on atraumatic needles effect hemostasis.

Postoperative Care

Refer to the postoperative care described under Cryptectomy (page 277).

FISSURECTOMY
Indications

Fissure-in-ano (anal ulcer) begins in an infected anal gland, usually at the posterior commissure. Here, the deep sphincter is fixed by the anococcygeal raphe and bears the brunt of the fecal stream. Fissures other than at the posterior commissure are more likely to be of specific origin. Fissures are removed if they are symptomatic and demonstrate the classic triad of sentinel pile, ulcer, and an infected papilla. Operation is advised before the complications of a blind or incomplete fistula, contraction of the anus, or recurrent constipation occur. It is rare to find an isolated fissure in the absence of other anorectal pathology. A careful examination will reveal one or more infected crypts, other enlarged anal papillae, internal and external hemorrhoids, some degree of anal contraction, and other evidences of infection. The most common cause of recurrence of an anal fissure is the failure to correct all of the anorectal pathology at the time of the fissurectomy.

Steps of the Operation

1. The internal edge of the fissure or the crypt from which it has arisen is identified by probing with a crypt hook. An outline of skin and mucosa adjacent to the fissure is made (Plate 38, *F*).

2. The anoderm, including the crypt, sentinel pile, and adjacent skin are widely excised. All of the infected tissue adjacent to the fissure is removed (Plate 38, *G*).

3. Several sutures are placed in the anoderm for hemostasis. An adequate clover leaf of skin is excised. A sphincterotomy of the subcutaneous external sphincter is performed, and the edges of the wound are left open (Plate 38, *H*).

Postoperative Care

Refer to the postoperative care described under Cryptectomy (page 277).

INCISION AND DRAINAGE OF ISCHIORECTAL ABSCESS
Indications and Surgical Principles

Incision and drainage of an ischiorectal abscess are indicated as soon as the diagnosis is made and the mass is fluctuant. Abscesses that extend above the levator sling or have extended higher are much more dangerous than those that are confined to the ischiorectal fossa.

All of the locules into which these abscesses divide are broken down, and a large segment of skin is removed. The wound heals by granulation from within outward, and the skin is not permitted to close over the external drainage site until the final step of the healing process.

Steps of the Operation

1. After induction of general or spinal anesthesia, an incision up to several inches in length is made in an anteroposterior direction over the area of fluctuation (Plate 38, *I*). The rectal sphincters are avoided in making the incision and in the subsequent evacuation of the abscess.

2. A hemostat is introduced into the abscess cavity and spread (Plate 38, *J*). This removes most of the pus. A finger is inserted into the cavity, and all of the locules are broken down to complete the drainage. The cavity is carefully palpated to determine whether the abscess has extended above the levator sling, since such extension would require deeper drainage.

3. A wide segment of skin is removed (Plate 38, *K*), and several drains are inserted into the depths of the cavity. When dressing the wound, a gloved finger or blunt instrument is passed into the cavity to open smaller abscesses that become sealed off before the wound has completely granulated from within outward.

Postoperative Care

Refer to the postoperative care described under Cryptectomy (page 277).

FISTULA-IN-ANO
Etiology and Pathologic Anatomy

The gynecologist sees a number of rectovaginal fistulas after surgical procedures on the perineum and posterior vaginal wall. They may follow incomplete healing of a complete laceration of the pelvis sustained at parturition. The majority of fistulas of unknown etiology have their primary opening at or near the anorectal line. It is not understood whether these tracts are congenital in origin or develop from a sinus in and about the anorectal line that eventually reaches the skin surface. Since a fistula-in-ano rarely manifests itself without abscess formation, it may be that an infection along the sinus tract with subsequent abscess

formation causes the tract to reach the skin surface. As with other lesions of the anus, the posterior half is the most common site of fistulas.

Surgical Principles

Successful fistula repair depends on visualization, débridement, and closure of the mucosal orifice from the anorectal approach. The entire tract and an adequate margin of normal tissue are excised. The drawings shown in Plate 39, *A* and *B*, were made during an operation for a combined vaginorectoperineal fistula. The secondary opening on the skin led to one tract with a primary opening in the vagina, while a second primary opening was near the anorectal line. This fistula followed the incision and drainage of a Bartholin's abscess and subsequent drainage of an ischiorectal abscess several years apart. Both had been done as office procedures and apparently with inadequate excision.

Steps of the Operation

1. Probes are used to follow the tract and, if possible, are passed through its entire length (Plate 39, *A*). The injection of dye in the tract is seldom of any help and obscures the field of operation. If probes can be inserted, a wedge-shaped excision of the tract is carried out (Plate 39, *A*). All of the infected tissue between the primary and secondary openings is removed. In Plate 39, *A*, the excision of the tract going from the vagina to the perineum is shown. Subsequently the entire tract from the primary opening near the anorectal line to the skin of the perineum is excised.

2. The anterior tract, after thorough and adequate excision from the vagina to the perineum, is closed with atraumatic interrupted sutures (Plate 39, *B*). After excision of the fistula-in-ano, several sutures are used to close the skin of the anoderm and invert it into the anal canal. Remnants of the rectal sphincter that can be approximated without tension are brought together with 0000 chromic catgut on atraumatic needles. A drain was inserted in the most dependent portion of the skin just lateral to the rectal sphincter (Plate 39, *B*).

Postoperative Care

Refer to the postoperative care described under Cryptectomy (page 277).

PLATE 39

VAGINORECTOPERINEAL FISTULA

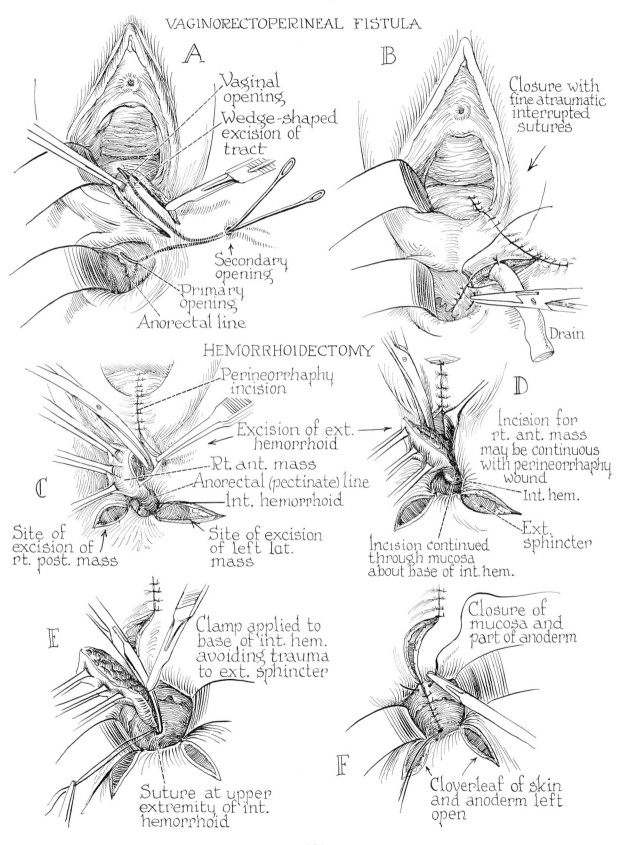

A

Vaginal opening

Wedge-shaped excision of tract

Secondary opening

Primary opening

Anorectal line

B

Closure with fine atraumatic interrupted sutures

Drain

HEMORRHOIDECTOMY

Perineorrhaphy incision

Excision of ext. hemorrhoid

Rt. ant. mass

Anorectal (pectinate) line

Int. hemorrhoid

C

Site of excision of rt. post. mass

Site of excision of left lat. mass

D

Incision for rt. ant. mass may be continuous with perineorrhaphy wound

Int. hem.

Incision continued through mucosa about base of int. hem.

Ext. sphincter

E

Clamp applied to base of int. hem. avoiding trauma to ext. sphincter

Suture at upper extremity of int. hemorrhoid

F

Closure of mucosa and part of anoderm

Cloverleaf of skin and anoderm left open

281

HEMORRHOIDECTOMY
Etiology and Pathologic Anatomy

Internal hemorrhoids are covered with columnar epithelium and arise in the lower inch of the rectum and upper part of the anal canal. They represent varices of the superior hemorrhoidal plexus. External hemorrhoids are lined with transitional epithelium of the anal canal or skin of the anus. They arise from the lower third of the anal canal and represent varices of the inferior hemorrhoidal plexus. Hemorrhoids are usually grouped in three main areas, designated as the left lateral, right anterior, and right posterior groups. They are aggravated by pregnancy, presence of large fibroids or other tumors of the pelvis, prolapse of the uterus, and particularly by malignancies higher in the rectum.

Symptoms and Diagnosis

Bleeding is the common symptom and the blood is bright red in color. Pain and pruritus are frequently annoying. The presence of hemorrhoids is obvious on inspection. A complete proctosigmoidoscopy, however, is done to avoid missing other anorectal pathology at a higher level.

Indications and Surgical Principles

Hemorrhoids are removed to relieve bleeding, pain, and rectal pruritus. In the usual hemorrhoidectomy, three ellipses of skin and mucous membrane, including the external and internal hemorrhoid, are removed. Small hemorrhoids, in addition to the main three ellipses, are uncapped. To prevent postoperative contracture, areas of perianal skin and mucosa are left in continuity to promote healing. It is better to leave some unresected hemorrhoidal tissue than to violate the above principle. The amount of tissue removed at the mucocutaneous junction is kept reasonably small in another attempt to prevent stricture. Incision of the subcutaneous sphincter posteriorly prevents contracture and postoperative pain. This technique reduces the resistance of the posterior segment of the rectal sphincters, against which the fecal stream is impacted. This helps prevent recurrence of the hemorrhoids or the development of fistulas, fissures, cryptitis, and papillitis. The following description applies to the semiclosed type of operation in which the skin is left open, while the anoderm is closed after ligation of any deep, bleeding vessels.

Preoperative Care and Anesthesia

The gynecologist prefers a general anesthesia if he is performing other vaginal surgery in addition to the hemorrhoidectomy. Low spinal or caudal anesthesia can be used for the operation. Local anesthesia can be used where there is distinct contraindication to the other forms of anesthesia.

Steps of the Operation

1. A hemorrhoidectomy following an extensive posterior vaginal plastic operation may proceed in the following manner. The incision from the perineorrhaphy is extended to include the right anterior mass of hemorrhoids, and the skin about the external hemorrhoid is incised (Plate 39, C). A suture ligature is placed inside the anorectal line at the uppermost portion of the internal hemorrhoid and tied. In the drawings, the sites of the excision of the right posterior and left lateral masses are shown as if they had already been done. The order in which they are removed is unimportant.

2. The external hemorrhoid is excised, with care being exercised not to traumatize the external sphincter. This causes severe postoperative pain. A mucosal incision is made around the internal hemorrhoid (Plate 39, D). Care is used to narrow the incision at the mucocutaneous line to prevent postoperative contracture.

3. As the hemorrhoidal mass is excised, Kelly clamps are placed around the base of the hemorrhoid and suture ligatures used to control bleeding (Plate 39, E). The sutures used to effect hemostasis in this manner do not close the skin of the anus when they are tied.

4. Several sutures of 0000 catgut on atraumatic needles are used to close the mucosa of the anoderm and mucosa of the rectum above the anorectal line (Plate 39, F). The clover leaves of skin and a portion of the anoderm are shown left open in Plate 39, F. Following this the subcutaneous sphincter is divided posteriorly to prevent contracture of the anal canal.

Postoperative Care

Refer to the postoperative care described under Cryptectomy (page 277).

COMPLETE LACERATION OF THE PERINEUM (LATE REPAIR)
Etiology and Pathologic Anatomy

A complete laceration of the perineum is most frequently the result of a tear during childbirth which has been inadequately repaired. The tear may follow a long labor, an excessively large infant, or a difficult breech delivery. Cephalopelvic disproportion, particularly with a narrow arch at the pelvic outlet, displaces the presenting part into the posterior sagittal diameter of the outlet and causes a considerable number of tears. This is not a recommendation for a lateral or mediolateral episiotomy but rather a plea for a careful anatomic approximation of the tissues in the repair of the episiotomy. With few exceptions, I personally would prefer to cut through the sphincter in the midline rather than perform a mediolateral episiotomy. The latter, regardless of the care with which it is repaired, is a distorting and unphysiologic incision. In healing, the vulva gapes and the pelvic floor is deformed. The cosmetic result is seldom as good as that of a midline incision. This is especially true if a wide mediolateral or lateral episiotomy is cut or crushed with a large, strong, bandage scissors. A midline episiotomy extending through the sphincter or deliberately cut through the sphincter heals with no more morbidity than an ordinary episiotomy, if it is repaired meticulously, with careful attention given to the gentle approximation of the tissues of the perineum. It requires no special attention during the post-partum period. Partial degrees of incontinence are caused by trauma and subsequent scarring of the sphincter muscles during anorectal surgery. A rare case results from injury to the rectovaginal septum and anal sphincter when the patient becomes impaled or straddled on some sharp object. The essential pathology of this condition is that the continuity of the external sphincter is interrupted. A complete tear disrupts the vaginal mucosa, skin, and subcutaneous tissue, the superficial and deep transverse perineal muscles, and the muscularis and mucosa of the rectum. The subcutaneous, superficial, and deep divisions of the external sphincter, together with the internal sphincter, are divided.

Symptoms and Diagnosis

The common complaint is the loss of control and continuous leakage of fecal material. It is particularly bad when the stool is loose, either from diet or some other cause of diarrhea. The diagnosis is made by inspection and examination. Characteristic sphincter pits representing the retraction of the external sphincter of the rectum are noticed on either side of the anus. On rectal examination, when the patient is asked to hold as if attempting to restrain the leakage, there is little movement of the muscle, and the characteristic clamping down of the sphincter on the examining finger is absent.

Surgical Anatomy and Principles

1. A proctosigmoidoscopic examination is done and also a barium enema if any disease of the colon above the perineal reflection is suspected.

2. The remnants of the sphincter are mobilized and approximated without tension.

3. The extent of the tear above the external sphincter is important. The higher in the vagina this has extended, the more retraction of the sphincter is to be expected.

4. The higher in the vagina the tear has extended, with the subsequent retraction and shrinkage of the edges, the larger the area to cover. In any plastic operation the greater the area to be covered, the more difficult the closure and the more necessary is an extensive mobilization of the flaps.

5. Extensions up the vagina are triangular in shape, with the base of the triangle just above the site of the approximation of the remnants of the external sphincter. Thus, the least viable edges of the mucosa, those farthest from the blood supply, must be approximated.

6. The surgeon does not forget that hemorrhoids and other minor anorectal pathology can be present with a complete laceration of the perineum. All anorectal pathology is corrected at the time of operation.

7. The incision selected in the repair removes all of the scar tissue. Scar tissue cannot heal firmly and is not included in any plastic flap.

8. Closure of the rectal wall above the anorectal line approximates some fibers of the internal sphincter and decreases the caliber of the anal canal. This increases resistance and improves postoperative control.

9. If the anterior thickened edge of the levator sling is approximated in the midline, it aids in postoperative control, particularly in those patients in whom the rectal sphincter has been almost completely destroyed.

10. Complete study of the lesion may indicate that a simple repair is inadequate because of the absence of sufficient sphincter or perineal musculature to close the defect. The use of fascial strips or the transplantation of the gracilis are to be considered for these patients.

11. Repair of a complete laceration of the perineum immediately post partum is a minor procedure and rarely presents any difficulties. The surgeon remembers that interrupted sutures are used to approximate the rectal sphincters and muscles of the perineum. He should avoid figure-of-eight, mattress, and other novelty sutures that vie for efficiency in strangulating tissue.

12. Bizarre types of running sutures have no place in either the immediate or late repair of a complete laceration of the perineum.

Preoperative Care and Anesthesia

The bowel is prepared according to the following routine: Three days prior to operation, citrate of magnesia, 240 ml., is given nightly. A cleansing enema is given each day, including the day of operation. Forty-eight hours prior to operation, neomycin, 1.0 Gm. every four hours, is started. The patient is given only clear liquids the day before operation, despite the fact that postoperatively a progressive diet is ordered. This prevents discomfort postoperatively, and it is better not to have a formed stool during the first seventy-two hours after operation. In complicated cases a preliminary defunctioning left inguinal colostomy is performed. This puts the lower sigmoid, rectum, and anus at rest during the postoperative period. General anesthesia is preferred by the gynecologist. Spinal or caudal anesthesia can be used.

Steps of the Operation

1. Traction sutures are placed outlining a triangular area to be denuded. The apex of this triangle is above any scar tissue in the vagina, while the angles of the base are over the sphincter pits (Plate 40, A). The incision is carried high enough so the full thickness of the vaginal wall over a rectocele or lateral vaginal wall relaxation can be mobilized to aid in the closure.

2. The dissection is continued until the full thickness of the vagina is mobilized and separated from the rectal wall and mucosa. The scar tissue in the vaginal and rectal walls is excised so that fresh edges are approximated, and the rectal and anorectal walls are inverted into the canal by interrupted sutures of 0000 catgut on atraumatic needles (Plate 40, B). These sutures extend just to the submucosa and precisely approximate the tissues.

3. The retracted ends of the external sphincter are located and mobilized sufficiently for approximation in the midline without tension (Plate 40, C). They are sutured together with interrupted sutures of 0000 catgut on atraumatic needles.

4. The medial edges of the bulbocavernosi and remnants of the transverse perineal muscles are used to build up the perineal body over and above the reunited external sphincter (Plate 40, D). The anterior edges of the levators are approximated in the midline to give additional support.

5. The full thickness of the vaginal wall and the skin of the perineum are closed by interrupted sutures (Plate 40, E). They are approximated without tension and inspected again so that scar tissue is not incorporated into the wound.

Postoperative Care

The patient is put on a regular diet and given an enema on the third day after operation. Preoperative bowel preparation avoids a hard, formed stool in the immediate postoperative period. A wide-spectrum antibiotic is given for four to five days postoperatively to prevent wound infection. The patient is kept as comfortable as possible with sedation and analgesic drugs. The operative area is kept clean and dry by the use of a mild astringent wash, and a heat lamp is directed to the operative area for ten minutes several times daily.

PLATE 40

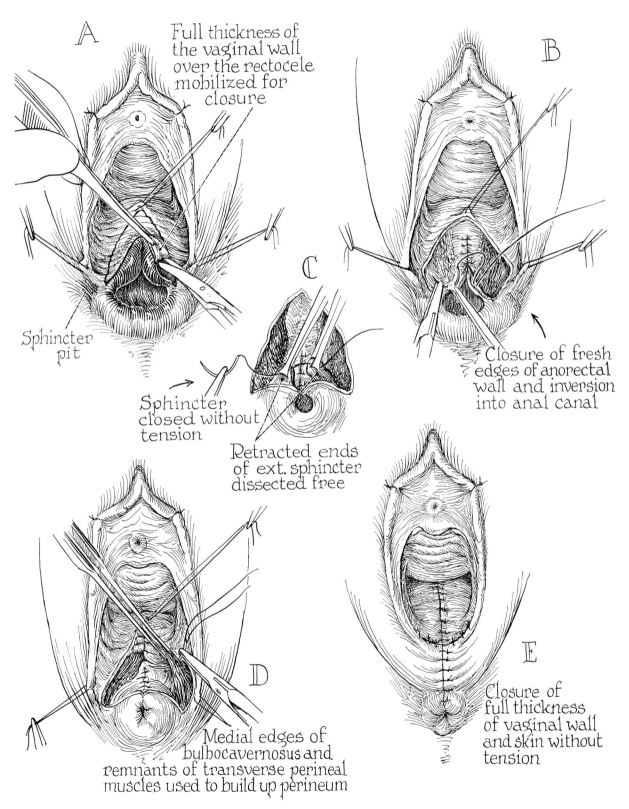

A — Full thickness of the vaginal wall over the rectocele mobilized for closure

Sphincter pit

B — Closure of fresh edges of anorectal wall and inversion into anal canal

C — Sphincter closed without tension

Retracted ends of ext. sphincter dissected free

D — Medial edges of bulbocavernosus and remnants of transverse perineal muscles used to build up perineum

E — Closure of full thickness of vaginal wall and skin without tension

285

OTHER ANORECTAL OPERATIONS ENCOUNTERED BY THE GYNECOLOGIST

RECTOVAGINAL FISTULA

The closure of a rectovaginal fistula with the external sphincter intact embraces all of the principles of closure of a complete laceration of the pelvic floor plus many of the principles elicited in the discussion of vesicovaginal fistulas (Chapter 11, page 277). Rectovaginal fistulas commonly follow surgical and obstetric procedures involving the perineum and posterior vaginal wall. In the healing of a complete laceration of the perineum, the lower end of the wound plus the approximation of the sphincters may remain intact, but incomplete healing may occur above. This may result in a small fistula just above the rectal sphincter. Other fistulas occur during the repair of a large enterocele or a high rectocele or during the course of a vaginal hysterectomy. Sutures to control bleeding, placed through both vaginal and rectal walls, may compromise the blood supply in a limited area. Some fistulas follow a high vaginorectal abscess, particularly if drainage results in perforation of both rectal and vaginal walls. Rectovaginal fistulas following radiation, radical surgery, and infiltration with malignant disease are common but usually require more extensive surgery than is to be discussed in the simple repair of a rectovaginal fistula. Rectovaginal fistulas are seen following pressure necrosis after a prolonged labor and difficult delivery. Patients are seen with rectovaginal fistulas following straddle wounds to the vagina and rectum. Fistulas in the course of lymphopathia venereum are special problems. The disease is treated systemically and the fistula closed during a quiescent phase. The surgical principles and technique of closure of vesicovaginal fistulas are followed here. Scar tissue and the tract between the rectum and the vagina are excised so that fresh edges of tissue are approximated. The rectum and vaginal walls are adequately mobilized. The rectum is closed in a longitudinal plane, with inversion of the mucosa into the rectal canal. The vagina is closed transversely or in a different sagittal plane than the rectal wall. The vaginal mucosa is inverted toward the vagina. With very large rectovaginal fistulas, particularly those due to radiation or specific granulomatous disease, a preliminary colostomy is indicated. Some rectal or sigmoidovaginal fistulas are approached from the abdomen. This approach is used when a bowel resection is anticipated.

STRICTURES OF THE RECTUM

Congenital strictures of the rectum are usually at the dentate line and are diagnosed during childhood. Acquired strictures frequently follow operative procedures about the anorectum and are the result of scar tissue contracture at the mucocutaneous junction. Fecal continence results from the action of the external sphincter plus the ability of the left colon to act as a large reservoir. The internal sphincter contributes little or nothing to retention of the fecal stream. When a stricture exists at the dentate line or at the mucocutaneous junction, the left colon is called upon to retain a large amount of fecal material. The distention of the colon causes the symptoms associated with a stricture such as rectal tenesmus, a bearing-down feeling accompanied by pain, or discomfort radiating toward the hollow of the sacrum. Ribbon stools are not commonly due to a hard, fixed, scarred anal canal but more frequently are due to spasm—the result of inflammatory reaction about the anorectum. Fibrous constrictions are more likely to result in bleeding as a symptom than cause the stool to be of small caliber. The same principles apply in the operative correction of such a constriction as in vaginal surgery. An anteroposterior incision is made through the constricting scar and continued beyond the scar into healthy-appearing tissue. The scar tissue about the incision is removed until healthy pliable edges of rectal mucous membrane are encountered. The rectal mucosa is undermined so as to mobilize the tissue and permit suture in a transverse direction without tension. If the subcutaneous portion of the external sphincter muscle is fibrotic and contracted, a sphincterotomy is performed in conjunction with the plastic repair of the rectal mucosa. The postoperative care following this procedure is the same as for other anorectal operations for benign disease.

PROLAPSE AND PROCIDENTIA OF THE RECTUM
Introduction

Decompensation of the pelvic floor is rarely isolated to one of the three organs that must pass through hiatuses to gain access to the exterior to perform their functions. While one organ may have sustained the major damage and prolapse of its walls, the others show some degree of relaxation. The pelvic floor, as has been repeatedly emphasized, must be assessed as a whole, and the surgeon must reduce all the herniations.

Surgical Anatomy and Pathology

Childbearing cannot be indicted as the major factor in rectal procidentia since the identical condition occurs in men. Studies of the etiology should therefore search for similar factors in both sexes but should be modified by the differences in the anatomy.

Simple prolapse and procidentia are distinguished by the layers of the rectum involved. Simple prolapse refers to the protrusion of the rectal mucosa in varying degrees. Hemorrhoidal masses are frequently prolapsed with the mucosa but are not the sole cause. Constant straining at stool with either constipation or diarrhea may cause the protrusion. Any cause of recurrent and violent increases in intra-abdominal pressure, such as coughing, vomiting, sneezing, and crying, may initiate protrusion of the mucosa. Children with their characteristically straight rectum and deep cul-de-sac of Douglas may develop the condition because of the direction of the forces impinging on the pelvic floor. The elderly patient with loss of tone and pliability is predisposed to the disease. All of these factors operate in both sexes. They play only an aggravating or accessory part in a true rectal procidentia.

A procidentia of the rectum is an intussusception of the terminal sigmoid and rectum into the already prolapsed and inverted lower rectum. Thus the full thickness of the walls of both are involved together with an anterior sac of varying size of the cul-de-sac peritoneum. The mechanics of the production of this herniation is complex with still unsolved factors.

Clinical observations have established several consistent findings. First, in the presence of a procidentia, the rectal sphincter is dilated, somewhat attenuated, and frequently incompetent. This, most will agree, is a result of, rather than a cause of, the problem. Second, a deep cul-de-sac hernia is found. This too could be considered a result, were it not that the most logical explanation of the pathologic processes that create the herniation have a deep cul-de-sac as one of the initial defects. Third, a long sigmoid colon is observed although seldom is a sigmoid seen that is so short that an intussusception could not occur. Fourth, the hiatus in the pelvic floor for the rectum is large and incompetent and fails to retain the obturator (the rectum). My own observations, which are difficult to prove by precise anatomic studies, are similar to those seen in congenital prolapse of the uterus. Namely, these patients seem to have an unusually low origin of the levator muscles. Observed in the lithotomy position, the pelvic floor seems to bulge out toward the observer, and palpation of the anterior edge of the levators (puborectali) reveals a thin, elongated structure in contrast to the thick, strong muscle felt in the female with a competent pelvic floor.

What then happens is a total incompetency of the pelvic floor as illustrated in Plate 41. Assuming that the one consistant finding, a cul-de-sac hernia, is the focal point of the herniation, the sequence of events could be this: If the direction of forces are such that the invagination occurs between the posterior vaginal wall and the rectum, the uterus is projected through its hiatus in the pelvic floor, pulling its anterior vaginal wall through the defect. If the direction of forces are such that the major impact is against the anterior rectal wall and the posterior vaginal wall, the rectal wall invaginates and finally draws the full thickness

PLATE 41

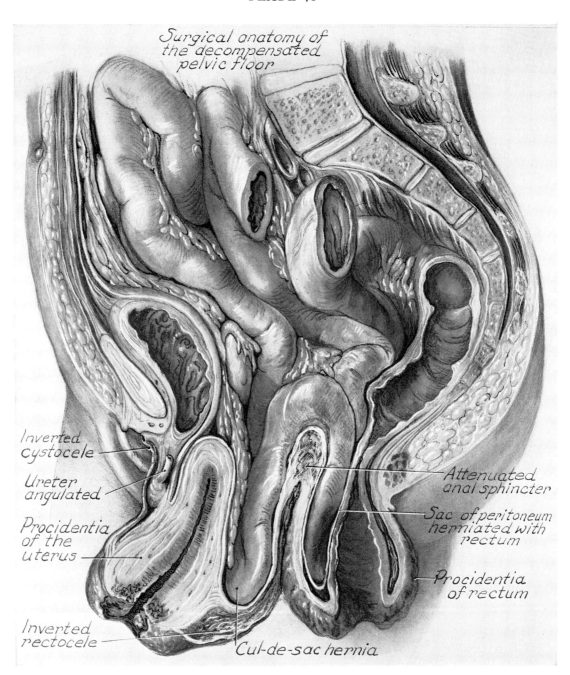

Surgical anatomy of
the decompensated
pelvic floor

Inverted
cystocele

Ureter
angulated

Procidentia
of the
uterus

Inverted
rectocele

Cul-de-sac hernia

Attenuated
anal sphincter

Sac of peritoneum
herniated with
rectum

Procidentia
of rectum

of the rectum through the incompetent hiatus. Into this a gradual intussusception of the terminal sigmoid colon occurs. If the pelvic floor is no longer able to sustain the intra-abdominal and pelvic pressures through all its obturators then the cul-de-sac hernia virtually straddles the anterior edge of the rectal sphincter and a procidentia of both the uterus (or vaginal vault) and the rectum occurs.

These observations do not lend themselves to precise experimental proof. One can only decide to what the accumulated facts point and then base his operation for repair of the pelvic floor on these clinical observations.

Principles of the Operation

Whatever the operation, and there have been well over twenty that have enjoyed a period of popularity, it will fail if the hiatuses in the pelvic diaphragm for vagina and rectum are not reduced in size to just accommodate the obturators (uterus or vaginal vault and the rectum). This is assured by attention to the following principles:

1. The hernial sac of the cul-de-sac peritoneum is isolated and obliterated.

2. The uterosacral thickenings are sutured in the midline to reduce the diameter of the vaginal and rectal hiatuses.

3. The everted, protruding rectal mucosa and wall must be excised with an end-to-end anastomosis, or the intussusception reduced by denudation and longitudinal suturing to shorten the prolapsed segment of bowel and create a larger obturator.

4. In general, bowel resection will be tolerated in younger patients, whereas the denudation type procedures are utilized for the elderly patient.

5. The distal rectum is further supported by suture of its lateral wall to the plicated uterosacral thickenings.

6. The incompetent external anal sphincter is repaired to reduce its caliber and help prevent a future simple mucosal prolapse.

On page 147 and Plate 20, *Q* through *HH*, is shown the author's technique for the correction of a complete decompensation of the

female pelvic floor. This case involved a combined procidentia of the vaginal vault as well as the rectum. Patients have to be individualized in this sphere of plastic surgery as elsewhere. Thus, the presence of the uterus or cervical stump would require their removal in the course of the repair, but this would be only incidental to the primary reason for surgery, the reconstruction of the pelvic floor.

Where the rectal procidentia is more pronounced than the relaxation of structures in the anterior half of the pelvic outlet, the posterior vaginal wall and cul-de-sac should be opened and repaired in the same manner in order to suspend the rectum and vaginal vault to the all-important uterosacral ligaments as described in the operation. Other modifications of this operation are certainly possible as the combination of defects in the pelvic floor are innumerable.

IMPALEMENT INJURIES AND FOREIGN BODIES OF THE PERINEUM, ANUS, AND RECTUM

The midline location of the vagina, rectum, and bladder plus the funnel of the female vulva directs foreign bodies and forces toward the midline. Most of the injuries involving these structures will also involve the vagina in the female, so these are discussed under Penetrating, Straddle, Coital, and Foreign Body Injuries (page 509).

POLYPS OF THE RECTUM AND COLON

In the course of gynecologic surgery, many polyps of the rectum and colon are excised not only for diagnosis, but also for prophylactic reasons. Pseudoinflammatory polyposis is most frequently the result of inflammation of the anal papillae that subsequently become hypertrophic. Many inflammatory polyps, not only at the anorectal line, but also above this line in the rectal ampulla, are seen with ulcerative colitis. Congenital polyposis is a distinct disease and requires frequent examination for removal of polyps that become inflamed or show signs of malignant degeneration. Solitary or discrete polyps may be pedunculated or may have a broad sessile base. They are most frequently found in the rectum and lower sigmoid and represent true neoplasms. They are prone to malignant degeneration and should be completely removed, since it is frequently difficult to determine from the histologic appearance whether a benign polyp has gradually crossed the barrier and become a malignant tumor.

RADIUM REACTIONS (FACTITIAL PROCTITIS)

Radium or factitial proctitis is an inflammatory reaction of the rectal mucosa following the use of intracavitary radium. Subsequently, due to endarteritis and contracture, the rectovaginal septum becomes fibrotic, and the rectal mucosa becomes more pale due to the decrease in its blood supply. The majority of patients recover from such an inflammatory reaction of the rectal mucosa except when an excessive dose of radium is administered and the process progresses to a rectovaginal fistula.

References

Anderson, R. E., and Witkowski, L. J.: Post-Partum Fistula-in-Ano: A Complication of Episiotomy, Surgery 41: 790, 1957.

Barter, R. H., Parks, J., and Tyndal, C.: Median Episiotomies and Complete Perineal Lacerations, Am. J. Obst. & Gynec. 80: 654, 1960.

Blaisdell, P. C.: A Simpler Yet More Effective Repair of the Incontinent Sphincter Ani, Surg., Gynec. & Obst. 112: 375, 1961.

Blaisdell, P. C.: Prevention of Massive Hemorrhage Secondary to Hemorrhoidectomy, Surg., Gynec. & Obst. 106: 485, 1958.

Block, I. R.: Repair of the Incontinent Sphincter Ani Following Operative Injury, Surg., Gynec. & Obst. 108: 111, 1959.

Buck, R. L.: Diverticulosis and Diverticulitis: Review of Cases at New Orleans Charity Hospital From 1950 to 1956: Discussion of Complications and Treatment, Dis. Colon & Rectum 1: 205, 1958.

Cohn, I.: Dangers of Intestinal Antisepsis, Dis. Colon & Rectum 3: 305, 1960.

Collins, D. C.: Extensive Colotomy for the Intraluminal Location of Elusive Polyps, Ulcers, and Tumors; a Preliminary Clinical Report, Am. J. Proct. 9: 47, 1958.

De Bernardis, F., and D'Ambrosio, G.: Lipomas of the Cecum (Contributo allo studio dei cieco), Arch. ital. mal. App. diger. 22: 251, 1956.

Deloyers, L.: Indications for the Surgical Treatment of Sigmoid Diverticulitis and Its Complications (Les indications du traitement chirurgical des diverticulites du sigmoide et de leurs complications), Acta chir. belg. 55: 396, 1956.

Eisenhammer, S.: The Evaluation of the Internal Anal Sphincterotomy Operation With Special Reference to the Anal Fissure, Surg., Gynec. & Obst. 109: 583, 1959.

Ferguson, J. A., and Heaton, J. R.: Closed Hemorrhoidectomy, Dis. Colon & Rectum 2: 176, 1959.

Graber, E. A., and O'Rourke, J. J.: Rectal Injuries During Vaginal Delivery, Am. J. Obst. & Gynec. 73: 301, 1957.

Hamandi, W. J., and Kratzer, G. L.: Management of Polyps of the Rectum and Colon, Dis. Colon & Rectum 4: 173, 1961.

Helwig, E. B.: Adenomas and the Pathogenesis of Cancer of the Colon and Rectum, Dis. Colon & Rectum 2: 5, 1959.

Holtz, F., and Schmidt, L. A.: Lymphoid Polyps (Benign Lymphoma) of the Rectum and Anus, Surg., Gynec. & Obst. 106: 639, 1958.

Hurwitz, A., and Solomons, E.: Diverticulitis, a Diagnostic Dilemma; Report of 5 Cases, Obst. & Gynec. 10: 128, 1957.

Jacobs, W., and Adams, B.: Midline Episiotomy and Extension Through the Rectal Sphincter, Surg., Gynec. & Obst. 111: 245, 1960.

Kaiser, L. H.: Rectal Stricture Complicating Labor. An Analysis of 48 Cases, Am. J. Obst. & Gynec. 46: 672, 1943.

Kratzer, G. L.: Recurrent Anal Fissure; Concept of Pathogenesis and Treatment, J. A. M. A. 153: 1165, 1953.

Kratzer, G. L.: Relaxation of the Internal Anal Sphincter in Anorectal Surgery, Dis. Colon & Rectum 2: 294, 1959.

LeBlanc, L. J.: An Appraisal of Radical Hemorrhoidectomy, Dis. Colon & Rectum 4: 125, 1961.

Lochridge, E. P., and Jackman, R. J.: Evaluation of Conservative Management of Certain Polypoid Lesions of the Lower Part of the Large Intestine, Dis. Colon & Rectum 1: 101, 1958.

McCune, W. S., Iovine, V., and Miller, D.: Resection and Primary Anastomosis in Diverticulitis of the Colon, Ann. Surg. 145: 683, 1957.

McElwain, J. W., and Gaines, T. L.: Single-Stage Treatment of Anorectal Abscesses and Fistulas, New York J. Med. 58: 2385, 1958.

McGregor, R. A., and Bacon, H. E.: Diverticular Disease of the Colon, Dis. Colon & Rectum 1: 197, 1958.

Marks, M. M.: Topical Treatment of Anorectal Inflammations With Hydrocortisone Acetate, Dis. Colon & Rectum 3: 250, 1960.

Ochsner, S. F., and Ray, J. E.: Submucosal Lipomas of the Colon: Experience With 12 Cases, Dis. Colon & Rectum 3: 1, 1960.

Ortmayer, M.: Management of Small Colonic Polyps, Gastroenterol. 31: 404, 1956.

Parkinson, E. D.: Surgery With Muscle Preservation for Anorectal Fistula, Dis. Colon & Rectum 2: 565, 1959.

Pickrell, K., Georgiade, N., Maguire, C., and Crawford, H.: Correction of Rectal Incontinence. Transplantation of the Gracilis Muscle to Construct a Rectal Sphincter, Am. J. Surg. 90: 721, 1955.

Rosensweig, J., and Horwitz, A.: Adenomatous Tumours of the Colon and Rectum. The Importance of Early Detection and Treatment, Am. Surgeon 24: 515, 1958.

Smalley, M. A., LoRusso, V., and O'Brien, J. E.: Sigmoidouterine Fistula Complicating Diverticulitis; Report of a Case, J. A. M. A. 165: 827, 1957.

Spratt, J. S., and Ackerman, L. V.: Pathologic Significance of the Polyps of the Rectum and Colon, Dis. Colon & Rectum 3: 330, 1960.

Swinton, N. W.: Polyps of Rectum and Colon, J. A. M. A. 154: 658, 1954.

Turell, R.: Treatment in Proctology, Baltimore, 1949, The Williams & Wilkins Co.

Turell, R.: Anal Fistula: Background and Surgical Treatment, New York J. Med. 58: 1473, 1958.

Warshaw, L. J., and Turell, R.: Occupational Aspects of Proctologic Disease, New York J. Med. 57: 3006, 1957.

Wittoesch, J. H., Woolner, L. B., and Jackman, R. J.: Basal Cell Epithelioma and Basaloid Lesions of the Anus, Surg., Gynec. & Obst. 104: 75, 1957.

15 · Major Rectocolonic Surgery and Conditions Complicating Gynecologic Disease

POSTERIOR PELVIC EXENTERATION

The most common indication for posterior pelvic exenteration is a primary cancer of the rectum that does not permit resection and end-to-end anastomosis from above. When the rectal lesion is at or near the peritoneal reflection, one or another of the pull-down operations is feasible. Such operations have been technically possible with higher lesions. The decision may frequently rest with the question of a perineal colostomy versus an abdominal colostomy, and many are convinced that the latter is easier to manage. Gynecologists perform this operation, together with a vaginectomy, for cervical cancer that has extended into the rectum. The bladder and ureters are free of disease. It may be infrequently indicated for a recurrent fundal cancer, an ovarian malignancy causing obstruction in the cul-de-sac, or a retroperitoneal tumor invading the rectum. Since these gynecologic lesions involving the rectum are too high up for any type of pull-down operation and since a complete lymphadenectomy must be done with the en bloc dissection which will not permit an end-to-end anastomosis with retention of any sort of blood supply, the usual procedure is an abdominoperineal resection with a vaginectomy, vulvectomy, and pelvic lymphadenectomy. Some lesions may be so confined as to permit clearance without the perineal phase of the operation, but the contralateral spread of disease through the perineal lymphatics must be remembered.

Steps of the Operation
Abdominal Phase

1. The abdomen is opened through a long left rectus incision extending above the umbilicus. The rectus muscle is split, the abdomen opened, and a thorough exploration done. Special reference is made to the palpation of the mesentery and metastatic stations ultimately draining the presacral and pararectal nodes.

2. The descending colon is drawn to the left and the inferior mesenteric artery palpated. An incision is made in the mesentery and a primary ligation of the inferior mesenteric artery done (Plate 42, A). The bowel is then observed and ultimately resected as near the splenic flexure as is necessary to ensure adequate collateral circulation from the middle colic artery.

3. During the dissection of the mesentery, the proximity of the left ureter must be remembered and injury avoided. The ureter will be exposed for a considerable portion of its length both in the abdomen and pelvis. However, since this operation is undertaken for a malignancy that started in the genital tract and subsequently extended posteriorly into the rectum, anything less than a complete dissection should not be done since it would only add mutilation to the patient's misery without the maximum chance of a cure.

4. In Plate 42, A, is shown a dotted outline for resection of the mesentery of the descending colon and rectosigmoid. This must be individualized for each patient, depending on the length of the sigmoid with a correspondingly longer mesentery. Branches of the superior hemorrhoidal and sigmoidal arteries must be ligated as encountered, since the collateral circulation through the middle hemorrhoidal vessels permits of considerable blood loss during the dissection despite the ligation of the inferior mesenteric artery.

PLATE 42

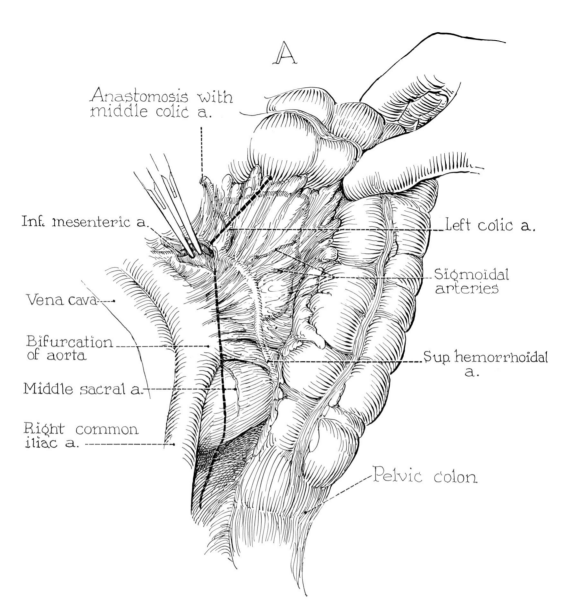

A

Anastomosis with middle colic a.

Inf. mesenteric a.

Left colic a.

Sigmoidal arteries

Vena cava

Bifurcation of aorta

Sup. hemorrhoidal a.

Middle sacral a.

Right common iliac a.

Pelvic colon

Primary ligation of the inf. mes. artery for left upper quadrant colostomy. This permits more thorough dissection of the mesentery of the sigmoid colon and metastatic stations draining the lower sigmoid

PLATE 42 (Continued)

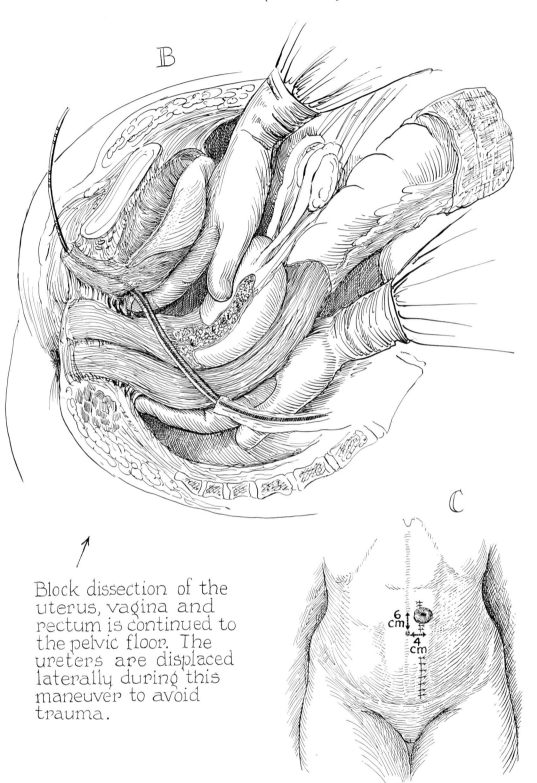

B

Block dissection of the
uterus, vagina and
rectum is continued to
the pelvic floor. The
ureters are displaced
laterally during this
maneuver to avoid
trauma.

C

6
cm

4
cm

Left upper quadrant colostomy

293

PLATE 42 (Concluded)

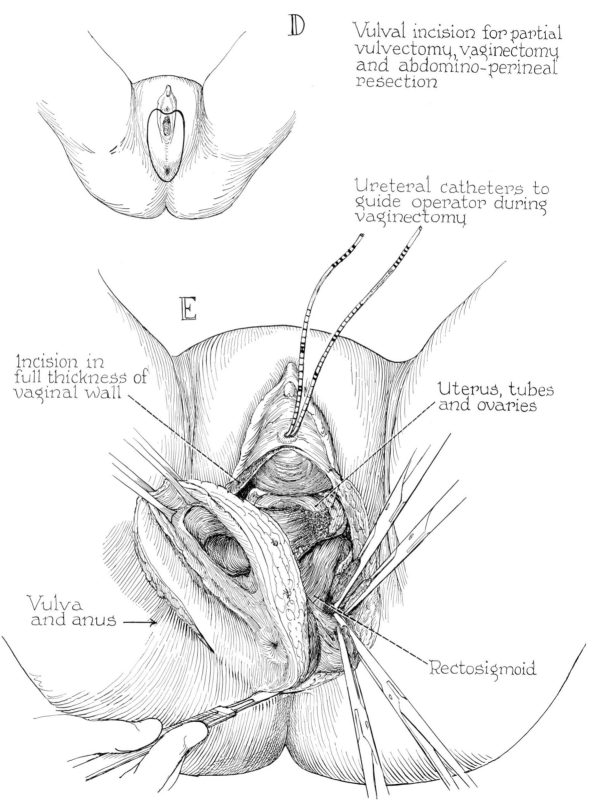

D

Vulval incision for partial
vulvectomy, vaginectomy
and abdomino-perineal
resection

Ureteral catheters to
guide operator during
vaginectomy

E

Incision in
full thickness of
vaginal wall

Uterus, tubes
and ovaries

Vulva
and anus

Rectosigmoid

5. Proceed now as for a radical hysterectomy and mobilize the ureters to the ureterovesical junction. Leave the parametrial thickenings lateral to the ureters attached for nourishment of the terminal ureter. Enter the vesicovaginal reflection of the peritoneum, and by sharp and blunt dissection separate the bladder base from the cervix and vagina to a point well below the lesion.

6. With the bladder and ureters retracted anteriorly, the rectosigmoid and rectum are mobilized as for an abdominoperineal resection (Plate 42, B). Large Kelly clamps are used to clamp the paracolpium and pararectal connective tissue flush with the pelvic side walls. Carry on this dissection by alternately clamping, cutting, and tying until the rectum is mobilized well below the lesion. Cut across the vagina and rectum and remove the specimen.

7. The terminal portion of the descending colon is now brought out of the upper part of the wound approximately 6 cm. above and 4 cm. to the left of the umbilicus (Plate 42, C). It should have good color and adequate length for the permanent colostomy. The ureteral catheters are then removed and an indwelling catheter left in the bladder.

Perineal Phase

1. If a perineal phase is required in this operation, the abdominal stage is terminated just before amputating the specimen. The ureteral catheters are left in place. After placing the patient in the lithotomy position, an incision is made encircling the anus and vagina (Plate 42, D). The vaginal incision curves to a point above the trigone of the bladder to avoid injury to the bladder or ureters.

2. The perineal phase as outlined by this incision will permit a partial vulvectomy (posterior), removal of segments of the levator ani, excision of the anus, anal sphincters, and the nerves, vessels, and lymphatics to the anus and lower rectum, and removal of the transverse perineal muscles and fascia, the origins of the bulbocavernosi and ischiocavernosi, and the vestibular bulbs, together with other minor structures making up the posterior part of the vulva. Involvement of the inguinal lymphatics from a lesion presumed to be limited to the posterior pelvic organs and their lymphatics would be unlikely, and evidence of metastatic spread to these nodes would require a radical groin dissection and more extensive exenteration if any surgery were indicated at all.

3. The incision in the vaginal wall is extended toward the vault until it joins with the dissection in the vesicovaginal septum performed during the abdominal phase of the operation (Plate 42, E). The ureters can then be palpated while the incision is extended laterally and anteriorly to reach the skin of the vulva at about the junction of the anterior and middle thirds. The index finger of the left hand palpates the course of the ureter on the patient's left side during the dissection and pushes it laterally to avoid damage. The same technique is used on the right side with the operator's hands reversed.

4. The index finger is then used to palpate and guide the resection of the levator ani, which is cut close to the pelvic side wall. The incision is then carried around the anus, through the ischiorectal fossa, and deep through the anococcygeal raphe to mobilize the rectum from the lower border of the sacrum and coccyx (Plate 42, E). The specimen is then removed, and any areolar or lymphatic tissue remaining on the sacrum or coccyx is excised.

5. The vagina is then closed with interrupted sutures, but it will now be represented by only a shallow groove—not a functional organ. The skin and fat of the remainder of the wound are approximated by interrupted sutures after placing multiple soft rubber drains in the lower end of the incision.

Postoperative Care

An indwelling catheter is inserted, since bladder function is not only impaired as with an ordinary abdominoperineal resection, but is further compromised by the vaginectomy and denudation of the ureters during the lymphadenectomy. Urinary antiseptics and antibiotic therapy are administered, electrolyte balance is maintained, and blood is replaced as previously outlined for any radical pelvic operation. (See Management of Electrolyte Abnormalities in Gynecologic Surgery, page 543, and Transverse and Permanent Left Inguinal Colostomy, Postoperative Care, page 597.)

References

Allen, A. W., and Donaldson, G. A.: Carcinoma of the Colon, Am. J. Gastroenterol. 30: 287, 1958.
Ault, G. W.: A Technique for Cancer Isolation and Extended Dissection for Cancer of the Distal Colon and Rectum, Surg., Gynec. & Obst. 106: 467, 1958.
Bacon, H. E.: Abdominoperineal Proctosigmoidectomy With Sphincter Preservation, J. A. M. A. 160: 628, 1956.

Bacon, H. E.: Cancer of the Colon, Rectum and Anal Canal, Am. J. Surg. 94: 567, 1957.

Bacon, H. E.: Major Surgery of the Colon and Rectum: Rehabilitation and Survival Rate in 2,457 Patients, Dis. Colon & Rectum 3: 393, 1960.

Bacon, H. E., and Berkley, J. L.: Refinements in Prevention of Recurrent Carcinoma Prior to and During Resection of the Colon and Rectum; Preliminary Report, J. Internat. Coll. Surgeons 30: 539, 1958.

Bacon, H. E., Lowell, E. J., Jr., and Trimpi, H. D.: Significance of Ureteral Studies in Colonic and Rectal Surgery, Am. J. Surg. 86: 572, 1953.

Best, R., R., and Rasmussen, J. A.: Results of Sphincter-Preserving Operations for Carcinoma of the Midrectum, J. A. M. A. 164: 739, 1957.

Blatt, L. J., and Cincotti, J. J.: In Vivo Visualization of Lymphatics; an Experimental and Clinical Study With Reference to the Rectum, Surgery 38: 373, 1955.

Block, I., and Enquist, I.: Lymphatic Studies Pertaining to Local Spread of Carcinoma of the Rectum in the Female, Surg., Gynec. & Obst. 112: 41, 1961.

Block, I. R.: A More Radical Perineal Phase for Abdominoperineal Resection of Rectum for Carcinoma, Surg., Gynec. & Obst. 107: 667, 1958.

Brunschwig, A.: Radical Surgical Management of Cancer of the Colon Spread to Tissues and Organs Beyond the Colon, Dis. Colon & Rectum 4: 83, 1961.

Burke, R. M., and Jackman, R. J.: A Modified Thiersch Operation in Treatment of Complete Rectal Prolapse, Dis. Colon & Rectum 2: 555, 1959.

Burns, F. J.: Volvulus of the Colon, Dis. Colon & Rectum 3: 403, 1960.

Burns, F. J., and Pfaff, J., Jr.: Vascular Invasion in Carcinoma of Colon and Rectum, Am. J. Surg. 92: 704, 1956.

Butcher, H. R., Jr., and Spjut, H. J.: An Evaluation of Pelvic Exenteration for Advanced Carcinoma of the Lower Colon, Cancer 12: 681, 1959.

Carroll, P, T.: Diverticula, Diverticulosis and Diverticulitis of the Colon: Indications for Operation and Refinement of Surgical Technic, Dis. Colon & Rectum 4: 88, 1961.

Cattell, R. B., and Swinton, N. W.: One-Stage Abdominoperineal Operation for Cancer of the Rectum, Dis. Colon & Rectum 2: 353, 1959.

Chapuis, P., and Dargent, M.: Treatment of Rectovaginal Fistulas Following Radium Therapy of Cancer of the Cervix (Traitement des fistules recto-vaginales survenant après radium-therapie du cancer du col), Sem. hop. Paris 32: 79, 1956.

Cohn, I., Langford, D., and Rives, J. D.: Antibiotic Support of Colon Anastomoses, Surg., Gynec. & Obst. 104: 1, 1957.

Cole, J. W., O'Hara, R. S., and Holden, W. D.: Observations on the Relationship of Benign Adenomatous Polyps of the Colon to the Natural History of Colonic Cancer, Surg., Gynec. & Obst. 107: 651, 1958.

Deddish, M. R., and Hertz, R. E.: Colotomy and Coloscopy in the Management of Neoplasms of the Colon, Dis. Colon & Rectum 2: 133, 1959.

Delarue, J., Mignot, J., and Bulliard, A.: Study on the Vascularization of Cancers of the Large Intestine, La presse méd. 64: 2164, 1956.

Dukes, C. E.: The Etiology of Cancer of the Colon and Rectum, Dis. Colon & Rectum 2: 27, 1959.

Edwards, M.: Multilocular Retrorectal Cystic Disease—Cyst-Hamartoma: Report of Twelve Cases, Dis. Colon & Rectum 4: 103, 1961.

Erich, J., Hill, J., and Schwartz, W.: Use of Pedicle Flaps of Skin for Closure of Perianal and Sacral Defects, Dis. Colon & Rectum 3: 481, 1960.

Fansler, W. A.: A Consideration of the Surgical Treatment of Cancer of the Colon and Rectum, Dis. Colon & Rectum 2: 32, 1959.

Gabriel, W. B.: The Treatment of Complete Prolapse of the Rectum by Rectosigmoidectomy (Auffret-Mikulicz-Miles Procedure), Dis. Colon & Rectum 1: 241, 1958.

Gilchrist, R. K.: Lymphatic Spread of Carcinoma of the Colon, Dis. Colon & Rectum 2: 69, 1959.

Goligher, J. C.: Correction of Complete Rectal Prolapse, Brit. J. Surg. 45: 323, 1958.

Goligher, J. C.: Extraperitoneal Ileostomy or Colostomy, Brit. J. Surg. 46: 97, 1958.

Hallenbeck, G. A.: Anterior Resection and Pull-Through Procedures for Cancer of the Rectum and Rectosigmoid, Dis. Colon & Rectum 2: 117, 1959.

Helwig, F. C.: The Association of Benign and Malignant Polyps of the Large Intestine, Dis. Colon & Rectum 3: 343, 1960.

Horava, A., and Von Haam, E.: Experimental Carcinoma of the Colon, Cancer Res. 18: 764, 1958.

Johnson, J. W., Judd, E. S., and Dahlin, D. C.: Malignant Neoplasms of the Colon and Rectum in Young Persons, A. M. A. Arch. Surg. 79: 365, 1959.

Kerr, J. G.: Complications of Surgical Procedures on the Colon and Rectum Occurring During the Immediate Postoperative Period, Dis. Colon & Rectum 3: 418, 1960.

Levy, S.: Adenomatous and Carcinomatous Polyps of the Large Intestine, Rev. brasil. gastroenterol. 10: 163, 1958.

Lewis, F. J., and Wangensteen, O. H.: Explorations Following Resection of the Colon, Rectum, or Stomach for Carcinoma With Lymph Node Metastases. In Surgical Forum: Proceedings of the Forum Sessions, Thirty-sixth Clinical Congress of the American College of Surgeons, Boston, Mass., Oct., 1950, Philadelphia, 1951, W. B. Saunders Co.

McGregor, R. A., and Bacon, H. E.: Surgical Management of Sigmoido-vesical and Sigmoido-uterine Fistula Complicating Diverticulitis, Dis. Colon & Rectum 3: 446, 1960.

McKay, J. L., and McMahon, W. A.: Management of Adenomas of the Colon and Rectum Showing Malignant Changes: Report of 44 Cases Treated by Local Removal, Dis. Colon & Rectum 2: 298, 1959.

McKittrick, L. S.: Resection of the Colon for Carcinoma, Dis. Colon & Rectum 2: 123, 1959.

Madden, J. L., and Amendola, F. H.: Radical Left Hemicolectomy, Dis. Colon & Rectum 1: 81, 1958.

Mayo, C. W.: Requirements of Adequate Cancer Operation on the Colon, Rectum and Anus, Surg., Gynec. & Obst. 110: 497, 1960.

Mayo, C. W., Laberge, M. Y., and Hardy, W. M.: Five Year Survival After Anterior Resection for Carcinoma of the Rectum and Rectosigmoid, Surg., Gynec. & Obst. 106: 695, 1958.

Morgan, C. N., and Griffiths, J. D.: High Ligation of the Inferior Mesenteric Artery During Operations for Carcinoma of the Distal Colon and Rectum Surg., Gynec. & Obst. 108: 641, 1959.

Palmer, J. A.: The Management of Massive Rectal Prolapse, Surg., Gynec. & Obst. 112: 502, 1961.

Peltier, L. F.: The Search for Lymph Node Metastases in Cancer of the Rectum, Surgery 30: 443, 1951.

Pickrell, K., and others: Correction of Rectal Incontinence. Transplantation of the Gracilis Muscle to Construct a Rectal Sphincter, Am. J. Surg. 90: 721, 1955.

Pickrell, K., and others: Gracilis Muscle Transplant for Rectal Incontinence, Surgery 40: 349, 1956.

Postlethwait, R., Adamson, J., and Hart, D.: Carcinoma of the Colon and Rectum, Surg., Gynec. & Obst. 106: 257, 1958.

Ray, J. Hines, M. and Hanley, P.: Postoperative Problems of Ileostomy and Colostomy, J. A. M. A. 174: 2118, 1960.

Remington, J. H.: Prevention of Ureteral Injury in Surgery of the Pelvic Colon, Dis. Colon & Rectum 2: 340, 1959.

Roof, W. R., Morris, G. C., and DeBakey, M.: Management of Civilian Colon Injuries, Dis. Colon & Rectum 4: 115, 1961.

Rosi, P. A., and Capos, N. J.: Colon. The Selection of

Operation for Carcinoma of the Colon, J. Kansas M. Soc. 57: 679, 1956.

Ruff, C. C., and others: Preoperative Radiation Therapy for Adenocarcinoma of the Rectum and Rectosigmoid, Surg,, Gynec. & Obst. 112: 715, 1961.

Scarborough, R. A.: The Relationship Between Polyps and Carcinoma of the Colon and Rectum, Dis. Colon & Rectum 3: 336, 1960.

Shann, H.: The Complete Prolapse or Procidentia of the Rectum, an Unsolved Surgical Problem, Internat. Abstr. Surg. 109: 521, 1959.

Smellman, B.: Complete Prolapse of the Rectum, Dis. Colon & Rectum 4: 199, 1961.

Sonneland, J., Anson, B. J., and Beaton, L. E.: Surgical Anatomy of the Arterial Supply to the Colon From the Superior Mesenteric Artery Based Upon a Study of 600 Specimens, Surg., Gynec. & Obst. 106: 385, 1958.

Stearns, M. W., and Deddish, M. R.: Five-Year Results of Abdominopelvic Lymph Node Dissection for Carcinoma of the Rectum, Dis. Colon & Rectum 2: 169, 1959.

Swinton, N. W.: Recent Trends in the Treatment of Cancer of the Colon and Rectum, Am. J. Surg. 92: 727, 1956.

Turnbull, R. B.: Carcinoma in Polyps of the Colon and Rectum: A Study of 86 Treated Patients, Dis. Colon & Rectum 2: 44, 1959.

Ulin, A. W., Ehrlich, E. W., and Shoemaker, W. C.: Transcecal Colostomy With Notes on Technique and Management, Surg., Gynec. & Obst. 107: 104, 1958.

Ulm, A. H., and Klein, E.: Management of Ureteral Obstruction Produced by Recurrent Cancer of the Rectosigmoid Colon, Surg., Gynec. & Obst. 110: 413, 1960.

Wangensteen, O. H.: The Surgeon's Approach to the Problem of Alimentary Tract Malignancy, Journal-Lancet 70: 411, 1950.

Waugh, J. M., and Turner, J. C.: A Study of 268 Patients With Carcinoma of the Midrectum Treated by Abdominoperineal Resection With Sphincter Preservation, Surg., Gynec. & Obst. 109: 777, 1958.

Wittoesch, J. H., and Jackman, R. J.: Results of the Conservative Management of Cancer of the Rectum in Poor Risk Patients, Surg., Gynec. & Obst. 107: 648, 1958.

Section VII · BENIGN TUMORS AND CYSTS

16 · Benign Tumors of the Vulva and Vagina

VULVA AND PERINEUM
Surgical Anatomy

The vulva (pudendum) includes the labia majora and minora, clitoris, vestibule, hymen, vestibular bulbs, and Bartholin's glands. Because of the proximity and frequent involvement in the same disease, the mons veneris, urethra, and Skene's glands are included in this description of the surgical anatomy. The vulva is traumatized by straddle injuries, all sorts of mechanical manipulations by inexperienced hands, and, in most adult females, by obstetric injuries. It is only a reflection of the remarkable blood supply of the vulva that the pelvic floor is seen as well preserved as it is in most patients. Few other parts of the body recover as remarkably and completely from injuries that are equivalents of major obstetric lacerations, hemorrhage, and compression necrosis of the soft parts.

The mons veneris is the rounded eminence over the symphysis pubis created by a collection of fat beneath the skin. The skin of the mons resembles that of the labia majora. The labia majora are prominent, longitudinal folds of skin which originate at the mons veneris and extend backward to the anterior boundary of the perineum. They form the urogenital cleft (rima pudendi), into which the urethra and vagina open. The labia majora are thicker at the anterior end, and posteriorly they turn inward toward the middle line, forming the pos-

terior commissure (posterior boundary of the vulva). A direct or indirect inguinal (inguinolabial) hernia follows the course of the round ligament but is infrequent in females as compared with femoral hernias. The protrusion of a sac and its intra-abdominal contents through the inguinal canal follows the course of the round ligament. If the internal inguinal ring is palpated in every female subjected to laparotomy, the existence of a small hernial sac along the round ligament is found rather frequently. This extension of the so-called canal of Nuck becomes symptomatic only when it reaches an appreciable size or strangulates its contents. Surgical anatomists in the past have described a pudendal hernia. This hernia was described as protruding between the vagina and the descending ramus of the pubis to present a large mass in the introitus. We know now that when the pelvic floor is decompensated, there are relaxation and protrusion laterally as well as the universally recognized cystocele and rectocele. If students of surgical anatomy had only studied and written about the hernias of the female pelvic floor as extensively as they have written about the simple, male, indirect inguinal hernia, the mechanics of the support of the abdominal and pelvic viscera would be better understood.

The perineum in its limited definition is the interval between the posterior commissure and the anus. It is lacerated or stretched during delivery, whether the patient be a primipara with a rigid perineum or a multipara with scarcely any muscle fibers left between the vagina and rectum. Such wounds are separated by the tension produced by the remains of the superficial transverse perineal, deep transverse perineal, and levator ani extensions when the laceration extends high enough. If these lacerations are not properly sutured, the obturators (vagina and rectum) are left to gape, and the pelvic aperture (puborectalis of the levator ani) remains weakened. The result or compensation for this defect, in the presence of an intact rectal sphincter, is the development of a rectocele with forward displacement of the remains of the transverse perineal muscles and fascia. The visible laceration of the perineal floor may not reflect the total damage, since hematomas within the muscles may further impair their subsequent function. Only a surgeon with considerable obstetric training can understand the complexities of the pelvic floor and a muscle group subjected to the passage of a solid object about 10 cm. in diameter as occurs with a term delivery.

The labia minora (nymphae) are double folds of skin parallel and internal to the labia majora. They are much narrower, and their posterior extremities fade into the medial surface of the labia majora except in young women, in whom they may be seen to join in the midline by a small fold called the fourchette (frenulum pudendi). Anteriorly each labium minus divides into two parts, a lateral and a medial. The lateral portions join over the glans clitoridis and form the prepuce of the clitoris. The medial portions join underneath the clitoris to form the frenulum. Posteriorly the depression between the hymen and the fourchette is called the fossa navicularis, which is obliterated by childbirth.

The clitoris is the organ of erectile tissue attached by two crura or roots to the rami of the os pubis and the ischium. The structure of the roots is very vascular (corpora cavernosa), and they are enclosed by a dense layer of fibrous membrane. The body of the clitoris is short and is concealed beneath the labia. The glans in the terminal end of the clitoris is usually concealed above by the prepuce and below by the frenulum (Plate 43, *A*).

The vestibule is the medial area of skin between the labia minora and the hymen. It thus contains the orifices of the urethra, vagina, Bartholin's glands, and, posteriorly, the depression called the fossa navicularis. The orifice of the urethra emerges just anterior to the vaginal orifice. Occasionally there are elevations of the mucous membrane of the vestibule on each side of the urethra containing the paraurethral glands. Just within the external urethral meatus may be found the openings of Skene's ducts.

The hymen is a membranous fold of variable shape around the orifice of the vagina. It is most commonly semilunar in shape, attached posteriorly with the concave margin pointing anteriorly. The hymen may be imperforate, in which event secretions and menstruum would be retained. It may be annular, cribriform, fimbriated, or semilunar in shape. With few exceptions, in the adolescent or adult female the hymen can be gently distended and a narrow speculum introduced to visualize the cervix. When this is not possible and the seriousness of the patient's symptoms warrant, she should be examined under anesthesia after a hymenotomy.

The vestibular bulbs are two small, piriform, erectile bodies on either side of the vestibule. They are behind the labia minora and bulbocavernosi and rest on the inferior layer of the urogenital diaphragm. Composed of an intricate plexus of veins and about 2.5 cm. in length, they communicate anteriorly to form the corpus spongiosum at the lower part of the root of the clitoris. Each bulb has a fibrous capsule derived from the urogenital diaphragm that may be ruptured as a result of injury and give rise to a pudendal hematocele.

Bartholin's glands (greater vestibular glands) are about the size of a bean and are situated in the lower vagina. They are overlapped by the posterior ends of the vestibular bulbs and are covered by the bulbocavernosus on each side. Their ducts open into the ves-

PLATE 43

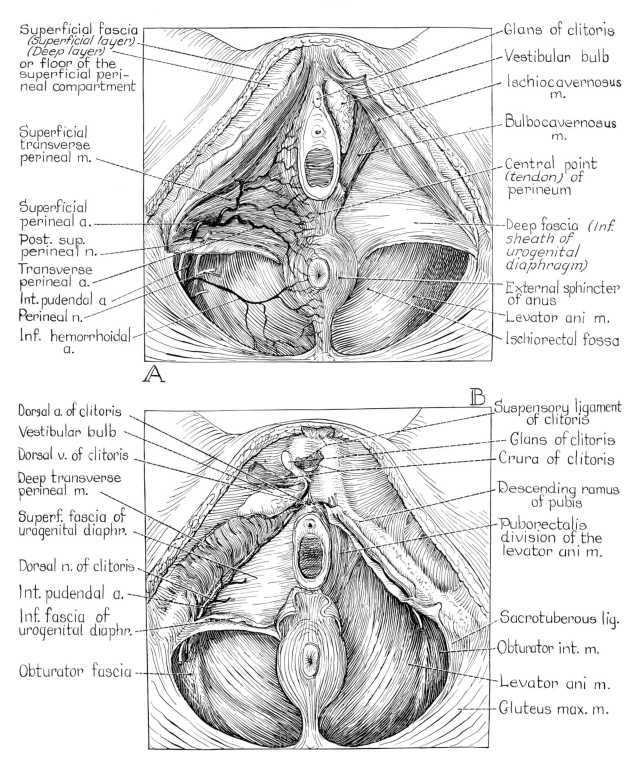

Superficial fascia
(Superficial layer)
(Deep layer)
or floor of the
superficial peri-
neal compartment

Superficial
transverse
perineal m.

Superficial
perineal a.

Post. sup.
perineal n.

Transverse
perineal a.

Int. pudendal a.

Perineal n.

Inf. hemorrhoidal
a.

Glans of clitoris

Vestibular bulb

Ischiocavernosus
m.

Bulbocavernosus
m.

Central point
(tendon) of
perineum

Deep fascia *(Inf.*
sheath of
urogenital
diaphragm)

External sphincter
of anus

Levator ani m.

Ischiorectal fossa

A

B

Dorsal a. of clitoris

Vestibular bulb

Dorsal v. of clitoris

Deep transverse
perineal m.

Superf. fascia of
urogenital diaphr.

Dorsal n. of clitoris

Int. pudendal a.

Inf. fascia of
urogenital diaphr.

Obturator fascia

Suspensory ligament
of clitoris

Glans of clitoris

Crura of clitoris

Descending ramus
of pubis

Puborectalis
division of the
levator ani m.

Sacrotuberous lig.

Obturator int. m.

Levator ani m.

Gluteus max. m.

tibule between the attachment of the labia minora and the hymen.

The blood supply of the vulva is derived from the internal pudic artery (Plate 43, *A* and *B*), which is the terminal branch of the hypogastric, and from branches of the femoral and the deep external pudic and superficial external pudic arteries. The internal pudic (pudendal) artery leaves the true pelvis through the greater sciatic foramen and, curving over the spine of the ischium, re-enters the pelvis through the lesser sciatic foramen, where it enters Alcock's canal. Alcock's canal is formed by fascial extensions of the obturator fascia and helps make up the outer wall of the ischiorectal fossa. A finger in the rectum or vagina can palpate this canal, which is a favorite site for anesthetic blocking of the pudendal nerve. The internal pudic artery then gives off the inferior hemorrhoidal artery, which courses medialward through the fat of the ischiorectal fossa and terminates in the lowermost two or three inches of the rectum and anus. It then gives some superficial branches to the skin of the labia and a perineal artery to the muscles in the superficial perineal compartment. Passing farther anteriorly in the deep perineal compartment, it terminates by short branches emerging near the midline to supply the erectile tissues, the artery to the bulb, the artery to the crus, and the dorsal artery of the clitoris.

The internal pudic (pudendal) veins are usually double and accompany their respective arteries except for the dorsal vein of the clitoris. The dorsal vein of the clitoris enters the pelvis through the subpubic space to help form the pudendal plexus, which lies below and behind the arcuate ligament of the symphysis. The pudendal plexus represents the commencement of the pudendal vein but communicates also with the uterovaginal plexus through the vesical plexus surrounding the floor of the bladder. The superficial and deep external pudic arteries supply the skin, subcutaneous tissues, and muscles of the labia mainly in the anterior portion.

The nerve supply of the vulva is derived from three sources: the pudic nerve, the posterior cutaneous nerve of the thigh (small sciatic), and the ilioinguinal nerve. The pudic nerve is formed from fibers from the second, third, and fourth sacral nerves. It accompanies the pudendal artery. The pudendal nerve divides into a perineal branch and the dorsal nerve to the clitoris. The nerve supply of the clitoris is greater than that of the penis when their relative sizes are considered. The perineal nerve sends a superficial branch to the skin of the labia and adjacent muscles. The deep branch sends fibers to the anterior half of the external sphincter ani. This should be spared in operations performed in this area if at all possible. A knowledge of the exact course of this nerve is essential in performing nerve-cutting procedures for intractable pruritus. The perineal branch of the posterior cutaneous nerve of the thigh passes medialward and, becoming subcutaneous over the pubic arch, supplies fibers to the skin of the labia. More anteriorly the labial skin receives fibers from the ilioinguinal nerve after it emerges from the inguinal canal. (Plate 43, *A* and *B*.)

The superficial inguinal glands are the only lymphatics draining the vulva. The superior group just below Poupart's ligament receive lymphatics from the lower vagina, vulva, perineum, and anus. There is a rich anastomosis from side to side. The inferior group about the fossa ovalis receive lymphatics from the perineum and lower extremity. It is a good practice to examine the patient's feet for fungus or other infections and the legs for ulcerations before becoming concerned with enlarged glands about the fossa ovalis and inguinal regions. A patient with varicose veins of the extremities frequently has vulval varicosities that complicate the situation and may be as symptomatic as the distended veins of the legs. From the superficial glands, efferents pass to the deep inguinal glands in the femoral canal and then to the common iliac chain. Lymphatics from the dorsal aspect of the clitoris may go directly to the deep glands. Clinically, enlargement of the superficial inguinal glands is caused by disease or malignancy of the vulva, lower vagina, perineum, anus, or lower extremities. Rarely a fundal malignancy involves these glands by lymphatics accompanying the round ligament to its insertion in the labia majora.

THE MUSCULAR AND FASCIAL STRUCTURES OF THE PERINEUM
Surgical Anatomy

The fascia of the perineum has its counterparts in the fascia of the thigh and abdomen. The superficial perineal fascia consists of two layers. A superficial layer of the superficial fascia (Camper's layer) is fatty and areolar and gives contour to the mons pubis and labia majora and fills the ischiorectal fossa. The deep layer of the superficial fascia (Scarpa's layer) is membranous and not fatty in character. This deep layer continues from the abdomen and thigh—where it overlies the fascia lata—and is attached to a fibrocartilaginous ridge on the ischiopubic ramus. It then extends to cover the structures in the superficial perineal compartment and thus forms the floor of the space. The deep layer of fascia of the abdomen (Colles' fascia), after attaching to the inguinal ligament, passes over into the thigh as the fascia lata. This deep layer has its counterpart in the perineum—the strong inferior sheath of the urogenital diaphragm. Together with the deep layer of the superficial fascia, it encloses the erectile and muscular structures in the superficial compartment (Plate 43, *A*).

The superficial transverse perineal muscles are small firm bands arising from the tuberosities of the ischium and inserting into the central point of the perineum. The central point (tendon) of the female perineum is a fibromuscular structure in the midline between the anus and vagina. It is made up of fibers derived from the superficial and deep transverse perineal muscles, the bulbocavernosi, and the external sphincter ani. The ischiocavernosi arise from the rami of the ischium and ensheath the crura of the clitoris. They help to produce erection of that organ through obstruction of the return flow of blood. The bulbocavernosi arise from the central point and pass forward

along either side of the vaginal orifice to be inserted into the body of the clitoris. Their action is to constrict the vagina and vestibular bulbs. The perineal division of the pudendal nerve supplies all three muscles of the superficial compartment. The pudendal artery supplies branches to these muscles. The crura of the clitoris, vestibular bulbs, and pars intermedia of the bulbs occupy the anterior portion of the superficial compartment. The clitoris itself extends beyond but receives, like the penis in the male, a firm fascial investment (Plate 43, *A*).

The urogenital diaphragm (triangular ligament) consists of two layers which enclose muscle, vessels, and nerves in what is known as the deep compartment. Its inferior layer has been described. Its superior layer is weak and is a continuation of the obturator fascia over the pubic arch. The urogenital diaphragm is perforated anteriorly to allow passage of the dorsal vein of the clitoris. The fascia thickens where this vessel passes and has been called the transverse perineal ligament. The diaphragm is hardly recognizable as it passes posteriorly, even in the dissecting room. It is pierced by the urethra and vagina and then extends slightly more posteriorly than the vagina, where it passes into the central tendon. The deep compartment contains the deep transverse perineal muscle and the pudendal vessels and nerves which perforate it to reach structures in the superficial compartment (Plate 43, *B*). A constrictor urethrae muscle or group of fibers is described as arising from the pubic rami and interweaving with fibers from the opposite side about the urethra. While these fibers can be identified by dissection or histologic studies, it is doubtful that they can act as a true external urethral sphincter as some insist. The deep transverse perineal muscles arise on either side from the pubic rami and ischium. Some fibers intermingle with the constrictor urethrae, while others pass to the central point of the perineum. Nerve and blood supply of these structures is from the pudendal nerve and vessels (Plate 43, *A* and *B*).

The detailed structure of the perineum with

its muscles, erectile tissues, vessels, and nerves is not recognizable at the operating table, particularly in multiparous women. In operations where muscles are transplanted (bulbocavernosus for urinary incontinence) or where fibers of the pudendal nerve are severed (during an undercutting operation for intractable pruritis), the structures must be identified, although their detailed anatomy may not be essential. In operations on the anterior vaginal wall the remnants of the urogenital diaphragm appear as strong bands on either side of the urethra near its meatus and extend to the pubic rami. Often they are scarred and retracted, causing distortion of the urethra and fixing it abnormally forward with a gaping meatus. The perineal body (collectively the central point, origins of muscles and fascial insertions) may not be recognizable as such after many lacerations of childbirth. As the perineum is dissected in performing a perineorrhaphy, the anterior edges of the puborectalis portions of the levators come into view as firm but thin masses of muscle directed obliquely in an anteroposterior direction. The anterior edges of the paired levators have usually been distorted by parturition but often can be utilized to strengthen the repair by suturing the leading edges anterior to the rectum.

BARTHOLIN'S ABSCESS
General Considerations

With the widespread use of antimicrobial therapy, infections of Bartholin's glands are infrequently of specific origin and are a less common complication of lower genital tract gonorrhea. The cultures rarely reveal only colonies of the gonococcus, and other pyogenic organisms such as the staphylococcus, streptococcus, or a mixed infection are found. The symptoms of a Bartholin's abscess are pain and swelling in one or both labia, together with a vaginal discharge. The abscess may induce symptoms from pressure on the anorectum or the urethra and cause pain on defecation or urination. Many abscesses rupture spontaneously or resolve with sulfonamide or antibiotic therapy. Incision and drainage of a Bartholin's abscess provide prompt relief and can be done under local anesthesia as an office procedure. Recurrence of the condition is almost a foregone conclusion. The procedure of choice is marsupialization, which results in a permanent cure in the majority of patients. This requires hospitalization and preferably general anesthesia.

MARSUPIALIZATION OPERATION FOR BARTHOLIN'S ABSCESS
Indications and Surgical Principles

The best results are obtained in marsupializing unilateral abscesses of nonspecific origin. These abscesses have thick walls that can be everted with remarkably little reaction in the surrounding tissue. Acute bilateral abscesses of gonorrheal origin, if not recurrent, can be treated by this eversion of the cyst wall, but the tissues are fragile and the procedure may accomplish little more than an incision and drainage.

Marsupialization permits healing from the depths of the abscess to the surface. Some observers feel that glands can regenerate and function to some degree. Distortion of the introitus is remarkably little with the operation, and whether a functional gland is obtained or not is of little import.

Steps of the Operation

1. An incision is made adjacent to the hymeneal ring of its remnants. The opening of Bartholin's duct has usually long since been obscured. The incision is carried down through the mucous membrane of the fourchette to the capsule of the gland. The incision will vary from 6 to 8 cm., depending on the size of the abscess (Plate 44, A).

2. An old, chronically recurring abscess will present a thick capsule. The mucous membrane is dissected from the wall of the abscess for a few millimeters. This permits their subsequent approximation with a broad area of contact (Plate 44, B).

3. An incision is then made into the abscess cavity. This is planned with each case, depending on the size and configuration of the abscessed gland, so that a maximal area of the cavity is everted (Plate 44, B).

PLATE 44

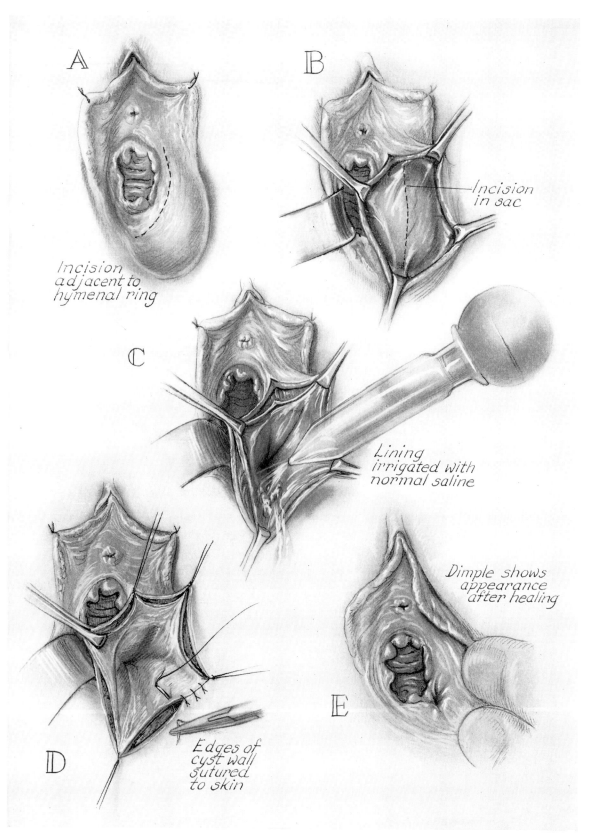

A

Incision
adjacent to
hymenal ring

B

Incision
in sac

C

Lining
irrigated with
normal saline

D

Edges of
cyst wall
sutured
to skin

E

Dimple shows
appearance
after healing

4. The cavity is irrigated with normal saline and thoroughly explored, so that any loculated areas, not connected with the main abscess cavity, could be overlooked and remained undrained. The sac is now everted and studied for approximation to the mucous membrane of the fourchette. The wall can be trimmed as indicated. This should evert the depths of the sac as seen in Plate 44, *C.*

5. The edges of the cyst wall are sutured to the skin by interrupted sutures of fine 000 chromic catgut. They should be placed less than a centimeter apart so that healing between cyst wall and skin and epithelization of the cyst wall is ensured (Plate 44, *D*).

6. The cavity is firmly packed with Vaseline gauze. Several sutures can be left long after tying and then criss-crossed over the pack to hold it in place for twenty-four hours.

7. Plate 44, *E,* shows the end result of a marsupialization operation. A small dimple results in the depths of which some functional glands may regenerate.

Postoperative Care

The sutures retaining the Vaseline gauze pack are cut the day after operation, the pack removed, and the cavity lightly packed with Vaseline gauze. A wide-spectrum antibiotic may be administered, particularly if the swelling was such that an indwelling catheter was necessary. In cases of long standing it is doubtful if any antimicrobials are necessary. The patient can usually be returned home on the second postoperative day. All packing is removed, and she is instructed to take sitz baths twice a day. She should be seen within four to six days after discharge, and the cavity probed to be sure that no loculations are sealed off and the wound is healing from the depths to the surface.

BARTHOLIN'S CYST
Etiology and Pathologic Anatomy

A Bartholin's cyst forms as a result of inflammation of Bartholin's gland, in which the duct is occluded and no longer serves as a method of drainage. As the gland enlarges, it tends to spread the labia minora on the same side over the cyst wall. It is seldom possible to identify the point of exit of Bartholin's duct in the posterior aspect of the vestibule of the vagina.

Symptoms and Diagnosis

In the absence of any inflammation, the patient complains of a painless swelling in one or the other labia. The distortion of the vulva and introitus may cause dyspareunia and the mucosa covering the cyst to become irritated from pressure and chafing as the patient walks.

Indications and Surgical Principles

A Bartholin's cyst is removed for the patient's comfort, and she is reassured that the swelling does not represent a tumor or malignant disease. The incision and operation are done so as to cause a minimum of distortion of the vulval cleft. For a rather simple procedure there is a great difference of opinion as to the position of the skin incision. An incision toward the vaginal introitus affords the best exposure and ensures removal of Bartholin's duct to prevent recurrence. If a scar forms in this area, however, it is more likely to give rise to dyspareunia than is an incision in the labia majora. Lateral incisions do not form a scar near the introitus but distort the external appearance of the vulva. The objective of the surgeon is to remove the entire cyst, cyst wall, and Bartholin's duct without the removal of tissue of the vestibular bulb and bulbocavernosus. If large segments of tissue are removed from these structures, the labia are distorted. A simple line of cleavage between the cyst wall and the surrounding tissues is difficult to define. Rupture of the cyst during the course of the procedure is common. Careful hemostasis is observed in this operation because of the vascularity of the area. The surgeon removes all segments of the duct to prevent recurrence of the cyst or the formation of a sinus.

Preoperative Care and Anesthesia

A general anesthetic is preferred to local infiltration. Local infiltration reduces the amount of bleeding during the procedure but obscures

PLATE 45

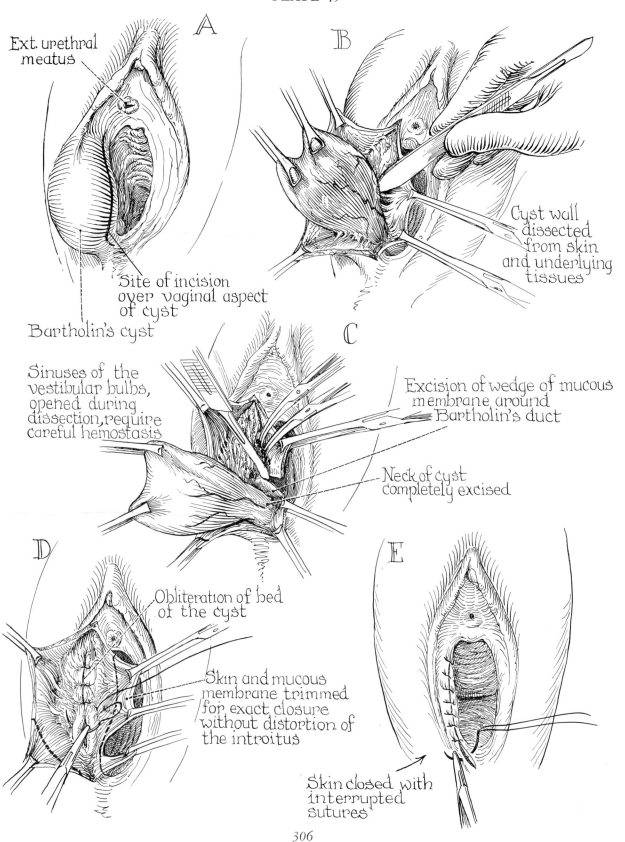

A

Ext. urethral
meatus

Site of incision
over vaginal aspect
of cyst

Bartholin's cyst

B

Cyst wall
dissected
from skin
and underlying
tissues

Sinuses of the
vestibular bulbs,
opened during
dissection, require
careful hemostasis

C

Excision of wedge of mucous
membrane around
Bartholin's duct

Neck of cyst
completely excised

D

Obliteration of bed
of the cyst

Skin and mucous
membrane trimmed
for exact closure
without distortion of
the introitus

E

Skin closed with
interrupted
sutures

small bleeding points that may later form a hematoma in the wound.

Steps of the Operation

1. A longitudinal incision is made in the skin of the vestibule over the medial aspect of the cyst (Plate 45, *A*). This incision is inside or corresponds to the inner aspect of the labia minora that is stretched over the cyst wall.

2. The fragile and easily ruptured cyst wall is dissected from the skin and underlying tissue (Plate 45, *A*). Perforation of the cyst does not add any complications to the healing of the wound. The cyst is grasped with Babcock clamps to aid the operator in removing the entire cyst wall (Plate 45, *B*).

3. There is seldom a definite line of cleavage between the cyst and adjacent tissues. Many sinuses of the vestibular bulbs are opened during the course of the dissection, and these bleeding points are clamped and ligated (Plate 45, *C*).

4. The entire cyst wall is mobilized and the neck of the cyst identified. The probable area where Bartholin's ducts emerge into the vestibule of the vagina is outlined. A wedge of mucous membrane around the area is excised to ensure the removal of the duct (Plate 45, *C*).

5. The bed formerly occupied by the cyst is obliterated with interrupted sutures of 00 chromic catgut (Plate 45, *D*). Meticulous hemostasis is obtained. The skin and mucous membrane that lay over the cyst are trimmed to give an exact closure and good cosmetic result (Plate 45, *D*).

6. The skin incision in the vestibule is closed with interrupted sutures of 00 chromic catgut (Plate 45, *E*). The sutures gently approximate the tissues without strangulation so that a minimum amount of scar and contraction results. The contents of the cyst are usually sterile. Drains are not necessary unless purulent material is found within the cyst.

Postoperative Care

A wide-spectrum antibiotic is administered for several days postoperatively. The immediate operative area is kept clean by washes with a mild antiseptic solution. On the second postoperative day the patient can sit in warm water. This affords considerable relief from pain. She is discharged on the third postoperative day if the wound is healing well.

EXCISION OF A FIBROMA OF THE LABIA MINORA
Indications and Surgical Principles

Benign tumors of the labia minora are removed when they distort the normal anatomy and interfere with the sexual function. They are removed for urinary symptoms as the result of pressure upon the external urethral meatus or distortion of the urethra. Although they seldom undergo carcinomatous change, they may reach a large size, become pedunculated, or ulcerate on the surface from pressure. The surgeon studies the size of the tumor and the structures that are distorted. He plans an incision and operation on the vulva that leaves the best possible cosmetic result. The tumors shell out readily and do not cause difficulty because of adherency to surrounding structures.

Steps of the Operation

1. In Plate 46, *A,* is shown a large fibroma of the labia minora that displaces the urethral meatus to the right. A catheter is placed in the urethra to outline this structure during the procedure. An incision is planned, as shown in Plate 46, *A,* to remove the excess mucous membrane covering the mass and permit an anatomic reapproximation of the tissues.

2. By sharp and blunt dissection the tumor and its capsule are shelled out (Plate 46, *B*). An assistant retracts the urethra to avoid injury (Plate 46, *B*). At the posterior margin the tumor receives its blood supply from branches of the pudendal artery. These require suture ligatures since they may be quite large.

3. The wound is closed in layers. Edges are trimmed to restore the contour of the labia minora. The urethra, displaced by the tumor, falls back to the midline (Plate 46, *C*). It may be necessary to employ a few sutures to draw the urethra to its normal position. Unless there are suggestive malignant changes in the gross appearance of the tumor, this operation may be combined with other vaginal plastic procedures.

Postoperative Care

The routine management of patients subjected to vaginal surgery is ordered. A pressure dressing, crisscrossed over the labia and wound, prevents the development of a seroma or hematoma.

PLATE 46

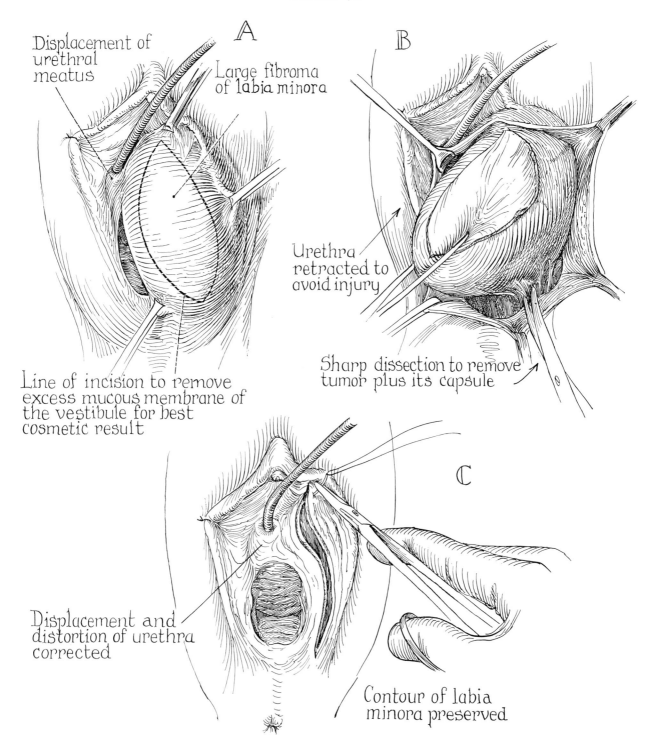

A

Displacement of urethral meatus

Large fibroma of labia minora

Line of incision to remove excess mucous membrane of the vestibule for best cosmetic result

B

Urethra retracted to avoid injury

Sharp dissection to remove tumor plus its capsule

C

Displacement and distortion of urethra corrected

Contour of labia minora preserved

Plastic Repair of a Constricted Introitus
Indications and Surgical Principles

Enlargement of the introitus by plastic repair is indicated for painful intercourse. A constricted introitus may result from a failure of the patient to resume normal sexual relations at an early date following a vaginal plastic operation. The surgeon may be at fault because of too enthusiastic trimming and a poorly planned repair of the pelvic floor. Many of the patients who complain of painful intercourse following vaginal plastic surgery have emotional reasons for not wishing to resume intercourse and readily adapt this excuse to avoid their marital obligations. The futility of surgery to resolve their marital difficulties is explained to the patient and she should be encouraged to make the necessary adjustments in her emotional problems. During the first four to six weeks after a plastic repair, if there is considerable contraction of the tissues and a constriction is impending, the use of vaginal dilators is recommended until regular sexual relations are resumed.

Many patients in the postmenopausal years, who are still sexually active, may have contraction subsequent to senile changes about the vagina and vulva. Where there is no contra-indication to local and systemic estrogen therapy, this will usually suffice to make the vagina and vulva more pliable. A few of these patients require surgery in addition to the use of estrogens. Vaginismus is a condition, emotionally instigated, with some aggravating, organic factors. Organic disease of the introitus that initiates a spasm of the levator sling, with painful intercourse, is corrected simultaneously with the instigation of appropriate psychotherapy. A constricted introitus may also follow a simple vulvectomy for benign disease or other vulval surgery where scar tissue contracts in and about the introitus or vagina.

Steps of the Operation

1. The area of contraction and scar tissue is outlined by Allis clamps and a longitudinal incision made to determine the depth of the scar (Plate 47, *A*).

2. The tissue about the area of contracture is excised. If this extends into the musculature of the perineum or, in the event of a higher stricture, into the musculature of the vaginal wall, the muscle and scar tissue are incised to release the constriction (Plate 47, *B*). The mucosa and skin of the perineum, if the constriction is at the introitus, are then mobilized to permit a transverse closure without tension (Plate 47, *C*). The vaginal circumference in this operation is reconstructed larger than normal to allow for some postoperative contracture.

3. The incision is closed with interrupted sutures of 00 chromic catgut, and the sutures are tied to approximate the edges without strangulation of the tissues (Plate 47, *C*).

Postoperative Care

Routine postoperative care is prescribed as for any vaginal plastic procedure. Appropriate vaginal plugs are given the patient to be inserted several times a day. This prevents subsequent retraction and constriction as the perineal wound is healing. In an elementary but convincing way it informs the patient that the organ can be penetrated without discomfort. Within the limitations of the patient's marital situation, the pleasure-pain principle should be directed toward the repression of the latter. Local and systemic estrogen therapy is given to postmenopausal patients and to those who have had a bilateral oophorectomy for other reasons.

Sliding Flap Operation for Constricted Introitus
Indications and Surgical Principles

Frequently the simple expedient of enlarging a constriction of the introitus by longitudinal incision, excision of scar tissue, and traverse closure will not prevent recurrence. Even at the time of operation, the surgeon may be dissatisfied with the degree of enlargement he has accomplished. Sliding flaps provide a method of moving normal, pliable skin into the area to prevent postoperative contracture.

Steps of the Operation

1. A longitudinal incision is made in the perineal body through scar tissue and muscle deep enough

PLATE 47

PLASTIC REPAIR OF CONSTRICTED INTROITUS

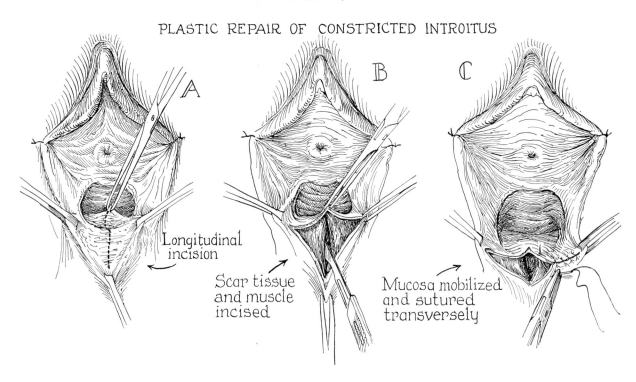

A

Longitudinal
incision

B

Scar tissue
and muscle
incised

C

Mucosa mobilized
and sutured
transversely

EXCISION OF LARGE VAGINAL INCLUSION CYST

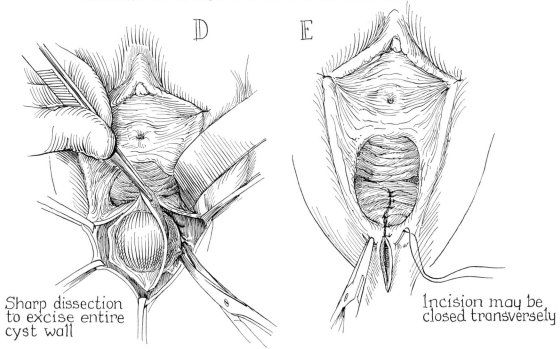

D

Sharp dissection
to excise entire
cyst wall

E

Incision may be
closed transversely

PLATE 48

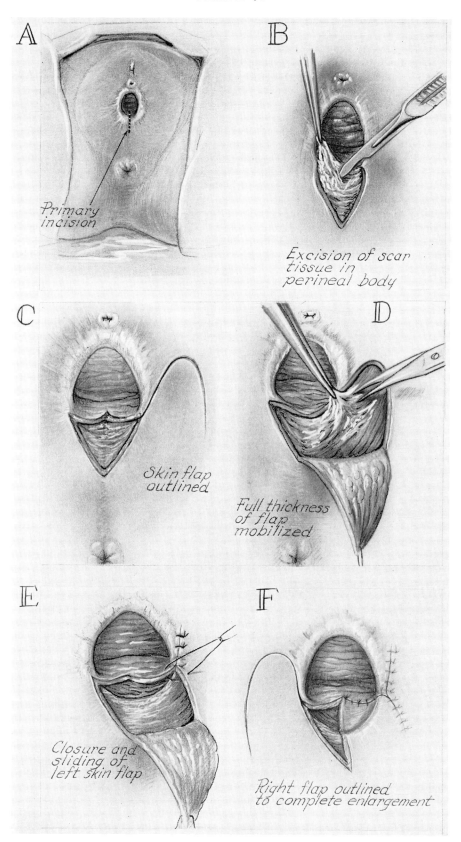

A

Primary incision

B

Excision of scar tissue in perineal body

C

Skin flap outlined

D

Full thickness of flap mobilized

E

Closure and sliding of left skin flap

F

Right flap outlined to complete enlargement

to recognize fibers of the external sphincter of the anus (Plate 48, *A*).

2. The scar tissue is excised, and the full thickness of the skin is undermined upward into the lower vagina and laterally and posteriorly for several centimeters (Plate 48, *B*).

3. Plate 48, *C,* shows one of many incisions that might be made in order to slide flaps of adjacent skin into the area.

4. Scar tissue may be found extending laterally in the perineal body and this is excised. The full-thickness flap of skin is turned back as shown in Plate 48, *D.* The edges are undermined for several centimeters or more until it is evident that the flap can be moved medially without difficulty. Since the base of the flap is so broad, the color and blood supply of the flap is excellent.

5. The edges of area from which the flap was displaced are closed in the usual Y-type approximation. Further undermining is done if at any time the surgeon feels there is any tension on the suture lines (Plate 48, *E*).

6. Plate 48, *F,* shows the left flap approximated to the vaginal mucosa just inside the introitus. As in any plastic surgery meticulous hemostasis should be secured since a hematoma or seroma under the flaps endangers their viability. Plate 48, *F,* also shows the right flap outlined to complete the enlargement.

7. If hemostasis has been good and the field is dry, it is not necessary to use any type of pressure dressing. Occasionally, since this is an extremely vascular area, one may elect to place a pack in the vagina, cover the area with sponges, and secure them with an elastic dressing. An indwelling catheter must be used if the area is compressed.

Postoperative Care

If the vagina is packed and an indwelling catheter used, the patient should receive a urinary antiseptic. The area is inspected daily, and the pack and compression dressings, if used, removed on the first postoperative day. If there is any evidence of accumulation of fluid in any part of the operative field, this is aspirated, or, if large, a small drainage site is established. The undermining would normally denervate most of the area, but, if it is still sensitive, local anesthesia is used. The patient is seen weekly after discharge from the hospital, and,

with the slightest evidence of contracture before normal sexual relations can be resumed, vaginal plugs are used prophylactically.

EXCISION OF A LARGE VAGINAL INCLUSION CYST
Indications and Surgical Principles

Vaginal inclusion cysts are removed if they are symptomatic or large enough that irritation and infection would complicate a relatively simple operation. They commonly result from a laceration of the perineum during childbirth. In healing, fragments of the mucosa are inverted beneath the surface. They may follow infected episiotomies or a perineorrhaphy where mucosa is inadvertently buried. It is possible that some of the cysts result from an inflammatory reaction about buried suture material. The cysts are lined by squamous epithelium to substantiate this point, and the fluid within them is usually clear and serous.

Steps of the Operation

1. A longitudinal incision is made over the cyst to include a portion of the adjacent vaginal wall and scar tissue.

2. By sharp and blunt dissection the cyst wall is systematically freed from the surrounding tissues so that squamous epithelium is not left behind to cause a recurrence (Plate 47, *D*).

3. If it does not cause a constriction, the incision may be closed longitudinally (Plate 47, *E*). Should it appear that a constriction will result, the edges are undermined and the wound is closed transversely. The operation may be incorporated with a vaginal plastic procedure, including both anterior and posterior walls and a perineorrhaphy.

Postoperative Care

No special postoperative care is necessary except to keep the area clean and dry during the postoperative period.

VAGINA
Surgical Anatomy

The anterior wall of the vagina is approximately three inches in length and the posterior wall an inch longer. As it encloses the vaginal portion of the cervix, it forms an anterior and posterior fornix, as well as two lateral fornices. The wall of the vagina is composed of an outer fibrous, a middle muscular, and an inner mucous coat. It makes a 90-degree angle with a normally anteverted uterus and is relatively small in its lower third, where it is surrounded by the musculature of the pelvic floor. The anterior and posterior walls are in approximation and in the lower third fold so as to form a broad letter H.

Exponents of the full-thickness operations for the correction of cystocele and rectocele do not subscribe to the existence of a distinct fascia surrounding the vagina—pubovesical fascia. A hollow viscus has an adventitia of loose areolar tissue, and this can be said for the bladder and vagina. This full thickness of vaginal wall can be dissected from the bladder base by entering the natural line of cleavage between the two. This line of cleavage disappears at the bladder neck, and here the urethra and anterior vaginal wall are intimately blended and sharp dissection is required to separate them. The posterior fornix of the vagina is in contact with the peritoneum of the pouch of Douglas, with the usual retroperitoneal connective tissue intervening. Between the vagina and rectum, a natural line of cleavage, the rectovaginal septum, exists from the posterior fornix to the area of insertion of fibers of the levator ani. The association of the two structures then becomes more intimate as the vagina passes through the urogenital diaphragm and is surrounded by the transverse perineal muscles and bulbocavernosi. The blending of fibers of the rectal sphincters and the central tendon and transverse perineal muscles again requires sharp dissection for their separation. This is even more true in patients requiring a perineorrhaphy in whom extensive scarring of the perineal body has occurred. The levator ani is the chief factor in the closure of the vaginal orifice. Gartner's ducts are embryonic remnants that extend downward in the lateral walls of the vagina and may give rise to vaginal cysts.

The blood supply of the vagina is, for the most part, derived from the inferior vesical artery (vaginal branch or independent vaginal artery), the vaginal branch of the uterine artery, the vaginal branches of the middle hemorrhoidal artery, and the branches of the internal pudendal artery. There is some confusion in the textbooks of anatomy regarding the inferior vesical artery and the vaginal artery. In this text they will be presumed to be the same vessel, although with the many variations of the pelvic vessels it should be realized that two separate arteries are possible. Neither of the two should be confused with the vaginal branch of the uterine artery. The veins form a plexus surrounding the vaginal wall and drain their blood into the tributaries of the hypogastric veins and pudendal veins. The lymphatics of the upper two thirds of the vagina join the hypogastric and sacral chains. The lymphatics of the lower third drain, for the most part, into the superficial inguinal glands, but the rich anastomosis between them must be appreciated by any surgeon operating for malignancy. The nerves of the vagina are derived from the uterovaginal plexus that in turn originated from the hypogastric plexuses. Some parasympathetic fibers probably come direct from the third and fourth sacral nerves.

Recall now the consistency, pliability, and distensibility of the upper vagina and adjacent bladder on one side and rectum on the other. After radiation how things have changed! The feel of a radiation shelf, the immobility of the postradiation vaginal vault, and a postradiation cervix flush with the vagina all would confuse the untrained and suggest a dire outcome were not the expected changes in the character of the tissue appreciated. Likewise there are changes after radical surgery. The depth of the vagina may now be the distance from the tip to the first joint of one's index finger. If the patient were not your own, such a discovery would reassure the examiner that an adequate operation had been done. The vault of the vagina after a radical hysterectomy is anemic, constricted, and fixed—no longer a sexual organ in its former capacity. The patient should be so informed and the method of sexual intercourse adjusted to the foreshortening of the vagina. Wounds of the vagina, especially during pregnancy, bleed vigorously. As is true elsewhere, the primary source should be located, clamped, and ligated securely. False security is the reward of vaginal packing to control such injuries.

BENIGN TUMORS OF THE VAGINA
General Considerations

The following two operations, excision of a fibroma of the vagina and the excision of a Gartner's duct cyst, demonstrate some of the principles of surgery in benign tumors of the vagina. Exclusive of lesions caused by specific disease, such as tuberculosis or the venereal diseases, there are multiple benign tumors and conditions that may require surgery in the vagina. A common lesion is an inclusion cyst at the site of a previous vaginal laceration or episiotomy. Such cysts may be multiple in number and attain a moderate size. Arising from the muscularis of the vagina are found fibromyomas, myomas, simple fibromas, and adenomyomas. The fetal remnants of the Wolffian ducts—Gartner's duct cysts—tend to occur along the anterolateral walls of the vagina. A papilloma of nonvenereal origin may require excision. Endometriosis can spread to the vagina, with endometrial cysts in the posterior vaginal wall. Dermoids and lymphosarcoma have been diagnosed by palpating a retroperitoneal mass vaginally.

EXCISION OF A FIBROMA OF THE VAGINA
Symptoms and Diagnosis

The symptoms caused by a fibroma of the vagina depend on the size of the tumor and the method by which it presents in the vagina. The patient notices a mass, feels a lump in the vagina when taking a douche, or notes some obstruction during sexual intercourse. The tumor may undergo ulcerative changes on the surface. Infection and bleeding bring the patient to a physician. The tumor may assume large proportions and cause pressure upon the bladder and rectum. Some of the lesions are exceedingly tender and cause severe dyspareunia.

Indications and Surgical Principles

Small inclusion cysts and small benign tumors that are asymptomatic need not be removed. Lesions distorting the vagina or those that are ulcerated and infected are removed. Tumors of the vagina may be removed through transverse or longitudinal incisions. The abundant blood supply of the vagina requires careful hemostasis to prevent a hematoma behind the operative area.

Steps of the Operation

1. In Plate 49, A, is shown a small fibroma of the posterior wall of the vagina. Traction sutures are placed on each side of the small tumor. A Jacobs tenaculum on the posterior lip of the cervix draws it anteriorly to expose the field of operation.

2. A transverse incision is made through the full thickness of the vaginal wall, and the edges are grasped with traction sutures or an Allis clamp (Plate 49, B).

3. Numerous methods can be used to make traction upon the tumor. In Plate 49, C, is shown the method of using a needle and needle holder to make traction upon a small fibroma while it is dissected free from the surrounding structures. The base and its capsule are excised from the adjacent vagina.

4. The vaginal incision is closed longitudinally by interrupted sutures of 00 chromic catgut. In this location a longitudinal closure of the incision preserves the depth of the posterior fornix of the vagina (Plate 49, D).

Postoperative Care

No special care is indicated. Sexual intercourse and douching are avoided for several weeks until the incision is healed.

EXCISION OF A GARTNER'S DUCT CYST
Indications and Surgical Principles

Gartner's duct cysts occur along the anterolateral wall of the vagina. If they remain small in size, they need not be removed. Many cysts occur in the fornix of the vagina and displace the cervix to one side or the other. In this location they may distort the course of the ureters. When they become large enough to distort the vagina and cause pressure on surrounding structures, they are removed before

PLATE 49

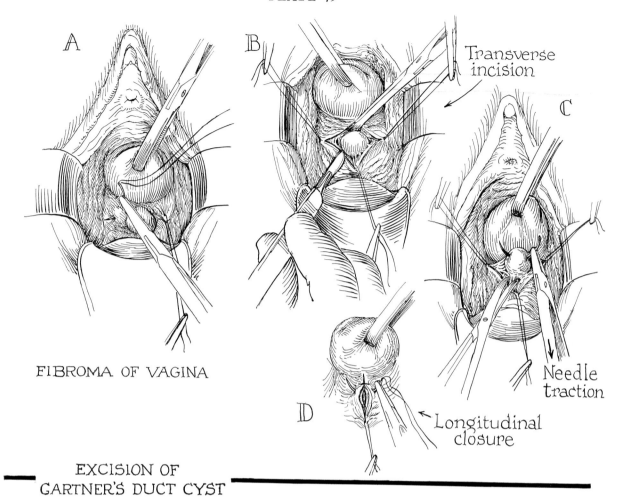

A

FIBROMA OF VAGINA

B Transverse incision

C

D Longitudinal closure

Needle traction

EXCISION OF
GARTNER'S DUCT CYST

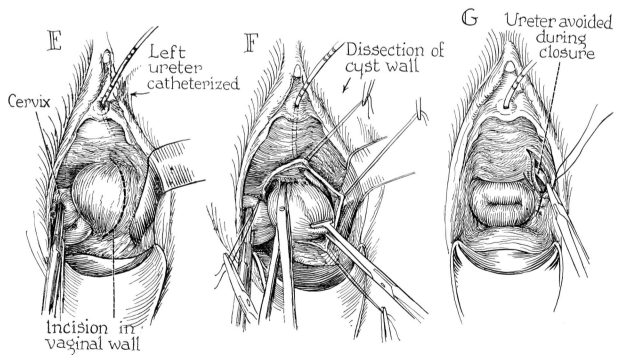

E Left ureter catheterized

Cervix

Incision in vaginal wall

F Dissection of cyst wall

G Ureter avoided during closure

they rupture or become infected. Their proximity to the ureter is shown in Plate 49, *E, F,* and *G.* The ureter is catheterized for positive identification as the cyst wall is excised. Simple drainage or marsupialization of a cyst may lead to recurrence and infection. The entire cyst wall should be removed.

Steps of the Operation

1. The ureter on the same side as the cyst is catheterized with a large ureteral catheter, and an incision is made in the anterior vaginal wall over the cyst (Plate 49, *E*). This is in an anteroposterior direction, although the size and presentation of the cyst may require a different type of incision. The incision is carried through the full thickness of the vagina until the wall of the cyst is identified.

2. Traction sutures are placed in the vaginal wall and the cyst grasped with an Allis clamp, a Babcock clamp, or a similar blunt type of instrument. The cyst wall is completely dissected from its bed (Plate 49, *F*). The operator palpates the course of the ureter at frequent intervals.

3. After the cyst is removed, the operative field is inspected for hemostasis. The ureter is palpated for evidence of distortion. Almost invariably the ureter is exposed with large cysts in the upper vagina. A thin layer of areolar tissue separates the ureter from the bed of the cyst. The vaginal wall is closed with interrupted sutures of 00 chromic catgut (Plate 49, *G*). A catheter is placed in the bladder and a light vaginal pack inserted.

Postoperative Care

Since the ureter has been catheterized and manipulated during the course of the dissection, urinary antiseptics are administered for five days.

References

Banner, E. A., and Winkelmann, R. K.: Glomus Tumor of the Vagina, Obst. & Gynec. 9: 326, 1957.
Bickel, D., and Bennett, J.: Rare Mesodermal Tumors of the Uterus and Vagina, Am. J. Obst. & Gynec. 67: 1257, 1954.
Birge, E. A., Cron, R. S., and Madden, W.: Paget's Disease of the Vulva, Obst. & Gynec. 12: 425, 1958.
Blakey, D. H.: The Treatment of Bartholin's Cysts by Marsupialization, Am. J. Obst. & Gynec. 65: 800, 1958.
Chiodi, N. E., and others: Granular-Cell Myoblastoma of the Vulva and Lower Urinary Tract, Obst. & Gynec. 9: 472, 1957.
Collins, C. G., and others: Vulvectomy for Benign Vulvar Disease: Indications, Complications, and Mortality in a Special and General Hospital Service, Am. J. Obst. & Gynec. 77: 503, 1959.
Danforth, W.: Sweat Gland Tumors of the Vulva, Am. J. Obst. & Gynec. 58: 326, 1949.
Deacon, A., and Taylor, C.: Hydradenoma of the Vulva, J. Obst. & Gynaec. Brit. Emp. 58: 64, 1952.
De Sousa, L. M., and Lash, A. F.: Hemangiopericytoma of the Vulva, Am. J. Obst. & Gynec. 78: 295, 1959.
Frith, K.: An Unusual Cause of Dyspareunia, J. Obst. & Gynaec. Brit. Emp. 67: 303, 1960.
Hoffman, B., and Grundfest, P.: Vaginitis Emphysematosa; a Case Report, Am. J. Obst. & Gynec. 78: 428, 1959.
Hyman, A. B., and Falk, H. C.: White Lesions of the Vulva: Discussion of Lichenification, Leukoplakia, Bowen's Disease, "Kraurosis Vulvae," Lichen Sclerosis et Atrophicus, and Senile and Essential Atrophies of the Vulva, Obst. & Gynec. 12: 407, 1958.
Kanter, A. E., and Strean, G. J.: Melanoma of the Vulva, Obst. & Gynec. 12: 516, 1958.
Lang, W. R., Israel, S. L., and Fritz, M. A.: Staphylococcal Vulvovaginitis, Obst. & Gynec. 11: 352, 1958.
Mastroianni, L., and Rock, J.: Introital Obstruction to Intromission, Obst. & Gynec. 9: 55, 1957.
Moghissi, K.: Myoma of the Vagina, Obst. & Gynec. 15: 235, 1960.
Norburn, L. M., and Coles, R. B.: Recurrent Erysipelas Following Vulvectomy, J. Obst. & Gynaec. Brit. Emp. 67: 279, 1960.
Oliphant, M. M., and Anderson, G. V.: Management of Bartholin-Duct Cysts and Abscesses, Obst. & Gynec. 16: 476, 1960.
Palmer, E.: Pilonidal Cyst of the Clitoris, Am. J. Surg. 93: 133, 1957.
Patterson, T. J., and Rodes, P.: Treatment of Stenosis of the Vagina by a Thigh Flap, J. Obst. & Gynaec. Brit. Emp. 65: 481, 1958.
Printer, K. D.: A Case of Chronic Hypertrophic Vulvitis, J. Obst. & Gynaec. Brit. Emp. 67: 478, 1960.
Ruch, R.: Dysontogenetic Tumors of the Female Lower Genital Tract, Am. J. Obst. & Gynec. 65: 1263, 1953.
Ruch, R. M., and Clayton, E.: Bartholin Cystectomy: Paraffin Technique, Am. J. Obst. & Gynec. 75: 1055, 1958.
Studdiford, W. E.: Vaginal Lesions of Adenomatous Origin, Am. J. Obst. & Gynec. 73: 641, 1957.
Sullivan, T., Malfetano, J., and Marsh, M.: Granular-Cell Myoblastoma of the Vulva, Am. J. Obst. & Gynec. 67: 687, 1954.
Woodruff, J. D., and Hildebrandt, E. E.: Carcinoma in Situ of the Vulva, Obst. & Gynec. 12: 414, 1958.
Woodruff, J. D., and Williams, T. F.: The Dopa Reaction in Paget's Disease of the Vulva, Obst. & Gynec. 14: 86, 1959.

17 · Operations on the Cervix and Fundus of the Uterus for Benign Disease

TRACHELORRHAPHY AND CERVICAL AMPUTATION
General Considerations

Operations limited to the cervix without consideration of the bladder, rectum, perineum, and pelvic floor are seldom utilized in modern definitive surgery. If the cervical lesion cannot be managed as an office procedure, it would be most rare to find the remainder of the genital tract so well preserved that a complete operation was unnecessary. An exception to this is the amputation of the cervix for intraepithelial cancer in a nullipara desirous of having her childbearing function preserved.

Etiology and Pathologic Anatomy

The cervix is bilaterally lacerated during delivery, and the healing of the lacerations varies with their severity and post-partum care. A severe laceration that is unattended during the patient's post-partum follow-up results in a gaping, everted, chronically infected cervix. Simple erosions of the cervix caused by the downgrowth of glandular epithelium beyond the normal squamocolumnar junction do not require surgery and are left alone unless it is felt that they contribute to an abnormal vaginal discharge. Smears and biopsies are indicated in the older patients or in those in whom the lesion looks suspicious. A plastic operation on the cervix for congenital atresia or stenosis following cautery or a surgical procedure is occasionally indicated. Preservation of the childbearing function in patients with an intraepithelial cancer has been

mentioned as an indication for conservative surgery.

Symptoms and Diagnosis

The symptoms bear no relation to the condition of the cervix. Foul, profuse, irritating discharges are seen in patients after total hysterectomy as well as in those with a chronic cystic cervicitis. A chronically infected cervix could conceivably contribute to low back pain, but a critical appraisal rarely proves the relationship. Diagnosis is made by inspection of the cervix. The surgical anatomy of the cervix and fundus is described together as they apply to this and subsequent operations.

Surgical Anatomy of the Cervix and Fundus of the Uterus

The uterus is a hollow, muscular, pear-shaped organ, flattened from before backward. Normally it is anteverted or directed forward in its relation to the horizontal. It is anteflexed in the relationship of the fundus (body) to the cervix. A retroversion may permit coils of the small intestine to lie between the bladder and the anterior surface of the uterus. This should be remembered when entering the vesicouterine reflection of peritoneum. With an anteverted uterus it is normal for coils of the small bowel to be in the pelvis. The dome-shaped fundus rests between the bladder and rectum and is movable both laterally and anteroposteriorly. Since the fundus of the uterus is mobile, distention of the bladder and rectum will modify its position in normal patients. The cervix may be divided into a supravaginal and infravaginal portion. The isthmus of the uterus is a poorly defined constriction between the fundus and cervix. It marks the level of the internal os.

The uterus, while varying markedly in size due to age, fibroids, or pregnancy, conforms to the following general dimensions in the adult: It is about 7.5 cm. in length, 5.0 cm. in breadth at its upper part, and about 2.5 cm. in thickness. It weighs around 30 to 45 grams. Years of experience in gynecology teach one to palpate the size of the uterus accurately, knowledge of which is so fundamental for clinical judgment. Judgment leads to knowledge, and knowledge leads to wisdom, and in the surgery of this organ, as in no other, do we need wisdom.

The cavity of the uterus is small in comparison to the thickness of its muscular walls. In sagittal section it is a long narrow cleft and averages about 7 cm. in length from the external os to the top of the cavity. The anterior and posterior walls are almost in opposition, and when viewed this way the cavity resembles a triangle with the base at the fundus. The cavity in the body of the uterus communicates with the cervical canal at the internal os. The cervical canal is spindle shaped, is flattened anteroposteriorly, and ends at the external os of the vaginal portion of the cervix.

The wall of the uterus is thickest in the fundus, particularly the posterior wall. It is composed of three coats. The serosa or peritoneal covering is firmly attached except on the posterior aspect near the internal os, where it is reflected onto the cul-de-sac of Douglas. This is important in culdoscopy and instances where one wishes to enter the vagina from the pelvis or the pelvis from the vagina. In performing a hysterectomy the fact that the posterior fornix is deeper than the anterior fornix of the vagina must be appreciated in determining whether the bladder and rectum have been adequately displaced to excise the cervix from the vaginal vault. This is usually done with the thumb and index finger palpating from in front and behind while strong upward traction is made on the uterus. When the anterior and posterior vaginal walls can be approximated by this maneuver distal to the cervix, the operator has reached well down in the vagina. Dense adhesions from pelvic inflammatory disease or endometriosis or the presence of a cervical fibroid may obscure the landmarks in this test.

Combined rectovaginal examination is a most revealing maneuver. Anteriorly the thickness of the perineal body is determined and infiltration, nodularity, or thickening of the rectovaginal septum realized. Higher up, anteriorly, the cervix can be palpated through the septum and its consistency, size, and mobility reaffirmed. Further, the posterior aspect of the cervix and lower part of the fundus are felt through the cul-de-sac. In a retroverted fundus the entire posterior aspect of the uterus may be explored by the examining finger. The condition of the uterosacral thickenings (ligaments) and the cardinal thickenings (ligaments)—after years of training—can be of the utmost prognostic value in both benign and malignant disease. The diagnostic points in palpating these structures will be amplified upon in the discussion of individual diseases. The ischial spine, sacrotuberous and sacrospinous ligaments, the falciform process of the sacrotuberous ligament, the coccyx, and structures on the pelvic side walls all are within reach of the gynecologist's finger. The finger in the rectum can be hooked around the falciform process of the sacrotuberous ligament as it curves upward along the ascending ramus of the pubis like the lacunar (Gimbernat's) ligament does as it inserts into the pubic tubercle.

The reflection of the peritoneum from the uterus to the bladder is mobile to permit filling of the bladder and displacement of the uterus. In any radical operation this plane of cleavage between the uterus and bladder is entered when the bladder is preserved.

The muscular layer (unstriped muscle), together with fibrous and elastic connective tissue bundles, comprises the bulk of the organ. There are really no definite anatomic layers of the muscular wall that may be useful in gynecologic surgery. The study of the musculature, anatomically and physiologically, of the human uterus is presently one of the most fascinating subjects of modern medicine. There is an ill-defined outer layer of longitudinal fibers, an intertwining, thick, circular middle layer, and an innermost thin layer of longitudinal and oblique fibers. Just how these layers play a part in labor or are involved in the lymphatic drainage of endometrial carcinoma, to cite a few problems, will require many studies. The endometrium is 2.0 to 5.0 mm. thick, is firmly attached to the underlying muscularis, and is composed of columnar epithelium and simple, tubular endometrial glands. The nonpregnant uterus is only rarely wounded due to its mobility and small size. The protection afforded by the bony pelvis and the thickness of its muscular walls minimize any injury sustained. The pregnant uterus presents a different problem and is dealt with in Chapter 28 (page 509).

The structure of the cervix is the subject of much research. Either the amount of muscular and fibrous tissue must vary or the methods of histologic study are in error to arrive at such conflicting conclusions. The cervix feels firmer than the uterus—this is the important clinical observation—and diseases of this organ must be interpreted with this in mind. The existence of infiltration, the nodularity, and the presence of retraction to one or the other side are all interpreted in terms of the normal feel of the cervix. The endocervix is lined with a columnar epithelium that forms compound racemose glands. At the external os there is a transition from the columnar epithelium of the endocervix to that of the squamous epithelium of the vagina.

Current thinking on the part played by the round, broad, and cardinal ligaments in the support of the uterus and a description of these ligaments are discussed in Chapter 8, The Statics of the Female Pelvic Viscera.

The blood supply of the uterus is from the uterine and ovarian arteries. The uterine artery arises from the visceral division of the anterior trunk of the hypogastric artery. It passes from the posterolateral wall of the pelvis toward the midline and somewhat forward to enter the base of the broad ligament. Here it arches over the ureter about 2 cm. from the uterus and reaches the cervix just above the lateral fornix of the vagina. It then divides into two branches: the vaginal branch of the uterine artery (a different artery than the vaginal artery which is the homologue of the inferior vesical artery in the male) and the main uterine artery. The uterine artery passes upward in the layers of the broad ligament, giving branches to the anterior and posterior aspects of the uterus, and finally anastomoses with the ovarian artery. The blood vessels of the uterus run transversely as they enter the musculature. Thus ligatures placed in the uterus, such as in the closure of a low transverse cesarean section, do not impair the circulation above the incision. The vaginal artery courses downward on the lateral vaginal wall, giving branches to the vagina. It is important to the gynecologic surgeon as the source of bleeding from the vaginal flaps after either abdominal or vaginal hysterectomy. The uterine artery, while seldom approached as a single entity to be ligated or otherwise dealt with, may be reached by incising the broad ligament between the Fallopian tube and round ligament. It is found in the loose areolar tissue deep in the broad ligament, with the ureter passing underneath. The ovarian arteries arise from the abdominal aorta below the renal arteries. They pass downward and laterally over the ureters and then over the external iliac vessels and enter the infundibulopelvic ligament, which is actually the posterolateral, upper portion of the broad ligament. Running in the broad ligament below the tube, branches are given off to the tube and ovary, and the artery terminates by anastomosing with the uterine artery. Surgically, the point of crossing of the ureter is a landmark in radical surgery and also a common point of kinking or stricture of the ureter, which is bound in a common mass of areolar tissue with the ovarian vessels at the point of crossing. The ligation of the infundibulo-pelvic pedicle includes both artery and vein. It has a tendency to retract so the pedicle should be carefully inspected for hemostasis after ligation. A retroperitoneal hematoma from these vessels can be large and extend around the kidney.

One or more uterine veins accompany the artery. These veins have no valves, so that massive varicosities of these veins are frequently seen, especially in the multipara. The free communication of the veins in the numerous venous plexuses of the pelvis is important clinically in thrombophlebitis and the ligation of major venous trunks. The ovarian veins arise in the hilum of the ovary, forming the pampiniform plexus, which lies between the layers of the broad ligament. There is extensive communication between this plexus and the uterovaginal plexus, which in turn communicates with the vesical and hemorrhoidal plexuses. Two ovarian veins emerge on each side to accompany the ovarian arteries. They fuse into one vein for each side, with the right vein emptying into the inferior vena cava and the left joining the renal vein on that side.

The nerve supply of the uterus is discussed in Chapter 19 (page 359) and the lymphatic drainage in Chapters 24 and 25 (pages 404 and 418).

The cul-de-sac of Douglas, in part separated from the examining finger by only two thicknesses of peritoneum plus some areolar tissue, lends itself admirably to the palpation of the contents of the lower pelvis. Prolapsed ovaries, endometriosis, malignant transplants, thickened and chronically infected tubes, adherent bowel, ascitic fluid, and other conditions present themselves to the trained finger in constant array. When the finger is uncertain, the same area can be opened and visualized or an endoscope introduced and the pelvic organs observed. Here, again, the training of the gynecologist in endoscopy reaps rich rewards.

TRACHELORRHAPHY
Indications and Surgical Principles

Trachelorrhaphy is an ill-advised procedure and would not be described were it not for my conviction that the length of the cervical canal may be important in some uteri, with a limited capacity for expansion, in preventing abortion and premature labor. Until the syndrome of the incompetent internal os is disproved or accredited, this operation could be done as an isolated procedure or combined with a revision of the internal os as described later. The sterility enthusiasts would have a cervicitis preventing subsequent conception by hostility to the sperm cast into the aggressive secretions of the cervix that agglutinate, dissipate, and destroy them. They do not explain how the happy, carefree, loving, grand multipara with a fish-mouth, gaping, chronically infected, prolapsed, and unhealthy cervix presenting at the introitus manages to have offspring after offspring in defiance of the sperm destruction theory. Studies of uterine muscle physiology, and particularly the capacity of the uterus to expand, nourish, and retain a term pregnancy, may modify plastic operations on the cervix so that they have some purpose.

Steps of the Operation

1. The infected tissue of the exocervix is denuded and the epithelium undermined to permit approximation of the flaps (Plate 50, *A*). Meticulous hemostasis is obtained throughout this procedure, since bleeding behind the flaps has been a common cause of disruption of the wound and a cervix—after resuturing and secondary closure —that is traumatized more than it was at parturition.

2. The distal few centimeters of the cervical canal are coned to remove any obviously infected tissue (Plate 50, *B*). This helps the surgeon justify the procedure on more than theoretical grounds.

3. The denuded and coned areas are covered by suturing the mucosal flaps of the exocervix transversely (Plate 50, *C*). The sutures are placed deep to include the fibromuscular tissue of the cervix and to prevent dead space where a hematoma may form and cause dehiscence of the flaps.

PLATE 50

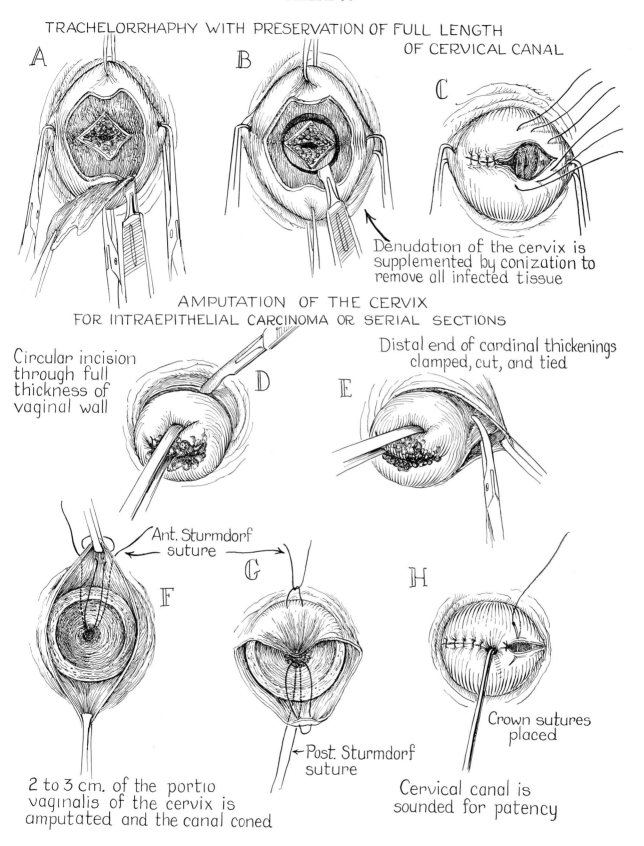

TRACHELORRHAPHY WITH PRESERVATION OF FULL LENGTH OF CERVICAL CANAL

A

B

C

Denudation of the cervix is supplemented by conization to remove all infected tissue

AMPUTATION OF THE CERVIX
FOR INTRAEPITHELIAL CARCINOMA OR SERIAL SECTIONS

Circular incision through full thickness of vaginal wall

D

Distal end of cardinal thickenings clamped, cut, and tied

E

Ant. Sturmdorf suture

F

G

H

Post. Sturmdorf suture

Crown sutures placed

2 to 3 cm. of the portio vaginalis of the cervix is amputated and the canal coned

Cervical canal is sounded for patency

CERVICAL AMPUTATION
Indications and Surgical Principles

A cervical amputation, without repair of the pelvic floor, is indicated for an intraepithelial cancer with preservation of the remainder of the female genital tract. Repeated suspicious smears or biopsies that do not differentiate an invasive from an intraepithelial malignancy may require removal of the major portion of the portio vaginalis of the cervix for serial section. A hypertrophic, infected cervix, requiring amputation, with no other visible damage to the pelvic floor, is an entity few gynecologists would accept. This excludes rare mycotic or venereal infections of the cervix that might require excision.

Steps of the Operation

1. The cervix is grasped with a Jacobs tenaculum and drawn sharply downward, and a circular incision is made through the full thickness of the vaginal wall distal to the bladder reflection (Plate 50, D).

2. The distal end of the cardinal thickenings is clamped, cut, and tied (Plate 50, E) and permitted to retract.

3. The cervix is amputated by an oblique circular incision that cones the canal at the same time. An anterior Sturmdorf suture is placed (Plate 50, F).

4. A posterior Sturmdorf suture is placed, and this and the anterior suture are tied (Plate 50, G). The lateral flaps can be trimmed if they are redundant. Absolute hemostasis in the vascular, fibromuscular tissue of the cervix is obtained by transfixion sutures before closure of the flaps of vaginal wall.

5. Lateral (crown) sutures are placed to approximate the flaps (Plate 50, H). They pass into the fibromuscular structure of the cervix so as to obliterate any dead space behind the flaps. The cervical canal is sounded for patency (Plate 50, H).

Postoperative Care After a Trachelorrhaphy or Amputation

A vaginal pack is seldom necessary after a trachelorrhaphy or amputation since careful hemostasis is required. An indwelling catheter is not needed. The patient is mobilized early but is not discharged from the hospital for at least six days and not until the cervix has been gently inspected and the flaps noted to be healing well. These operations are notorious for postoperative bleeding from the flaps, and the patient should be warned to report any bleeding so an alarming hemorrhage can be interdicted.

VAGINAL MYOMECTOMY
Etiology and Pathologic Anatomy

Two types of cervical myomas may be removed by a vaginal myomectomy. The first type is a submucous myoma that is pedunculated, and with attempts of the uterus to expel the tumor, the pedicle becomes elongated, allowing the myoma to present at the external os. The second type of cervical myoma is a true tumor arising in the substance of the cervix below the point of entrance of the uterine artery. This presents a considerably different surgical problem than the first type and may or may not be best removed by the vaginal route, depending on the size and location of the tumor and whether there are other indications for removing the entire uterus. A true cervical myoma may impact in the pelvis and efface or obliterate the normal features of the cervix. Such a tumor may extend into the broad ligament and be mistaken for a tumor of ovarian origin. A presumptive diagnosis of a solid ovarian tumor is made. The position of the ureters in a true cervical myoma is characteristic. Tumors arise below the level of the uterine artery and almost invariably displace the ureter laterally and anteriorly. With a large tumor the ureter runs over the anterior surface of the growth, as do the uterine artery and vein. Appropriate cystoscopic studies are done prior to surgery, and it is useful to place an indwelling catheter in one or both ureters regardless of whether the tumor is approached from the vaginal aspect or is removed in conjunction with an abdominal hysterectomy.

Symptoms and Diagnosis

Menometrorrhagia that fails of medicinal management, accompanied by a bearing-down pain, suggests the presence of a pedunculated submucous myoma that the uterus is attempting to expel. Frequently the pain is referred posterior to the rectum, as during a spontaneous abortion. The cervix may be patent and readily admit a large dilator. A hysterogram, using anterior, posterior, and oblique films, helps identify the origin of the tumor and the approximate location of its pedicle. Large, true cervical myomas may give rise to the above symptoms plus those resulting from pressure on the bladder, ureters, and rectum.

Indications and Surgical Principles

Cervical myomas are removed whenever the growth is discovered unless it is totally asymptomatic and there are other contraindications to surgery. They become symptomatic by growth, degeneration, bleeding, and infection. In the event a large, pedunculated submucous myoma, polyp, or other tumor cannot be removed through the internal os or if the cervical canal warrants more thorough exploration, an anterior vaginal trachelotomy (hysterotomy) is done. This saves the patient a laparotomy and the surgeon the embarrassment of missing a moderately large pedunculated tumor that contemptuously avoids the curette and ovum forceps. In removing a large cervical myoma, the course of the ureters is identified by the use of ureteral catheters.

PEDUNCULATED CERVICAL MYOMA
Steps of the Operation

1. The anterior lip of the cervix is grasped with a Jacobs tenaculum, and the distortion of the cervical canal by the tumor is studied (Plate 51, A).

2. The canal is sounded and dilated sufficiently to either visualize or palpate the base of the pedicle (Plate 51, B).

3. In Plate 51, C, the width of the pedicle is determined by the examining finger. It is possible to remove tumors with a sessile pedicle through a widely dilated cervix.

4. If the pedicle is thin, a tonsil snare provides an excellent instrument for removal. The snare is placed over the body of the tumor up to the

base of the pedicle (Plate 51, D). The snare crushes the base and controls bleeding. The base is observed to be sure that it has been entirely removed. It may be necessary to expose the base to control bleeding from vessels that have not been occluded by the snare technique.

5. With larger tumors the base of the pedicle is dissected out by sharp dissection (Plate 51, E). The entire base is removed, and bleeding about the base of the pedicle is controlled by suture or cautery. Active bleeding from the base of the pedicle is seldom controlled by use of a pack. Tumors that present at the external os and that the uterus has been attempting to expel frequently have nutrient vessels in the pedicle that have undergone considerable thrombosis, and bleeding is not excessive.

ANTERIOR VAGINAL TRACHELOTOMY
(HYSTEROTOMY)
Indications and Surgical Principles

Some tumors arise by a broad pedicle in the lower uterine segment, even though the body of the tumor presents at the external cervical os. It is inadvisable to remove these tumors blindly, since the entire base may not be excised and there is insufficient exposure to control active arterial bleeding. An anterior vaginal trachelotomy or hysterotomy, if it need be extended higher in the fundus of the uterus, is performed.

Steps of the Operation

1. An incision is made in the midline, extending several centimeters on the anterior vaginal wall from the vesicle reflection (Plate 51, F). The full thickness of the vaginal wall is dissected laterally and anteriorly to expose the base of the bladder. The bladder is pushed well off the cervix and lower uterine segment and retracted out of the field of operation. An incision is made through the anterior wall of the cervix and lower uterine segment into the cervical canal and cavity of the uterus (Plate 51, F). The walls are retracted laterally and the pedicle of the tumor followed to its origin. The tumor is excised and bleeding controlled at its base. Following this, a very careful exploration of the remainder of the uterine cavity is done so that other lesions are not overlooked.

2. The cervix and the lower uterine segment are closed by interrupted sutures of 00 chromic cat-

PLATE 51

PEDUNCULATED CERVICAL MYOMA

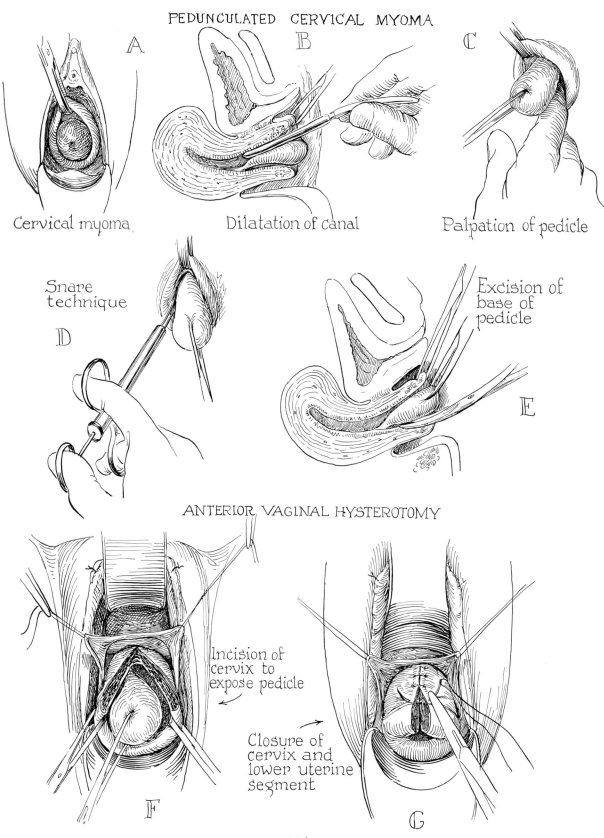

A

Cervical myoma

B

Dilatation of canal

C

Palpation of pedicle

Snare technique

D

Excision of base of pedicle

E

ANTERIOR VAGINAL HYSTEROTOMY

Incision of cervix to expose pedicle

Closure of cervix and lower uterine segment

F

G

gut (Plate 51, *G*). Care is exercised not to stenose the cervical canal. The vaginal wall is closed with interrupted sutures and a pack placed in the vagina.

Postoperative Care

An indwelling catheter is necessary for twenty-four hours until the vaginal pack is removed. The cervix is inspected on the fifth postoperative day and, if it is healing well, the patient may be discharged from the hospital. Urinary antiseptics are prescribed to prevent a urinary tract infection from the displacement and manipulation of the bladder.

VAGINAL MYOMECTOMY (TRUE CERVICAL MYOMA)
Surgical Principles

The method of presentation of a cervical myoma requires modifications of the operation for each patient. Cervical myomas are best removed vaginally unless they are very large or are adherent to vital structures high in the pelvic cavity or to the major vessels on the pelvic side wall. Ureteral catheters are inserted in both ureters, and the distortion of the bladder base and the course of the ureters is noted. Adequate exposure is obtained and a tenaculum used to make traction on the myoma. A sound should be placed in the cervical canal to determine its direction, for it may be greatly distorted or completely effaced by the tumor. The position of the bladder reflection may be abnormal, and a sound passed into the bladder aids the operator in determining that portion of the bladder base that is over the tumor. An incision is made at the bladder reflection and the bladder identified. It is retracted out of the field of operation. Likewise, the points of reflection of the lateral and posterior fornices of the vagina upon the tumor mass are identified and incisions made in these locations. If it is desirable to save the cervix, the point of origin of the tumor from the cervix is determined by following the capsule of the tumor until the cervical canal is reached. Not infrequently the tumor obliterates all semblance of the wall of the cervix on one or the other side, in which event this has to be reconstructed after the tumor is removed. With very large tumors the growth is morcellated to facilitate its removal without injury to adjacent structures. As in any myomectomy, the capsule of the tumor is identified, and by sharp and blunt dissection the structures impinging upon the tumor mass are separated along the line of cleavage of the capsule of the tumor. Following removal, the cervix is reconstructed and the vaginal walls are closed in such a way as to reconstruct the anterior and posterior fornices and the lateral sulci of the vaginal vault. If there is any oozing that cannot be controlled by direct ligation of bleeding points, a pack is left in the vagina and an indwelling catheter placed in the bladder until the pack is removed on the first postoperative day.

TOTAL ABDOMINAL HYSTERECTOMY
Indications

The most common indications for a total abdominal hysterectomy are myomas (fibroids) of the uterus. Of the vast majority of women who have fibroids, only a small fraction ever require a hysterectomy. This percentage depends on the conservative attitude of the surgeon and the position and symptoms caused by the fibroids. The size of the tumors becomes a factor if the uterus exceeds the dimensions of a three months' pregnancy and appears to be growing rapidly. In this event the uterus should be removed, even though the symptoms caused by the tumors are minor. The more common indications for removal of fibroids are as follows: (1) the presence of bleeding that cannot be controlled by medical or expectant treatment—this constitutes the bulk of the indications for surgery; (2) much less frequently, the presence of pain or urinary and rectal symptoms; (3) an intraligamentary tumor which compresses the ureter on one side or the other and requires removal before a hydronephrosis develops. Not infrequently the uterus has to be removed because the rapid growth of the fibroids may suggest that they are undergoing degeneration or hemorrhage. A pedunculated myoma may twist on its pedicle, and some have become parasitic and adherent to bowel or omentum. In some instances the size and number of the fibroids will obscure the pelvic examination, even if done under anesthesia, so that a solid ovarian tumor cannot be excluded without a laparotomy. The use of radium and x-ray in the management of fibroid tumors has been discarded by most pelvic surgeons. The secondary effects of the radium on the base of the bladder, vagina, and vulva may be more serious than the morbidity attendant upon a hysterectomy, even in a "poor-risk" patient. The limitations of x-ray and radium, namely, the presence of large tumors or the presence of submucous tumors that may slough and become infected, contraindicate the use of these agents in many patients. With anesthesia administered by a capable anesthetist, a hysterectomy can be performed with less risk to the patient than she might suffer from radiation sickness and late radiation reactions.

A hysterectomy may be indicated because of endometriosis or adenomyosis that is far advanced in its destructive course. The young patients on whom conservative surgery cannot be done for endometriosis are rare indeed. However, in the older age group or in those patients in whom involvement of the bowel and bladder is seriously impairing the vital functions of the urinary and gastrointestinal tracts, a hysterectomy and bilateral salpingo-oophorectomy may have to be done, despite the desire of the surgeon to preserve the child-bearing and menstrual functions.

Chronic pelvic inflammatory disease formerly was a common indication for hysterectomy. The advent of antimicrobial therapy has reduced the number of patients requiring this operation for pelvic infections. When recurrent pelvic inflammatory disease has compromised the health of a patient and has involved other vital structures in the pelvis, a total hysterectomy is indicated, with conservation of ovarian tissue if she is premenopausal.

There are a group of indications on the basis of chronic uterine bleeding in which the surgeon is unable to demonstrate the presence of submucous myomas, polyps, hyperplasia, or other organic disease. After failure to control the bleeding by hormonal methods and two or more curettages, a hysterectomy is the last resort for dysfunctional uterine bleeding. In the surgery of malignant ovarian tumors, the uterus and cervix are removed at operation. Some of the less common indications for hysterectomy are as follows: Cesarean hysterectomy is indicated if the uterus fails to contract and the patient continues to bleed. A fibroid uterus in an older multigravida may be removed at the time of section. The cesarean section should be indicated for appropriate obstetric reasons. Hysterectomy has sometimes been done as a means of therapeutic abortion when there are other gynecologic indications for removal of the uterus in addition to the termination of the pregnancy. A hysterectomy may have to be done in the treatment of a septic abortion, for a chronic pyometra, or for chronic inversion of the uterus. I do not feel that a simple total hysterectomy is adequate surgery for fundal malignancy, and the type of operation recommended for this condition will be described later.

Twenty-Nine Surgical Principles and Refinements in Technique

1. A high Trendelenberg position is essential to exposure in this operation. As the operator incises the skin, he should direct the anesthetist to lower the patient approximately 10 degrees at a time. When the peritoneum is incised, the patient is in the desired position for the pelvic surgery.

2. The size of the tumor has little to do with the technical difficulties of the operation. Large, uncomplicated fibroids are easily elevated out of the pelvis and seldom complicate the performance of a hysterectomy.

3. In the choice of incisions, a Pfannenstiel type is adequate for simple operations. If the upper abdomen must be explored or other difficulties are anticipated with the bowel, a midline or rectus incision that can be extended is preferable.

4. The incision should be adequate since some fibroid uteri will just fill a small incision, making it difficult for the operator to work in and about the tumor.

5. When a vaginal plastic procedure is done prior to an abdominal hysterectomy, which is indicated on some occasions, a retrograde dissection of the rectocele and cystocele from the introitus toward the cervix should be done. This minimizes the operative trauma and edema about the vaginal vault that is approached later from the abdominal aspect.

6. Endometriosis and pelvic inflammatory disease make a hysterectomy difficult, and it is for these dissections that ureteral catheters are inserted and not necessarily for large, freely movable tumors.

7. The practice of freeing and scooping up the adnexa to begin a hysterectomy in patients with old inflammatory disease or endometriosis is to be condemned not only because of its crudeness, but also because of the risk to the ureters. The operation can and should proceed without complete mobilization of the uterus and adnexa. This need not be done blindly and dangerously. When the stage of the operation is reached where mobilization of the uterus and adnexa is necessary, namely, the clamping of the uterine arteries and the resection of the base of the broad ligaments, meticulous dissection will accomplish the mobilization without injury to ureters, bladder, and rectum.

8. The direction of traction on the uterus for exposure is an art. Alternately the surgeon should make traction himself—as it aids him in the dissection—or pass the uterus and instruments for traction to his assistant, indicating the direction and force to apply on the uterus.

9. Not only traction but also rotation of the uterus facilitates a hysterectomy. For instance, rotation to the right and posteriorly, with traction toward the left sacroiliac joint, makes the right round ligament and anterior sheath of the broad ligament prominent. Rotation to the left and anteriorly makes the right ovarian artery and vein, the tube, and ovarian ligament more accessible. While traction and rotation of the uterus is a useful technique, the surgeon should remember that both of these maneuvers occlude vessels that may bleed actively after release of the traction and rotation.

10. Pelvic surgeons—for speed, efficiency, and teaching—develop a routine technique to perform this operation. One should not be so rigid in following the routine that the operation cannot be modified for special situations.

11. Pedicles are clamped, cut, and tied as they are encountered. The field of operation is not clut-

tered with clamps should the operator have unexpected difficulty.

12. Without distortion from disease, the vesicouterine reflection of the peritoneum is at or near the internal os. Just distal to this the peritoneum is incised to reflect the bladder from the cervix. Underneath the peritoneum, at this level, is a thin areolar layer of the vesicovaginal septum. Posteriorly it attaches firmly to the uterus (perimetrium), and anteriorly it becomes adherent to the bladder wall. These anatomic facts are appreciated so that the natural plane of cleavage is not entered in displacing the bladder.

13. The veins of the broad ligament may be large, varicose, and pampiniform in arrangement. These facts should be appreciated in the removal of intraligamentary fibroids or cysts. They can cause alarming bleeding.

14. The finger-spreading technique to displace the ureters, illustrated later, can be done gently and will not rupture varicose veins in the broad ligament.

15. Direct catheterization of the ureter at the pelvic brim is a useful technique and is employed during a hysterectomy when ligation, perforation, or kinking of the pelvic ureters is suspected (see Section IX, Gynecologic and Obstetric Injuries and Emergencies, page 357). This is the time to recognize and deal with this complication. With the catheter as a guide, the condition can be corrected with relative ease compared with the extensive urologic studies and subsequent surgery necessary if an injured ureter is overlooked at the primary operation. One may rarely elect to catheterize the ureters from the pelvic brim before proceeding with the dissection of the base of the broad ligament or excision of the cervix when the technical difficulties were not anticipated preoperatively.

16. The position of the uterus, as determined on bimanual examination, gives useful information to the operator as to where he may anticipate adhesions of the small bowel in dealing with pelvic inflammatory disease or endometriosis. Retroversion permits coils of the small bowel to become adherent between the bladder and anterior surface of the uterus. With an anteverted uterus the adhesions of the small bowel are more likely to be on the posterior surface of the uterus and in the cul-de-sac.

17. When multiple bleeding points about the angle of the vault resist several attempts at hemostasis by suture ligature, the uterine artery should be

ligated at its origin from the hypogastric artery as is done in a radical hysterectomy. This reduces the brisk bleeding, and other vessels can be controlled with less risk to the ureter.

18. Intraligamentary fibroids almost invariably displace the ureter laterally and anteriorly. If these tumors are dissected from the uterus toward the lateral pelvic wall, staying close to the capsule of the tumor, the risk to the ureter is minimized.

19. A recalcitrant branch of the uterine artery in the vesicovaginal septum that bleeds despite repeated ligation invites the operator to place sutures that may compromise the ureter or penetrate the full thickness of the bladder wall, with the possibility of a ureterovaginal or a vesicovaginal fistula. The operator should dissect the bladder from the vagina at the angle of the vault as he does for a radical hysterectomy. With the structures clearly seen, bleeding can be controlled without danger.

20. A finger placed behind the base of the cardinal thickening to push the tissues anteriorly facilitates the identification of the uterine artery.

21. The veins of the bladder base that drain into the space of Retzius and plexus of Santorini are larger laterally than in the midline of the bladder base. Likewise, the vesical veins drain laterally, making the edge of the bladder a frequent site of bleeding. In addition, the vaginal plexus with its abundant anastomoses, both in the vagina and to the superior middle and inferior hemorrhoidal vessels, drains the vagina from the lateral aspect. This causes more venous bleeding on the lateral edges than in the midline of the vagina.

22. A large uterus with multiple fibroids in the lower segment may be first myomectomized and a subsequent hysterectomy done. Frequently it becomes necessary to do a subtotal hysterectomy first and subsequently remove the stump.

23. To perform a total abdominal hysterectomy of a uterus with a large cervical fibroid, enter the vagina anteriorly and identify the landmarks distorted by the mass. Under direct vision the distortion of the vaginal vault is less of a technical problem, and the vagina is dissected from the tumor after proper orientation.

24. A side-to-side amputation of the uterine fundus, performing a subtotal hysterectomy first, is a useful device when there is a large, adherent intraligamentary fibroid that extends to the side wall of the pelvis. The course of the uterine artery may be distorted by this mass. Start on the free side and amputate the fundus of the uterus across the

midline, and identify the uterine artery on the tumor side by this approach. Remove the cervical stump after the fundus.

25. The identification of the rectovaginal septum and uterosacral ligaments can be difficult or impossible when the cul-de-sac is obliterated by endometriosis, or pelvic inflammatory disease, or cancer. Enter the vagina anteriorly and, as the cervix is amputated from the vaginal vault, draw it posteriorly and perform the dissection of the uterosacral ligaments from the vaginal aspect. This permits identification of anatomic landmarks and completion of the dissection with less risk of rectal injury. I prefer to enter the vagina from the anterior aspect as a routine approach. To do this, the bladder is displaced well off the upper vagina, automatically removing the ureters from the field of operation.

26. A total abdominal hysterectomy may be indicated in a patient with pelvic floor relaxation. The urgency of the hysterectomy and the patient's condition may not permit a prolonged procedure with repair of the bladder and rectal hernias from below. Some support can be gained by resecting a wedge of peritoneum in the cul-de-sac and uniting the uterosacral thickenings in the midline. A wedge of the posterior vaginal vault is also removed. This extends the support of the pelvic floor posteriorly, where it is needed, and may prevent prolapse or retain the pelvic contents adequately. Subsequent surgery is avoided.

27. The attachment of the round ligaments to the cervical stump after a subtotal hysterectomy—aside from the performance of this ill-advised and incomplete procedure—draws the cervical stump toward the symphysis and directs the intrapelvic pressure into the cul-de-sac. Should the operator have been forced to perform a hysterectomy without regard for the support of the pelvic floor, this maneuver aids the development of a cul-de-sac hernia. This same erroneous technique has been done in the performance of a total hysterectomy, which only compounds the felony. The surgeon might have strengthened the pelvic floor by a midline union of the uterosacral condensations of the visceral connective tissue.

28. Before entering the vagina, the operator palpates the portio vaginalis of the cervix to determine whether the rectum and bladder have been sufficiently displaced. This is best done with the thumb and index finger palpating the cervix through the vaginal wall. When a cervical fibroid obviates this maneuver, the technique of entering the vagina anteriorly and resecting the specimen under direct vision is advised.

29. Patients with mild stress incontinence are helped by an anterior plication of the bladder neck and a suprapubic urethral suspension. This is done during closure of the abdominal incision. It corrects the condition in mild cases (see Stress Incontinence, page 184).

Steps of the Operation

1. The bladder is emptied by catheterization, and a preliminary dilatation and curettage are performed. If no grossly suspicious tissue or other unexpected findings occur, the patient is positioned for laparotomy.

2. Most gynecologists prefer to operate from the patient's left side when performing a simple hysterectomy. The description of this operation and the illustrations sketched by the artist at the operating table were done from the patient's left side. Some surgeons prefer to operate in the pelvis from the patient's right side, even though they are right-handed.

3. The choice of laparotomy incisions is individualized. A liberal left rectus incision in the case of an obese patient with a deep, funnel pelvis gives excellent exposure. A midline incision often suffices but may sometimes have to be extended to one side of the umbilicus when the distance from the latter to the symphysis is short. In most instances a low transverse (Pfannenstiel) incision is adequate but should be large enough to permit thorough exploration of the upper abdominal organs. Often it is desirable to remove an unsightly scar from previous surgery or to correct a hernia or fascial defect in such a scar. In any event, provide yourself with adequate room lest a simple operation be made an ordeal. If your operating table will tilt, rotate it to your side.

4. In the course of entering the abdomen, have the anesthetist lower the head of the table 10 degrees at a time, so that when the peritoneum is reached, the patient will be in a 45-degree or more Trendelenberg position.

5. Advise the anesthetist that you are going to enter the peritoneal cavity and explore the abdomen. A preliminary appraisal of the pelvic findings is made after dampening the glove of the exploring hand. The cecum, appendix, and ascending colon are palpated to the hepatic flexure of the colon. The liver and gall bladder are explored, and the latter is emptied by gentle pressure. The index finger is inserted into the foramen of Winslow, and the common duct and the pyloric region of the stomach are palpated. The right kidney, stomach, and transverse colon are felt. In the left upper abdomen the spleen and left kidney are palpated, and then the exploration continues along the descending colon, sigmoid, and into the pelvis. The root of the mesentery is palpated, and if injury to the small bowel, obstruction, or other lesion is suspected, the small bowel should be run from the ligament of Treitz to the ileocecal valve, or vice versa. The bowel is adequately packed off out of the field.

6. The pelvic pathology is more thoroughly evaluated and the plan for hysterectomy decided. One should have a routine of doing this operation to gain speed. It should be capable of easy modification as necessary.

7. One school of thought advocates that the pelvic organs be completely mobilized prior to the actual hysterectomy. This frequently leaves large denuded areas to bleed and be exposed for some time before they come into the immediate field of operation. I believe the field of operation immediately in advance of the various operative steps should be mobilized. This makes the landmarks clearer as the operation proceeds and avoids the temptation to scoop the uterus and adnexa up out of the pelvis and forcibly detach them from adhesions and other structures to which they may be firmly adherent.

8. The ensuing series of illustrations show the performance of this operation for a simple fibroid uterus. The round ligament is grasped with an Allis clamp midway between the uterus and the internal inguinal ring (Plate 52, A). A Kelly hemostat is seated about 2 cm. distant on the uterine side (Plate 52, A, right side). A suture ligature of medium silk is placed on the round ligament between the clamps and the Allis clamp removed. The round ligament is now cut and the anterior sheath of the broad ligament incised with Metzenbaum scissors (illustrated in Plate 52, A, left side, although the right side would have been done). In the absence of active pelvic inflammatory disease, I prefer the use of medium silk for suture ligatures on pedicles and fine silk for ties for other bleeding points encountered in the course of the operation up to and including the ligation of the uterine arteries. Absorbable material is used about the vaginal vault. Surgeons who prefer catgut may elect to use 0 chromic in place of medium silk and 00 chromic in place of fine silk.

9. The assistant makes gentle traction on the round ligament by means of the tagged suture ligature, and the operator makes traction on the uterus to the opposite side (Plate 52, B). The

Text continued on p. 337.

PLATE 52

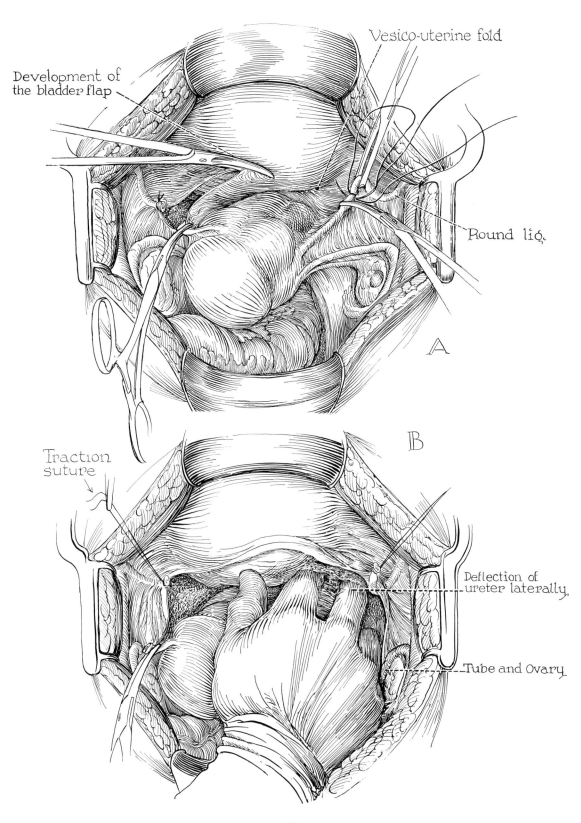

Development of
the bladder flap

Vesico-uterine fold

Round lig.

A

B

Traction
suture

Deflection of
ureter laterally

Tube and Ovary

PLATE 52 (Continued)

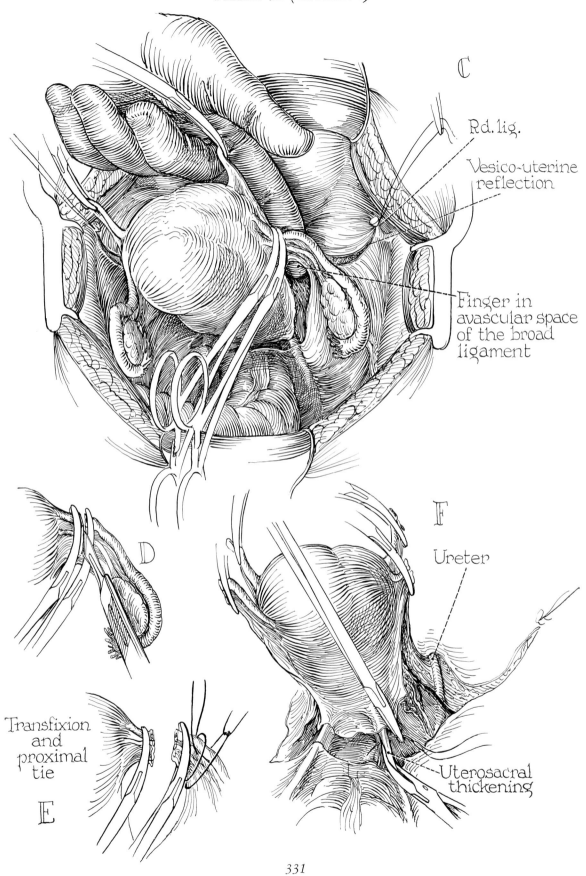

C

Rd. lig.

Vesico-uterine reflection

Finger in avascular space of the broad ligament

D

F

Ureter

Transfixion and proximal tie

E

Uterosacral thickening

PLATE 52 (Continued)

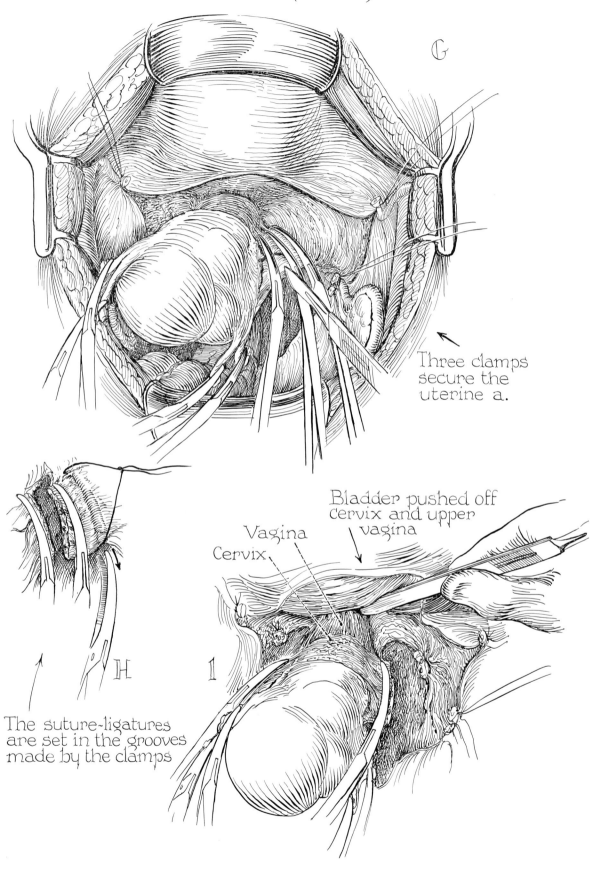

G

Three clamps
secure the
uterine a.

The suture-ligatures
are set in the grooves
made by the clamps

H

1

Bladder pushed off
cervix and upper
vagina

Vagina

Cervix

PLATE 52 (Continued)

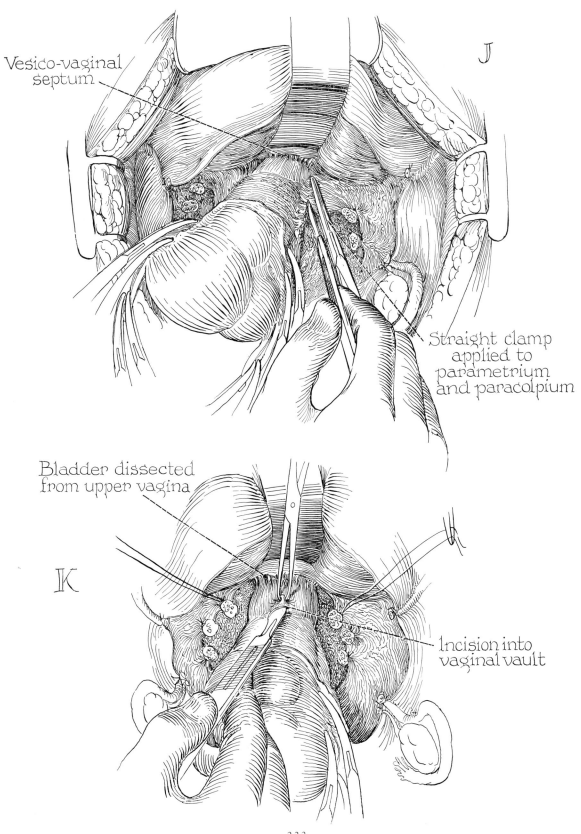

Vesico-vaginal
septum

J

Straight clamp
applied to
parametrium
and paracolpium

Bladder dissected
from upper vagina

K

Incision into
vaginal vault

PLATE 52 (Continued)

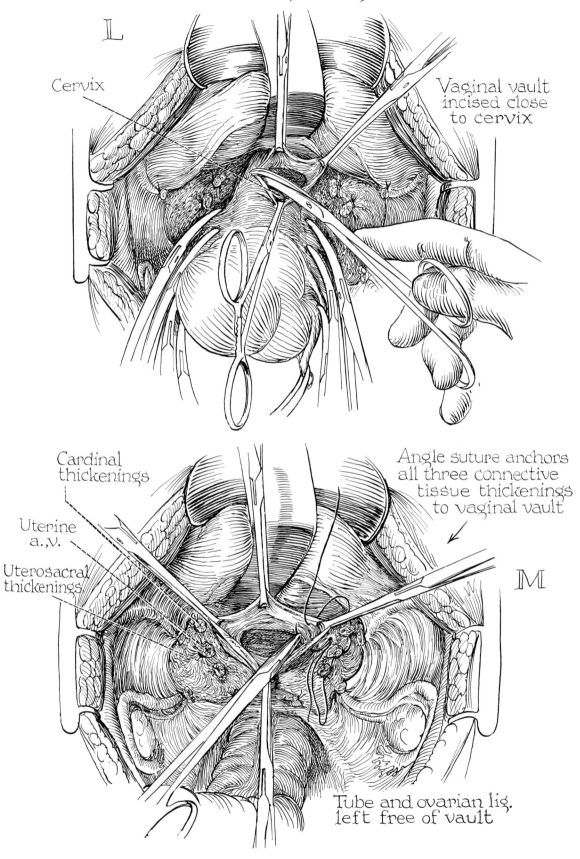

L

Cervix

Vaginal vault
incised close
to cervix

Cardinal
thickenings

Uterine
a.,v.

Uterosacral
thickenings

Angle suture anchors
all three connective
tissue thickenings
to vaginal vault

M

Tube and ovarian lig.
left free of vault

PLATE 52 (Continued)

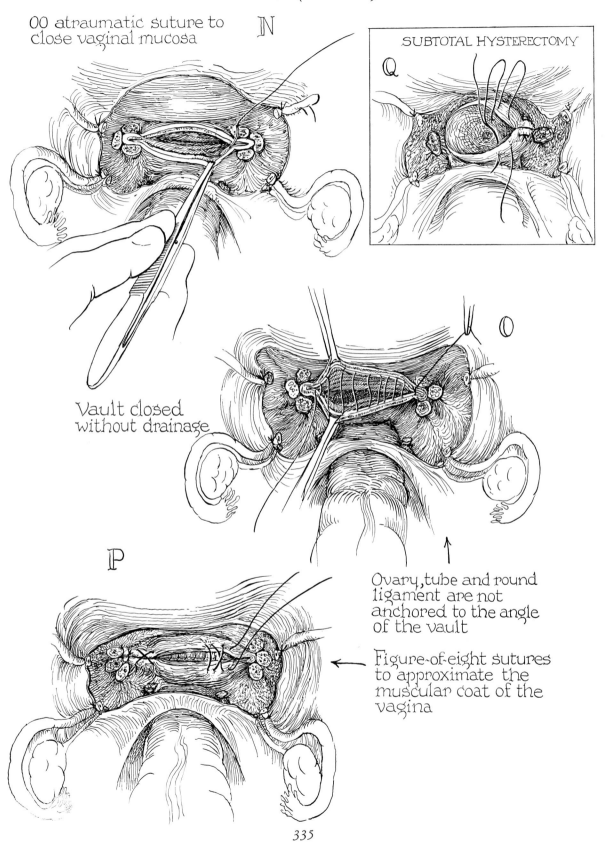

OO atraumatic suture to close vaginal mucosa

N

SUBTOTAL HYSTERECTOMY

Q

Vault closed without drainage

O

P

Ovary, tube and round ligament are not anchored to the angle of the vault

Figure-of-eight sutures to approximate the muscular coat of the vagina

335

PLATE 52 (Concluded)

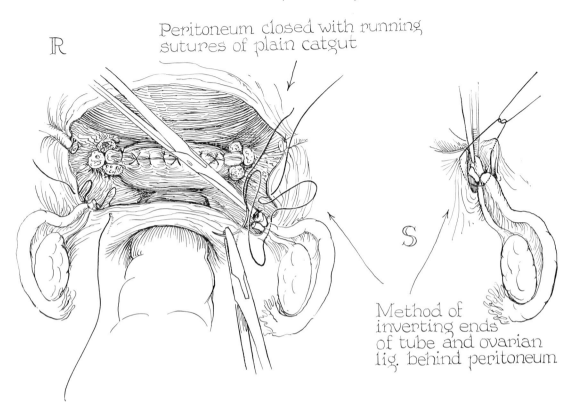

R

Peritoneum closed with running sutures of plain catgut

S

Method of inverting ends of tube and ovarian lig. behind peritoneum

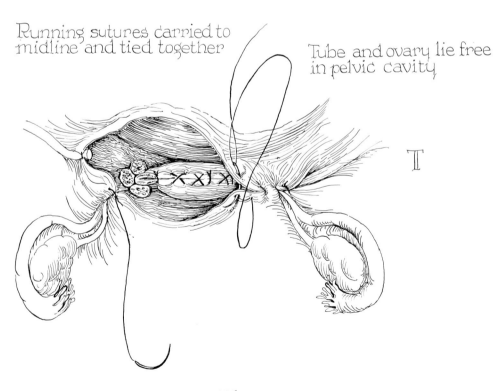

Running sutures carried to midline and tied together

Tube and ovary lie free in pelvic cavity

T

index and middle fingers are then inserted anteriorly under the sheath of the broad ligament. With a scissors motion of the index and middle fingers, the sheath is spread open. The uterine vessels may now be seen, while at the same time this maneuver tends to displace the ureter laterally (Plate 52, B). The same technique is used on the other side. Small vessels are occasionally ruptured. If bleeding is slight, a tagged sponge can be left behind the flap until the surgeon returns to this site later. Definite bleeding points are clamped and tied.

10. The index finger is then inserted under the anterior sheath, through the avascular area of the broad ligament, and through the posterior sheath (Plate 52, C). This area is above the uterine vessels and lateral to the ascending branches of the latter. Rather than forcing a finger through, it is better technique to cut through the posterior sheath by incising it while stretched over the operator's index finger. When the tubes and ovaries are preserved, Kelly clamps are placed on the tube and ovarian ligament. A curved Kocher clamp can be substituted for the Kelly clamp nearest the uterus and the uterine stump of the round ligament included so as to eliminate the clamp on this structure. The tube and ovarian ligament are cut and a suture ligature placed as shown in Plate 52, D and E. The clamp should be flashed as the suture is seated and tied. A free tie is placed proximal to this to avoid a hematoma in the pedicle. This may happen from perforation of a vessel by the fixation ligature. An identical step is performed on the opposite side.

11. The uterus is now pulled strongly forward and the posterior sheath of the broad ligament incised at about the level of the internal os. This has the effect of further skeletonizing the uterine vessels and exposing the uterosacral thickenings. These are clamped with curved Kocher clamps, cut, and ligated with a suture ligature of medium silk. Insert a finger between the rectum and cervix and push the rectum off if it is adherent. Usually the posterior fornix of the vagina can be readily palpated by a finger inserted behind the cul-de-sac peritoneum. Plate 52, F, shows this stage of the operation and the relationship of some of the structures. The ureters lie a few centimeters lateral to the uterosacral thickenings, so direct the point of your needle to the midline as further assurance against damage. If in doubt, isolate the ureter and draw it laterally out of the way with a vein retractor.

12. The uterine artery and veins are now triply clamped with curved Kocher clamps (Plate 52, G). The vessels are divided, leaving two clamps on the proximal pedicle. These are doubly ligated with suture ligatures set in the grooves made by the clamps as shown in Plate 52, H. The uterine vessels are similarly treated on the left side. If you are using medium silk, these are the last pedicles ligated with this material, and subsequent ligatures will be of 0 chromic catgut since they are near the vaginal vault.

13. The bladder is now pushed off the cervix and upper vagina by the method shown in Plate 52, I. Gentle strokes of the knife locate the thin areolar layer between the cervix and vagina on the one hand and the bladder on the other. This procedure is alternated with pushing the bladder down and laterally with the knife handle. Some operators prefer to perform this dissection by pushing the bladder free of the cervix by means of a folded sponge grasped by a Kelly clamp or ovum forceps. This creates more bleeding than does sharp dissection.

14. Make strong traction on the uterus a little to the opposite side of the midline from the side on which you are working. An Ochsner clamp is used to clamp the cardinal ligament and a portion of the paracolpium (Plate 52, J). The cardinal ligament is cut close to the cervix and the paracolpium close to the lateral vaginal fornix and the pedicle is carefully ligated since it contains the descending or vaginal branch of the uterine artery. The same maneuver is done on the left side as described for the right.

15. A Deaver retractor is placed anteriorly and the bladder strongly retracted. The upper vagina and cervix can then be palpated. An Allis clamp is placed on the vagina just beyond the cervix and the vagina incised between the clamp and cervix (Plate 52, K). The full thickness of the vaginal wall is then grasped with the Allis clamp or with an Ochsner clamp.

16. An Ochsner or Allis clamp is placed on the anterior lip of the cervix or just behind it to maneuver the cervix during this dissection (Plate 52, L). The completion of the amputation of the cervix from the vagina is done with a Metzenbaum scissors.

17. The uterus has been removed and is being opened by the pathologist or other person available. Unexpected findings may change the course of your operation, but, assuming a benign lesion, preparations are made for closure of the vaginal vault. Active bleeders are clamped and tied and clamps placed at both angles of the vault (Plate 52, M).

18. The angle suture illustrated in Plate 52, *M,* attaches the vessels and their connective tissue thickenings to the angle of the vault. Starting from the vaginal aspect of the angle of the new vault, the suture passes through the vagina, into the cardinal ligament distal to its hemostatic ligature, into the bundle containing the uterine artery and again distal to its hemostatic ligature, is anchored to the uterosacral pedicle, and then passes back into the vagina at the posterolateral angle of the vault. It is thus tied on the vaginal aspect.

19. A running suture of 00 chromic catgut is now used to approximate vaginal mucosa to vaginal mucosa (Plate 52, *N*). The use of drains or suturing around the vaginal wall for hemostasis and leaving part of it open into the vagina has no part in an uncomplicated hysterectomy. Such measures may be indicated under unexpected circumstances, such as uncontrollable bleeding of systemic etiology, pelvic abscesses, bladder or ureteral injuries, or rectal complications. These special situations will be discussed separately. In Plate 52, *N,* the closure of the vault has begun. Ideally, the suture closing the vaginal vault should run in the submucosa of the vagina (Plate 52, *O*). If a fine, atraumatic, continuous suture is used, this is frequently possible and provides the best opportunity for primary healing without granulation tissue.

20. The number of sutures placed in the muscularis of the vagina will vary according to the amount of relaxation and the dimensions of the vaginal vault. Sufficient sutures are placed to form a firm and muscular vault in appreciation of its function as a supporting structure in the mechanics of the pelvis considered as a whole. Attachment of the round ligaments to the vaginal vault contributes nothing to its support. If the proximal ends of the round ligaments are sutured to the vaginal vault, they form an artificial bridge of tissue under the bladder base and may cause persistent urinary tenesmus in some patients. Likewise, the attachment of the ovaries to the angles of the new vault may only give rise to dyspareunia in the sexually active patient and stretch and compromise the vascular pedicle supplying these structures. The figure-of-eight sutures placed in the vaginal muscularis make the vault of the vagina firm and help this structure to resist subsequent prolapse (Plate 52, *P*).

21. The field of operation is inspected for hemostasis before the peritoneum is closed over the bladder, vaginal vault, and rectum. The ovarian pedicle is inverted behind the peritoneum by the method shown in Plate 52, *R* and *S.* An Allis clamp grasps the pedicle and pushes it behind the peritoneum. The suture is continued to the midline, and an identical running suture is placed from the left side (Plate 52, *T*). They are tied in the midline after the completion of the peritonealization. The sigmoid should be placed in the pelvis, a better place for it than the small bowel. The omentum is drawn down over the bowel after removal of the laparotomy pads and prior to closure of the abdominal incision.

Postoperative Care

The patient is mobilized early, and fluids and nourishment are started as soon as tolerated. Parenteral fluids may be required for the first postoperative day or longer if the operation was complicated. Sulfonamides or antibiotics are not routinely given but are reserved for specific indications.

SUBTOTAL (SUPRACERVICAL) HYSTERECTOMY

Subtotal hysterectomy is seldom indicated in modern gynecology. Most pelvic surgeons would have to stop and think about the technique of the procedure, which might take longer than removing the cervix. It might be done in emergencies to terminate a procedure for shock or cardiac arrest. In hopeless abdominal carcinomatosis the operation could be done in conjunction with the removal of the primary tumor in the ovary. One might find a benign condition in which the cervix would be left behind, such as endometriosis, where it was technically impossible to remove the entire uterus. After the uterine arteries are tied, the corpus is amputated and the stump closed with interrupted sutures. The pelvis is reperitonealized as in the total operation. Plate 52, *Q,* shows the operation.

ABDOMINAL MYOMECTOMY
Indications

A myomectomy is indicated for a variety of reasons concerned with the conservation of the uterus. In young patients the menstrual and childbearing functions are preserved. The tumors may be removed for infertility or habitual abortion. Frequently, a myomectomy is performed in the course of other pelvic surgery as a prophylactic measure. Subserous myomas can be removed at the time of cesarean section.

Surgical Principles

Bonney advocated the development of a peritoneal flap at the vesicouterine reflection and the removal of practically all the tumors through an incision later to be covered by this peritoneum. This is ideal in many situations, but each procedure has to be individualized. Excision of tumors of the posterior wall by transversing the endometrial cavity is logical provided that the intramural portion of the tube is identified and protected from accidental ligation or destruction.

The use of clamps or tourniquets on the uterine vessels for hemostasis violates several surgical principles in the handling of the tissue of an organ that the surgeon is trying to restore to a normal anatomic and functional state. The ovarian arteries continue to keep up the pressure in the uterine vessels above the clamp or tourniquet, defeating, to some extent, the whole idea. Further, it seems unreasonable to traumatize vessels that are subsequently going to be needed to revascularize the suture lines and the reconstructed uterus. Finally, the presence of hematomas or seromas between the opposing surfaces of any incision is the most common cause of nonunion, and it is no different in the uterus. Yet, mechanical hemostasis may mask bleeding points in the field. The use of Pitocin does not have these objections, since it reduces bleeding during the initial dissection and its effects are worn off by the time of closure, when all bleeding points can be surgically controlled. The use of synthetic Pitressin for this purpose is under study.

Steps of the Operation

This operation is not done without a preliminary dilatation and curettage, for a simple endometrial polyp or other benign lesion may be responsible for the patient's symptoms.

1. The case selected to illustrate the technique of a myomectomy is that of a left intraligamentary fibroid that had distorted the bladder, had displaced the ureter in its bed, had altered the course of the round ligament and tube, and had pushed the uterus to the right side of the pelvis (Plate 53, A). A myomectomy requires appreciation of the basic techniques of plastic surgery, and the position and contour of the tumors are studied before incising the uterus. The incisions used to remove one or more tumors are conceived at laparotomy, and a decision is made as to how to do the operation with the best possible cosmetic result.

2. A No. 6 ureteral catheter has been inserted in the left ureter. After exposing the uterus, 4 minims of Pitocin are injected into the fundus to contract the musculature.

3. In Plate 53, A, the round ligament has been doubly clamped. A bullet tenaculum grasps the fibroid tumor. The broad ligament must be opened widely to determine the exact course of the ureter and to free the bladder, which may extend over the tumor. To do this the round ligament is clamped, cut, and tied. The dissection continues anteriorly to free the bladder, which may be riding up over this tumor. An incision is made to remove the excess perimetrium over the tumor (Plate 53, B).

4. By alternately using the finger, knife, and knife handle, the tumor is shelled from its bed with minimal disturbance of the uterine musculature (Plate 53, C). The dissection is done within the capsule of the myoma, particularly near the tube, so as not to disturb the continuity of the latter (Plate 53, C). Often several myomas can be removed through the same incision. The number of variations in this operation is limitless, and the surgeon can pride himself on his selection of incisions that allow the removal of many tumors while at the same time allowing a functional uterus to be reconstructed. Often a twisting motion of the tenaculum will tend to delineate the capsule of the fibroid.

5. Plate 53, D, shows the intraligamentary fibroid almost removed from its bed. The dissection has now exposed the ureter and uterine artery and its accompanying veins. With the ureter catheterized, its course is easily followed, and it can be displaced laterally as the tumor is enucleated from its bed.

6. Interrupted sutures of 00 chromic catgut are now used to reconstruct the uterus. Many tumors may be removed and several incisions used. The objective of all this is to have a functional organ,

PLATE 53

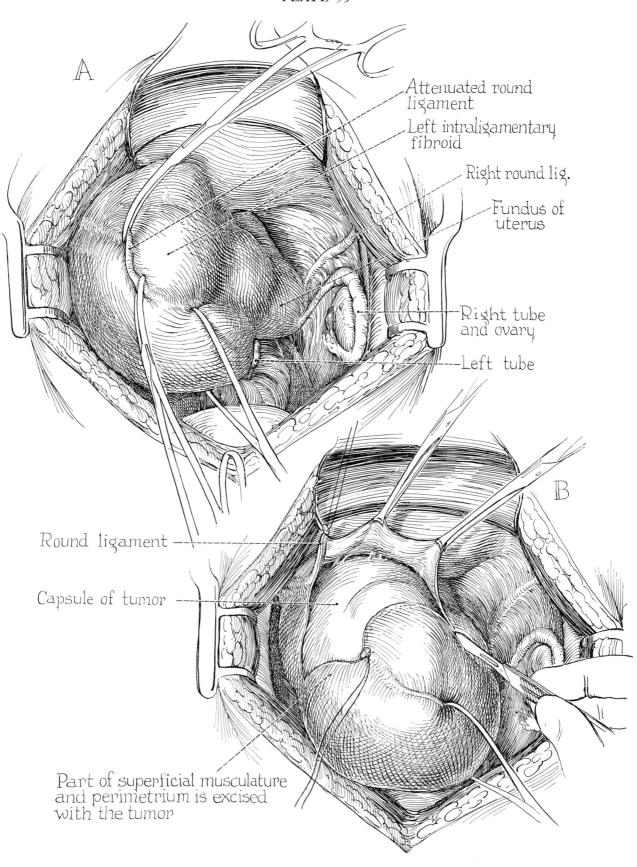

A

Attenuated round ligament

Left intraligamentary fibroid

Right round lig.

Fundus of uterus

Right tube and ovary

Left tube

B

Round ligament

Capsule of tumor

Part of superficial musculature and perimetrium is excised with the tumor

PLATE 53 (*Continued*)

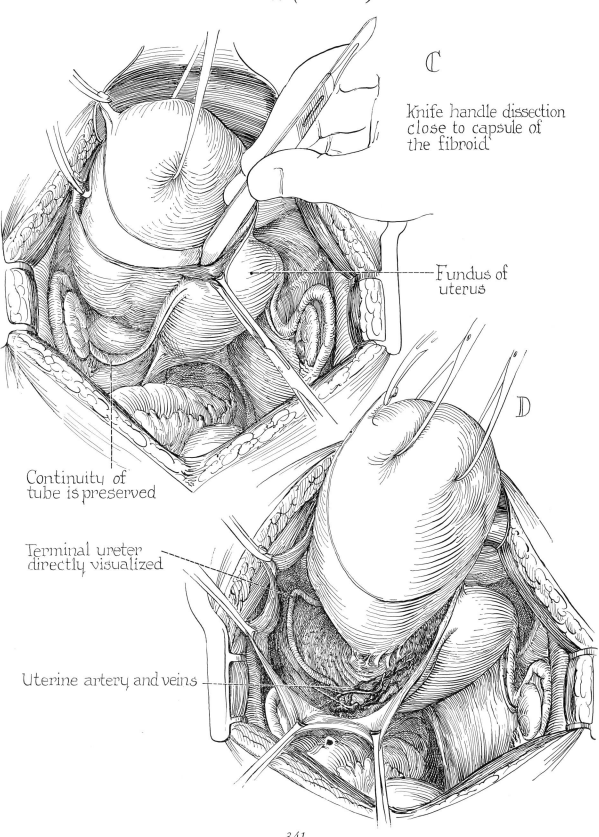

C

Knife handle dissection
close to capsule of
the fibroid

Fundus of
uterus

D

Continuity of
tube is preserved

Terminal ureter
directly visualized

Uterine artery and veins

PLATE 53 (Concluded)

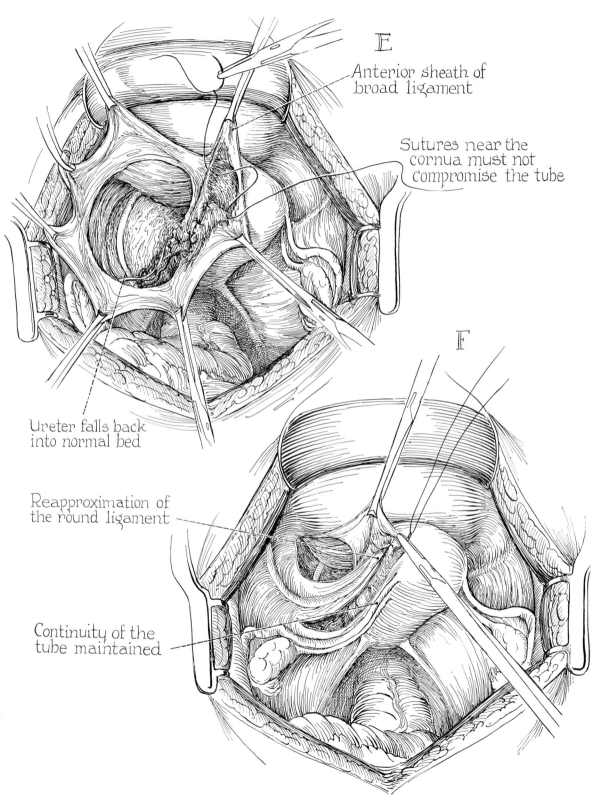

E

Anterior sheath of
broad ligament

Sutures near the
cornua must not
compromise the tube

Ureter falls back
into normal bed

F

Reapproximation of
the round ligament

Continuity of the
tube maintained

342

and to this end the fewer sutures used, the less will be the scarring. As shown in Plate 53, *E,* interrupted sutures are placed to approximate but not strangulate the uterine musculature. They should be tied without cutting into the tissue. If there is any doubt concerning the condition of the interior of the uterus, a retrograde exploration of the uterus is done. With adequate antibiotic therapy this adds no morbidity to the procedure.

7. The round ligament is reapproximated by several interrupted sutures. The ureter is allowed to fall back into its normal bed, and the anterior sheath of the broad ligament is closed. The perimetrium is closed over the operative site, with care being exercised not to constrict or angulate the Fallopian tube (Plate 53, *F*).

Postoperative Care

The postoperative care previously described under Total Abdominal Hysterectomy (page 338) is applicable here.

References

Abell, M. R.: Cervicocolpitis (Vaginitis) Emphysematosa, Surg., Gynec. & Obst. 107: 631, 1958.

Black, E. F. E., and McFarlane, C. J.: Torsion of the Uterus Causing Infarction of a Fibromyoma, Am. J. Obst. & Gynec. 77: 513, 1959.

Bonney, V.: The Technic and Results of Myomectomy, Lancet 220: 171, 1931.

Branscomb, L.: Habitual Premenstrual Spotting Following Electrocauterization of the Cervix: A Newly Observed Phenomenon, Am. J. Obst. & Gynec. 79: 16, 1960.

Buerger, P., and Petzing, H.: Congenital Cysts of the Corpus Uteri, Am. J. Obst. & Gynec. 67: 143, 1954.

Cody, M. J., and Wall, H. A.: Submuous Uterine Myoma Causing Postpartum Complications, Obst. & Gynec. 7: 304, 1956.

Corey, E. L., McGaughey, H. S., and Thornton, W. N.: Electromyography of the Human Uterus, Am. J. Obst. & Gynec. 74: 473, 1957.

Demetrakopoulos, N. J., and Greene, R. R.: Lymph Follicles in the Cervix Uteri, Surg., Gynec. & Obst. 106: 729, 1958.

Dill, L. V., and Jeffrey, J. E.: Wedge Resection of the Uterine Fundus in the Therapy of Intractable Menorrhagia, Am. J. Obst. & Gynec. 80: 472, 1960.

Dunn, R.: The Pathological Normal Uterus, Tr. Pacific Coast Obst. & Gynec. Soc. 27: 13, 1959.

Everett, H., and Sturgis, W.: The Effect of Some Common Gynecological Disorders Upon the Urinary Tract, Urol. & Cutan. Rev. 44: 638, 1940.

Farrar, H. K., and Nedoss, B. R.: Benign Tumors of the Uterine Cervix, Am. J. Obst. & Gynec. 81: 124, 1961.

Fleming, A. R.: Advantages of Cold Conization, J. A. M. A. 168: 886, 1958.

Fluhmann, C. F.: The Developmental Anatomy of the Cervix Uteri, Obst. & Gynec. 15: 62, 1960.

Fluhmann, C. F.: The Glandular Structures of the Cervix Uteri, Surg., Gynec. & Obst. 106: 715, 1958.

Fluhmann, F. F.: The Nature and Development of the So-Called Glands of the Cervix Uteri, Am. J. Obst. & Gynec. 74: 753, 1957.

Fluhmann, C. F.: The Squamocolumnar Transitional Zone of the Cervix Uteri, Obst. & Gynec. 14: 133, 1959.

Gardner, G. H., Greene, R. R., and Peckham, B.: Tumors of the Broad Ligament, Am. J. Obst. & Gynec. 73: 536, 1957.

Gerbie, A., Hirsch, M., and Greene, R.: Vascular Tumors of the Female Genital Tract, Obst. & Gynec. 6: 499, 1955.

Goldberg, B., and Jones, H.: Some Characteristics of the Acid Phosphatase of the Human Endometrium, Obst. & Gynec. 4: 426, 1954.

Golden, M. L., and Betson, J. R.: Hysterectomy in 861 Selected Cases, Surg., Gynec. & Obst. 110: 182, 1960.

Graham, D., and Hill, R.: Inversion of Nonpuerperal Uterus; Report of a Case Associated With Fibromyomata Uteri, Obst. & Gynec. 16: 667, 1960.

Hamperl, H., and Kaufmann, C.: The Cervix Uteri at Different Ages, Obst. & Gynec. 14: 621, 1959.

Henry, J. H., Jr., and Latour, J. P. A.: Glycogen in the Squamous Epithelium of the Cervix Uteri, Am. J. Obst. & Gynec. 74: 610, 1957.

Hershey, S. J.: Enterouterine Fistulas: Report of a Case of Cervicosigmoidal Fistula, Obst. & Gynec. 14: 234, 1959.

Hester, L. L., and Read, R. A.: An Evaluation of Cervical Conization, Am. J. Obst. & Gynec. 80: 715, 1960.

Hofmeister, F., and Gorthey, R.: Benign Lesions of the Cervix, Obst. & Gynec. 5: 504, 1955.

Ingelman-Sundberg, A., and others: The Spontaneous Motility of Uterine Fibromyomata and Their Responses to Pharmacological Stimuli, Acta obst. et gynec. scandinav. 36: 263, 1957.

Kroger, W. S., and DeLee, S. T.: Use of Hypnoanesthesia for Cesarean Section and Hysterectomy, J. A. M. A. 163: 442, 1957.

Lamb, E., Fucilla, I., and Greene, R.: Basement Membranes in the Female Genital Tract, Am. J. Obst. & Gynec. 79: 79, 1960.

Lardaro, H.: Extensive Myomectomy; Review of 157 Cases, Am. J. Obst. & Gynec. 79: 43, 1960.

Mayo, W.: Some Observations on the Operation of Abdominal Myomectomy for Myomata of the Uterus, Surg., Gynec. & Obst. 12: 97, 1911.

Melody, G. F.: Obstructed Cervix: A Study of 100 Patients, Obst. & Gynec. 10: 190, 1957.

Meyer, R.: In Henke, Friedrich, and Lubarsch, Otto (editors): Handbuch der speciellen pathologischen Anatomie und Histologie, Part 1, Berlin, 1930, Julius Springer.

Miller, N., Ludovici, P., and Dontas, E.: The Problem of the Uterine Fibroid, Am. J. Obst. & Gynec. 66: 734, 1953.

Molumphy, P. E., and others: Cold Knife Conization of the Cervix, Obst. & Gynec. 14: 398, 1959.

Mondina, R.: The Significance of Mast Cells in Fibromyoma of the Uterus (Presenza delle mastzellen nei fibromiomi dell' utero), An. ostet. ginec. 78: 437, 1956.

Morrison, J. K.: The Ureter and Hysterectomy; Including the Effects of Certain Gynaecological Conditions on the Urinary Tract, J. Obst. & Gynaec. Brit. Emp. 67: 66, 1960.

Munnell, E., and Flick, F.: The Surgical Diagnosis and Management of Dysfunctional Uterine Bleeding, Surg., Gynec. & Obst. 106: 321, 1958.

Nichols, D. H., and Hayes, L. W., Jr.: Cervical Fibroid in Pregnancy and Delivery, Obst. & Gynec. 2: 180, 1953.

Novak, E. R.: Postmenopausal Endometrial Hyperplasia, Am. J. Obst. & Gynec. 71: 1312, 1956.

Offen, J. A., and Ferguson, J. H.: Cold Conization of the Cervix, Obst. & Gynec. 15: 396, 1960.

Pedowitz, P., Felmus, L. B., and Grayzel, D. G.: Hemangiopericytoma of the Uterus, Am. J. Obst. & Gynec. 67: 549, 1954.

Perl, J. I., and Milles, G.: Hydrocolpos After Total Hysterectomy, Am. J. Obst. & Gynec. 73: 1125, 1957.

Radman, H.: Blood Dyscrasia as a Causative Factor in Abnormal Uterine Bleeding, Am. J. Obst. & Gynec. 79: 1, 1960.

Richardson, E.: A Simplified Technic for Abdominal Pan-hysterectomy, Surg., Gynec. & Obst. **48**: 248, 1929.

Robson, T. B.: Hysterectomy–a Comparison of Indications, Complications, and Mortality in a Special and General Hospital Service, Am. J. Obst. & Gynec. **77**: 503, 1959.

Salm, R.: Cavernous Lymphangioma of the Uterus, Am. J. Obst. & Gynec. **80**: 365, 1960.

Schneider, G. T., and Weed, J. C.: Hysterectomy for Benign and Malignant Disease. Analysis of 2,284 Consecutive Cases, South. M. J. **51**: 561, 1958.

Schneppenheim, P., and others: The Relationship Between Columnar and Squamous Epithelium in the Uterine Cervix During the Life Span of Women (Die Beziehungen des Schleimepithels zum Plattenepithels an der Cervix Uteri im Lebenslauf der Frau), Arch. Gynäk. **190**: 303, 1958.

Scott, J., Welch, W., and Blake, T.: Bloodless Technique of Cold Knife Conization (Ring Biopsy), Am. J. Obst. & Gynec. **79**: 62, 1960.

Seaman, A., and Benson, R.: Coagulation Studies of Patients With Abnormal Uterine Bleeding, Am. J. Obst. & Gynec. **79**: 5, 1960.

Stander, R. W.: Irradiation Castration: A Follow-up Study of Results in Benign Pelvic Disease, Obst. & Gynec. **10**: 223, 1957.

Taylor, A. B.: Sarcoidosis of the Uterus, J. Obst. & Gynaec. Brit. Emp. **67**: 32, 1960.

Watts, W. F., and Kimbrough, R. A., Jr.: Hysterectomy; Analysis of 1000 Consecutive Operations, Obst. & Gynec. **7**: 483, 1956.

Welch, J. S.: Surgical Treatment of Uterine Myomas, S. Clin. North America **37**: 1101, 1957.

Williams, G. A., and Richardson, A. C.: Conization Biopsy of the Cervix, Obst. & Gynec. **10**: 60, 1957.

Woodruff, J. D., and Peterson, W. F.: Condylomata Acuminata of the Cervix, Am. J. Obst. & Gynec. **75**: 1354, 1958.

Zeigerman, J. H.: Vascular Tumors of the Uterus: Benign or Malignant; Their Significance in Our Daily Practice, J. A. M. A. **176**: 486, 1961.

Zeigerman, J. H., Valdes-Dapena, A. M., and Fettig, L.: Submucous Myoma in the Normal-Sized Uterus, Am. J. Obst. & Gynec. **73**: 1286, 1957.

Zettergren, L.: The Histogenesis of Uterine Myomas, Acta obst. et gynec. scandinav. **35**: 366, 1956.

18 · Adnexal Surgery for Benign Disease

General Considerations

Adnexal surgery for benign disease is rarely difficult unless complicated by adhesions to surrounding structures. An extensive knowledge of ovarian function and pathology is necessary to decide at the operating table the extent of the tissue that should be removed. The age of the patient is an important consideration, since castration of a young woman is undesirable.

Etiology and Pathologic Anatomy

Functional cysts make up a large majority of the ovarian enlargements. The total size of the cyst, plus the remaining ovarian tissue, is rarely larger than 6 cm. in diameter. Follicle cysts are the most common. They may be noted to increase and decrease in size if observed over a period of several months. Functional cysts develop in the corpus luteum, particularly if a hemorrhage has taken place into one of these structures. The corpus luteum cysts seen in the presence of an hydatidiform mole or a chorionepithelioma are much larger than other functional cysts. The true epithelial tumors of the ovary represent new growths. They have the potentiality of malignant change. More than half of the true tumors are serous cystadenomas and pseudomucinous cystadenomas. A higher percentage of the serous cystadenomas become malignant as compared with the pseudomucinous type of tumor. Their malignant counterpart will be considered in Chapter 26, Cancer of the Fundus, Tube, and Ovary (page 493). About 10 per cent of all primary ovarian tumors are derived from cells with a variable potential for growth. The most frequent of these is a dermoid cyst that may be filled with hair, teeth, cartilage, or bone. The cystic areas are filled with fatty material and desquamated epithelium. A true teratoma of the ovary contains elements of all three germ plasm layers. Many such tumors are malignant in one area, usually forming an adenocarcinoma of some type. A rare type of tumor contains thyroid tissue and has been called struma ovarii. A rare group of tumors, some of which have specific hormonal activity, are thought to arise from the ovarian stroma. Granulosa and theca cell tumors may be functional and result in an increased secretion of estrogen. About 25 per cent of granulosa cell tumors are malignant. A dysgerminoma is a solid tumor of the ovary that is an analogue of a similar testicular tumor. Many dysgerminomas are highly malignant. They have not been shown to have any hormonal activity. An arrhenoblastoma is a tumor with pronounced masculinizing effects. About 25 per cent of such tumors are malignant. A fibroma of the ovary is benign and is often accompanied with ascites and a hydrothorax. This is not specific for a fibroma of the ovary and may occur with other solid tumors. A Brenner cell tumor is usually discovered accidentally when the ovary is removed for some other reason. It does not grow to a large size or become symptomatic. The surgeon should be always alert to the possibility of metastatic disease in the ovary even though the patient has no symptoms attributed to the primary site.

Symptoms and Diagnosis

The symptoms of an ovarian cyst or tumor are variable, and the patient may harbor a large tumor that is discovered at a routine general physical examination. Menstrual dysfunction, in the form of amenorrhea, polymenorrhea, or menometrorrhagia, is more commonly found with the functional cysts. Pain is not a constant symptom, and it is only when there is sufficient distention or peritoneal irritation that the cyst causes pelvic pain. The patient may note an unexplained enlargement of the abdomen. A twisted ovarian cyst gives rise to a more definite sequence of symptoms. A long pedicle lends to mobility and possible twisting. When the pedicle becomes twisted, pain is cramplike in nature and tends to radiate toward the midline. Late in the course of the illness, after ischemic necrosis has set in, there is adjacent peritoneal reaction, and the pain will be continuous in character and associated with localized tenderness. A volvulus of the cecum is extremely rare but has occasionally confused the picture. Nausea and vomiting are common symptoms of a twisted cyst. On bimanual examination cysts are felt in one or both adnexa, and usually the uterus can be outlined distinct from the tumors. Large fibroids tend to displace the cervix up under the symphysis, whereas large cysts tend to displace the uterus into the hollow of the sacrum. The position of the cervix may help distinguish between large fibroids and a large ovarian cyst. An examination under anesthesia or a laparotomy may be necessary to make a differential diagnosis.

Indications and Surgical Principles

Some basic rules have been established over the years in regard to the management of ovarian tumors. They are not universally applicable to every patient but do provide a guide to surgeons so that unnecessary pelvic surgery is not done.

1. A cystic ovarian tumor, 6 cm. or more in diameter, that enlarges after an observation period extending through at least two menstrual periods requires exploration. If the examination suggests that the tumor is solid, it is investigated immediately.

2. Any ovarian tumor in the menopausal age group is investigated surgically without delay, and this may be done through an exploratory colpotomy or by means of a laparotomy.

3. All ovarian tumors in the postmenopausal age group are removed and submitted for histologic study.

4. Persistent pain in the presence of an ovarian enlargement, after pelvic inflammatory disease has been excluded, is an indication for further investigation.

5. Precocious puberty in a child may require exploration to rule out the presence of a granulosa cell tumor.

6. If an x-ray shows that a small tumor is a dermoid by the presence of teeth, bone, or cartilage, the tumor is removed before it displaces and destroys adjacent normal ovarian tissue or undergoes torsion.

7. Benign ovarian cysts and tumors are managed by conservative surgery. It is a lack of knowledge of ovarian pathology that prompts some surgeons to inadvertently remove normal ovarian tissue together with a small benign cyst.

8. The delivery of an extremely large cyst, particularly in an individual with a short distance between the costal margin and the symphysis, can present serious difficulties. Even with what I call a "battle-field exploration incision," namely, from the symphysis to the xiphoid, some tumors cannot be delivered without considerable manipulation. Some students of ovarian pathology feel that the aspiration of a tumor should never be carried out because of the risk of spillage of malignant cells and the subsequent inoculation of the peritoneal cavity and omentum. That this can happen still lacks conclusive experimental and clinical evidence. We, likewise, do not know whether the manipulation of a large tumor, that may subsequently be proved malignant, forces tumor cells into the regional lymphatics, with the same disastrous results. If it would appear that the delivery of a tumor of large size is going to require considerable stretching, pulling, and manipulation to be delivered intact, the cyst is collapsed by the insertion of a trocar and aspiration of its contents until it can be delivered. This cannot be done without some spillage of contents of the cyst. The surgeon may as well palpate the inside of the lining for excrescences, since he may now be faced with the decision of removing the entire pelvic contents and omentum. He may decide that the tumor is malignant and prepare the patient for the use of intraperitoneal radioactive isotopes or nitrogen mustard to prevent extension of the

disease or to destroy tumor cells in the lymphatics.

9. In the immediate post-partum period, be especially alert for the torsion of a cyst. Freedom of movement, newly acquired after the evacuation of the uterus, makes this more probable. Operation should not be deferred.

10. Operation on benign ovarian cysts during pregnancy is deferred until the sixteenth week, when abortion is less likely to occur.

11. Torsion of an ovarian tumor may produce thrombi in the veins of the pedicle. Some surgeons advocate clamping of the pedicle prior to untwisting. This is to prevent a pulmonary embolus from thrombotic vessels. This complication is managed in the same manner as a volvulus of the bowel. If the tumor is obviously gangrenous throughout, the pedicle is immediately clamped and the tumor removed. In less-advanced cases of torsion, strangulation is reduced and the tumor observed for any salvageable ovarian tissue that may become evident after the circulation is restored. As with a volvulus of the bowel, an observation period of twenty minutes or more may produce changes in some segment of the tumor where a fragment of ovarian tissue can be preserved.

Surgical Anatomy of the Tubes and Ovaries

The Fallopian tubes are paired muscular tubes, 10 to 12 cm. in length, which extend from the cornu of the uterus to the tubal extremity of the ovary. Each tube may be divided into four sections. The interstitial (uterine section of the tube) part begins at the upper angle of the uterine cavity, is less than a millimeter in thickness, and extends through the muscular wall to the cornu of the uterus. The next part is the isthmic section—narrow and cordlike—that forms about one third of the extrauterine part of the tube. The outer two thirds of the tube becomes wider in diameter and more thin walled. The tube then ends in the trumpet-shaped infundibulum, with its fingerlike projections, the fimbriae. The longest fimbria, the ovarian fimbria, extends along the free border of the mesosalpinx to the ovary. The mesovarium just beneath the tube seems to be shorter than the tube itself, and this causes numerous twists and kinks.

The tubes extend downward and backward from the cornua of the uterus and then rise slightly before the fimbriated extremity curves downward once more to the ovary. The position of the tube, as well as the ovary, is determined by the state of anteflexion and anteversion of the uterus. Diseased tubes frequently sink down in the pelvis behind the uterus.

The wall of the tube is composed of three layers: peritoneal, muscular, and mucosal. The muscular layer has an outer longitudinal coat and an inner circular coat. The muscular layer is thinner in the outer portion of the tube. The mucosa contains ciliated and nonciliated cells but no glands. Toward the fimbriated end the simple folds seen at the uterine end become more branched and complicated to form villi, which almost obliterate the lumen of the tube. In operating on the tubes, the surgeon must remember that they are richly supplied with elastic tissue, blood vessels, and lymphatics. The ciliated columnar epithelium has been observed by some to undergo cyclic changes with the menstrual cycle, so that plastic operations may be affected by this fact, although this remains to be studied further. Diverticula have been observed in the tube, which might account for some ectopic pregnancies in what appear to be normal tubes. When diseased tubes become adherent in the pelvis, the infundibulopelvic pedicle holds them along the course of the ureter. This should be remembered by surgeons who subscribe to the technique of freeing up adherent tubes by the scooping-out method before ligating the infundibulopelvic pedicle and prior to removing a tubo-ovarian mass. Infection in the right tube may be the result of an acute appendicitis, or a periappendicitis may result from extension of infection from the right tube to the appendix.

The parovarium is a vestigial structure representing the remains of the Wolffian body and duct. When the broad ligament (mesosalpinx and mesovarium) are examined in good light, several vestigial structures are seen. Several small tubules arise near the hilum of the ovary and pass up toward the Fallopian tube to join a longitudinal duct, which is usually closed at

347

both ends. This duct may be prolonged mesially in the broad ligament as Gartner's duct and also down along the lateral vaginal wall. The hydatid of Morgagni is a pea-sized, pedunculated cyst of Müllerian origin that is attached to the mesosalpinx near the fimbriated end of the tube. The parovarium is important as the source of broad ligament cysts, while Gartner's duct may give rise to vaginal cysts.

The ovaries are paired, solid structures and are normally about 3.75 cm. in length, 2 cm. in width, and about 8 mm. thick. They each weigh about 4 to 8 grams, but their size and weight vary markedly with age, pregnancy, and the presence of functional cysts. The ovary is suspended from the back of the broad ligament by an extension or fold of that ligament called the mesovarium. It is also attached to the peritoneum of the lateral pelvic wall by the infundibulopelvic ligament (suspensory ligament of the ovary) and to the uterus by a muscular cord from 1 to 3 cm. in length, the ovarian ligament. The position of the ovary varies so greatly, depending on the uterus and attenuation of its ligaments, that a description of borders and surfaces is impractical. Frequently one or the other of the ovaries is prolapsed in the cul-de-sac, where it is readily palpable on combined rectovaginal examination. The length of the sigmoid colon and its mesocolon may affect the left ovary. Grossly it must be appreciated that ovarian tissue is easily cut through with sutures, so gentleness is essential in the approximation of its tissue. The nerve, blood, and lymphatic supply will be detailed where they have a specific bearing on a certain disease.

What is the composition of the pedicle of most ovarian cysts? Unless they originate in the hilus of the ovary and extend into the broad ligament, the following structures are usually found: the much-elongated Fallopian tube, a thickened and elongated upper portion of the broad ligament, the mesovarium and its blood vessels, the infundibulopelvic ligament (ovarian artery, veins, and nerves, together with their connective tissue extensions from the parietal connective tissue), the ovarian ligament, occa-sionally the round ligament, and the vestigial structures, some identifiable and some not, that occupy the mesosalpinx or are found in the parovarium.

A cyst originating in the broad ligament may have no pedicle or, like those of the hilum of the ovary, may have a very sessile one. Its gross characteristic is that of a cyst with the tube extended over its surface and the ovary hanging freely on its posterior side.

OOPHORECTOMY AND OOPHOROCYSTECTOMY
Steps of the Operation

1. An incision believed to be adequate to deliver the cyst is made either in a longitudinal or a transverse direction. At times this incision may extend from the symphysis to the xiphoid process.

2. In Plate 54, *A*, the delivery of a moderately large ovarian cyst with a twisted pedicle was drawn by the artist. The cyst was delivered intact and was not necrotic, although the circulation was impaired.

3. The technique of aspirating a large cyst that cannot be delivered without undue manipulation and the possibility of rupture is shown in Plate 54, *B* and *C*. A purse-string suture is placed in the cyst wall and a trocar introduced in the center. The suture is tied about the trocar as the fluid is aspirated. Should the surgeon feel it necessary to palpate for excrescences within the tumor, this is done with every precaution to prevent the leakage of the contents (Plate 54, *C*). The surgeon is responsible for the decision as to the extent of the operation indicated by the pathologic findings.

4. After delivery of the tumor illustrated, portions of the pedicle and the tube were cyanotic and had to be observed for viability.

5. After untwisting the pedicle, observation of the tube revealed the circulation to be adequate so that the tube could be preserved (Plate 54, *D*). No functional, normal ovarian tissue was observed. If even a fragment of normal ovarian tissue can be preserved, an oophorocystectomy, in a young patient with a benign lesion, is preferable to loss of the entire ovary.

6. The mesovarium is clamped, cut, and ligated in small segments to prevent kinking (Plate 54, *G*). Since this patient was very desirous of having children, great care was exercised to prevent any injury to the tube, despite the fact that no ovarian tissue could be preserved.

PLATE 54

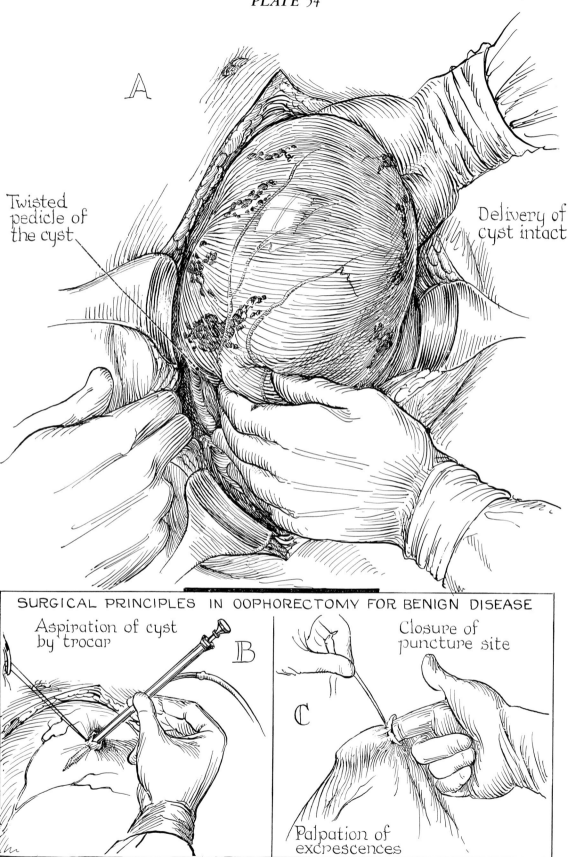

A

Twisted pedicle of the cyst

Delivery of cyst intact

SURGICAL PRINCIPLES IN OOPHORECTOMY FOR BENIGN DISEASE

Aspiration of cyst by trocar

B

Closure of puncture site

C

Palpation of excrescences

349

PLATE 54 (Continued)

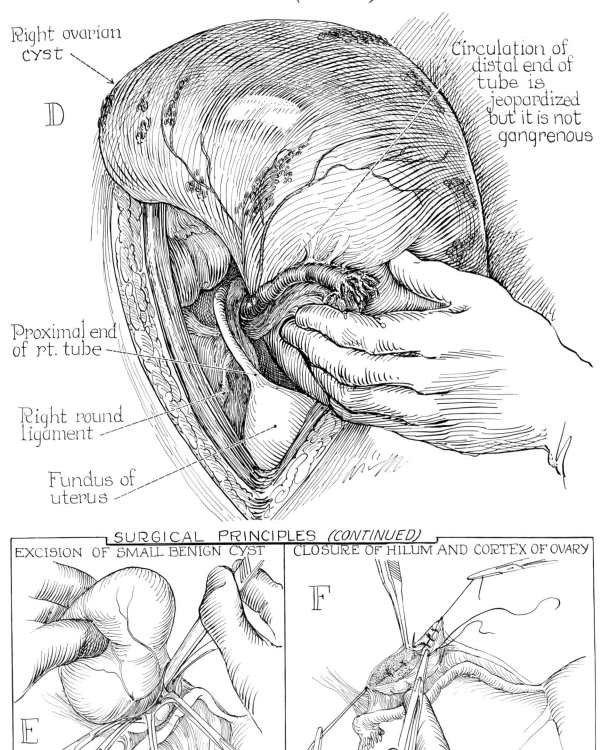

Right ovarian cyst

Circulation of distal end of tube is jeopardized but it is not gangrenous

D

Proximal end of rt. tube

Right round ligament

Fundus of uterus

SURGICAL PRINCIPLES *(CONTINUED)*

EXCISION OF SMALL BENIGN CYST

CLOSURE OF HILUM AND CORTEX OF OVARY

E

F

350

PLATE 54 (*Concluded*)

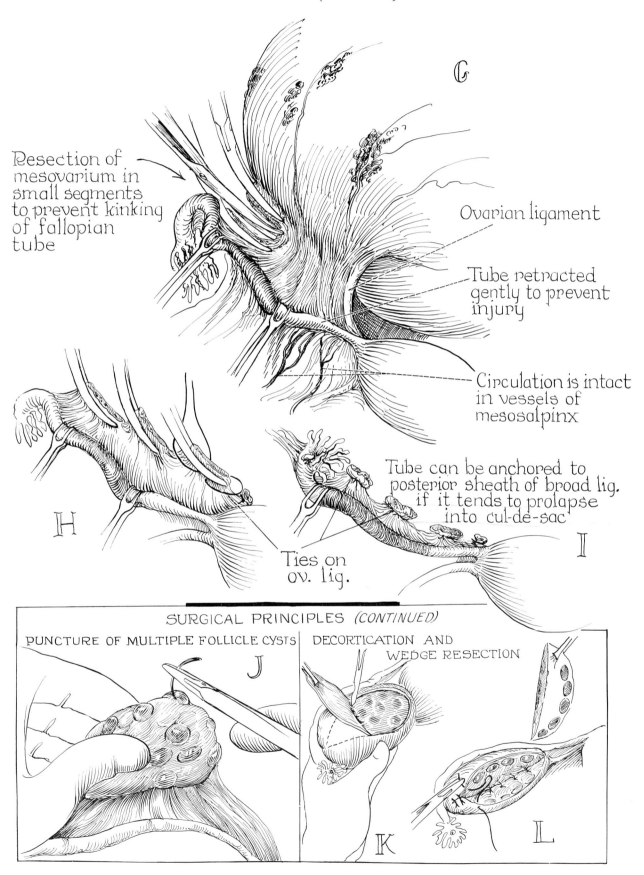

G

Resection of
mesovarium in
small segments
to prevent kinking
of fallopian
tube

Ovarian ligament

Tube retracted
gently to prevent
injury

Circulation is intact
in vessels of
mesosalpinx

Tube can be anchored to
posterior sheath of broad lig.
if it tends to prolapse
into cul-de-sac

H

Ties on
ov. lig.

I

SURGICAL PRINCIPLES (*CONTINUED*)

PUNCTURE OF MULTIPLE FOLLICLE CYSTS

J

DECORTICATION AND
WEDGE RESECTION

K

L

7. The ties on the mesovarium are of fine chromic catgut, which cause only a minimum of reaction (Plate 54, *H*).

8. If the tube tends to prolapse into the cul-de-sac, it is anchored to the posterior sheath of the broad ligament so that it remains near its normal position (Plate 54, *I*).

EXCISION OF SMALL BENIGN CYSTS (OOPHOROCYSTECTOMY)

Many small benign cysts are removed, with preservation of normal ovarian tissue. The surgical principles in this operation are shown in Plate 54, *E* and *F*. An incision is made along the base of the cyst between its wall and normal ovarian tissue. The cyst wall is carefully dissected from normal ovarian tissue. The contents of a dermoid cyst produce irritation if spilled in the peritoneal cavity, so the field of operation is protected with laparotomy pads. Bleeding points in the ovarian stroma are ligated, and the ovary is closed by interrupted sutures of fine chromic catgut. A minimum number of sutures consistent with adequate closure and hemostasis are employed.

PUNCTURE OF MULTIPLE FOLLICLE CYSTS

Many ovaries contain multiple follicle cysts. If the ovary appears tense and the multiple cysts are impairing the circulation, this may be improved by puncturing the cysts (Plate 54, *J*). The end results of this dawdling are difficult to assess. Since these cysts do not produce mature ova, the procedure can do no harm.

DECORTICATION OF THE OVARY AND WEDGE RESECTION

Enlarged ovaries with a smooth capsule and multiple microfollicular cysts are seen in the Stein-Leventhal syndrome. Function of these ovaries has been restored by decortication and wedge resection. The principles of this operation are shown in Plate 54, *K* and *L*. A large segment of the ovarian cortex opposite the hilum of the ovary is removed. The cysts are punctured and collapsed. A large wedge of ovarian stroma extending *deep into the hilum* is resected. The cortex of the ovary is closed

with interrupted sutures of fine chromic catgut on atraumatic needles. The procedure relieves tension within the ovary, and, in many instances, subsequent ovulation is proved by endometrial biopsy.

BROAD LIGAMENT CYSTS

Large broad ligament cysts arise from the ovary near the hilum and grow between the sheaths of the broad ligament. There is some evidence that some of these cysts develop from accessory ovarian tissue. They may become quite large and displace the uterus to the opposite side and impinge upon the ureter and vessels on the lateral pelvic wall. They rarely become malignant and can be enucleated without difficulty. Attention to the position of the ureter is necessary so that it is not compromised.

SALPINGECTOMY

Primary indications for salpingectomy are most frequent because of inflammatory disease (see Chapter 5, Venereal Diseases, page 81). Ectopic pregnancy, endometriosis, and a rare malignancy are other specific diseases that may require excision of the tube. When the ovary is preserved, the mesosalpinx is clamped close to the tube. This prevents impairment of the circulation to the ovary.

VAGINAL SALPINGO-OOPHORECTOMY
Indications and Surgical Principles

Gynecologists who are adamant in removing the tubes and ovaries during the course of an abdominal hysterectomy in women over a certain age should likewise remove the tubes and ovaries when performing a vaginal hysterectomy upon the same patient. Obviously in the course of a vaginal hysterectomy a diseased tube or ovary should be removed. As has been described under Exploratory Colpotomy (page 28), the cul-de-sac approach can be used for removal of diseased adnexa or tubal ligation without a vaginal hysterectomy. This approach can be used to perform a bilateral oophorectomy in carcinoma of the breast provided an abdominal exploration is not indicated.

PLATE 55

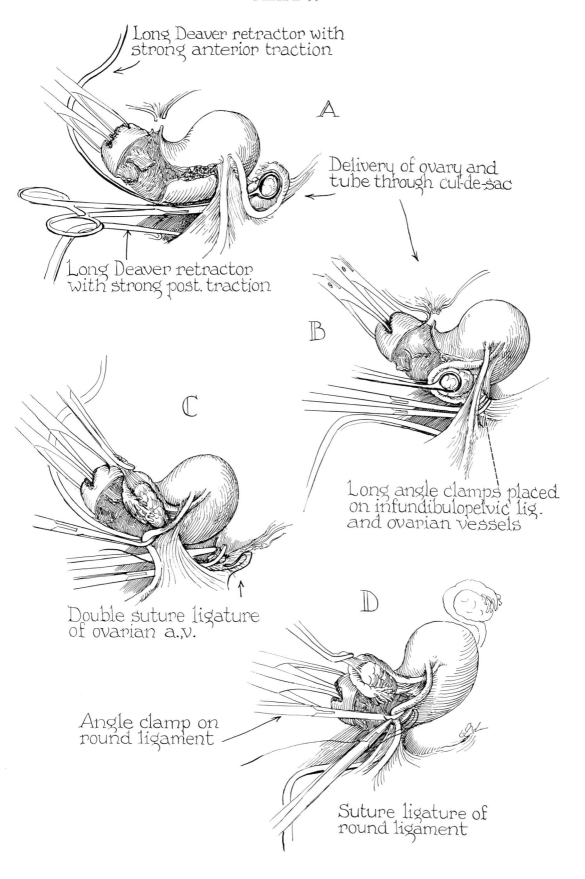

Long Deaver retractor with strong anterior traction

A

Delivery of ovary and tube through cul-de-sac

Long Deaver retractor with strong post. traction

B

Long angle clamps placed on infundibulopelvic lig. and ovarian vessels

C

Double suture ligature of ovarian a.,v.

D

Angle clamp on round ligament

Suture ligature of round ligament

Steps of the Operation

1. The tubes and ovaries may be removed attached to the uterus, or the uterus alone can be removed and the tubes and ovaries removed individually. The technical difficulties in the individual case will decide which procedure is most rational. If the tubes and ovaries are to be removed together with the uterus, the vaginal hysterectomy proceeds to the point where it remains only to section the infundibulopelvic pedicle and the round ligament. At this time the operator further explores the adnexa for adhesions to surrounding structures and their accessibility through the cul-de-sac. The uterus is drawn strongly to one side or the other, and an ovum forceps is used to grasp the ovary, which is drawn with gentle traction into the field of operation (Plate 55, *A*). It is important to handle the structures gently so as not to rupture any vessels in the infundibulopelvic pedicle which may subsequently retract and cause annoying bleeding. During the course of this procedure, the use of a long Deaver retractor and long instruments of each type greatly facilitates the removal of the structures.

2. Long angle clamps are then placed on the infundibulopelvic pedicle (Plate 55, *B*), securing both the ovarian artery and vein. A third clamp may subsequently be placed on the uterine side of the pedicle and the vessels sectioned between clamps.

3. The infundibulopelvic pedicle is then doubly ligated with 00 chromic catgut (Plate 55, *C*). One clamp should be left attached to the distal end of the ligated pedicle and then released to visualize the pedicle for evidence of any bleeding.

4. An angle clamp is placed on the round ligament, a suture ligature is used, and the ligament is resected (Plate 55, *D*). If vaginal salpingo-oophorectomy immediately follows a vaginal hysterectomy, the round ligament, the ovarian ligament, and the tube will have been ligated close to the uterus. The ends of these pedicles are then used to make traction, and the operation is performed in the same way. In the closure of the vault after vaginal hysterectomy and vaginal salpingo-oophorectomy, only the round ligament is incorporated in the angle suture. The infundibulopelvic pedicle retracts and would be under considerable tension if brought down to the angle of the vaginal vault.

PRIMARY UTERINE SUSPENSION
General Considerations

Every few years, in a gynecologic service with several thousand admissions per year, there seems to be a patient who has an adequate indication for a uterine suspension as a primary operation. Every method of therapy in gynecology, psychiatric evaluation and analysis, and orthopedic studies, with a long trial of corrective exercises and months in the physiotherapy department, will have preceded the decision to suspend the uterus. The patient will consistently report relief from reposition of the uterus and the insertion of a pessary and complain of back pain when the pessary is out and she thinks it is in. For the benefit of colleagues who may be faced with this situation, a method of sewing the round ligaments of the uterus toward the bladder is suggested.

Surgical Principles

The round ligaments are shortened by one method or another. The least time-consuming technique is to draw the elongated round ligament through the inguinal canal and suture it to the aponeurosis of the external oblique muscle, simultaneously obliterating the external ring. A segment of the round ligament near the internal ring that brings the uterus forward without tension is selected. This operation obliterates the inguinal canal and probably has prevented many potential hernias or cured hernias not recognized as such from the peritoneal aspect.

References

Amromin, G. D., and Haumeder, E. M.: Feminizing Ovarian Gynandroblastoma, Am. J. Obst. & Gynec. 77: 645, 1959.

Angervall, L., and Knutson, H.: Heterotopic Ovarian Tissue, Acta obst. et gynec. scandinav. 38: 275, 1959.

Arey, L. B.: The Origin and Form of the Brenner Tumor, Am. J. Obst. & Gynec. 81: 743, 1961.

Averbach, L. H., Promin, D., and Hanna, G. C.: Brenner Tumor of the Ovary: A Case of Unusually Large Size, Am. J. Obst. & Gynec. 74: 207, 1957.

Ayerst, R. L., and Johnson, C. G.: Dysgerminoma, Obst. & Gynec. 14: 685, 1959.

Beck, R. P., and Latour, J. P. A.: Review of 1019 Benign Ovarian Neoplasms, Obst. & Gynec. 16: 479, 1960.

Berkheiser, S. W.: Hilus-Cell Tumor of the Ovary, Am. J. Obst. & Gynec. 73: 429, 1957.

Bolton, R. N., and Hunter, W. C.: Adenomatoid Tumors of the Uterus and Adnexa, Am. J. Obst. & Gynec. 76: 647, 1958.

Brady, D. F.: Torsion of a Previously Normal Fallopian Tube, A. M. A. Arch. Surg. 81: 329, 1960.

Brantley, W. M., and others: Rupture of a Silent Pyosalpinx Following a Hysterosalpingogram; Report of a Case, Obst. & Gynec. 16: 483, 1960.

Braunstein, P. W., Ryan, B. J., and McCormick, R.: Isolated Torsion of the Fallopian Tube, New York J. Med. 61: 1268, 1961.

Brewer, J. I., and Guderian, A. M.: Diagnosis of Uterine-Tube Carcinoma by Vaginal Cytology, Obst. & Gynec. 8: 664, 1956.

Bungard, R. J., and Haug, W. A.: Bilateral Brenner Tumors of the Ovaries, Am. J. Obst. & Gynec. 77: 660, 1959.

Costantini, O.: Fibroma of the Fallopian Tubes (Contributo allo studio del fibroma tubarico), Clin. obst. ginec. 60: 33, 1958.

DiMasi, F. T., and Grogan, R. H.: Proliferative Ovarian Tumors, Obst. & Gynec. 15: 315, 1960.

Dougherty, C. M.: Four Unusual Pelvic Tumors (Discussion by Hertig, A. T., Jaques, W., Sternberg, W., and Dockerty, M. B.), Obst. & Gynec. 9: 656, 1957.

Dougherty, C. M., Thompson, W. B., and McCall, M. L.: Hilus-Cell and Granulosa-Cell Tumors in the Same Ovary, Am. J. Obst. & Gynec. 76: 653, 1958.

Evans, T. N., and Riley, G. M.: Polycystic Ovarian Disease; a Clinical and Experimental Study, Am. J. Obst. & Gynec. 80: 873, 1960.

Evans, T. N., and Riley, G. M.: Polycystic Ovarian Disease (Stein-Leventhal Syndrome): Etiology and Rationale for Surgical Treatment, Obst. & Gynec. 12: 168, 1958.

Feinberg, R.: Ovarian Estrogenic Tumors and Diffuse Estrogenic Thecomatosis in Postmenopausal Colporrhagia, Am. J. Obst. & Gynec. 76: 851, 1958.

Foraker, A., Celi, P., and Denham, S.: Dehydrogenase Activity; I. In the Ovary, Obst. & Gynec. 2: 407, 1953.

Frost, I.: The Significance of Abnormal Uterine Bleeding Due to Ovarian Dysfunction, New York J. Med. 53: 2459, 1953.

Frymire, L. J.: Arrhenoblastoma With Two Subsequent Pregnancies; Report of a Case, Obst. & Gynec. 17: 248, 1961.

Gemmell, A.: Some Incidents in Surgery of the Ovary, J. Obst. & Gynaec. Brit. Emp. 65: 392, 1958.

Hughesdon, P. E.: Thecal and Allied Reactions in Epithelial Ovarian Tumours, J. Obst. & Gynaec. Brit. Emp. 65: 702, 1958.

Ince, J. G. H., and Salm, R.: A Very Large Brenner Tumor; With Comments on Certain Points in Histogenesis, Am. J. Obst. & Gynec. 77: 1351, 1959.

Ingersoll, F. M.: Indications for Wedge Resection, Obst. & Gynec. 14: 748, 1959.

Israel, S. L., and Mutch, J. C.: Endocrinologic Effects of Certain Ovarian Tumors, Surg., Gynec. & Obst. 104: 166, 1957.

Jackson, R. L., and Dockerty, M. B.: The Stein-Leventhal Syndrome: Analysis of 43 Cases With Special Reference to Association With Endometrial Carcinoma, Am. J. Obst. & Gynec. 73: 161, 1957.

Joel, R., and Foraker, A.: Fate of the Corpus Albicans: A Morphologic Approach, Am. J. Obst. & Gynec. 80: 314, 1960.

Jonas, E. G.: Functioning Brenner Tumour of the Ovary. A Clinico-pathological Case Report, J. Obst. & Gynaec. Brit. Emp. 66: 141, 1959.

Kallio, H.: Medullary Resection of the Ovaries in Treatment of the Stein-Leventhal Syndrome; Report of 11 Cases, Acta obst. et gynec. scandinav. 40: 16, 1961.

Kaufman, R. H., Abbott, J. P., and Wall, J. A.: The Endometrium Before and After Wedge Resection of the Ovaries in the Stein-Leventhal Syndrome, Am. J. Obst. & Gynec. 77: 1271, 1959.

Kendall, B., and Bowers, P. A.: Bilateral Brenner Tumor of the Ovaries; Case Report and Review of the Literature, Am. J. Obst. & Gynec. 80: 439, 1960.

Lees, D. H., and Paine, C. G.: Lipoid Masculinizing Tumours of the Ovary, J. Obst. & Gynaec. Brit. Emp. 65: 702, 1958.

Leventhal, M. L.: The Stein-Leventhal Syndrome, Am. J. Obst. & Gynec. 76: 825, 1958.

Lowi, R. N. P.: Uterine Tube Physiology; a Review of the Literature, Obst. & Gynec. 16: 322, 1960.

Lygonis, C.: Torsion of Fallopian Tube, J. Obst. & Gynaec. Brit. Emp. 67: 1005, 1960.

MacFarlane, K. T.: Rational Ovarian Surgery, Am. J. Obst. & Gynec. 80: 683, 1960.

McNulty, J. R.: The Ovarian Serous Cystadenofibroma; a Report of 25 Cases, Am. J. Obst. & Gynec. 77: 1338, 1959.

Maurer, E. R.: Complete Extirpation of the Thoracic Duct; Its Use in the Management of the Primary Benign Tumor Producing Spontaneous Chylothorax, J. A. M. A. 161: 135, 1956.

Muller, W., Schubothe, H, and Elert, R.: Hemolytic Anemia With Dermoid Cyst (Die haemolytische Anaemie als Begleiterkrankung bei Dermoidzysten), Geburtsh. u. Frauenh. 18: 723, 1958.

Novak, E. R., and Mattingly, R. F.: Hilus Cell Tumor of the Ovary, Obst. & Gynec. 15: 425, 1960.

Novak, E. R., and Williams, T. J.: Autopsy Comparison of Cardiovascular Changes in Castrated and Normal Women, Am. J. Obst. & Gynec. 80: 863, 1960.

Pryor, J. H.: Haemorrhage Into Bilateral Cysts Related to the Ovarian Veins in Association With a Large Uterine Fibromyoma, J. Obst. & Gynaec. Brit. Emp 67: 142, 1960.

Quinto, P.: Contribution to the Study of Virilizing Tumors of the Ovary (Contributo allo studio dei tumori virilizzanti dell'ovaio), Riv. ital. ginec. 39: 245, 1956.

Randall, C.: Indications for the Surgical Treatment of the Ovary, Obst. & Gynec. 5: 591, 1955.

Roddick, J., and Greene, R. R.: The Relation of Non-malignant Postmenopausal Endometrial Changes to Ovarian Morphology, Am. J. Obst. & Gynec. 75: 235, 1958.

Rothman, D., and Blumenthal, H. T.: Serous Adenofibroma and Cystadenofibroma of the Ovary, Obst. & Gynec. 14: 389, 1959.

Sarason, E. L., and Prior, J. T.: Acute Abdominal Pain Due to Torsion and Infarction of a Normal Ovary, Surg., Gynec. & Obst. 109: 771, 1958.

Schein, C. J., and Ferreira, R.: The Use of Autogenous Arterial Grafts for the Experimental Reconstruction of Fallopian Tubes, Am. J. Obst. & Gynec. 71: 206, 1956.

Schneider, G. T.: Functioning Ovarian Tumors, Am. J. Obst. & Gynec. 79: 921, 1960.

Shaaban, A. H., Abdine, F. H., and Youssef, A.: Functioning Brenner Tumour of the Ovary, J. Obst. & Gynaec. Brit. Emp. 67: 138, 1960.

Stein, I., Cohen, M., and Elson, R.: Results of Bilateral Ovarian Wedge Resection in 47 Cases of Sterility, Am. J. Obst. & Gynec. 58: 267, 1949.

TeLinde, R. W., and Wharton, L. R.: Ovarian Function Following Pelvic Operation; an Experimental Study on Monkeys, Am. J. Obst. & Gynec. 80: 844, 1960.

Wallingford, A. J.: Ascites in Gynecology With Special Reference to a Possible Hormonal Origin of Meigs' Syndrome, New York J. Med. 55: 221, 1955.

Whitelaw, R. G.: Pathology and the Conserved Ovary, J. Obst. & Gynaec. Brit. Emp. 66: 413, 1959.

Woodruff, J. D., and Markley, R. L.: Struma Ovarii, Obst. & Gynec. 9: 707, 1957.

Woodruff, J., Swan Bie, L., and Sherman, R.: Mucinous Tumors of the Ovary, Obst. & Gynec. 16: 699, 1960.

Zellner, K. E.: Meigs' syndrom und struma ovarii, Acta obst. et gynec. scandinav. 40: 40, 1961.

19 · Dysmenorrhea and Pelvic Endometriosis

PRIMARY DYSMENORRHEA
Etiology and Pathologic Anatomy

The etiology of primary dysmenorrhea is the subject of many fascinating studies. The older concepts of a menstrual toxin, low pain threshold, and sensitiveness of the cerebral cortex to pain impressions have been replaced by studies that cast more light on the physicochemical changes. The psychosomatic aspects of primary dysmenorrhea may one day be correlated with the physicochemical changes. Two basic observations have been studied. (1) there is an increase in the excitability of the myometrium and (2) an angiospasm similar to the pain of angina pectoris or intermittent claudication takes place. The hormonal dysfunction responsible for these changes probably involves the pituitary gland, as well as the ovary and the two important regulators of menstrual function, estrogen and progesterone. Progesterone is essential to functional dysmenorrhea, since pain is absent in proved anovulatory cycles.

Medical Management

A bilateral attack upon the somatic manifestations of this symptom and the psychosomatic problems of the patient is necessary. The inevitability of the pain each month and other symptoms such as nausea and vomiting, malaise, irritability, premenstrual tension, and bloating is interrupted, if possible, by one of several methods. The clinician should evaluate each patient and what has been done by previous consultants before selecting a regimen of treatment. Many patients can have the vicious cycle modified by salt restriction, mild analgesic drugs, and psychotherapy. More disturbed patients with a history of dysmenorrhea of longer duration may require the interruption of ovulation by the use of large doses of estrogen or by androgen therapy. Finally, if the situation is very pressing, the patient is incapacitated and suffering an economic loss each month, and the patient meets all of the requirements for surgical interruption of the sympathetic pathways to the internal os, a prelumbar sympathectomy is considered. A slow dilatation of the cervix preceding the presacral neurectomy is done. Resection of the uterosacral ligaments after an exploratory colpotomy gives considerable relief to many patients. Sufficient data have not been accumulated to properly assess this surgical approach to the problem.

PELVIC ENDOMETRIOSIS
Etiology and Pathologic Anatomy

Pelvic endometriosis is divided into internal endometriosis (adenomyosis) and external endometriosis, in which ectopic endometrium is widely distributed in the tissues of the pelvis and in some extrapelvic locations. Adenomyosis is a histologic diagnosis and may exist to a minor degree or may cause a diffuse enlargement of the uterus. Since it does not produce a characteristic clinical picture and indication for surgery, this discussion is confined to the external type of endometriosis and its management.

The histogenesis of pelvic endometriosis has interested gynecologic pathologists for many years. The various theories dealing with regurgitation of endometrium through the tubes, theories that endometriosis develops in situ from local tissues, and the concept that both factors act in the development of the disease explain in a general way the pathologic findings.

Javert's theory of *benign metastatic disease* is the hypothesis that today provides a sound approach to the surgical management of endometriosis. He has shown that this disease, in the advanced stages, spreads like and simulates endometrial cancer but stops short of destroying the host. Endometriosis should then be attacked by searching for all the contiguous and metastatic areas of spread when it is desired to eradicate the disease without castrating the patient by bilateral oophorectomy.

The organ most frequently involved in this disease is the ovary, and this may vary from a small area a few millimeters in diameter to a large chocolate cyst replacing all but a shell of the normal ovarian tissue. The posterior portion of the uterus and the cul-de-sac, including the uterosacral ligaments, are the next most common sites. Following these, the remaining organs in the pelvis, including the peritoneum over the bladder, rectum, sigmoid, and appendix, are involved. The disease spreads through the regional lymphatics and is readily demonstrated in the nodes draining the pelvic organs. Unmistakable endometrial glands have been found in the kidney, in abdominal wounds, and in the alveoli of the lungs.

Symptoms and Diagnosis

Some observers estimate that 12 per cent of all women in the childbearing age have some endometriosis. The symptomatology of this disease presents many incongruities—extensive destructive lesions giving few symptoms and small lesions causing severe pain. In some characteristics the disease may be compared to a hydronephrosis. With a hydronephrosis the distention of the kidney pelvis is painful when the structure is intact and tends to be less symptomatic when the pelvis and calyces become dilated, saclike, and atonic. Minimal endometriosis may cause annoying pain to a sensitive peritoneum, ovary, or adjacent ligaments. With further destruction of tissue,

pain may not be so severe, and patients with advanced disease are seen with mild or no symptoms. Early in the disease the ovary may become adherent to surrounding structures. With each menstrual period the endometrial implants or endometriomas become active and more blood or pigment is added. This may cause a progressive type dysmenorrhea that is unrelieved by the usual measures. To this may be added menorrhagia or metrorrhagia, particularly if there is adenomyosis. Involvement of the cul-de-sac causes dyspareunia and pain on defecation. Complete obstruction of the rectosigmoid has occurred. Infrequently a large chocolate cyst ruptures and produces an acute abdomen.

The involvement of the urinary and gastrointestinal tracts with endometriosis presents symptoms so specific and management so varied that they are considered separately. I feel that many complaints in the presence of this disease, concerned with the tubes and ovaries, the uterus, and the adjacent connective tissue extensions (ligaments) to the pelvic organs, may have a more logical explanation when direct involvement of bladder or rectum is considered. Diseases not confined to one organ system tend to be interpreted and explained in each speciality in terms of the specific speciality rather than the total effects on the patient. This is wrong. Endometriosis may have its etiology in the genital organs, but its main consequences may be in the urinary or gastrointestinal tract.

Medical Management

Pregnancy is advised when the circumstances permit. This should not be deferred. In addition, the patient should nurse her infant as long as possible to delay the return of menstruation. Symptomatic treatment consists of the use of analgesics and antispasmodic preparations to alleviate the pain and discomfort that increase as the menstrual period approaches. Propadrine hydrochloride, 25 mg., can be combined in a capsule with one or more of the analgesic drugs. Salt restriction and the use of diuretic drugs for premenstrual

357

antihistamine

bloating and tension are useful measures. The hormonal approach to therapy involves the use of massive estrogen therapy or the administration of an androgenic hormone. The success of either form of therapy is probably dependent on the production of an anovulatory cycle, and as long as this is continued the patient has some relief. The exact mechanism by which this occurs is not known, but it probably is the result of a depression of the anterior pituitary gland and an interruption of the follicle-stimulating and luteinizing hormones. Parenteral administration of the hormones is unnecessary, since the same results can be obtained by administration in tablet form. With estrogen therapy any one of several preparations is used. The objective is to start with a small dose to prevent a gastric upset and gradually to increase the schedule until relief is obtained. If the patient has vaginal bleeding, the dosage must again be increased to control the metrorrhagia. With stilbestrol this may be started as 1 mg. three times a day and increased to as high as 50 mg. three times a day over a period of months. The patient may experience some tenderness in the breasts and ankle edema with doses of this magnitude. Androgen therapy is given in the equivalent of 300 mg. of methyltestosterone as a total dose in one month. It is customarily started during menstruation or in the early part of the cycle before ovulation takes place. The patient is observed for signs of masculinization, which is one disturbing factor in this type of therapy. Evaluation of the results of therapy must place strong emphasis on the psychosomatic considerations. Numerous reports show wide variations in the results and enthusiasm of medical management. The symptomatic results must be appraised with proper regard not only for the psychosomatic considerations, but also for the measures and diagnostic means that were used to prove the patient had endometriosis in the beginning.

Progestational Hormones

Another advance in the medical management of endometriosis has resulted from the use of the progestational hormones. The suppression of ovulation and pregnancy simulation by these agents arrests the progress of the disease just as would a normal pregnancy. Some patients tolerate the progestational hormones well regardless of the indication for administration. Others do not. When the side effects of the administration of these hormones do not overweigh the positive benefits, an extended trial is indicated.

The induction of hormonal-controlled, intermittent, withdrawal bleeding has immediate gratifying results in many patients. But what of the patient in her early twenties with bilateral chocolate cysts encroaching on the remnants of her functional ovarian tissue. Just how does this therapy reverse this advance pathologic process? Does this therapy, since it inhibits ovulation, contribute anything to the patient with endometriosis whose objective is to conceive? The patient must conceive during ovulation, and, if this is stopped, her chances are nil. For the patient whose greatest concern is her inability to have children, the relief of pelvic pain is little compensation. She wants to have a child, and the suspension of ovulation for varying periods of time with the anticipation of some rebound phenomenon that suddenly makes her more fertile has yet to be proved.

Indications and Surgical Principles

Surgery is undertaken when the severity of symptoms cannot be controlled by medical management or when the progression of the disease suggests it may permanently damage vital structures. The fundamental point in the management of this disease is the fact that the adherent endometrium, like the lining of the uterus itself, is controlled by the ovary. Therefore, as long as functional ovarian tissue remains, regardless of the presence or absence of the uterus, there can be persistence and extension of the process. The absence of the uterus may slow down the rate of progression of the disease, but it has not been conclusively shown that the presence of the uterus is necessary for survival of endometrial implants. Even though both ovaries are reduced to the state of thin-walled chocolate cysts, a young woman is not castrated. The shell of an ovary can be preserved in the most advanced cases, and not infrequently the patient will menstruate and conceive in defiance of what appears to be extensive pelvic involvement. One result of surgery, difficult to prove statistically, is the apparent increase in fertility following the resection of endometrial implants. Where midline dysmenorrhea, particularly radiating into the hollow of the sacrum and into the rectum, is a prominent symptom, a prelumbar sympathectomy is done as an essential part of a conservative operation. It is not expected that this will relieve all of the symptoms from areas that are not denervated. If it appears that the uterus will fall back in the cul-de-sac and become adherent, the round ligaments can be shortened by one method or another. How much this contributes to the relief of pain or the prevention of any recurrence of the disease is questionable. Even the most enthusiastic exponents of the regurgitation theory hesitate to indict a retroverted uterus as responsible for the spillage of endometrium fragments into the peritoneal cavity.

The *uterine nerve block test* provides additional information for prognosticating the results of a lysis of the uterosacral ligaments. Indirectly it indicates the pain relief that may be expected from a prelumbar sympathectomy. During the height of a patient's dysmenorrhea, with all medication and supportive measures withheld, the uterosacral ligaments and base of the cardinal ligaments are infiltrated with 1 per cent Xylocaine or procaine. About 5 ml. are injected on each side after raising a wheal over the ligaments in the vaginal wall of the posterior fornix. The patient who will be appreciatively benefited by surgery experiences almost complete relief of pain for several hours, and some patients remain relatively symptom-free for the remainder of their menstrual cycle.

PRELUMBAR SYMPATHECTOMY
(Presacral Sympathectomy or Neurectomy, Superior Hypogastric Sympathectomy)
Surgical Anatomy

The presacral plexus is not presacral in location. On the lateral wall of the abdominal aorta from the superior mesenteric trunk to the inferior mesenteric artery are seen the intermesenteric nerves. They have frequent oblique anastomoses from side to side and receive branches from the lumbar sympathetic chains. At the level of origin of the inferior mesenteric artery, two plexuses are formed: the inferior mesenteric plexus and the presacral plexus. The presacral plexus lies entirely on the lower border of the fourth lumbar vertebra, the intervertebral disc, and the fifth lumbar vertebra. It is misnamed and should be called the prelumbar plexus.

An easily definable trigone is formed by the two common iliac arteries as the sides and the promontory of the sacrum as the base. The apex of this trigone is the bifurcation of the aorta. The common iliac veins are under their respective arteries, with the right vein lateral to the artery and the left almost parallel to its artery at the level of the promontory. The prelumbar plexus lies in this trigone under the peritoneum and over the middle sacral artery and its homonymous veins. In this location the subperitoneal connective tissue, ordinarily loose and areolar, becomes compact and thicker, binding the nerves together. They are easily separated from the periosteum, peritoneum, and vessels because of this. The ureters cross the lateral aspect of the interiliac trigone near its base. The right ureter is easily identifiable, but the left is hidden by the pelvic mesocolon (Plate 56, *A* and *B*).

The prelumbar plexus has many variations. Elaut, after studying the plexuses of fifty cadavers, found four principal types. The most common was a plexus type (58 per cent), the second, a single nerve type (24 per cent), the third, a parallel type (16 per cent), and the fourth, an arch-shaped type (2 per cent). The implantation and position of the pelvic mesocolon are variable and depend on the length of the sigmoid. Between the leaves of the mesocolon pass the sigmoidal arteries and the superior hemorrhoidal artery, that is, the terminal branch of the inferior mesenteric artery. Usually the pelvic mesocolon implants on the left upper surface of the sacrum and arches gently over the promontory toward the right.

It thus covers the left ureter at this point and also the left common iliac artery and vein. It may rarely extend to the right of the aorta. The implantation and position of the pelvic mesocolon are carefully studied in this operation and the many variations appreciated (Plate 56, *A*). Note the position of the superior hemorrhoidal and sigmoid vessels as they lie over the field of operation and the left common iliac vein and artery. I have only once had to be satisfied with an incomplete presacral neurectomy. In this patient the technical difficulties prevented complete resection. At the age of 5 years she had had a hernia repair of a left indirect inguinal hernia, in the sac of which was incarcerated left tube and ovary that were inadvertently removed. At the age of 21 she had severe dysmenorrhea, more on the right, with midline pain and backache. Urologic studies revealed a left pelvic kidney, small but with some function, and no hydronephrosis. At operation the pelvic kidney had a substantial amount of parenchyma—more than was presumed on x-ray—and a contemplated nephrectomy was not done. The blood supply to this ectopic kidney prevented a thorough neurectomy except with undue risk to the patient. The vessels to the kidney arose from the bifurcation of the aorta and passed directly over the fifth lumbar vertebra and promontory. The superior hemorrhoidal artery crossed anterior to the renal artery and vein but was almost in the midline. Two sigmoidal arteries passed over the ectopic kidney, that lay on the sacro-iliac synchrondrosis, to enter the colon. The sigmoidal arteries and the superior hemorrhoidal artery were retracted from their beds without difficulty. The renal vessels were short and could be partially mobilized. It was possible to resect most of the plexus but not the portions on the patient's extreme left without a rather difficult nephrectomy and possible damage to the aorta and vena cava. This, together with the realization that the pelvic kidney was functional and otherwise normal, led to abandonment of the resection of the nerves on the left side.

Indications and Surgical Principles

A prelumbar sympathectomy is indicated for intractable dysmenorrhea of the midline type, particularly with radiation of pain to the sacrum and accompanied by low backache. The degree of disability that warrants this procedure is such that the patient is unable to do her work and is confined to bed for several days during the course of menstruation. She may have nausea, vomiting, and fainting spells at intervals. Menstrual pain that is lateral or ovarian in origin is not helped by the procedure. The mechanism of relief is not clearly understood by neurologists. It is probable that the operation interrupts afferent pain fibers in the superior hypogastric plexus, while efferent vasoconstricting fibers are also interrupted. The latter possibly produce some type of vasoconstriction of the uterus that results in dysmenorrhea. The operation may be combined with a lysis of the infundibulo-pelvic pedicle and resection of fibers in the broad ligament to give some relief from ovarian pain. A periarterial sympathectomy of the ovarian arteries has been suggested by some surgeons. This is technically difficult in an artery of this size. Follow-up of patients who have had a lysis of the infundibulopelvic pedicles has not revealed any deleterious effect upon the ovaries. Resection of the superior hypogastric plexus in the female has no deleterious effects on libido or bladder function. The uterus does not become engorged because of the interruption of the efferent vasoconstrictive fibers. The psychosomatic aspects are carefully weighed. A patient will, of course, have had considerable general medical and supportive therapy, including attention to water retention and the use of various antispasmodic drugs, before surgery is considered. Two cycles of the menstrual period should be interrupted by large doses of estrogenic substance or testosterone. If the induction of these anovulatory cycles is accompanied by pain or pain with withdrawal bleeding after estrogenic therapy, it is probable that the psychosomatic aspects of the disease are playing a prominent part.

Too much stress cannot be laid on the variability of the presacral plexus. When the bulk of the nerve tissue is in the midline over the fifth lumbar vertebra, a thorough resection of all the fibers can be done. The extensive stretching of nerve elements over the promontory of the sacrum necessitates that the dissection be carried down to the periosteum to remove all the fibers. Some factors work in the operator's favor. The usually loose, areolar, subperitoneal connective tissue becomes rather compact in the region of the plexus. This holds the nerves together like a webbed foot and permits the operator to raise the plexus from the periosteum in a fan-shaped ensemble or flat ribbon (Plate 56, B).

Steps of the Operation

1. A preliminary dilatation and curettage are done as is customary with most gynecologic procedures. The incision preferred is a right rectus incision, with the operator working from the patient's right side. However, the operation can be performed with any number of incisions that allow access to the bifurcation of the aorta. After the pelvis has been explored and other corrective surgery in the pelvis performed, including preliminary preparations for a uterine suspension in a retroverted, retroflexed, adherent uterus, the bowel is packed well away in the upper abdomen. The bifurcation of the aorta, plus an area at least 5 to 6 cm. cephalad to this, is exposed.

2. If the appendix has not been removed, this is done at this time. The position of the appendix may necessitate some mobilization of the cecum to perform the appendectomy, and this will further expose the right lateral margin of the operative field for the neurectomy.

3. The surgeon studies the implantation and position of the pelvic mesocolon. Depending on his findings, the posterior peritoneum is incised in the midline for a variable distance above and below the promontory of the sacrum. This incision is curved to the right when the sigmoid mesocolon is unusually long or extends across the midline of the aorta.

4. The peritoneum, together with its subperitoneal connective tissue, is elevated. The condensation of connective tissue in the plexus will hold it together; however, the underside of the peritoneum is inspected for any nerve fibers elevated with the parietal peritoneum during this phase of the operation.

5. The right ureter is retracted to the right by means of a vein retractor, and when the position of the ureter is accurately ascertained, a traction suture is placed on the edge of the peritoneum and left to hang over the side of the patient in order to facilitate the exposure (Plate 56, A).

6. Beginning as far laterally as any nerve fibers can be identified, the nerves of the plexus are dissected from the surface of the aorta and inferior vena cava and drawn toward the midline. This not infrequently results in the inclusion of the lower lumbar sympathetic ganglion. This may have a transient effect on the temperature in the legs but no serious consequences in the female as compared with a male who might have some impairment of sexual function after sympathectomy at this level.

7. The terminal branches of the inferior mesenteric artery are identified and, by gentle traction, they are lifted laterally without compromising the supply to the bowel. The operator is constantly alert for the presence of anomalous vessels. Vessels that are inadvertently opened are clamped and tied immediately so that the field of operation is not cluttered with clamps. In Plate 56, A, is shown the dissection of the root of the sigmoid mesentery. The lowermost sigmoidal artery and also the superior hemorrhoidal artery can be seen. While interruption of these arteries to control bleeding would probably not interfere with the circulation to the bowel, it is best to preserve them rather than to have to deal with any bowel complications. If they are cut and tied off, the sigmoid colon is observed for a period of time to note that the collateral circulation is maintaining the viability of the bowel.

8. By the alternate use of angle clamps, Metzenbaum scissors, and small peanut sponges, the nerve fibers are teased away from the left common iliac artery and vein. They are brought to the midline in one mass, with the remainder of the plexus dissected from the right side (Plate 56, B).

9. At the completion of this dissection the left ureter, which has heretofore been protected by the root of the sigmoid mesentery, will come into view (Plate 56, B). The ureter is retracted as needed to complete the dissection.

10. The plexus is then elevated from the periosteum of the fifth lumbar vertebra beyond the promontory of the sacrum (Plate 56, B). In doing so, the middle sacral artery and several of

PLATE 56

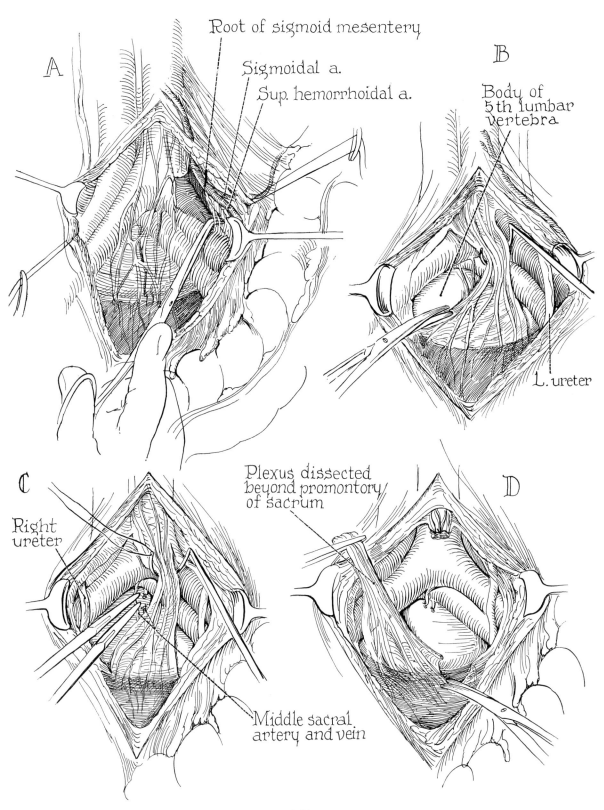

A

Root of sigmoid mesentery

Sigmoidal a.

Sup. hemorrhoidal a.

B

Body of 5th lumbar vertebra

L. ureter

C

Right ureter

Plexus dissected beyond promontory of sacrum

D

Middle sacral artery and vein

its accompanying veins may be opened (Plate 56, C). These can be controlled by compression until the plexus is completely elevated, after which they are specifically tied off.

11. An aneurysm needle is passed underneath the plexus and a ligature of medium silk drawn through (Plate 56, C). This is tied 3 or 4 cm. above the bifurcation of the aorta and the plexus resected just distal to the tie. In Plate 56, C, the middle sacral artery and vein are being ligated close to their origins from the bifurcation of the aorta and the origin of the inferior vena cava.

12. The upper end of the plexus is used for traction and drawn anteriorly (Plate 56, D). All of the nerve fibers are dissected free down to the periosteum and beyond the promontory of the sacrum. When the point is reached where the plexus is dividing to form the two hypogastric plexuses, a medium silk ligature is placed around the plexus and the bundle of nerves resected proximal to this ligature. The field is inspected for hemostasis and the parietal peritoneum closed by a running suture of plain catgut or by interrupted sutures of fine black silk.

13. The entire bundle of nerves is sent to the laboratory with a request that the pathologist section the specimen transversely and roughly count the number of large nerve bundles included.

Postoperative Care

The operation itself requires no special postoperative care. Orders for catheterization are left, since patients may have a retention of urine for the first twenty-four to thirty-six hours. Should they have a large amount of residual urine for several days, appropriate antibiotic therapy is administered. Prolonged bladder dysfunction is rare following prelumbar nerve resection.

ENDOMETRIOSIS OF BLADDER AND URETER

Many of the symptoms of pelvic endometriosis are due to involvement of the urinary tract. Review of several large groups of patients with proved endometriosis shows that, when such minor involvement such as implants on the bladder peritoneum are recorded, about 40 per cent of patients can be said to have urinary tract lesions. This may seem high, but one must also consider the number of urinary tract lesions that are missed because of inadequate urologic work-up of the patient.

Etiology and Pathologic Anatomy

Reflux of viable endometrial cells from the tubes probably accounts for the implants on the bladder peritoneum and over the pelvic ureters. Patients with urinary tract involvement will also be found to have had previous pelvic surgery more frequently than those without this complication. Endometriomas of the bladder or ureter may occur from direct extension of the process in the paracervical and parauterine connective tissue. Retrograde lymphatic metastases to the bladder wall through the common lymphatic channels probably occur especially when a seemingly isolated endometrioma is found some distance from other lesions.

Involvement of the vesicovaginal septum by direct implantation after vaginal hysterotomy for prophylactic abortion has been repeatedly demonstrated. Pelvic endometriosis is not uncommon after an abdominal hysterotomy in which endometrial or decidual cells are spilled during the operation.

Symptoms and Diagnosis

The patient frequently gives a history of previous pelvic surgery. A positive diagnosis of endometriosis may or may not have been made at that time. The signs and symptoms tend to be cyclic and increase in intensity toward the latter half of the menstrual cycle. Cyclic frequency, dysuria, hematuria, and suprapubic pain should prompt the surgeon to perform a complete urologic work-up. Involvement of the ureter gives rise to cyclic pain radiating into the groin and medial aspect of the thigh. Should obstructive urinary tract disease with hydroureter, hydronephrosis, or pyelonephritis develop, the symptoms and signs common to these conditions are found. The location of the lesions rather than the extent of the disease frequently determines the severity of the urologic symptoms.

On bimanual examination nodules may be felt in the vesicovaginal septum. If the patient is examined in the immediate premenstrual period, these nodules may be distinctly more tender than they were earlier in the cycle. Palpation of nodules in the cardinal and uterosacral connective tissue extensions and the thickening and retraction of these structures may confirm a suspicion of ureteral involvement on one side or the other. The patient may have evidence of widespread involvement of the adnexae in conjunction with the findings relative to the urinary tract. With extensive disease the pelvis may be frozen with the uterus adherent and the tubes and ovaries firmly adherent to the pelvic side walls or posterior sheath of the broad ligament.

Cystoscopy and urography may confirm the diagnosis. Very few lesions penetrate through the bladder mucosa and give frank hematuria during menstruation. However, lesions that have deeply involved the musculature close to the mucosa have a suggestive appearance that, I am sure, is frequently interpreted as varicosities in the bladder base. Cystic areas in a bladder endometrioma filled with old menstrual blood, as magnified by the cystoscope, are easily mistaken for dilated veins. Just before menstruation the raised, congested endometrioma projects into the bladder with a granular, irregular surface interrupted by small blue-domed cysts surrounded by the typical, dark, powderburn effects caused by lesions just underneath the transitional epithelium of the bladder.

Surgical Principles

If the patient is to be castrated, there is rarely any problem concerning the urinary tract lesions. Occasionally, an obstructive endometrioma of the ureter might have to be resected to preserve the kidney. Subsequently, the lesions after bilateral oophorectomy become quiescent and, unless responding to extra-ovarian sources of estrogen, become inactive. Where the menstrual function and the childbearing function are to be preserved, this is a complex problem.

No one ever duplicates the remarkable results of the pure endocrinologist without surgical background. It is worth a trial, but how eight or even twelve months of suppression of ovulation and a substitution of with-

drawal bleeding by the use of the progestational hormones are going to reverse advanced lesions of the urinary tract is not quite clear. The retraction of the surrounding tissues, the fibrosis in response to the ectopic endometrium and its stroma, the distortion of the ureter in particular, all may be considered damage done. Isolated, nonobstructive lesions will remain quiescent. But what does one do when the patient wishes to menstruate again or have children? The patients must be individualized, and, where the induction of anovulatory, withdrawal bleeding-type cycles by hormones is felt to only postpone the inevitable surgical approach, the latter should be done as soon as possible to prevent further destruction of normal tissues. In the urinary tract this would be manifested in the case of obstructive disease by repeated urinary tract infections.

An endometrioma of the bladder is removed by a segmental resection of the bladder. At the same time the pelvis is explored, and any coincident lesions resected. Endometriosis of the ureter as a result of contiguous spread requires mobilization and release from the tissues causing obstruction. Rarely, an endometrioma of the wall of the pelvic ureter may require resection and end-to-end anastomosis. A segmental resection of the bladder is illustrated to show some of the urinary complications of this disease.

SEGMENTAL RESECTION OF THE BLADDER
Steps of the Operation

1. The vesicouterine reflection of peritoneum is identified preparatory to mobilizing the bladder base (Plate 57, *A*). With a lesion in the bladder base the ureters should be catheterized either cystoscopically or directly after performing a cystotomy. In Plate 57, *A,* the right uterine artery is ligated to mobilize more adequately the right ureter and retract it out of the field of operation.

2. A preliminary cystotomy is done to directly ascertain the extent of the lesion (Plate 57, *B*). This incision can then be extended to the bladder base to excise the endometrioma. Plate 57, *B,* shows both ureters exposed and the lesion as it appears from the outside of the bladder. In this patient it was immediately adjacent to the intramural ureter.

Text continued on p. 370.

PLATE 57

SEGMENTAL RESECTION OF THE BLADDER

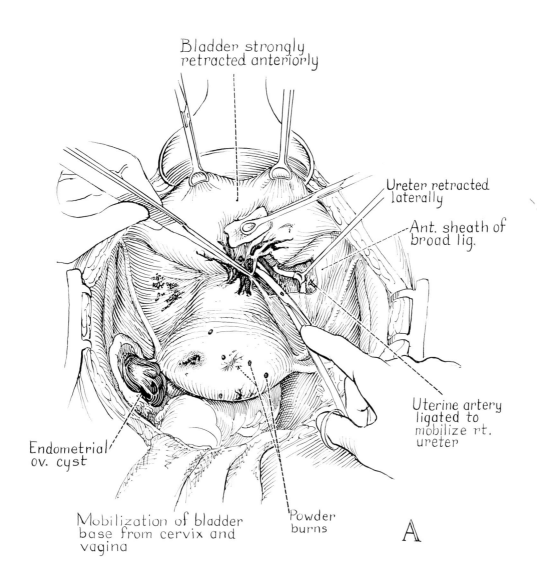

Bladder strongly
retracted anteriorly

Ureter retracted
laterally

Ant. sheath of
broad lig.

Uterine artery
ligated to
mobilize rt.
ureter

Endometrial
ov. cyst

Mobilization of bladder
base from cervix and
vagina

Powder
burns

A

PLATE 57 (Continued)

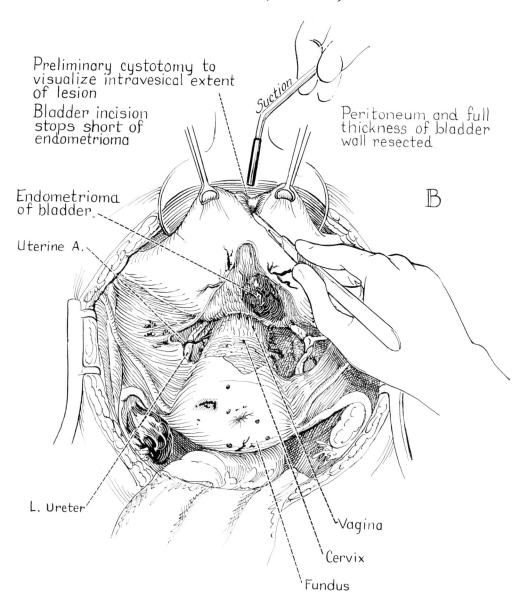

Preliminary cystotomy to
visualize intravesical extent
of lesion
Bladder incision
stops short of
endometrioma

Suction

Peritoneum and full
thickness of bladder
wall resected

Endometrioma
of bladder

B

Uterine A.

L. Ureter

Vagina

Cervix

Fundus

PLATE 57 (Continued)

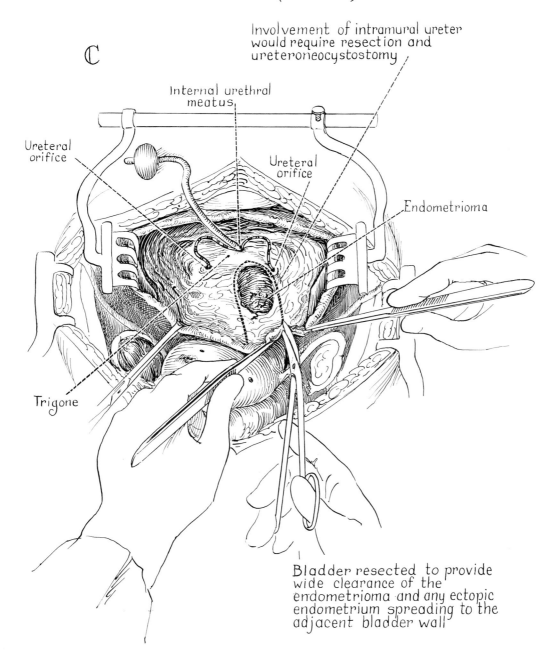

C

Involvement of intramural ureter would require resection and ureteroneocystostomy

Internal urethral meatus

Ureteral orifice

Ureteral orifice

Endometrioma

Trigone

Bladder resected to provide wide clearance of the endometrioma and any ectopic endometrium spreading to the adjacent bladder wall

PLATE 57 (Continued)

Flap of bladder retracted to identify
and protect the intramural ureter during
the resection

D

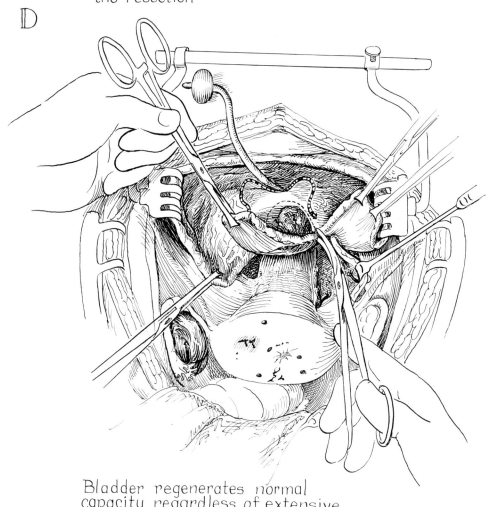

Bladder regenerates normal
capacity regardless of extensive
resection

PLATE 57 (Concluded)

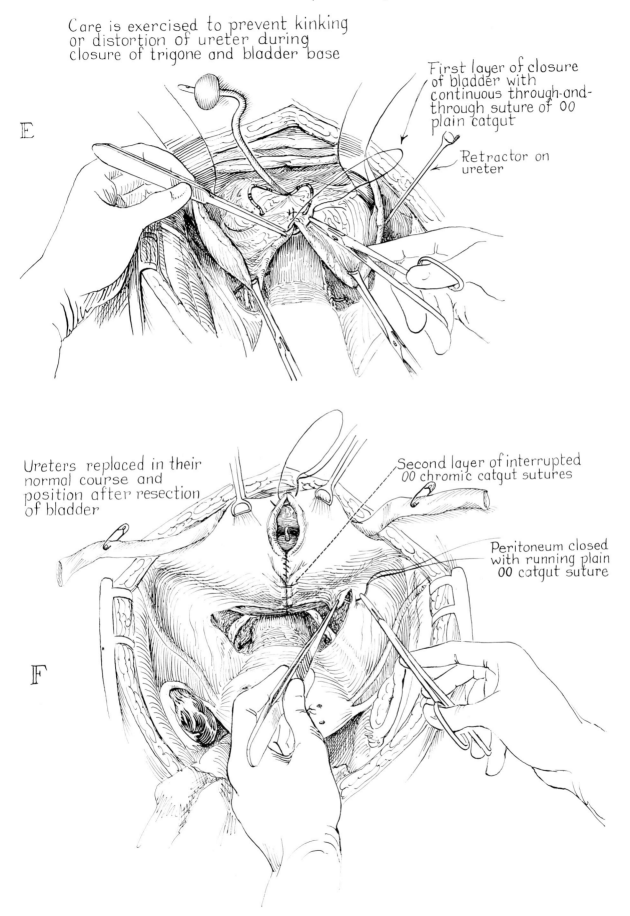

Care is exercised to prevent kinking or distortion of ureter during closure of trigone and bladder base

E

First layer of closure of bladder with continuous through-and-through suture of 00 plain catgut

Retractor on ureter

Ureters replaced in their normal course and position after resection of bladder

F

Second layer of interrupted 00 chromic catgut sutures

Peritoneum closed with running plain 00 catgut suture

3. The bladder base is widely exposed, and the anterolateral walls retracted (Plate 57, C). The full thickness of the bladder wall is resected with adequate clearance of the lesion. If the intramural ureter is involved, it is resected with the lesion and a ureteroneocystostomy performed.

4. The ureteral catheter inserted in the right ureter is palpated frequently to determine proximity of the intramural ureter to the line of resection. The bladder will regenerate a normal capacity regardless of the extent of the resection (Plate 57, D).

5. A through-and-through suture of 00 plain catgut is used to close the bladder wall. During the closure, care is exercised to prevent kinking or distortion of the ureter (Plate 57, E). One or more continuous sutures may be needed for the first layer if the bladder has been widely opened.

6. A second layer of 00 interrupted sutures of chromic catgut is used to reinforce the first layer. The ureters now fall into their normal bed (Plate 57, F). The peritoneum of the anterior sheath of the broad ligament and the vesicouterine reflexion is closed with a running suture of 00 plain catgut.

7. When the endometrioma is in the bladder base, as was the case in the patient from whom the artist drew the illustrations, a suprapubic cystostomy is the preferred method of drainage. However, if the incisions in a given case are in such a position that the indwelling urethral catheter would not rest on them, this route may be used.

8. One or more drains are placed in the lateral recesses of the space of Retzius. The wound is closed in layers.

Postoperative Care

The ureteral catheters are removed before the patient goes to the recovery room. The surgeon may elect to leave one or the other as a splinting catheter if a ureter had to be anastomosed or transplanted. The cystostomy catheter is connected to straight drainage and irrigated as often as necessary to remove clots of blood. It may be removed on or about the eighth postoperative day. Urinary antiseptics known to control any organisms cultured preoperatively are administered. If the urine had been sterile preoperatively, one antibacterial agent, either of the sulfonamide group or wide-spectrum antibiotic group, is given prophy-

lactically. The drains are removed either on the first or second postoperative day, depending on the amount of drainage. An intravenous pyelogram is done on the fourth or fifth postoperative day to confirm the status of the urinary tract.

ENDOMETRIOSIS OF THE GASTROINTESTINAL TRACT
Introduction

Endometriosis of the gastrointestinal tract was reported shortly after the turn of the century by Robert Meyer. Patients with obstruction of both large and small bowel by endometrial implants were recognized. Gynecologists and radiologists are alert to this possibility when a female patient in the childbearing age group presents herself with cyclic gastrointestinal symptoms.

Etiology and Pathologic Anatomy

The theories of origin and spread of the disease have been discussed, but nowhere does Sampson's theory of tubal regurgitation find greater support. The majority of lesions involving the gastrointestinal tract are in the cul-de-sac of Douglas where viable cells extruded from the tube would be expected to lodge. Further, in the cul-de-sac there are opposing peritoneal surfaces for the nutrition of such transplanted cells.

The gross lesions are usually puckered areas of scarring with purplish discoloration secondary to pigment deposition. Small, blood-filled cysts may be seen among bowel adhesions. Diffuse **mulberry spots** or **powder burns** may be observed on many lopes of bowel. The lesions may be nodular and approach a cartilaginous consistency due to fibrous tissue. Contraction of these lesions is the cause of partial or occasionally complete bowel obstruction. These nodules may resemble carcinoma grossly but grow from the serosal surface inward, seldom reaching the mucosa of the bowel.

Symptoms and Diagnosis

A history of previous pelvic surgery, especially if a positive diagnosis of endometriosis had been made, should alert the surgeon investigating a patient with cyclic gastrointestinal symptoms. The most common symptom is pain occurring immediately prior to or during menses. The location is deep in the midline or the lower abdomen although pain in the lower lumbar area and sacrum is frequently found. Bowel malfunction of various degrees is common. Pain at stool, constipation, diarrhea, and abdominal distention worsening premenstrually is pathognomic of extensive endometriosis involving the bowel. Cyclical rectal bleeding is a rarity since the process seldom passes the barrier of the rectal mucosa.

Obstruction of the small or large intestines is manifested by the signs and symptoms of obstruction by this or other diseases. Abdominal pain, nausea, vomiting, dehydration, paralytic ileus, and shock would be seen with a sudden acute obstruction high in the small bowel. The onset of symptoms of obstruction would be less acute with the more common obstructions of the sigmoid colon.

Pelvic examination almost always reveals convincing evidence of endometriosis. The uterosacral ligaments may be nodular and fixed, the adnexa adherent, or the pelvis frozen by widespread disease. Annular constricting lesions at the level of the peritoneal reflexion in the cul-de-sac of Douglas may prevent passage of a sigmoidoscope past this level. The barium enema and gastrointestinal study may show the lesion which, combined with other evidence of endometriosis, confirms the diagnosis. On roentgenologic examination the lesions may simulate those of primary carcinoma or chronic perforation of a diverticulum of the colon. The significant findings are an intact mucosa, fixation of the segment of the bowel to the surrounding bowel or omentum (since this is a lesion starting on the serosa rather than the mucosa), a concentric stenosing lesion, and involvement of the bowel relatively short in length and sharply demarcated. This extraluminal origin of the lesion reflects these differences radiologically from carcinoma of the colon.

Medical and Surgical Principles of Treatment

Acute obstruction of the bowel requires emergency measures just as obstruction from other causes. After the bowel lesion has been dealt with, the patient's age and desires regarding the menstrual and reproductive functions are considered. In general, once having encountered symptomatic involvement of the bowel, the surgeon would tend to be more radical. When the genital functions must be preserved, the lesions on the bowel are resected or the bowel itself resected, the major cysts and implants removed from the ovaries and other structures, and the patient treated medically with the progestational hormones for six to eight months postoperatively.

Should a subacute obstructive lesion of the bowel exist in a patient in whom the genital organs must be preserved, the question of resection of the lesion and closure of the bowel to enlarge the lumen or bowel resection with end-to-end anastomosis may arise. With the anticipation of ovarian stimulation at some time in the future in most instances, it is well to remove the endometriotic lesion completely by bowel resection.

References

Allen, M., Lowell, F., and Campbell, Z.: Clinical and Experimental Endometriosis, Am. J. Obst. & Gynec. 68: 356, 1954.

Androutsopoulos, N. A., and Sommers, S. C.: Postmenopausal Endometriosis, Obst. & Gynec. 14: 245, 1959.

Antoine, T.: The Hormonal Dependency of Endometriosis, (La regulation hormonale de l'endometiose), Bull. féd. soc. gynéc. et obst. 133: 12, 1960.

Baldwin, R. M., Whalley, P. J., and Pritchard, J. A.: Measurements of Menstrual Blood Loss, Am. J. Obst. & Gynec. 81: 739, 1961.

Beahrs, O. H., Hunter, J. S., and Sloss, P. T.: Intramural, Obstructing Endometriosis of the Ureter, Proc. Staff Meeting, Mayo Clin. 32: 73, 1957.

Brewer, J., and Maher, F.: Conservatism in Endometriosis, Am. J. Obst. & Gynec. 68: 549, 1954.

Chamblin, W. D., and Corbit, J. D.: Chlorpromazine and Chlorpromazine Combinations in the Treatment of Dysmenorrhea, Am. J. Obst. & Gynec. 73: 419, 1957.

Chinn, J., Horton, R. K., and Rusche, C.: Unilateral Ureteral Obstruction as Sole Manifestation of Endometriosis, Tr. West. Sect. Am. Urol. A. 23: 174, 1956.

Culver, G. J., Pereira, R. M., and Seibel, R.: Radiographic Features of Rectosigmoid Endometriosis, Am. J. Obst. & Gynec. 76: 1176, 1958.

Doyle, J.: Paracervical Uterine Denervation by Transection of the Cervical Plexus for the Relief of Dysmenorrhea, Am. J. Obst. & Gynec. 70: 1, 1955.

Duson, C., and Zelenik, J.: Vulvar Endometriosis, Obst. & Gynec. 3: 76, 1954.

Elaut, L.: The Surgical Anatomy of the So-called Presacral Nerve, Surg., Gynec. & Obst. 55: 581, 1932.

Felson, H., McGuire, J., and Wasserman, P.: Stromal Endometriosis Involving the Heart, Am. J. Med. 29: 1072, 1960.

Gardner, G. H., Greene, R. R., and Ranney, B.: The Histogenesis of Endometriosis, Am. J. Obst. & Gynec. 78: 445, 1959.

Goldenberg, I. S., and Alderman, D. B.: Neurofibroma Following Presacral Neurectomy, Am. J. Obst. & Gynec. 76: 1204, 1958.

Golub, L. J., Menduke, H., and Lang, W. R.: Semi-objective Criteria of Teen-Age Dysmenorrhea, Obst. & Gynec. 14: 179, 1959.

Golub, L. J., and others: Therapeutic Exercises for Teen-Age Dysmenorrhea, Am. J. Obst. & Gynec. 76: 670, 1958.

Gottlieb, T.: Endometriosis in the Vaginal Scar Following Hysterotomy for Therapeutic Abortion, Acta obst. et gynec. scandinav. 36: 194, 1957.

Halban, J.: Hysteroadenosis metastatica. Die lymphogene Genese der sogenannten Adenofibromatosis heterotopica, Arch. F. Gynäk. 124: 457, 1925.

Hood, W. E., and Bond, W. L.: Enovid Therapy for Premenstrual Tension, Obst. & Gynec. 14: 239, 1959.

Javert, C. T.: Spread of Benign and Malignant Endometrium in Lymphatic System With Note on Co-existing Vascular Involvement, Am. J. Obst. & Gynec. 64: 780, 1952.

Johnson, C. G., Coppola, A. F., and Moll, C. F.: Complications of Endometriosis of the Sigmoid Colon, South. M. J. 50: 893, 1957.

Jungck, E. C., Barfield, W. E., and Greenblatt, R. B.: Chlorothiazide and Premenstrual Tension, J. A. M. A. 169: 112, 1959.

Kempers, R., and others: Significant Postmenopausal Endometriosis, Surg., Gynec. & Obst. 111: 348, 1960.

Kirkland, J. A.: Abdominal Menstrual Fistula, Am. J. Obst. & Gynec. 78: 1292, 1959.

Kistner, R. W.: Conservative Therapy for Endometriosis, Postgrad. Med. 24: 505, 1958.

Kistner, R. W.: The Use of Newer Progestins in the Treatment of Endometriosis, Am. J. Obst. & Gynec. 75: 264, 1958.

Kohout, E.: Mucocele of the Appendix Caused by Endometriosis, Am. J. Obst. & Gynec. 15: 1181, 1960.

Lane, R. E.: Endometriosis of the Vermiform Appendix, J. Urol. 79: 372, 1958.

Lash, S. R., and Rubenstone, A. I.: Adenocarcinoma of the Rectovaginal Septum Probably Arising From Endometriosis, Am. J. Obst. & Gynec. 78: 445, 1959.

Lebherz, T. B., and Fobes, C. D.: Management of Endometriosis With Nor-Progesterone, Am. J. Obst. & Gynec. 81: 102, 1961.

Lichtenheld, F. R., McCauley, R. T., and Staples, P.: Endometriosis Involving the Urinary Tract; a Collective Review, Obst. & Gynec. 17: 762, 1961.

MacFarlane, C. A., and others: Urological Complications of stromal Endometriosis, J. Urol. 79: 436, 1958.

McGavack, T. H., and others: The Treatment of Premenstrual Tension With a Combination of an Antihistaminic and a Theophylline Derivative, Am. J. Obst. & Gynec. 72: 416, 1956.

Niswander, K. R.: Inguinal Endometriosis; Report of Two Cases, Am. J. Obst. & Gynec. 75: 279, 1958.

Novak, E. R., and Hoge, A. F.: Endometriosis of the Lower Genital Tract, Obst. & Gynec. 12: 687, 1958.

Overton, D. H., Wilson, R. B., and Dockerty, M. B.: Primary Endometriosis of the Cervix, Am. J. Obst. & Gynec. 79: 768, 1960.

Paulson, M. J.: Psychological Concomitants of Premenstrual Tension, Am. J. Obst. & Gynec. 81: 733, 1961.

Phaneuf, L.: Presacral Neurectomy in Intractable Dysmenorrhea, J. Mt. Sinai Hosp. 14: 553, 1947.

Roddick, J. W., Conkey, G., and Jacobs, E. J.: The Hormonal Response of Endometrium in Endometriotic Implants and Its Relationship to Symptomatology, Am. J. Obst. & Gynec. 79: 1173, 1960.

Sampson, J. A.: Ovarian Hematomas of Endometrial Type (Perforating Hemorrhagic Cysts of the Ovary) and Implantation Adenomas of Endometrial Type, Boston M. & S. J. 186: 445, 1922.

Scott, R.: Malignant Changes in Endometriosis, Obst. & Gynec. 2: 283, 1953.

Scott, R., TeLinde, R., and Wharton, L., Jr.: Further Studies on Experimental Endometriosis, Am. J. Obst. & Gynec. 66: 1082, 1953.

Scott, R., and Wharton, L., Jr.: The Effects of Excessive Amounts of Diethylstilbestrol on Experiment Endometriosis in Monkeys, Am. J. Obst. & Gynec. 69: 573, 1955.

Svennerud, S.: Dysmenorrhoea and Absenteeism, Acta obst. et gynec. scandinav. 38: 6, 1959.

Taylor, H.: Pelvic Pain Based on a Vascular and Autonomic Nervous System Disorder, Am. J. Obst. & Gynec. 67: 1177, 1954.

Taymor, M. L.: Laboratory and Clinical Effects of Nortestosterone. II. The Endometrial Response, Am. J. Obst. & Gynec. 81: 95, 1961.

Voulgaris, D. M.: Dysmenorrhea: Treatment With Isoxsuprine, Obst. & Gynec. 15: 220, 1960.

Wickman, W., and Lamphier, T. A.: The Present Status of Endometriosis, Postgrad. Med. 23: 598, 1958.

Wolfe, S. A.: Endometriosis of the Vagina, Obst. & Gynec. 15: 612, 1960.

Wolfe, S. A., Mackles, A., and Green, H. J.: Endometriosis of the Cervix; Classification and Analysis of 17 Cases, Am. J. Obst. & Gynec. 81: 111, 1961.

Section VIII · MALIGNANT TUMORS, RADIATION, and RADICAL SURGERY

20 · Experimental Gynecologic Cancer and Virus Studies

The induction of tumors of the female genital tract of laboratory animals was studied shortly after the carcinogenic properties of crude tar were recognized. Recognition of the benzanthracene nucleus led to the synthesis of many related compounds with active carcinogenic properties. Synthetic and physiologically produced estrogens were found to have carcinogenic action limited to the genital organs and accessory tissues such as the breasts. While the immediate clinical usefulness of these studies may not be apparent or may seem far distant, gynecologists should be familiar with the step-by-step progress of cancer research.

Recent studies by von Haam and Scarpelli, that compare the cytology and histology of experimentally induced cervical cancer in C3H mice, shed interesting data on the perennial argument as to whether intraepithelial carcinoma of the cervix is a precursor of the invasive type. Their cancers were induced by painting the cervix of the mice twice weekly with 3,4-benzpyrene, 1 per cent, in acetone. A cotton-tipped wire loop, conforming to the axis of the vagina, was used to reach the cervix. They found that a cervical cancer produced in this manner, in this strain of mice, was characterized by four definite stages, leading to an invasive tumor when such occurred: (1) acute and chronic inflammation, (2) epithelial dysplasia, (3) noninvasive cancer, and (4) invasive carcinoma. Cytologic studies during the induction of cervical malignancies of this type and under these conditions showed the development of invasive cancer to progress from epithelial dysplasia to carcinoma in situ and finally to tumors fulfilling all the requirements of malignancy. The individual cells of a noninvasive cancer could not be distinguished from those invading the stroma.

HeLa, a rapidly dividing hypotetraploid stock of human epithelial cells derived from a carcinoma of the cervix, is characterized by a high frequency of abnormal mitoses. Moorhead and Hsu, studying this strain by means of time-lapse, phase contrast cinematography, found a positive correlation between increased duration of mitotic time and aberrancy. While there was a wide spread in plotting the data, such studies give the clinician pause to consider, since one always thinks of cancer as growing wildly and the adjacent tissue remaining comparatively static. In contrast to these observations on the HeLa strain, Grand and Ayre have studied the behavior of cervical neoplastic cells by tissue culture methods and conclude that the more anaplastic the cervical tissue cells, the greater their activity in culture and the shorter the time for epithelial cell migration and cell division. These contrasting observations are probably the result of variables in the experiments and technique but are significant when one considers the importance of the observations, which, when repeated and the basic facts established, will have an enormous influence on the management of the disease clinically.

The role of viruses in cancer has been the subject of speculation and research for decades. Recently the effectiveness of viruses in destroying cancer has come under investigation. Studies in progress at the National Institutes of Health have shown the ability of APC viruses (adenoidal, pharyngeal, conjunctival) to partially destroy cervical cancer. Prior to this, several workers learned that APC viruses grown in HeLa cells could destroy the host. The viruses were injected directly into the cervical lesion, with partial destruction of the malignant mass. It appears that antibodies soon develop and terminate the effect of the viruses. If the effect of the viruses could be prolonged or if they could be modified to propagate in a selected type of cancer, it could be considered a major breakthrough in research.

Production of cytotoxic antisera against the human strain of cervical cancer, HeLa, provides many basic observations on the behavior of cervical cancer. Tissue culture techniques exclude many other events that are taking place in vivo, such as cellular defense, vascular reactions, infection, clotting, and other responses of the host as a whole. This does not exclude these techniques from the study of the problem, since the isolation of a few or even a single event for study permits more accurate interpretation of the findings. Miller and Hsu recently reported further observations on the action of cytotoxic antisera. A suspension of ground HeLa cancer cells was injected into rabbits or roosters to produce the antiserum. The cytotoxic antiserum produced had cytopathogenic effects on HeLa cells, normal human cells, and other cultures of malignant cells.

The limitations of this type of study are evident, for in order to develop a cancer-specific antiserum, one must first have an antigen specific for the malignancy concerned. This is the hope of the devoted men in this field of research.

The seeding of cancer cells in operative wounds during the course of radical surgery is frequently unavoidable. Smith and Hilberg studied washings from incisions made for radical operations. At the conclusion of the procedure the wounds were washed with saline solution and the washings mixed with a fixative and centrifuged. Smears and fixed sections were made. Thirty-six wounds were studied by the method. The washings from ten wounds were positive for malignant cells, and five contained suspicious cells. Three of these wounds developed recurrences in the incision, and two cases of local recurrence occurred where the limitations of the method did not demonstrate cells at the time of the primary operation. The conclusion to be drawn is that operative wounds must be frequently seeded with malignant cells, although they do not necessarily survive. More important is the concept of immediate chemotherapeutic or radiologic attack when the seeding of a wound is inevitable. One should not hesitate to use agents directly if there is any prospect that they may be cancerocidal for the particular tumor and do not otherwise harm the host.

LYMPHANGIOADENOGRAPHY IN RADICAL CANCER SURGERY

Lymphangioadenography (lymphography), while as yet an experimental technique, promises to have practical uses in cancer surgery of the female genital tract. By this method the extent of metastases may be more accurately determined, involvement of deep nodes suspected where they cannot be palpated, and therapy altered because of this additional information. During surgery the nodes in the field of operation can be made to stand out by use of dyes, thus adding another refinement to surgical technique.

Technique of Lymphography

The four intermetatarsal web spaces of the foot are injected, using a No. 27 gauge needle with 0.25 ml. of a mixture of Xylocaine and Patent Blue V-F (Alphazurine2-G). The mixture contains 0.5 ml. of Xylocaine and 1.5 ml. of an 11 per cent aqueous solution of Patent Blue V-F. The same injection is repeated in the other foot. A blue discoloration develops locally, and, when the dye is picked up by the lymphatics draining the area, these also stand out.

The extremities are immobilized by splints for the cannulization of the lymph vessel and to prevent disturbance of the needle while roentgenograms are being taken. A site is selected near the ankle where several lymphatic channels can be seen under the skin. Under local anesthesia, a 4 to 6 cm. transverse incision is made through the deep fascia with great care until several lymph vessels in the subfascial plane stand out. No attempt is made to dissect out the lymphatic. It is best left in its bed supported by the surrounding connective tissue. Small venules may also stain blue, and a preliminary x-ray will be done later to exclude an accidental catheterization of a vein and the subsequent injection of oil into the blood stream.

The lymph vessel is cannulated with a No. 27 or No. 30 gauge needle connected by a polyethylene catheter (Clay Adams Pe 280, 15 inches long). An automatic apparatus with 20 ml. syringes and permitting a controlled rate of injection is preferred. Hand syringes may be used. Ethiodol (an ethyl ester of iodized poppy seed oil containing 37 per cent iodine) is used as the radiopaque medium.

One or two milliliters of the Ethiodol is injected on each side. An x-ray of the lower extremities is taken to confirm an intralymphatic injection and to exclude an intravenous injection or local extravasation. After it is confirmed that the cannulization is satisfactory, 12 ml. of the solution is injected into each extremity. This is done at a rate of 0.2 ml. per minute, but the rate may be faster if the solution is warmed and the caliber of the catheter permits. Transient pain in the legs may be observed. If the purpose of the cannulization is to outline nodes at the time of operation, dye as well as the radiopaque medium is injected.

Roentgenograms of the legs, thighs, abdomen, and chest are taken. A miliary pattern may be seen in the lungs several hours after injection from minor interstitial deposition of the Ethiodol. It is of no clinical significance. The x-rays are repeated twenty-four to forty-eight hours later when the architecture of the nodes is shown to better advantage. Laterals, obliques, stereopairs, and laminograms can also be done to aid in the study. Since the nodes remain radiopaque for six to eight weeks, x-rays can be repeated to follow the course of therapy whether by surgery, radiotherapy, or chemotherapy.

Metastatic lymph nodes show up normal, enlarged, or irregular of shape with marginal filling defects. The afferent vessels to them are normal or dilated. Unfortunately nodes that have been completely replaced by tumor have their afferent channels blocked so they do not pick up the dye and are not visualized. However, adjacent nodes that are visualized would probably give the surgeon the clinical information he desires. Nodes replaced completely by tumor would certainly be identified in most instances at the time of operation if the method is used for this purpose.

References

Ackerman, L. V., and Wheat, M. W.: The Implantation of Cancer—an Avoidable Surgical Risk? Surgery 37: 341-356, 1955.

Allen, E., and Gardner, W.: Cancer of the Cervix of the Uterus in Hybrid Mice Following Long-continued Administration of Estrogen, Cancer Res. 1: 359, 1941.

Bonini, L. D'I.: The Local Effects of an Antimitotic Preparation, Substrance F, on Malignancies of the Uterine Cervix and of the Vulva (Gli effetti locali di un antimitotico, sostanza F, sulle malignita della cervie uterina e della vulva), Ann. obstet. ginec. 78: 943, 1956.

Borelli, J., and others: A Starlike Pattern Observed in Cervical Mucus Smears Obtained From Patients With Breast Cancer and Endocrine Disorders, J. Nat. Cancer Inst. 25: 1, 1960.

Chun, L., Gong, G., and Roddick, J. W.: The Epithelium of the Uterine Tube and Cervix in Patients With Endometrial Carcinoma: A Search for Estrogenic Effect, Am. J. Obst. & Gynec. 78: 174, 1959.

Craig, A. B., and Waterhouse, C.: Body-Composition Changes in Patients With Advanced Cancer, Cancer 10: 1106, 1957.

Damon, A.: Host Factors in Cancer of the Breast and

Uterine Cervix and Corpus, J. Nat. Cancer Inst. 24: 483, 1960.

Dao, T., and Moore, G.: Clinical Observations of Conditions Which Apparently Enhance Malignant Cell Survival, Surg., Gynec. & Obst. 112: 191, 1961.

De Alvarez, R., Figge, D., and Brown, D.: Long-Range Studies of the Biologic Behavior of the Human Uterine Cervix; II. Histology, Cytology, and Clinical Course of Cervical Disease, Am. J. Obst. & Gynec. 74: 769, 1957.

DeAlvarez, R. R., and others: Long-Range Studies of the Biologic Behavior of the Human Uterine Cervix; III. Squamous Metaplasia, Am. J. Obst. & Gynec. 75: 945, 1958.

Dunn, J. E., and Buell, P.: Association of Cervical Cancer With Circumcision of the Sexual Partner, J. Nat. Cancer Inst. 22: 749, 1959.

Eichner, E., and Rubinstein, L.: Cervical Stump Lymphatics: An in Vivo Study, Obst. & Gynec. 12: 521, 1958.

Everson, T., and Cole, W. H.: Spontaneous Regression of Cancer, Preliminary Report, Ann. Surg. 144: 366, 1956.

Fennell, R. H., and Vazquez, J. J.: Immunocytochemical Study of the Sensitization Response (SR) in Vaginal Epithelium, Cancer 13: 555, 1960.

Figge, D. C.: Growth Characteristics of Human Endometrium in Tissue Culture, Obst. & Gynec. 16: 269, 1960.

Furth, J.: A Meeting of Ways in Cancer Research: Thoughts on the Evolution and Nature of Neoplasms, Cancer Res. 19: 241, 1959.

Gardner, W. U., and Ferrigno, M.: Unusual Neoplastic Lesions of the Uterine Horns of Estrogen-Treated Mice, J. Nat. Cancer Inst. 17: 601, 1956.

Gellhorn, A., Hyman, G., and Ultmann, J.: The Mechanism of the Anemia of Cancer, New York J. Med. 13: 614, 1957.

Gey, G., Bank, F., and Gey, M.: Responses of a Variety of Normal and Malignant Cells to Continuous Cultivation, and Some Practical Applications of These Responses to Problems in the Biology of Disease, Ann. New York Acad. Sc. 58: 976, 1954.

Gey, G. O., Bang, F. B., and Gey, M. K.: An Evaluation of Some Comparative Studies on Cultured Strains of Normal and Malignant Cells of Animals and Man, Texas Rep. Biol. & Med. 12: 805-827, 1954.

Goldberg, I. D., and others: The Probability of Developing Cancer, J. Nat. Cancer Inst. 17: 155, 1956.

Goldstein, M. N., Hiramoto, R., and Pressman, D.: Comparative Fluorescein Labeling and Cytotoxicity Studies With Human Cell Strains HeLa, Raos, and 407-Liver and With Fresh Surgical Specimens of Cervical Carcinoma, and Normal Adult Liver, J. Nat. Cancer Inst. 22: 697, 1959.

Grace, J T, and Kondo, T: Investigations of Host Resistance in Cancer Patients, Ann. Surg. 148: 633, 1958.

Grand, C., and Ayre, J.: Studies of Developing Cervical Neoplasms, Obst. & Gynec. 4: 411, 1954.

Gross, S. J., Kinzie, G., and Chang, N.: Histochemistry of Gynecologic Cancer, Obst. & Gynec. 14: 43, 1959.

Guthrie, M. J.: Tumorigenesis in Ovaries of Mice After X Irradiation, Cancer 11: 1226, 1958.

von Haam, E., and Scarpelli, D.: Experimental Carcinoma of the Cervix: a Comparative Cytologic and Histologic Study, Cancer Res. 15: 449, 1955.

von Haam, E., and Menzies, P.: Experimental Studies in Exfoliative Cytology, Proc. Am. A. Cancer Res. 1: 22, 1953.

Helwig, F. C.: Changing Ratio of Cervical to Corpus Carcinoma; a 32 Year Survey, Am. J. Obst. & Gynec. 81: 277, 1961.

Hertz, R., Lipsett, M., and Moy, R.: Effect of Vincaleukoblastine on Metastatic Choriocarcinoma and Related Trophoblastic Tumors in Women, Cancer Res. 20: 1050, 1960.

Hreshchyshyn, M., Sheehan, F., and Holland, J.: Visualization of Retroperitoneal Lymph Nodes; Lymphongiography as an Aid in the Measurement of Tumor Growth, Cancer 14: 205, 1961.

Hsu, T.: Cytological Studies on HeLa, a Strain of Human Cervical Carcinoma. I. Observations on Mitosis and Chromosomes, Texas Rep. Biol. & Med. 12: 843-846, 1954.

Hsu, T.: Mammalian Chromosomes in Vitro. VI. Observation on Mitosis With Phase Cinematography, J. Nat. Cancer Inst. 16: 691, 1955.

Kaminetzky, H.: Human Cervical Epithelial Changes Produced by Podophyllin, Am. J. Obst. & Gynec. 80: 1055, 1960.

Kaminetzky, H. A., McGrew, E. A., and Phillips, R. L.: Experimental Cervical Epithelial Dysplasia, Obst. & Gynec. 14: 1, 1959.

Kidd, J.: A Distinctive Substance Associated With the Brown-Pearce Carcinoma. Properties of the Substance: Discussion, J. Exper. Med. 71: 351, 1940.

Kullander, S., and Kallen, B.: The Fibrinolytic Activity of Human Endometrium Studied in Tissue Culture. Part I, Normal Endometrial and Decidual Tissue, Acta obst. et gynec. scandinav. 40: 1, 1961.

LeRoy, L., and others: Cancer Cells in Blood, A. M. A. Arch. Surg. 80: 910, 1960.

Long, M. E., Doko, F., and Taylor, H. C.: Nucleoli and Nucleolar Ribonucleic Acid in Nonmalignant and Malignant Human Endometria, Am. J. Obst. & Gynec. 75: 1002, 1958.

Luria, S. E.: Viruses, Cancer Cells and the Genetic Concept of Virus Infection, Cancer Res. 20: 677, 1960.

McDonald, G. O., Gines, S. M., and Cole, W. H.: Wound Irrigation in Cancer Surgery, A. M. A. Arch. Surg. 80: 920, 1960.

Malmgren, R. A., and others: A Method for the Cytological Detection of Tumor Cells in Whole Blood, J. Nat. Cancer Inst. 20: 1203, 1958.

Maturova, M., Malinsky, J., and Santavy, F.: The Biological Effects of some Podophyllin Compounds and Their Dependence on Chemical Structure, J. Nat. Cancer Inst. 22: 297, 1959.

Merriam, J. C., and others: Experimental Production of Endometrial Carcinoma in the Rabbit, Obst. & Gynec. 16: 253, 1960.

Miller, B. J.: A Phenomenon of Induced Local Reactivity in Experimental Tumors, Surg., Gynec. & Obst. 108: 195, 1958.

Miller, D., and Hsu, T.: The Action of Cytotoxic Antisera on the Strain of Human Carcinoma, Cancer Res. 16: 306, 1956.

Moertel, C. G., Dockerty, M. B., and Baggenstoss, A. H.: Multiple Primary Malignant Neoplasms. I. Introduction and Presentation of Data, Cancer 14: 221, 1961.

Moertel, C. G., Dockerty, M. B., and Baggenstoss, A. H.: Multiple Primary Malignant Neoplasms. II. Tumors of Different Tissues or Organs, Cancer 14: 231, 1961.

Moertel, C. G., Dockerty, M. B., and Baggenstoss, A. H.: Multiple Primary Malignant Neoplasms. III. Tumors of Multicentric Origin, Cancer 14: 238, 1961.

Momigliano, E.: Experimental Metaplasia of the Endometrium, Am. J. Obst. & Gynec. 75: 249, 1958.

Monis, B., and Rutenburg, A. M.: Alkaline Phosphatase Activity in Neoplastic and Inflammatory Tissues of Man, Cancer 13: 538, 1960.

Montgomery, J. A.: The Relation of Anticancer Activity to Chemical Structure: A Review, Cancer Res. 19: 447, 1959.

Moore, G. E.: The Significance of Cancer Cells in the Blood, Surg., Gynec. & Obst. 110: 360, 1960.

Moore, G. E., and Grace, J. T.: Cancer Immunity, Surg., Gynec. & Obst. 110: 234, 1960.

Moore, G. E., and others: Assessment of the Exfoliation of Tumor Cells Into the Body Cavities, Surg., Gynec. & Obst. 112: 469, 1961.

Moorhead, P., and Hsu, T.: Cytologic Studies of HeLa, a Strain of Human Cervical Carcinoma. III. Durations and Characteristics of the Mitotic Phases, J. Nat. Cancer Inst. 16: 1047, 1956.

Olch, P. D., Eck, R. V., and Smith, R. R.: An Experimental Study of the Effect of Irradiation on the Dissemination of Cancer, Cancer Res. 19: 464, 1959.

Papanicolaou, G. N., and Maddi, F. V.: Further Observations of the Behavior of Human Endometrial Cells in Tissue Culture, Am. J. Obst. & Gynec. 78: 156, 1959.

Patterson, W. B., Patterson, H. R., and Chute, R. N.: Transplantable Human Cancers, Cancer 10: 1281, 1957.

Potter, J. F., and others: The Relationship of Tumor Type and Resectability to the Incidence of Cancer Cells in Blood, Surg., Gynec. & Obst. 110: 734, 1960.

Reagan, R. B., Reagan, J. W., and Schoenberg, M.D.: The Mucins of the Normal and Cancerous Uterine Mucosa, Cancer 12: 215, 1959.

Reid, B. L., and Singh, S.: Deoxyribonucleic Acid Values (Feulgen Microspectrophotometry) in Epithelium of Human Ectocervix, Normal and Cancerous, J. Nat. Cancer Inst. 25: 1291, 1960.

Reimann, S. P.: Highways and Byways of Cancer Research, Cancer Res. 13: 493, 1953.

Rhoads, C. P. E.: The Experimental Method and the Cancer Problem, Bull. N. Y. Acad. Med. 27: 606, 1951.

Roberts, S., and others: The Isolation of Cancer Cells From the Blood Stream During Uterine Curettage, Surg., Gynec. & Obst. 111: 3, 1960.

Rubin, A.: The Histogenesis of Carcinosarcoma (Mixed Mesodermal Tumor) of the Uterus as Revealed by Tissue Culture Studies, Am. J. Obst. & Gynec. 77: 269, 1959.

Sandberg, A. A., and others: The Frequency of Tumor Cells in the Marrow and Blood, Cancer 11: 1180, 1958.

Saphir, O.: The Transfer of Tumor Cells by the Surgical Knife, Surg., Gynec. & Obst. 63: 775-776, 1936.

Scherer, W., Syverton, J., and Gey, G.: Studies on the Propagation in Vitro of Poliomyelitis Viruses. IV. Viral Multiplication in a Stable Strain of Human Malignant Epithelial Cells (Strain HeLa) Derived From an Epidermoid Carcinoma of the Cervix, J. Exper. Med. 97: 695-710, 1953.

Shope, R. E.: Koch's Postulates and a Viral Cause of Human Cancer, Cancer Res. 20: 1119, 1960.

Smith, R. R., and Gehan, E. A.: Effect of Formaldehyde Wound Wash on Development of Local Wound Recurrences, J. Nat. Cancer Inst. 23: 1339, 1959.

Smith, R., and Hilberg, A. W.: Cancer-Cell Seeding of Operative Wounds, J. Nat. Cancer Inst. 16: 645, 1955.

Smith, R. R., Thomas, L. B., and Hilberg, A. W.: Cancer Cell Contamination of Operative Wounds, Cancer 11: 53, 1958.

Southam, C.: Relationships of Immunology to Cancer: A Review, Cancer Res. 20: 271, 1960.

Ullery, J. C., and Hollenbeck, Z. J. R.: Early Diagnosis and Treatment in a Cancer Survey Program, Am. J. Obst. & Gynec. 76: 1083, 1958.

Ultmann, J. E., Koprowska, I., and Engle, R. L.: A Cytological Study of Lymph Node Imprints, Cancer 11: 507, 1958.

Van Rymenant, M., and Robert, J.: Enzymes in Cancer, Cancer 12: 1087, 1959.

Watne, A. L., Hatiboglu, I., and Moore, G. E.: A Clinical and Autopsy Study of Tumor Cells in the Thoracic Duct Lymph, Surg., Gynec. & Obst. 110: 339, 1960.

Zeidman, I.: The Fate of Circulating Tumor Cells. I. Passage of Cells Through Capillaries, Cancer Res. 21: 38, 1961.

Zeidman, I.: Experimental Studies of the Spread of Cancer in the Lymphatic System. IV. Retrograde Spread, Cancer Res. 19: 1114, 1959.

Zitcer, E. M., and Dunnebacke, T. H.: Transformation of Cells From the Normal Human Amnion Into Established Strains, Cancer Res. 17: 1047, 1957.

21 · Hormonal Factors in the Genesis and Control of Gynecologic Cancer

Induction of Gynecologic Cancer

The most striking clinical observation of the effect of hormones on a female genital cancer is the increased incidence of endometrial cancer in association with a feminizing tumor of the ovary. This is consistently observed in each series of clinical reports. Further studies of patients developing granulosa and theca cell tumors reveal an increased incidence of endometrial hyperplasia, uterine fibromyomas and malignancies of the breast. Cortical stromal hyperplasia of the ovary is manifested by an increased thickness and cellular density in the cortical stroma, with interlacing fascicles dipping irregularly into the cellular eosinophilic medullary stroma. The nuclei of these stromal cells are enlarged and take a fat stain, suggesting that they may be estrogen secreting. Studies of the ovaries removed from patients with endometrial and breast cancer, compared with those from controls in the same age groups, show a significant incidence of stromal hyperplasia in those patients with malignancies. It has been suggested that patients with breast cancer who experience a remission following castration have ovaries with cortical stromal hyperplasia.

A significant advance in the study of the hormonal factors in the genesis of gynecologic cancer, although in animal experiments, is reported by Moon and his co-workers, that prolonged administration of the growth hormone of the pituitary gland may induce in intact rats of the Long-Evans strain solid tumors of the ovaries and atypical hyperplasia of the ovarian follicles that are suggestive of granulosa cell tumors. The treated animals also developed fibroadenomas of the breast more often than the untreated controls. The relationship of the adrenal glands to the development of malignancies from the growth hormone of the pituitary gland is equally significant. Many of the treated animals developed adrenal cortices showing nodular changes. The medullae were hypertrophic and proliferative, with areas of neoplastic cells invading and displacing the cortex. The pituitary glands of these animals contained smaller, less granular, and fewer acidophils than those of the controls, while the basophils were increased in number. Hypophysectomized rats did not develop tumors on prolonged administration of the growth hormone. Again, these are observations in laboratory animals, but the experimental studies on adrenalectomy and hypophysectomy in the control of human malignancies will soon provide tissues and data for comparison.

Alteration of the Sensitivity of Pelvic Cancers

The possibility that a cancer of the female genital organs can be primed by hormones for other definitive therapy is under investigation. Nieburgs has administered massive doses of diethylstilbestrol to patients with carcinoma of the cervix in whom there were bleeding, necrosis, and purulent discharge. Some had had radiation therapy with local recurrence, some were under therapy, and some had advanced Stage IV lesions. They received doses of 200 to 500 mg. per os each day and suppositories in doses of 25 to 100 mg. daily. This regimen was found to be helpful in hemostasis and epithelization of the lesions. The favorable change in the gross appearance of the cervix can be considered an alteration of sensitivity only in the broadest definition, although the same criteria are frequently used to assess the effectiveness of radiation therapy.

In contrast, Ruth and John Graham have followed the effects of radiation on a few patients receiving testosterone and alpha-tocopherol. Their study represents an attempt to project well-known facts in the modification of responses of animals to total body radiation. Using their method of observing normal cells to determine the effectiveness of radiation, they studied five patients cytologically who received male hormone at some time during a course of radium and radiation therapy delivered by their modification of the accepted methods. Testosterone propionate, 25 mg., was given every other day to four patients. Alpha-tocopherol, 100 mg. every day intramuscularly for ten days and thereafter by mouth in the same dosage, was given to a fifth patient during the course of radiation. They felt that cytologically the hormones favorably altered the response in these instances.

Modification of Malignancies of the Parasexual Organs

Oophorectomy, adrenalectomy, and hypophysectomy have been used to modify the course of recurrent or metastatic breast cancer. The results are unpredictable, so the operations are not done indiscriminately. If the breast cancer appears to be estrogen dependent and the patient is premenopausal, the gynecologist may be consulted regarding a bilateral oophorectomy. The uterus and cervix are removed at the same time. Adrenalectomy has been performed to modify the course of pelvic cancers and malignancies of the parasexual organs. The results are not consistent enough to be included among the standard methods of therapy. Accessory adrenal tissue is quite common in the female genital tract, and this may modify the effects of adrenalectomy. Nonneoplastic adrenocortical nodules in the broad

ligament are frequently seen if a routine search is made for them during laparotomies. The nodes are found in the infundibulopelvic pedicle anywhere from its junction with the mesosalpinx to the lateral pelvic wall. It would seem they might be found anywhere along the course of the ovarian vessels. They are just beneath the peritoneum and contiguous with the ovarian vein. To detect them, slip the ovarian vessels and their connective tissue extensions between the fingers and look for some firm, discrete, yellow discs. They contain the three cortical layers, and evidence of active function is demonstrable.

References

Allen, E., and Gardner, W.: Cancer of the Cervix of the Uterus in Hybrid Mice Following Long-continued Administration of Estrogen, Cancer Res. 1: 359, 1941.

Arons, M. S., Ketcham, A. S., and Mantel, N.: The Effect of Growth Hormone and ACTH on a Transplanted Tumor, Cancer 14: 507, 1961.

Banner, E., and Dockerty, M.: Theca Cell Tumors of the Ovary, Surg., Gynec. & Obst. 81: 234, 1945.

Barnes, A.: The Production of ACTH in the Patient Undergoing Gynecologic Surgery or Receiving Pelvic Irradiation, Am. J. Obst. & Gynec. 65: 758, 1953.

Barnes, A. C.: ACTH and Cortisone in Obstetrics and Gynecology, Obst. & Gynec. 3: 322, 1954.

Brayer, F. T., Glasser, S. R., and Howland, J. W.: Hormones and Radioactivity in Cancer Therapy, New York J. Med. 56: 905, 1956.

Brody, S., and Westman, A.: Ovarian Hormones and Uterine Growth; Effects of Estradiol and Progesterone on Cell Growth and Cell Division in the Rabbit Uterus, Acta obst. et gynec. scandinav. 39: 557, 1960.

Christopherson, W., and Broghamer, W.: Progression of Experimental Cervical Dysplasia in the Mouse, Cancer 14: 201, 1961.

Dockerty, M., and Mussey, E.: Malignant Lesions of Uterus Associated With Estrogen-Producing Ovarian Tumors, Am. J. Obst. & Gynec. 61: 147, 1951.

Emerson, K., Jr., and Jessiman, A. G.: Hormonal Influences on the Growth and Progression of Cancer, New England J. Med. 254: 252, 1956.

Gardner, W., and others: Carcinoma of the Cervix of Mice Receiving Estrogens, J. A. M. A. 110: 1182, 1938.

Gluchsmann, A.: Relationships Between Hormonal Changes in Pregnancy and the Development of "Mixed Carcinoma" of the Uterine Cervix, Cancer 10: 831, 1957.

Graham, J., and Graham, R.: A Method of Enhancing the Effectiveness of Radiotherapy in Cancer of the Uterine Cervix, Cancer 6: 68, 1953.

Graham, J., Graham, R., and Liu, W.: Prognosis in Cancer of the Uterine Cervix Based on the Vaginal Smear Before Treatment; SR—the Sensitization Response, Surg., Gynec. & Obst. 99: 555, 1954.

Graham, R.: The Prognosis of Cancer of the Cervix by Vaginal Smear; Correlation With Five-Year Results, Surg., Gynec. & Obst. 93: 767, 1951.

Graham, R., and Graham, J.: A Cellular Index of Sensitivity to Ionizing Radiation; the Sensitization Response, Cancer 6: 215, 1953.

Greenstein, J., and Haddow, A.: Advances in Cancer Research, New York, 1954, Academic Press, Inc.

Haddow, A., Watkinson, J., and Paterson, E.: Influence of Synthetic Oestrogens Upon Advanced Malignant Disease, Brit. M. J. 2: 393, 1944.

Herman, G. G., Hughes, H. E., and Gusberg, S. B.: The Endocrine Basis for the Sensitization Response, Surg., Gynec. & Obst. 108: 463, 1959.

Hertig, A. T.: Endocrine Ovarian Cancer Relationships, Cancer 10: 838, 1957.

Hesseltine, H. C., Loth, M. F., and Smith, R. L.: Observations on the Use of ACTH in Certain Obstetric and Gynecologic Conditions, Am. J. Obst. & Gynec. 72: 777, 1956.

Jones, G. S., and Howard, J. E.: The Use of ACTH and Cortisone Therapy in Obstetrics and Gynecology, New York J. Med. 53: 2463, 1953.

Kistner, R. W.: Histological Effects of Progestins on Hyperplasia and Carcinoma in Situ of the Endometrium, Cancer 12: 1106, 1959.

Kofman, S., and others: The Use of Prednisolone in the Treatment of Disseminated Breast Carcinoma, Cancer 11: 226, 1958.

Lunell, N.: A Method for Determination of 11-Oxy-17-Hydroxy-Corticosteroids in Urine, Acta obst. et gynec. scandinav. 39: 698, 1960.

MacAlpin, R. N., and others: The Effects of Long Term Administration of Prednisolone and Growth Hormone on the Growth of Transplanted Mammary Adenocarcinoma in C3H Mice, Cancer 11: 731, 1958.

McKelvey, J., Stenstrom, K., and Gillam, J.: Results of an Experimental Therapy of Carcinoma of the Cervix, Am. J. Obst. & Gynec. 58: 896, 1949.

Moon, H., and others: Neoplasms in Rats Treated With Pituitary Growth Hormone; Pulmonary and Lymphatic Tissues, Cancer Res. 10: 297, 1950.

Moon, H., and others: Neoplasms in Rats Treated With Pituitary Growth Hormone; Adrenal Glands, Cancer Res. 10: 364, 1950.

Moon, H.: Neoplasms in Rats Treated With Pituitary Growth Hormone: Reproductive Organs, Cancer Res. 10: 549, 1950.

Myers, W. P. L.: Cortisone in the Treatment of Hypercalcemia in Neoplastic Disease, Cancer 11: 83, 1958.

Nelsen, T., and Dragstedt, L.: Adrenalectomy and Oophorectomy for Breast Cancer, J. A. M. A. 175: 397, 1961.

Nieburgs, H.: The Effect of Excessive Doses of Diethylstilbestrol on Carcinoma of the Cervix, Obst. & Gynec. 2: 213, 1953.

Richardson, F. L.: Incidence of Mammary and Pituitary Tumors in Hybrid Mice Treated With Stilbestrol for Varying Periods, J. Nat. Cancer Inst. 18: 813, 1957.

Richardson, F., and Hall, G.: Mammary Tumors and Mammary-Gland Development in Hybrid Mice Treated With Diethylstilbestrol for Varying Periods, J. Nat. Cancer Inst. 25: 1023, 1960.

Smith, G.: Carcinoma of the Endometrium, New England J. Med. 225: 608, 1941.

Smith, G., Johnson, L., and Hertig, A.: Relation of Ovarian Stromal Hyperplasia and Thecoma of the Ovary to Endometrial Hyperplasia and Carcinoma (Abstract), New England J. Med. 226: 364, 1942.

Sommers, S., and Teloh, H.: Ovarian Stromal Hyperplasia in Breast Cancer, A. M. A. Arch. Path. 53: 160, 1952.

Woll, E., and others: The Ovary in Endometrial Carcinoma, Am. J. Obst. & Gynec. 56: 617, 1948.

22 · Radiation and Isotope Methodology in Gynecologic Cancer

General Considerations

Dr. George E. Pfahler, the late dean of American roentgenologists, quotes Pierre Curie who, a half century ago, said, "in criminal hands, radium might become dangerous . . . is humanity ripe enough to profit by learning the secrets of nature, or might not that knowledge prove harmful?" Dr. Pfahler said, "I believe that humanity will obtain *more good than evil* from future discoveries." We are now in the era of supervoltage therapy, particle-accelerating beams, precision targeting, rotational therapy, induction of tumor susceptibility, and an almost endless number of isotopes with their unlimited potential for diagnosis and therapy. Isotope methodology is marking a new epoch in medical progress and has already produced much that is good and little or none of some of the predicted evils.

Genetic Effects and Physical Carcinogenesis

The problem of mutations, sterility, and tumor development in human generations far removed from those receiving various forms of radiation becomes a matter of serious concern when animal experiments are interpreted in terms of the possible similarity in human beings. Dr. Jacob Furth, working at the Cornell Medical Center, years ago induced ovarian tumors in mice with radiation as the physical agent. His students and subsequent workers have expanded this fundamental discovery.

Deringer and co-workers have studied hybrid mice exposed to whole body radiation, to whole body radiation with the ovaries shielded, and to radiation to the ovaries only. He found that females with ovaries only exposed to total doses of 300 to 500 r. produced one smaller than normal litter and were sterile thereafter. With 50 to 200 r. to ovaries only, they had multiple litters of somewhat smaller size. The mice exposed to 100 to 400 r. to the whole body produced a single litter of reduced size except for a few mice in the 100 r. group. When the ovaries were exteriorized and protected with lead shields, these mice bred like the control group. Ovarian tumors occurred in all animals receiving total doses of 300 to 500 r. to ovaries only and total doses of 100 to 400 r. to the whole body. Some tumors occurred with less radiation. No effect was apparent when the whole body excluding the ovaries was irradiated other than that ascribed to the operation itself.

Tolerance Limits of Exposure

The tolerance limit is expressed in terms of energy absorbed in the body. The roentgen is used for x-rays and gamma rays, the roentgen-equivalent-biologic unit for beta rays, protons, slow neutrons, and alpha particles, and the roentgen-equivalent-man (rem) unit for fast neutrons. The presently accepted tolerance level for x-rays and gamma rays has been 0.1 r. per eight-hour day, or 12.5 milliroentgens per hour. When the genetic effects, now unknown for man, are more clearly defined, this level may be high. Tolerance levels in roentgen-equivalent-physical (rep) are determined from the biologic effectiveness of each particular type.

Ionization chambers of special design, calibrated to the roentgen, are used for the most part. Pocket chambers can be used to measure gamma ray exposures, which include slow neutrons as far as they produce induced activities emitting gamma rays. For integrating exposures over a long period, photographic films worn on the person are used. These must be carefully calibrated and developed and the sensitivity of the emulsions checked to avoid gross errors.

The frightening possibilities raised by the studies of mutations caused by radiation cannot be definitely ascertained for human beings until several generations of radiated human beings have been observed. Anyone who radiates the ovaries to stimulate ovulation may give pause to consider. Radiation alters the structure of the chromosomes without, in every instance, causing the death of the cell or its ability to reproduce. Mutation changes are irreversible—there is no recovery. The effects of radiation are cumulative, and if a certain dose causes a certain percentage of mutations, it does not matter whether this dose is absorbed at one time or over a protracted period. The percentage of mutations is dependent and proportional to the dose, and the irreversibility of the change makes the genetic effects of radiation cumulative.

Nature of Radiation Injuries

The injury to living cells by any radiation is directly proportional to the ionization produced in the structure of the cells. It will vary according to the different types of ionization. The intense local ionization produced by alpha particles and protons is more damaging than the less densely localized ions produced by gamma rays. The effect of total body radiation as compared with radiation on an individual group of cells brings in the factor of replacement of destroyed cells by some tissues and not by others. Parts of the eye, muscular tissue, and brain cannot regenerate new cells to supplant those destroyed.

The radiation effects of atomic bombs and the radioactive fall-out may not be known for generations. The obstetricians may well be faced with the problem of what to do with the thousands of women whose early conceptions have been exposed to varying doses of atomic radiation. The radiation effects in the adults observed at Nagasaki and Hiroshima bear a tragic similarity to those observed in animals after exposure to experimental atomic detonations. The process may be compared to premature aging. Cataracts develop, infection is poorly tolerated, the hair becomes gray, albinism or leukemia occurs, and pituitary and other tumors are more common. There may develop vascular changes in the kidney simulating nephrosclerosis, and renal failure is not uncommon.

Evidence of Radiation Injury

The gynecologist must be familiar with the general effects of radiation injury as well as the more familiar local pelvic complications of radiation therapy. The advent of isotopes and radiomimetic compounds that may be used in gynecologic cancer necessitates more attention to the general systemic effects. These effects vary with the type of radiation, its penetrating power, the patient, the method of radiation, whether local or total, plus other factors of administration. Injuries range from a slight erythema of the skin or mucous membranes to severe osteitis. Aplastic anemia may preclude further treatment. Leukopenias are commonly associated with heavy doses of x-rays or gamma rays during a short time. The biologic effects of super-energy radiations are under study, and new effects either in degree or kind may produce new problems.

Substances Emitting Alpha Radiation

Alpha radiation is a densely bombarding and powerful source of ionization that is particularly dangerous at close range. The radium poisoning of radium dial painters is the classic example of ingestion of material emitting alpha radiation. Fatalities resulted when 2 to 100 mg. of radium were deposited in the skeletal tissues. Radium in the body is measured and detected by the radon in the exhaled breath. It can also be detected by Geiger-Müller counters, but this is less reliable. Some radioisotopes do not produce radon and have no strong gamma rays (polonium and plutonium) and are therefore difficult to detect in the human body. Radioactive cleanliness is the only protection from injurious amounts, and the lowest possible exposure limit should be placed on elements that emit alpha radiation.

Gamma Ray Protection

Gynecologists are familiar with the general methods of reducing exposure to gamma radiation due to their handling of radium and use of diagnostic radiation in pelvic disease. The inverse square law provides the soundest principle of protection, and the operator remains as far from the field of radiation as possible regardless of the source. Lead protectors are used, and the insertion of radium or contact with other substances is done as quickly as possible.

In June, 1956, the National Academy of Sciences published the results of a comprehensive study of the effects of radioactivity. The report found that most of the American public was using up about one third of the safety limit of exposure in the routine use of diagnostic x-ray and dental equipment. The mutagenic effects of radiation on human beings will not be evident for many generations. Dr. Hermann J. Muller, distinguished geneticist and Distinguished Service Professor of Zoology at the University of Indiana, has outlined some basic rules for anyone using radiation, whether in therapy, research, or industry:

(1) Keep the dose as low as possible and use much smaller doses for thin tissues. (2) Screen the reproductive organs whenever they fall in the line of stray beams. This is particularly important in young children who have yet to pass through their reproductive years. (3) Shutter down the field to the immediate region under investigation. In obstetrics and gynecology, pyelograms, hysterosalpingography, and pelvimetry deliver a large dose of radiation to the gonads. Pelvimetry is particularly dangerous, since it delivers a dose to the gonads of both the mother and the child. Despite its great field of usefulness, pelvimetry probably should be limited to a select group at

term. With a history of a difficult, traumatic delivery, pelvimetry could be done in between pregnancies. With subsequent conceptions, a single exposure for cephalometry would cut down the exposure of the infant. (4) Use a high voltage for deep areas and lower voltage for superficial areas to reduce the time of exposure. (5) Personnel working with radiation and even those receiving considerable radiation for diagnostic reasons should keep a record of their exposure. This is particularly true when fluoroscopes and dental equipment are used. As is well known among gynecologists, Dr. Muller regards as indefensible the use of radiation to stimulate ovulation. He believes that an ovum that matures after such radiation represents injured tissue and may subsequently cause mutations generations later.

GAMMA EMITTERS AND ROENTGENTHERAPY
General Considerations

Female pelvic cancer requiring radiotherapy would be ideally managed by the combined efforts of a gynecologist, radiotherapist, radiophysicist, and radiopathologist. Since radium application and roentgentherapy are still the standard treatment for cancer of the cervix and feature in the management of other genital malignancies, a method of utilizing the combined knowledge of each of the above-mentioned specialists should be worked out for each center undertaking the care of patients with pelvic cancer. It is futile to describe a standard method of therapy, since each hospital has different facilities and agents available. The minimum requirements are a deep x-ray therapy unit (200 to 250 kv.) and sources of a gamma emitter such as radium or radioactive cobalt (cobalt[60]) with either a standardized colpostat for insertion or an adequate improvisation.

RADIUM AND RADON; RADIOACTIVE COBALT; RADIOACTIVE IRIDIUM

Radium has a half-life of 1,590 years, while its gaseous product of degeneration, radon, has a half-life of 3.6 days. The short half-life of radon is considered in the prepared tables for calculating the millicurie hours. Alpha and beta components of these sources are readily screened out by 0.5 mm. or more of platinum or its equivalent. Since radioactive cobalt is less familiar to some gynecologists, its properties will be described in more detail.

Physical Properties of Radioactive Cobalt

Radioactive cobalt has radiologic properties that make it readily adaptable to cancer therapy. It has a half-life of 5.3 years that is relatively stable for isotope therapy. Its radiation consists of a soft beta ray that is easily filtered out and a homogeneous gamma radiation of 1.16 and 1.31 mev. The intensity of any piece of cobalt, when activated, can be predetermined by the length of time the cobalt is exposed to the reactor. Barnes and associates point out that residual activity can be "warmed up" in the reactor—that there are no gaseous radioactive daughters, leakage is impossible, and the regrouping of units of activity is facilitated. The cobalt remains magnetic after activation which makes its handling by magnets a desirable feature. Since cobalt can be activated in any shape or form and suitable alloys—not activated at the same time—are available, the entire procedure is relatively inexpensive. Cobanic, the nickel-cobalt alloy, can be activated as well as the pure cobalt metal. It is usually submitted as small diameter wire for some techniques of interstitial radiation. With radioactive cobalt the isodose curve about the end of the cylinders is not so flat as that measured for radium cylinders or needles. This should be taken into account in the placing of the cylinders.

Method of Action of Radioactive Cobalt

The physical effects of radioactive cobalt on malignant and normal cells has not been shown to differ qualitatively from the effects of radium or its emanations. Like radium, the calculated tissue dose may be varied by the number of units used and the length of exposure. The amount of shielding needed to exclude the beta radiation is much less than radium, so that thinner sources can be made up and a more homogeneous radiation delivered. As in any form of radiation, the objective is to deliver a cancerocidal dose to the tumors and their metastatic deposits without critically injuring the host.

Dosage for Gamma Emitters (Radium and Radioactive Cobalt)

The standard unit of radiation dosage now in use is the roentgen and is defined as follows: The roentgen shall be the quantity of x-radiation or gamma radiation such that the associated corpuscular emission per 0.001293 gram of air produces in air, ions carrying one electrostatic unit or quantity of electricity of either sign. Dosage expressed in milligram-element hours indicates the dose emitted by the source or sources but means little regarding the dose delivered to a tumor area or point in the pelvis. The dose delivered to a point in the pelvis is the sum total delivered by all the gamma sources and depends on their distribution, the length of the sources, the distance from a point in the pelvis, and the length of time the agent remains in the body.

In terms of roentgens, 1 milligram-element hour of radium with an 0.5 platinum filter delivers 8.47 gamma roentgens 1 cm. from a point source. The length of the applicators and their make-up must be known to calculate the gamma roentgens from prepared tables for linear sources. One or more points in the pelvis are selected for measurement. For cancer of the cervix, a point 2 cm. above the lateral fornix and 2 cm. lateral to the cervical canal (Manchester Point A) and a second point 2 cm. above the lateral fornix and 5 cm. lateral to the cervical canal (Manchester Point B) have frequently been used. These points are subject to so much variation among patients that it is more accurate to calculate the dose at centimeter intervals from the sources to the pelvic side wall after pelvimetry with the radium or cobalt[60] in place. In practice, each hospital or therapist must calculate the dose delivered to the pelvic side wall from his own gamma sources and technique and add this to the roentgens delivered by external radiation. This brings up the problem of the dose absorbed, which varies with the wave length of the rays. The biologic effect of gamma roentgens and roentgens from a 200 kv. apparatus cannot be added. Nor can the gamma roentgens from cobalt[60] be added to other gamma sources, since the cobalt has to be calibrated from time to time and its original emission depends on the length of time it was left in the pile.

Technique of Application of Radium and Radon

Radium has been used for surface application when large quantities are available for a teletherapy bomb. This will undoubtedly be replaced by cobalt bombs or other cheaper gamma emitters as they are brought into practical use. The common use of radium is by intracavitary techniques. All of the techniques for intracavitary radiation strive for a distribution of the sources to obtain the maximum tumor dose to the lateral pelvic wall or, basically, to the primary and secondary metastatic stations and the routes of contiguous spread of malignancies from the female genitalia. At the same time, the bladder, ureters, and rectum must be spared a necrotizing dose. The "Curie" technique utilizes a tandem in the uterine cavity and a variety of colpostats against the cervical os and lateral fornices. The "Stockholm" technique distributes the sources in the vaginal vault by a uterine tandem and a series of boxes designed to extend from side to side for parametrial radiation. A "bomb" technique has been used, with the open end of a lead cylinder placed against the cervix for both surface and deep radiation. Corscaden and Butz have developed a group of Lucite plaques and plugs, plastic tubes of various lengths, and a series of springs to hold the devices not only in the uterine cavity and cervical canal, but also in the vaginal vault, so the sources remain perpendicular to the axis of the cervical canal. This can be shown by x-ray measurements and calculations to give an excellent tumor dose to the pelvic side wall. Bishop has devised a rubber, positive-spread colpostat that provides adequate distribution of the sources in the vaginal vault insofar as the anatomic features permit. In Plate 58, *A,* is illustrated an Ernst applicator which, for surgeons and radiotherapists who have not had extensive experience with radium therapy and thereby invented their own applicator, provides a device that ensures a reasonable application of the sources to the cancer. It is by no means foolproof, nor does it ensure the maximum efficiency and tumor dose that can be obtained by the experienced radium therapist.

The Ernst applicator consists of a central tandem, divided in sections, in which gamma sources are placed. From one to three can be placed in the uterine cavity, depending on the length of the uterine cavity. Three mechanically operated metal tubes are available on each side of the central tandem. They are arranged so as to be perpendicular to the axis of the cervical canal and are mechanically spread to extend to the lateral fornices for radiation of the parametrium and pelvic side wall. This device can be used in the majority of patients, but since it is one size, places the sources in one direction, limits the number of sources to its construction, and requires linear sources of a length to fit in the containers, it has the limitations that vaginal vaults are not one size, cervical canals do not point in a standard direction, a greater number of sources may be desirable, and every institution may not have its sources made up by the Bureau of Standards to be accommodated by the device.

In practice the applicator is inserted with the maximum number of sources included and the spreader adjusted to distend the lateral fornices. A Lucite plug is introduced to steady the device after the handle is removed. Anteroposterior and lateral x-ray films are taken before the patient is awake and the position of the applicator determined. The bladder is distended with 250 ml. of radiopaque solution to delineate its proximity to the sources of ionization. Using the tables for linear sources and an isometric technique or other means of pelvimetry, the probable dose in gamma roentgens de-

PLATE 58

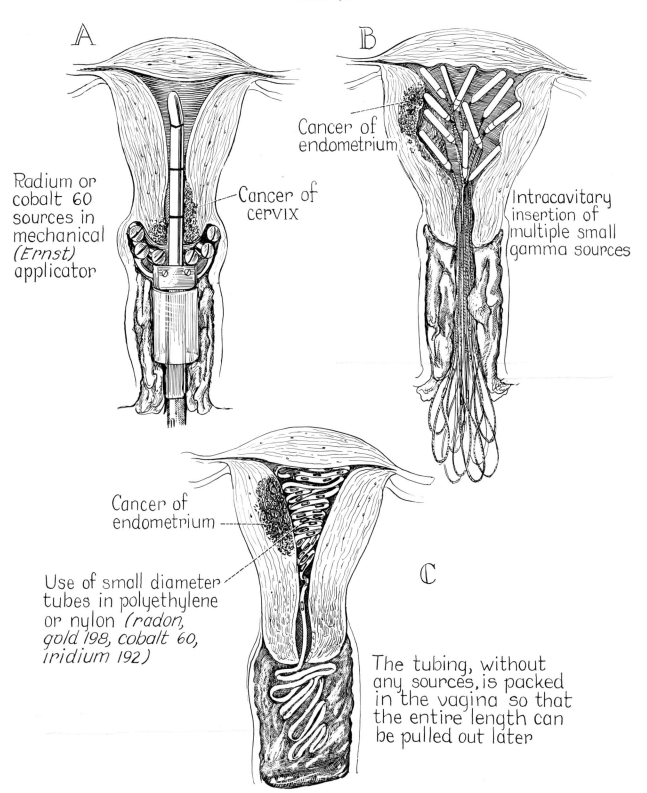

A

Radium or cobalt 60 sources in mechanical (*Ernst*) applicator

Cancer of cervix

B

Cancer of endometrium

Intracavitary insertion of multiple small gamma sources

Cancer of endometrium

Use of small diameter tubes in polyethylene or nylon (*radon, gold 198, cobalt 60, iridium 192*)

C

The tubing, without any sources, is packed in the vagina so that the entire length can be pulled out later livered to one or more points in the pelvis is calculated. This is added to the calculated dose in roentgens delivered by external radiation to determine if a cancerocidal dose has been delivered. This may be presumed to be 6,000 r. for a squamous cancer. It is realized that this addition is not of roentgens of the same quality or biologic activity but is better than prescribing a dose in air for external therapy or a milligram-hours expression for radium sources.

Plate 58, B, shows a method of intracavitary radiation for lesions of the uterine fundus. Multiple small containers are packed into the cavity in an attempt to uniformly radiate the uterus. The law of inverse squares limits the dose that can be delivered by this method much beyond 2 cm. A discussion of the merits of management of cancer of the endometrium combining surgery and radiation is found in Chapter 26 (page 494).

Plate 58, C, shows another method of intracavitary radiation for fundal lesions, utilizing polyethylene or nylon tubing as containers for small gamma sources. This method is adaptable to radon, gold[198], cobalt[60], and iridium[192]. An approximate calculation of the dose emitted can be calculated from tables giving the emission of the particular gamma source used. It would be almost impossible to calculate the dose to a given point from the uterine cavity packed with several dozen small sources by this method.

Interstitial Radiation

Interstitial radiation in gynecologic cancer is a major operative procedure, requiring an extensive knowledge of the pelvic anatomy and wide experience with the method. Needles with an active length varying from 1 to 6 cm., containing radium or cobalt[60], or seeds containing radium are introduced into the parametrium and about the cervix with the objective of obtaining a cancerocidal dose to the primary lesion and its contiguous spread. The interstitial technique is also applicable to cancers of the urethra, vagina, vulva, and retroperitoneal masses. Waterman and Reid have perfected this operation and obtained excellent results in an extensive experience with gynecologic cancer. The pattern of distribution to effectively radiate each cancer is studied before operation. A tandem containing 30 mg. of radium is placed in the cervical canal and lower part of the uterine cavity in the treatment of a cervical cancer. Needles containing 2 mg. of radium in an active length of 2 cm. are placed in a stockade about the central tandem. As many as eight can be placed in the average cervix. Needles are then directed into the parametrium and lateral pelvic wall at 1.5 cm. intervals and in two or more sagittal planes. Longer needles are needed for deep insertion laterally and may contain 5 mg. radium in a 5 cm. effective length. The ureters, as well as the rectum and bladder, are avoided. This requires a fine mastery of the female pelvic anatomy. Calculation of the dose emitted is done from the standard tables. Accurate calculation of the dose delivered to the pelvic side wall is difficult.

Iridium[192]

Iridium[192] has proved to be the most satisfactory isotope for use in any of the ribbon techniques for interstitial therapy. It has a half-life of 74 days, so storage and accidental loss is not so serious as with radium and cobalt[60]. Its gamma activity can be calibrated against radium in milligram-radium-equivalents for each day the sources are used. This permits the use of tables in existence for radium to calculate more accurate dosimetry for iridium[192]. The techniques for handling this isotope are being worked out to make the ribbons commercially available.

Special Uses and Properties of Radioactive Cobalt

The properties of cobalt lend themselves to various forms of interstitial radiation in the form of needles and nylon tubes. Cobalt lends itself to use by all the well-known techniques employed with radium and radon, and many of the forms of colpostats designed for radium could be adapted to radioactive cobalt or cobanic. The use of radioactive cobalt in nylon tubes is useful in inoperable tumors near bone or large vessels. The radioactive threads can be inserted into any area accessible by malleable needles or an aneurysm guide. The cobalt sutures are spaced about 1 cm. apart throughout the tumor tissue. Radioactive cobalt will find a larger use in irregular tumor masses, for no other form of interstitial radiation can be so readily applied. Preliminary observations indicate that it is less destructive to bone than is radium and is better tolerated in deep tissue previously exposed to maximum external radiation. This is possible because there is no selective absorption of the hard gamma ray in bone. Certainly no other method allows for palliative radiation for metastatic cancer in the retroperitoneal lymph nodes surrounding major vessels.

Treatment of Carcinoma of the Cervix With Radioactive Cobalt

Barnes and others have used a uterine tandem, at times with a colpostat (Paris type technique), for early carcinoma of the cervix or for local central palliation. The cylinders they used were 10 mm. long and 4 mm. in diameter and could be loaded in various arrangements, depending on the space afforded in the vaginal vault. They attempted to irradiate the parametrium beyond the limits of palpable extension of the tumor. As is well known, they felt that the upper third of the vagina should be given a cancerocidal dose to take care of any vaginal extension in the submucosa not palpable on examination. Interstitial needles, held in place by templates, were used in some patients. In some patients the radioactive cobalt was placed in plastic tubing that could be wrapped around invaded tissue. The radioactive cobalt was preceded in most instances by medium voltage deep x-ray therapy.

ROENTGENTHERAPY
Vaginal Cone Roentgentherapy

Radiation of the cervix by a vaginal cone was revived by del Regato, and he devised several modifications. Using low or medium voltage deep x-ray units, a lead-lined cone of various dimensions is introduced into the vagina and directed by a periscopic attachment in the direction of the cervix. The cone is shifted and the beam directed into one or other of the lateral fornices. Provided the patient is motionless during the therapy, the bladder and rectum empty and static, no cystocele or rectocele to bulge in front of the beam, and the patient can tolerate this painful therapy, 500 r. per treatment can be delivered in air to the region or regions to which the beam is directed. If the patient is extremely cooperative, a dose of 6,000 r. measured in air can be beamed in the general direction of the cervix in the course of twelve treatments. With the use of a low voltage unit, to avoid damage to the rectum or a rectocele that often ends up in the center of the target, a severe erythema of the vaginal vault results. With a medium voltage unit an excellent calculated tumor dose is possible, but the technical difficulties resist solution and better means are now available.

Deep External Roentgentherapy

Deep external radiation is produced by bombardment of a target in a vacuum tube. The electrons bombarding the target may be generated by voltages ranging from 50 kv. to many millions. With the usual therapy unit of 200 to 250 kv., electromagnetic waves of a length of 10^{-8} to 10^{-10} are produced. A harder or shorter ray is produced as the voltage is increased up to about 1,000 kv., when physical laws diminish the hardness that can be achieved. Cobalt bombs and cesium[137] units deliver therapy equivalent to several million volts and are being used more extensively because of the small cost as compared to the supervoltage units necessary to produce the same quality of radiation. Isotope units permit rotational teletherapy, delivering a large depth or tumor dose through an extensive portal of entry.

The technique of treatment of the pelvic organs varies, depending on the equipment available, but is more or less standardized. Portals 10 to 15 cm. are outlined anteriorly and posteriorly, the bladder or rectum is shielded by a lead strip, and 2,000 to 2,200 r. measured in air are delivered in divided doses (fractional-protracted method) to each of the portals in the course of five to six weeks. Some therapists use lateral or oblique portals to make six areas. The therapy is directed to the pelvic side wall, since a gamma emitter is used to destroy the cancer in the cervix and adjacent 2 to 3 cm.

A cancer of the cervix treated by x-ray and radium is managed by a course of external therapy and one or more insertions of radium during the course of the deep therapy. Most gynecologists insert the radium after each external portal has received 800 r. A second insertion is done later to give a combined total of 6,000 r. to the pelvic side wall. This is a calculation in which the gamma roentgens are added to roentgens, although the difference in the quality of the radiation is acknowledged.

Baclesse, at the Fondation Curie in Paris, is treating cancer of the cervix by the use of external radiation alone. He utilizes multiple external portals, including perineo-obturator and sciatic, as well as the standard anterior and posterior portals. Madame Baud, at the same institution, has continued the standard Paris technique with the addition of teleradium for supplementary radiation. A comparison of the results of therapy by these two distinguished radiotherapists is being made.

BETA EMITTERS
RADIOACTIVE GOLD
General Considerations

J. H. Müller (Zurich), in 1945, applied an artificial radioactive isotope, in liquid form, intraperitoneally for extensive abdominal carcinomatosis. He used radioactive zinc (Zn^{63}) that was cyclotron-produced in limited quantities. The radioactive material was in a chemically insoluble form (sulfide) and was suspended in an isotonic pectin solution. The radioactive zinc was given in ten doses of 100 mc. for a total of 1 curie. With the advent of radioactive gold, which has a longer half-life (2.7 days), the use of radioactive zinc was abandoned for the gold, which is easier to handle.

Physical Properties

Radioactive gold is produced in a nuclear reactor by slow neutron bombardment. The gold[197] foil is exposed for seven to fourteen days with the resultant formula: Au^{197} plus n $\rightarrow$ Au^{198} plus gamma ray. The Abbott Laboratories then incorporated the resultant gold with gelatin to form the brownish-red radioactive gold. The pH of this solution was between 5.5 and 6.5, and the specific activity between 20 and 30 mc. per milliliter. The colloidal particles average 0.003 micron in diameter.

The physical properties of Au^{198} are responsible for its therapeutic uses. It has a short half-life of 2.7 days, and at the end of eleven days 95 per cent of all its radiation has been emitted. Of the energy it gives off, 95 per cent is composed of soft beta rays, which have a maximum energy of 0.98 million electron volts. Radioactive gold decays into stable mercury. The range in tissues of the beta radiation given off by the radioactive gold is limited. The gamma radiation is on the order of 0.44 million electron volts. The predominance of the beta radiation gives it an excellent local effect, and, in addition, the metallic form in use is nontoxic both chemically and physiologically. The isotope has a maximum range in tissue of 3.8 mm., and 50 per cent travels only 0.38 mm. It is an agent that must be used for its effect in the first few millimeters of the tissue it bathes. The small amount of harder, more penetrating gamma radiation given off by the radioactive gold can be detected outside the body and be used to determine the distribution of the colloidal solution within the serous cavity concerned. Some commercially available solutions are made up to contain 3 to 4 mc. per milligram of gold. Thus, if 25 mg. of gold is introduced with strength of 4 mc. per milligram, the total radiation deposited in the cavity would be 100 mc. Schick and Bloor use an initial dosage of 125 mc. when treating the peritoneal cavity. The delivered dose defies accurate calculation as to the number of roentgens over any area of the peritoneal, omental, liver, or bowel surfaces. Estimates based on the calculated surface area of the peritoneum and other surfaces within the abdomen presume that if the deposition was equal throughout between 3,000 and 20,000 equivalent roentgens per 100 mc. of gold may be delivered.

Since the half-life of Au^{198} is 2.7 days, any plan of treatment must of necessity deliver the radioactive gold to the tumor or lymphatics within hours or the radiation will be dissipated. Berg and associates studied this in the lymphatics of the bronchial tree in dogs. After submucosal injection in various bronchi and subdivisions, nodes and tissue were studied by an end-window Geiger-Müller counter and later by autoradiographs. They found a high level of activity in the hilar nodes in four hours, but it was patchy when the entire hilar nodal system was considered. Within the nodes it was also patchy, and this is discouraging. Unfortunately it is probable that the patchy areas not showing activity in the autoradiographs were in the part of the node containing tumor.

The female bladder is so intimately involved in pelvic disease that its reaction to the administration of radioactive gold governs, as in other methods of radiation, the use of the agent involved. Radioactive gold injected into the dome of the bladder in dogs resulted in local necrosis at the site of injection. The radioactivity was found high in the trigone within five to fifteen days after injection; in addition, there was considerable activity in the regional nodes. The bladder drains through the same lymphatics as the female genital organs, and radical surgery involves the same structures. Radioactive gold picked up in any of the pelvic organs will cause a histologic response in the regional nodes. This should not be discounted, since anything that interrupts the dissemination of malignant cells should be employed until we have something better.

Method of Action

Radioactive gold is a useful palliative substance in the control of serous effusions in the chest and abdomen. Its use is limited to patients in reasonably good condition who have symptomatic effusions. The second of two applications is more effective than the first, and the entire process by which it reduces the ascites is probably one of simple fibrosis of the peritoneal or pleural surface by the radiation.

The site or histologic type of tumor has not as yet been important in the degree of palliation resulting from the administration of radioactive gold. The mode of action has been studied by Sherman and co-workers when it was injected interstitially. Various amounts of the colloidal solution were injected into the parametrium of patients with cervical cancer. The tissues removed after radical hysterectomy and pelvic lymphadenectomy were then studied. The sites of injection showed the usual radiation effects. The obturator, hypogastric, and iliac nodes, representing true metastatic stations, contained gold deposits. It was not possible to determine whether malignant cells were destroyed in these nodes by the radioactive gold absorbed along the same channels.

The use of colloidal gold in the therapy of tumor masses would have to be based on the existence of lymphatics in the tumor tissue if the radioactive gold were to be distributed by virtue of its pickup by the lymphatic system. Zeidman, using cancerous nodes and tumor outside the nodes in rabbits that had been induced by V_2 cancer cells, used radioactive gold and Berlin blue as tracers to determine whether metastatic cancer has lymphatic drainage. The result was the finding of the tracers in the lymphatics but none in solid, intranodal tumor tissue that was immediately adjacent. Radioautographs to identify the gold isotope, compared with routine hematoxylin and eosin sections, showed that the gold failed to concentrate in solid cancer nodules. While many clinicians felt that this would be found, it still supports the use of a thorough lymphadenectomy as our best—though obviously temporary, means of dealing with metastatic cancer in the nodes draining the primary and secondary lymphatic stations of a pelvic cancer. Even attempts at retrograde injection of dye back into the tumor mass were unsuccessful, showing that the tumor nodule not only lacked afferent lymphatics, but also efferent channels.

Protection of the Therapist

Unless the personnel engaged in the management of the patients are extremely careless, and this could scarcely happen since all have to undergo the necessary training, the exposure to radioactivity is small. The physicians administering the gold receive less than 5 milliroentgens during the average procedure, which is small compared with the 50 to 100 milliroentgens received while taking a standard chest film. The maximum permissible isodose distance from the patient, the distance from the patient at which a reading of 6.25 milliroentgens per hour is obtained, is observed. All nursing procedures are expeditiously done and personnel are carefully rotated.

Intraperitoneal Application

The radioactive gold is delivered to the therapist in sealed, sterile units. The normal precautions for handling any radioactive substance are observed, and the containers are moved about by long-handled forceps and are kept behind lead. An ionization chamber is used to check the activity of the shipment. One millicurie reads 0.24 milliroentgen per hour at 1 meter, with an error of measurement within 10 per cent. The colloidal suspension is then placed in a lead container and inlet and outlet needles are introduced. With the use of 100 mc., the activity is less than 5 milliroentgens per hour at the outside surface of the container and 14 milliroentgens per hour over the slot where the tubes emerge. A system of stopcocks is then arranged to permit the displacement of the colloidal gold from the bottle in which it is received to the peritoneal cavity by the injection of saline solution into the system and forcing the gold solution out. Up to 500 ml. of saline solution may be used with this method, and the saline solution tends to ensure more uniform distribution of the active material within the peritoneal cavity. (Plate 59, *A* to *E*.)

In most patients with abdominal carcinomatosis the fluid is thin in consistency and is not loculated in spite of the frequent presence of an omental cake. The therapy is contraindicated in the presence of viscid fluid and multiple loculations, for here the colloid becomes pocketed and may cause necrosis of the bowel. The presence of intraperitoneal abscesses from previous tappings, with perforation of the bowel, must be kept in mind, for attempts to introduce the gold in such locations would do more harm than any possible good when it is remembered that this is only palliative therapy. Where adhesions or some loculation interferes with the introduction by the simple trocar method, the colloid may be introduced through a laparotomy incision. Rose and associates use an epigastric incision, and, after evacuating the ascitic fluid and excising any major metastatic masses and freeing up any loculations, they place a No. 16 or No. 18 urethral catheter in each lumbar gutter. Holes are made along the length of the catheter that is intraperitoneal to help more uniform distribution of the gold. The catheters are led into the peritoneal cavity by an offset stab wound, which closes readily when they are withdrawn. An "offset stab wound," whether through the abdominal wall and peritoneum or in another location to reach a hollow viscus, allows drainage or the passage of a tube and closes more readily than the fistula of a direct drainage tube. The radioactive gold is introduced into the peritoneal cavity after the patient has been returned to her room. Spillage might tie up the operating room for some time.

The extent of spread of the radioactive material in the peritoneal cavity is determined by whatever monitor is available to count the gamma radiation. The changing of the position of the patient and the use of an oscillating bed both help to distribute the material throughout the peritoneal cavity. The direct catheter method undoubtedly gives better distribution but requires surgery with its effects on an already debilitated patient.

The dosage of radioactive gold is determined by several factors: the amount of stable gold

PLATE 59

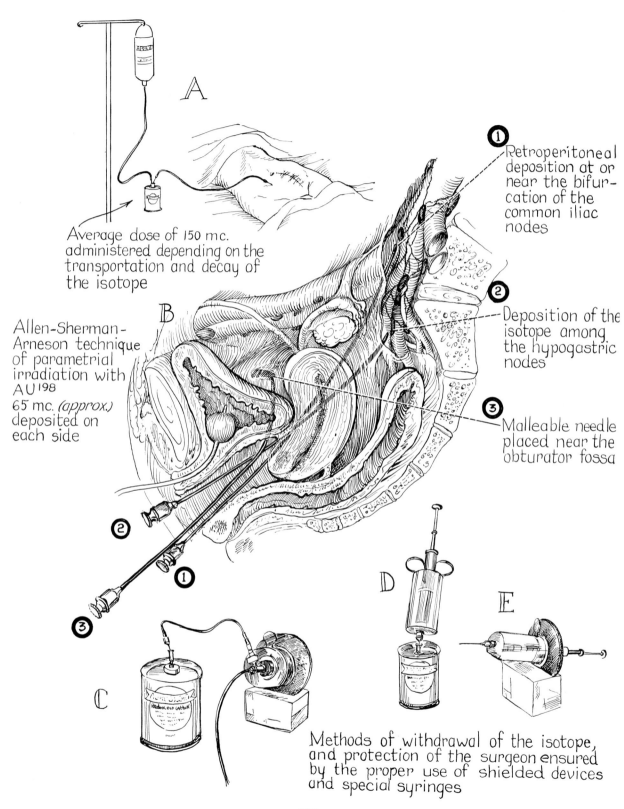

A

Average dose of 150 mc. administered depending on the transportation and decay of the isotope

Allen-Sherman-Arneson technique of parametrial irradiation with AU198

65 mc. (approx.) deposited on each side

B

① Retroperitoneal deposition at or near the bifurcation of the common iliac nodes

② Deposition of the isotope among the hypogastric nodes

③ Malleable needle placed near the obturator fossa

C   D   E

Methods of withdrawal of the isotope, and protection of the surgeon ensured by the proper use of shielded devices and special syringes injected, the radioactivity in millicuries injected, and the approximate radiation dose to the tissues. For every 100 mc. of radioactive gold, there are approximately 20 mg. of stable gold. Robert O. Gorson and R. H. Chamberlain of the University of Pennsylvania have estimated tissue dose in terms of millicuries injected and the resultant radiation dose within tissue levels beneath the serosal surface. According to their estimates, "the beta absorbed dose at a depth of 0.1 mm. is approximately 620 rads per millicurie per 1000 cm.^{2} and decreases to about 80 rads at a depth of 1.0 mm. The absorbed dose for distances less than 0.1 mm. cannot be specified accurately because it depends critically upon the distribution, specific activity, and thickness of the gold particles or their aggregates on the serosal surface. The peritoneum may have an area of 30,000 cm.^{2} and under these circumstances could receive a beta dose of 2100 rads at a depth of 0.1 mm. if 100 mc. were injected, if distribution were uniform. Theoretically, as the surface of an infinitely thin plane beta source is approached, the dose becomes infinite. In practice there are always finite sources whose distribution is far from uniform and the dose varies greatly. If the gold layer was .005 mm. thick and uniform, for example, the beta dose at the surface could be calculated at approximately 1800 to 1900 rads/μc/cm.^{2} When the thickness and distribution are unknown, these calculations have little meaning. The dose is very high immediately adjacent to any gold particle or aggregate. The total body integral gamma ray dose would be about 3×10^6 gram rads, resulting in an *average* gamma ray absorbed dose of 40 to 50 rads per 100 mc. injected."

Results of Intraperitoneal Therapy

One of the first effects that may be noted is the disappearance of blood from the ascitic fluid. The therapy of a patient in desperate need of palliation does not permit studies that will satisfy the exacting statistician regarding the survival of the treated cases as compared with the untreated. There are some remarkable survivals for a year or more among those who walk out of the clinic and refuse the therapy offered. The presence of large masses of cancer will render ineffectual the superficially penetrating beta rays delivered by radioactive gold. But in the diffuse metastatic disease, with small implants, the gold is superior to external radiation because it allows a substantial dose to be delivered to the cancer without a corresponding radiation sickness in the patient. Realizing the total number of roentgens (calculated physical equivalents) that are delivered by the colloidal solution as compared with the dosage in air necessary to produce the same effect, it would seem that this therapy has some substantial advantages over deep x-ray therapy; the latter, however, is more universally applicable.

Therapy of Carcinoma of the Cervix

The colloid is injected into the parametrium and the amount of radiation and its effects evaluated by direct measurement with a scintillation counter at the time of surgery and by counting the radioactivity of tissues and lymphatics removed at the time of radical hysterectomy. The tissues removed are studied histologically for evidence of radiation reaction. The calculated dose that can be delivered by this method is much greater than that possible by radium or deep x-ray therapy. The intense beta radiation in the immediate site of deposition of the colloid may reach 75,000 roentgen-equivalent-physical units. The gamma radiation from the radioactive gold, although only a small part, can be calculated to deliver 2,000 to 3,000 r. in the pelvis. The gold particles are rapidly phagocystosed and carried to the regional lymphatics, but it is not to be presumed that they are selective and migrate to nodes containing cancer. It has been suggested that they may even go to the normal nodes before the invaded lymphatics, since the latter are plugged up and static.

Allen and co-workers are now using 130 mc. of radioactive gold in the preoperative radiation of cancer of the cervix for control of nodal metastases (Plate 59, *B*). They operate about five weeks later. Sixty-five millicuries are deposited on both sides, with about equal amounts in the obturator, hypogastric, and external iliac group of nodes. Radium or radioactive cobalt controls the lesion in the cervix and any immediate extension by continuity.

Therapy of Carcinoma of the Vulva

The reaction of gold injected beneath the skin surface in vulval cancer can be followed with a counting chamber, and it soon diffuses beneath the skin surface. An erythematous reaction and epilation in the area draining the site of injection can be noted. Effects upon tumor cells in the region of phagocytosed gold particles have been noted.

Therapy of Tumor Masses

Direct intratumor infiltration with radioactive gold has been used in treatment of gynecologic cancer. It has been possible to achieve some local regression by this means. Direct infiltration of tumors of the female genital tract has been done for the ovary, cervix, vulva, vagina, and groin. The results are difficult to assess from these early studies.

Radiation Reactions

Herve and Closon demonstrated in rabbits that the intraperitoneal injection of Au[198] resulted in distribution of the isotope "chronologically, topographically, and quantitatively very similar to that of intravenous administration." Significant amounts of the isotope were found in the bone marrow, liver, spleen, and lungs within twenty-four hours. Botsford and co-workers found evidence of bone marrow destruction in six autopsies while at the same time identifying the presence of gold particles in the marrow. They used the Elftman technique for staining the marrow. This should be considered when giving this therapy to patients whose marrow may have already been depressed by other agents. A transitory leukopenia develops within four to six weeks after therapy. Pre-existing anemia from the malignancy itself must be kept in mind. The usual reactions that would normally follow radiation of the upper abdomen have not been a problem with intraperitoneal gold therapy in the dosages used. Some nausea, diarrhea, and occasionally a mild ileus are seen and are treated symptomatically.

References

Abrahamson, R. H.: Radiation Ileitis, A. M. A. Arch. Surg. 81: 553, 1960.

Agnew, A. M., Fidler, H. K., and Boyes, D. A.: Evaluation of Radiation Response, Am. J. Obst. & Gynec. 79: 698, 1960.

Agnew, C. H.: Radioisotopes in Obstetrics and Gynecology, Texas J. Med. 54: 706, 1958.

Allen, J. G., and others: Studies on the Causes of Death From Total Body Irradiation, M. Science 1: 40, 1957.

Allen, W., Sherman, A., and Arneson, A.: Carcinoma of the Cervix. Results Obtained From the Irradiation of the Parametrium With Radioactive Colloidal Gold, Am. J. Obst. & Gynec. 68: 1433, 1954.

Allen, W., Sherman, A., and Arneson, A.: Further Results Obtained in the Treatment of Cancer of the Cervix with Radiogold: A Progress Report, Am. J. Obst. & Gynec. 70: 786, 1955.

Allen, W. M., Sherman, A. I., and Camel, H. M.: Radiogold in the Treatment of Cancer of the Cervix, Radiology 70: 523, 1958.

Arneson, A. N.: The Clinical Relationship of Radiology and Gynecology in the Treatment of Cervical Cancer, Radiology 66: 327, 1956.

Bacq, Z., and Alexander, P.: Fundamentals of Radiobiology, New York, 1955, Academic Press, Inc.

Bane, H. N., Conrad, J. T., and Tarnowski, G. S.: Combination Therapy of Malignant Tumors With Ionizing Radiations and Chemicals: a Review, Cancer Res. 17: 551, 1957.

Barnes, A.: Experimental Nonsurgical Therapy of Pelvic Malignancies, Am. J. Obst. & Gynec. 65: 550, 1953.

Barnes, A.: Therapy of the Lateral Pelvic Nodes in Cervical Carcinoma, Am. J. Obst. & Gynec. 68: 489, 1954.

Barnes, A., Morton, J., and Callendine, G., Jr.: The Use of Radioactive Cobalt in the Treatment of Carcinoma of the Cervix, Am. J. Obst. & Gynec. 60: 1112, 1950.

Barnes, D. W. H., and Loutit, J. F.: The Radiation Recovery Factor: Preservation by the Polge-Smith-Parkes Technique, J. Nat. Cancer Inst. 15: 901, 1955.

Bases, R. E.: Modification of the Radiation Response Determined by Single Cell Technics: Actinomycin D, Cancer Res. 19: 1223, 1959.

Bishop, P.: A Flexible Rubber Applicator With a Positive Spread for Radium Treatment of Cancer of the Uterine Cervix, Am. J. Roentgenol. 71: 267, 1954.

Blahey, P.: Optimum Radium Distribution in the Treatment of Cancer of the Cervix, Obst. & Gynec. 16: 679, 1960.

Brues, A. M.: Late Effects of Radiation, Proceedings; Conference on Research on the Radiotherapy of Cancer, American Cancer Society, Inc., University of Wisconsin, Madison, Wis., June 16-18, 1960.

Burton, M., and Chang, J. Y.: Effect of Radiation on Organic Compounds, Proceedings; Conference on Research on the Radiotherapy of Cancer, American Cancer Society, Inc., University of Wisconsin, Madison, Wis., June 16-18, 1960.

Chamberlain, R.: Modern Therapeutic Measures in Cancer and Their Effectiveness: Radiology, Bull. New York Acad. Med. 31: 746, 1955.

Christy, N., and others: The Pathogenesis of Uterine Lesions in Virgin Mice and in Gonadectomized Mice Bearing Adrenal Cortical and Pituitary Tumors, Cancer Res. 11: 413, 1951.

Churchill-Davidson, I.: Oxygen Effect on Radiosensitivity, Proceedings; Conference on Research on the Radiotherapy of Cancer, American Cancer Society, Inc., University of Wisconsin, Madison, Wis., June 16-18, 1960.

Colcock, B. P., and Hume, A.: Radiation Injury to the Sigmoid and Rectum, Surg. Gynec. & Obst. 108: 306, 1959.

Cooper, G., and Williams, K.: Radiation Dosage to Female Gonads During Diagnostic Roentgenographic Procedures, J. A. M. A. 170: 766, 1959.

Copeland, W. E., Nelson, P. K., and Payne, F. L.: Intrauterine Radium for Dysfunctional Bleeding; a Long-Term Follow-up Study, Am. J. Obst. & Gynec. 73: 615, 1957.

Corscaden, J., and Butz, R.: Intracavitary Radium Technique in Treatment of Cancer of Cervix Uteri, Am. J. Roentgenol. 68: 47, 1952.

Cosbie, W. G.: The Contribution of Radiotherapy to the Modern Treatment of Female Pelvic Cancer, J. Obst. & Gynaec. Brit. Emp. 66: 843, 1959.

Cron, R., and others: Surgery and Radioactive Gold Treatment for Carcinoma of the Ovary, Am. J. Obst. & Gynec. 70: 910, 1955.

Dargent, M., and Guillemin, G.: The Treatment of Operable Cancer of the Cervix by the Combination of Radiation and Surgery, Cancer 8: 53, 1955.

Dean, R. E., and Taylor, E. S.: Surgical Treatment of Complications Resulting From Irradiation Therapy of Cervical Cancer, Am. J. Obst. & Gynec. 79: 34, 1960.

del Regato, J.: Role of Roentgen Therapy in Treatment of Cancer of Cervix Uteri, Am. J. Roentgenol. 68: 63, 1952.

Dennis, J. M., Workman, J. B., and Bauer, R. E.: Radioactive Colloidal Gold in the Control of Malignant Effusions; Report and Analysis of 60 Patients, Am. J. Roentgen. 75: 1124, 1956.

Deringer, M., Lorenz, E., and Uphoff, D.: Fertility and Tumor Development in (C57LXA) F₁ Hybrid Mice Receiving X-Radiation to Ovaries Only, to Whole Body, and to Whole Body With Ovaries Shielded, J. Nat. Cancer Inst. 15: 931, 1955.

Ernst, E.: Probable Trends in Irradiation Treatment of Carcinoma of Cervix Uteri With Improved Expanding Type of Radium Applicator, Radiology 52: 46, 1949.

Elftman, H., and Elftman, A.: Histological Methods for the Demonstration of Gold in Tissues, Stain Technol. 20: 59-62, 1945.

Finder, J. G., and Post, M.: Spontaneous Femoral Neck Fracture Following Pelvic Irradiation; Report of Three Cases, A. M. A. Arch Surg. 81: 545, 1960.

Fletcher, G. H.: Present Status of Cobalt⁶⁰ Teletherapy in the Management of the Cancer Patient, J. A. M. A. 164: 244, 1957.

Fletcher, G. H.: The Role of Supervoltage Therapy, Proceedings; Conference on Research on the Radiotherapy of Cancer, American Cancer Society, Inc. University of Wisconsin, Madison, Wis., June 16-18, 1960.

Frick, H. C., and others: A Study of Complications in the Surgical and Radiation Therapy of Cancer of the Cervix, Surg., Gynec. & Obst. 111: 493, 1960.

Furth, J., and Boon, M.: Induction of Ovarian Tumors in Mice by X-rays, Cancer Res. 7: 241, 1947.

Garcia, M.: Host Factors Affecting the Radiation Response in Carcinoma of the Cervix, Proceedings; Conference on Research on the Radiotherapy of Cancer, American Cancer Society, Inc., University of Wisconsin, Madison, Wis., June 16-18, 1960.

Glasser, O., Quimby, E., Taylor, L., and Weatherwax, J.: Physical Foundations of Radiology, ed. 2, New York, 1952, Paul B. Hoeber, Inc.

Gray, L. H.: The Modification by Chemical Agents of Biological Response to Irradiation, Proceedings; Conference on Research on the Radiotherapy of Cancer, American Cancer Society, Inc., University of Wisconsin, Madison, Wis., June 16-18, 1960.

Gray, M. J., and Kottmeier, H. L.: Rectal and Bladder Injuries Following Radium Therapy for Carcinoma of the Cervix at the Radiumhemmet, Am. J. Obst. & Gynec. 74: 1294, 1957.

Gusberg, S. B.: A Consideration of the Problems of Radiosensitivity in the Cancer of the Cervix, Bull. Sloane Hosp. for Women 3: 1, 1957.

Guttmann, R. J.: Dose Distribution and Results in Carcinoma of the Cervix; a Comparison of Conventional High Voltage Therapy Including Vaginal Cone Therapy With Supervoltage Therapy, Am. J. Roentgen. 77: 803, 1957.

von Haam, E., Hendricks, C., and Morton, T.: Cytological Studies on Patients With Carcinoma of the Cervix Treated With Co⁶⁰ (abstract), Cancer Res. 12: 303, 1952.

Hahn, G. A.: An Evaluation of Supervoltage Irradiation Therapy in the Treatment of Pelvic Malignancy, Am. J. Obst. & Gynec. 73: 626, 1957.

Hahn, P.: A Manual of Artificial Radioisotope Therapy, New York, 1951, Academic Press, Inc.

Hahn, P. F., and Meng, H. C.: Internal Irradiation of Dogs With Radio-Active Colloidal Gold: Synergistic Effect of Iron, Cancer 11: 591, 1958.

Handbook 41: Medical X-ray Protection Up to Two Million Volts, United States Department of Commerce, National Bureau of Standards.

Hankins, F., and Hockin, J.: Radium Treatment of Cancer of the Uterine Cervix by the Manchester System; Use of Plastic Vaginal Applicators, Am. J. Roentgenol. 68: 272, 1952.

Hames, I.: A New Method in the Use of Radon Gold Seeds, Am. J. Surg. 38: 235, 1937.

Henschke, U., James, A., and Myers, W.: Radiogold Seeds for Cancer Therapy, Nucleonics 11: 46, 1953.

Herve, A., and Closon, J.: Apropos de la Distribution dans L'organisme de l'or Colloidal Radioactif, Schweiz. med. Wchnschr. 82: 522, 1952.

Heyman, J.: Thoughts on Forty Years of Radiation Treatment of Carcinoma of the Uterine Cervix, Am. J. Obst. & Gynec. 68: 480, 1954.

Heyman, J.: Some Problems of Current Interest Relating to Classification and Treatment of Uterine Carcinoma, Am. J. Obst. & Gynec. 69: 502, 1955.

Hine, G. J., and Friedman, M.: Problems of Dosimetry of New Modes of Radiation, Proceedings; Conference on Research on the Radiotherapy of Cancer, American Cancer Society, Inc., University of Wisconsin, Madison, Wis., June 16-18, 1960.

Hinman, F., Jr.: Experience With Intracavitary Radiocobalt for Bladder Tumors, J. Urol. 73: 285, 1955.

Hofmann, D.: Radiation Treatment of Malignant Tumors of the External Genitalia (Zur Strahlenbehandlung boesartiger Geschwuelste der aeusseren Genitale), Geburtsh. u. Frauenh. 17: 725, 1957.

Jacobs, M. L.: Radioactive Colloidal Chromic Phosphate to Control Pleural Effusion and Ascites, J. A. M. A. 166: 597, 1958.

Johanson, C., Ostling, G., and Gasstrom, R.: Treatment of Uterine Cancer With Radioactive Cobalt (Co⁶⁰), Acta radiol. 36: 324, 1951.

Johns, H. E.: Newer Radiotherapeutic Sources of Radiation and the Distributions that They Produce in Biological Materials, Proceedings; Conference on Research on the Radiotherapy of Cancer, American Cancer Society, Inc., University of Wisconsin, Madison, Wis., June 16-18, 1960.

Jones, H. W., and others: Cellular Changes in Vaginal and Buccal Smears After Radiation: An Index of the Radiocurability of Carcinoma of the Cervix, Am. J. Obst. & Gynec. 78: 1083, 1959.

Kaplan, H.: Influence of Ovarian Function on Incidence of Radiation-Induced Ovarian Tumors in Mice, J. Nat. Cancer Inst. 11: 175, 1950.

Kaplan, H. S.: New Horizons in Radiotherapy of Malignant Disease, J. A. M. A. 171: 133, 1959.

Keettel, W., and Elkins, H.: Experience With Radioactive

Colloidal Gold in the Treatment of Ovarian Carcinoma, Am. J. Obst. & Gynec. 71: 553, 1956.

King, E.: The Use of Radioactive Colloidal Gold (Au198) in Pleural Effusions and Ascites Associated With Malignancy, Am. J. Roentgenol. 68: 413, 1952.

Kligerman, M. M.: The Role of Combination Radiation and Chemotherapy, Proceedings; Conference on Research on the Radiotherapy of Cancer, American Cancer Society, Inc., University of Wisconsin, Madison, Wis., June 16-18, 1960.

Kligerman, M., and Habif, D.: The Use of Radioactive Gold in the Treatment of Effusion Due to Carcinomatosis of the Pleura and Peritoneum, Am. J. Roentgenol. 74: 651, 1955.

Kottmeier, H. L.: Irradiation for Carcinoma of the Cervix, Am. J. Obst. & Gynec. 76: 243, 1958.

Lange, R., Shields, J., and Rozendaal, H.: Colloidal Radioactive Chromic Phosphate in the Control of Malignant Effusions, New York J. Med. 56: 1928, 1956.

Leissner, H., and Kjellgren, O.: Radium Reactions in the Bladder, Acta obst. et gynec. scandinav. 38: 544, 1959.

Lich, L., Kirschbaum, A., and Mixer, H.: Mechanism of Induction of Ovarian Tumors by X-rays, Cancer Res. 9: 532, 1949.

Looney, W., and Colodzin, M.: Late Follow-up Studies After Internal Disposition of Radioactive Materials, J. A. M. A. 160: 1, 1956.

Martin, C. L.: The Approximation Technique in Treatment of Cancer of the Cervix With Irradiation, Am. J. Roentgen. 77: 388, 1957.

Merrill, J. A., Wood, D. A., and Zippen, C.: Radiosensitivity-Testing Procedures in Cancer of the Cervix, Proceedings; Conference on Research on the Radiotherapy of Cancer, American Cancer Society, Inc., University of Wisconsin, Madison, Wis., June 16-18, 1960.

Meschan, I., and Nettleship, A.: Comparative Effects of Cobalt 60 and Radium When Utilized in Identical Doses on the Skin of Rabbits, Am. J. Roentgenol. 71: 306, 1954.

Meschan, I., Oddie, T., and Regnier, G.: A Method of Dosimetry for Carcinoma of the Cervix Utilizing a Modified Manchester Technic With Cobalt 60, Radiology 64: 546, 1955.

Miller, N. F., and others: Irradiation Sensitivity of Cervix Cancer, Am. J. Obst. & Gynec. 76: 1071, 1958.

Mizutani, M., and others: Changes in Model Values of Chromosomes After Irradiation of Human Amnion Cells, Proceedings; Conference on Research on the Radiotherapy of Cancer, American Cancer Society, Inc., University of Wisconsin, Madison, Wis., June 16-18, 1960.

Mole, R. H.: On Wasted Radiation and the Interpretation of Experiments With Chronic Irradiation, J. Nat. Cancer Inst. 15: 907, 1955.

Moore, V.: Radioactive Chromic Phosphate in Treatment of Urological Tumors, J. Urol. 73: 410, 1955.

Morton, J., and others: Irradiation of Cancer of the Uterine Cervix With Radioactive Cobalt 60 in Guided Aluminum Needles and in Plastic Threads, Am. J. Roentgenol. 69: 813, 1953.

Morton, J., Callendine, G., Jr., and Myers, W.: Radioactive Cobalt-60 in Plastic Tubing for Interstitial Radiation Therapy, Radiology 56: 553, 1951.

Muller, H. J.: Genetic Damage Produced by Radiation, Science 121: 837, 1955.

Müller, J. H.: Further Development of the Therapy of Peritoneal Carcinomatosis in Ovarian Carcinoma by Means of Artificial Radioactivity (Au198), Gynecologia 94: 289, 1950.

Nickson, J. J.: The Role of Electron Therapy in the Treatment of Patients With Cancer, Proceedings; Conference on Research on the Radiotherapy of Cancer, American Cancer Society, Inc., University of Wisconsin, Madison, Wis., June 16-18, 1960.

Nolan, J. F.: Postoperative Radiotherapy of Carcinoma of the Cervix, Am. J. Obst. & Gynec. 79: 892, 1960.

Nolan, J. F.: Response of Carcinoma in Situ of the Cervix to Radiation Therapy, Am. J. Obst. & Gynec. 79: 914, 1960.

Norwood, W. D.: Common Sense Approach to the Problem of Genetic Hazard Due to Diagnostic Radiology, J. A. M. A. 167: 1928, 1958.

Oddie, T., and Meschan, I.: The Physical Aspects of the Utilization of the Tripartite Rigid Cobalt 60 Applicator for the Treatment of Carcinoma of the Cervix, Radiology 64: 560, 1955.

Oster, I. I.: Radiation Effects on Genetic Systems, Proceedings; Conference on Research on the Radiotherapy of Cancer, American Cancer Society, Inc., University of Wisconsin, Madison, Wis., June 16-18, 1960.

Parlee, S. S.: Radiation Hazards in Obstetrics and Gynecology, Am. J. Obst. & Gynec. 75: 327, 1958.

Payne, F. L.: Radiation Safety in Obstetric-Gynecologic Practice, Am. J. M. Sc. 240: 782, 1960.

Putzki, P. S., and Varden, L. C.: Bowel Complications Due to Intraperitoneal Radioactive Gold; Report of 2 Cases, Obst. & Gynec. 16: 398, 1960.

Quastler, H.: Time-Dose Relations in Radiation Effects, Proceedings; Conference on Research on the Radiotherapy of Cancer, American Cancer Society, Inc., University of Wisconsin, Madison, Wis., June 16-18, 1960.

Quimby, E.: Dosage Table for Linear Radium Sources, Radiology 43: 572, 1944.

Quimby, E.: The Radioisotope Program in the General Hospital, J. A. M. A. 154, 449, 1954.

Rassmussen-Taxdal, D., Ward, G., and Figge, F.: Fluorescence of Human Lymphatic and Cancer Tissue Following High Doses of Intravenous Hematoporphyrins, Cancer 8: 78, 1955.

Rothschild, M. A., and Schreiber, S. S.: The Use of Radioisotopes in Research, Diagnosis, and Therapy, (Part 11), New York J. Med. 58: 2676, 1958.

Ruch, R. M., and others: Cervical Cancer in Aortic Lymph Nodes Treated With Radioactive Gold; Report of a Case, Obst. & Gynec. 10: 388, 1957.

Rutledge, F. N., and Fletcher, G. H.: Transperitoneal Pelvic Lymphadenectomy Following Supervoltage Irradiation for Squamous-Cell Carcinoma of the Cervix, Am. J. Obst. & Gynec. 76: 321, 1958.

Sands, R. H.: The Role of "Free Radicals" in Radiation, Proceedings; Conference on Research on the Radiotherapy of Cancer, American Cancer Society, Inc., University of Wisconsin, Madison, Wis., June 16-18, 1960.

Schmitz, H. E., Smith, C. J., and Fetherston, W. C.: Effects of Preoperative Irradiation on Adenocarcinoma of the Uterus, Am. J. Obst. & Gynec. 78: 1048, 1959.

Senn, A., and Lundsgaard-Hansen, P.: Diagnosis and Treatment of Radiation Damage of the Gastrointestinal Tract, Schweiz. med. Wchnschr. 86: 1015, 1956.

Sherman, A. I.: The Role of Combined Surgery and Radiation in the Treatment of Cancer of the Reproductive System, Proceedings; Conference on Research on the Radiotherapy of Cancer, American Cancer Society, Inc., University of Wisconsin, Madison, Wis., June 16-18, 1960.

Siegel, E. P., and others: Radioyttrium (Y90) for the Palliative Treatment of Effusions Due to Malignancy, J. A. M. A 161: 499, 1956.

Silk, M. H., Hawtrey, A. O., and MacIntosh. I. J. C., Indirect Effects During X-Radiation of Malignant Tumors, Cancer Res. 18: 1257, 1958.

Storaasli, J. P., and Schoeniger, E.: Present Status of Radioactive Isotopes in the Treatment of Cancer, Proceedings; Conference on Research on the Radiotherapy of Cancer, American Cancer Society, Inc., University of Wisconsin, Madison, Wis., June 16-18, 1960.

Thistlethwaite, J. R., Spencer, W. A., and Albert, S. N.: Blood Volume Fluctuations Determined by Radioisotopes of Chromium and Radio-Active Iodinated Serum Albumin, Surg., Gynec. & Obst. 103: 34, 1957.

Ullery, J. C., and Holzaepfel, J. H.: Radio-Isotopes in Gynecology as Applied in Pelvic Malignancies, Dept. of Obst. & Gynec., College of Medicine, Ohio State University, Columbus, Ohio.

Veldhuis, A. H., Swinehart, L. A., and Preuss, L. E.: Use of Radioactive Gold in Treatment of Cancer of the Cervix, Henry Ford Hosp. M. Bull. 4: 144, 1956.

Vermooten, V.: Use of Radioactive Cobalt in Nylon Sutures for Bladder Carcinoma, J. Urol. 73: 280, 1955.

Warren, S.: Carcinogenesis by Radiation, Cancer Res. 17: 1, 1957.

Warren, S.: The Pathological Effects of Small Doses of Radiation, Bull. New York Acad. Med. 34: 633, 1958.

Waterman, G., and Reid, W.: Place of Deep External X-ray Irradiation in the Treatment of Carcinoma of the Cervix by Long Element Needles, Radiology 52: 34, 1949.

Waterman, G. W., and Reid, W. A.: End Results of Radium Treatment for Non-Malignant Conditions of the Uterus, Tr. New England Obst. & Gynec. Soc. 11: 101, 1948.

Windeyer, B. W.: Discussion on Radiotherapy in Modern Treatment of Female Pelvic Cancer, J. Obst. & Gynaec. Brit. Emp. 66: 849, 1959.

Zeidman, I.: Recent Advances in Our Knowledge of the Spread of Cancer, Pennsylvania M. J. 58: 595, 1955.

Zeigerman, J. H., Tulsky, E. G., and Makler, P.: Post-radiation Nephritic Syndrome, Obst. & Gynec. 9: 542, 1957.

23 · Chemotherapy in Gynecologic Cancer

General Considerations

This chapter is not written to inform the practicing gynecologist of new drugs that will perform miraculous cures in female genital cancer. It is written because the regional gynecologic surgeon deals with a large percentage of the cancers that afflict women, and although the basic scientists may not be ready to give us the clinical materials today, their inroads into the understanding of malignant disease are promising enough to make it the duty of every clinician to prepare himself for the day when it becomes his task to test some therapy on statistically significant numbers of human patients.

A new orientation is necessary, for the clinician must now review his basic science, although he is not expected to become a theoretical chemist or physicist. Some basic principles come to mind. They will be ever more important when widespread clinical trials of compounds become a common occurrence. Drugs, enzymes, or combinations have a pharmacodynamic action (on the host) and a chemotherapeutic action (on the cancer), and the latter is the action that may make them valuable. Clinicians will more and more have to pin themselves down as to what is cause and effect—a fine distinction. Action of an agent refers to the site and mode, whereas effect of an agent deals with the ultimate results of the therapy and may involve a group of changes. As clinicians, we have often failed to make this clear in our writing and in our reporting of simple, statistical, clinical observations.

The objective in cancer chemotherapy is to find substances that have a toxic, selective action on a cancer with little or no deleterious effect on the host. This has been achieved in the laboratory with certain cancer strains in tissue culture. This is revolutionary, for in no other way have we been able to attack a cancer cell by a selective agent and leave normal cells immune in the same medium. We must soon learn to use some simple curves in measuring the action of a drug such as the standard frequency curve that plots the response against the dose or stimulus. We cannot, in the research that is soon to come, record the simple percentages of the occurrence of something in the hospital, as noted in the annual report, and accept these simple compilations with the same authoritativeness as a controlled, scientific investigation. Such percentages rarely take into consideration that "more than one event" may be occurring—that "more than one factor" may be operating. When we do a simple clinical experiment and compare two agents and their effect on something in the female genital tract, we have frequently seen significantly nonparallel response curves. It is probable that the two agents were acting quite differently and never should have been the object of clinical comparison.

We may soon be called upon to evaluate the results of combined therapy, which may be one of the most promising roads of endeavor, for now it is evident that drugs with an entirely different mode of action may be combined with a complementary effect upon each other. Indeed, even the route of administration may affect the result of a certain drug or its combined action with another agent in tumor inhibition. We are all familiar with the results of combined antibiotic and sulfonamide therapy. Is it not reasonable that the same mechanisms, although probably more complex, may be applied to the therapy of cancer? One agent enters one body system or cellular component and not another. The clinician, with the opportunity to explore the human patient, observe and assess the results, and suggest avenues to the treatment of human beings, may soon find himself duty bound to know the basic science and research preceding his endeavors.

Cancer research has advanced to the point where, in some few isolated types, it can now fulfill the postulates of Koch to prove the etiology of a disease. Rhoads points out the similarity of the stromal reaction about cancer cells to the tissue response to an invading bacteria. Koch's second postulate requires that the etiologic agent be cultivated in pure form in tissue cultures or experimental animals. This has been done for many cancers, including those of the cervix. The third postulate requires that the cultivated organism be reinoculated into the normal subject and cause the disease. At the Sloan-Kettering Institute for Cancer Research, cells maintained for months in pure culture have been reimplanted into the patient from whom they were originally obtained (with the patient's consent and full knowledge of the experiment) with subsequent propagation of the cancer cells. A successful transplant of metastatic epidermoid cancer of the cervix removed from an inguinal node was also achieved.

The use of hormones, especially estrogens, progesterone, and chemicals with adrenocortical action has modified the course of some cancers. The nitrogen mustards and similar substances with a radiomimetric effect may cause an inhibition of some rapidly growing types of cancer. The principle of the heterogeneity of nucleic acid anabolism, upon which the antifolic acid compounds depend for their cancerocidal function, has been established. These chemical functions may be very specific for each type of cell, and therefore cancer, in the body. Selective cancer restraint can be shown in the body as well as the test tube. One example of this is the compound 6-mercaptopurine (6-MP), or Purinethol, synthesized by Hitchings. This

chemical is useful in the restraint of the acute leukemias both in children and adults. It has induced remissions in the chronic myelocytic leukemias. Yet, it seems to have little effect upon Hodgkin's disease, chronic lymphatic leukemia, and other neoplasms.

Studies in the selective absorption of certain chemicals have been carried out by Peck and associates and Rassmussen-Taxdal and co-workers in the case of the hematoporphyrins. These substances have a tendency to accumulate in tissues that are neoplastic, embryonic, or regenerating from recent trauma. They thus accumulate in tissues with a high mitotic index, such as the lymphatics. The method used involves a skin test and a test for tolerance to the material injected intravenously. Then, hematoporphyrin hydrochloride (recrystallized) is dissolved in varying amounts in 600 ml. of 0.166 M sodium lactate. Up to 1,000 mg. was given in some patients during the course of six to ten hours. Search for fluorescence is made with a near-ultraviolet spotlight, such as the General Electric reflector spot quartz mercury-arc light, medical unit. The surgical specimen and tissue in situ in the patient can be photographed. This technique may sometimes assist the cancer surgeon in delineating neoplastic tissue during radical surgery. This type of investigation is mentioned because of the importance of selectivity in the agent or agents that will one day come under study in gynecologic cancer.

RADIOMIMETIC AGENTS IN GYNECOLOGIC CANCER
NITROGEN MUSTARD (HN₂)

Nitrogen mustard, methylbis (β-chloroethyl)amine HCl (HN₂), is a vesicant agent that is injected intravenously for its ability to simulate total body radiation. It has three fields of application in gynecologic cancer: (1) intravenous administration for widespread metastatic disease, (2) intra-arterial administration in the palliative treatment of selected tumor masses, and (3) intraperitoneal injection for the control of serous effusions due to pelvic cancer. The possibility that it may potentiate radiation therapy warrants a trial by intravenous administration in conjunction with radiation to a specific area of recurrent cancer. The total dose is 0.4 mg. per kilogram of body weight intravenously. It is administered in a dilution of 1 mg. of the drug per milliliter of saline solution. The drug may be given in a single dose or may be divided in four or more injections. Nausea and vomiting occur within a few hours of injection in any event. If the patient has a normal white cell count, this is depressed within a week and indicates that an adequate dose has been administered. The progress of the cancer may be retarded for several weeks with this combination therapy.

With bony metastases or other pelvic recurrent and inoperable cancer, intra-arterial nitrogen mustard has been tried. A fine catheter is threaded up the femoral artery into the aorta or into the femoral arteries on both sides. The location of the residual and recurrent tumor masses determines the technique. Depending on previous therapy and the depression of the bone marrow, 0.1 mg. per kilogram of body weight can be injected for a concentrated effect. Spotty relief of pain has been achieved, depending on the distribution of the agent. The systemic toxic manifestations are evident as with the usual intravenous administration.

Nitrogen mustard is administered intraperitoneally to cause adhesive obliteration of the visceral and parietal peritoneum and reduce the formation of ascitic fluid in abdominal carcinomatosis. A single injection of 0.4 mg. per kilogram of body weight is introduced through a trocar, a No. 18 needle, or a polyethylene catheter threaded into the peritoneal cavity. Sufficient ascitic fluid is left in the abdomen or saline solution is injected to allow for a free distribution of the drug. Several days before therapy, chlorpromazine (Thorazine) is administered in the dose of 25 mg. every six hours. This helps control some of the nausea and vomiting. The results are comparable to the use of radioactive gold in that better than 50 per cent of the patients have a reduction in the amount of fluid, fewer taps, and a short remission, during which they feel better.

TEM, one of the nitrogen mustard analogues, is used in ovarian cancer when surgery or radiation has failed to control the disease. Its cancerocidal properties have been assessed only in human beings with extensive masses of tumor, cachexia, and ascites. It causes less nausea and vomiting than HN_2 and can be administered by mouth. The dose of TEM, orally, is 5 mg., at intervals of a few days as tolerated, for a total dose of 20 to 40 mg. in one month. It has produced a decrease in the size of the tumor masses and subjective improvement in 25 per cent of the patients. Many other chemicals are being screened for cancerocidal activity and will periodically be presented to the gynecologist for clinical trial.

CHORIOCARCINOMA AND RELATED TUMORS OF TROPHOBLASTIC ORIGIN

Chemotherapy has offered little, heretofore, in the way of palliative therapy or cure to the gynecologist treating cancer of the female genital tract. Ironically, the first drug to show specificity for a tumor of this or any other organ system with a cancerocidal effect, at least in the initial course of therapy, should be against one of the rarest tumors of the female genitals. Nevertheless, the possibilities are exciting, and gynecologists treating a volume of pelvic malignancies feel encouraged to pursue the treatment of pelvic cancer with the new mediums.

METHOTREXATE

Methotrexate is another folic acid antagonist, amethopterin (Methotrexate–MTX). Its efficacy is limited by the time it causes ulcerations of the tongue and digestive tract in addition to the bone marrow depression and the usual sequence of hematologic sequelae. By contrast with many chemotherapeutic agents, this drug can be evaluated by its effect on a laboratory test. The response to therapy can be roughly evaluated by reduction in the urinary gonadotropin titer. Clinically, palpable masses in the pelvis, pulmonary lesions seen on x-ray, symptoms from intracranial metastatic disease, and the general condition of the patient can be seen to improve in those with a favorable response.

Methotrexate can be administered orally in doses of 2.5 to 5.0 mg. a day until signs of toxicity appear. After the patient recovers from all signs of toxicity, the course of therapy can be repeated one or more times, depending on the clinical response. Another regimen is to administer the drug intramuscularly or intravenously with a daily dose of 15 to 30 mg. in five-day courses. The stomatitis, skin reactions, and intestinal complications are observed before another five-day course is administered. Few patients tolerate more than fifteen such courses of Methotrexate therapy. The effects on the liver and kidneys are evaluated clinically and by laboratory tests of hepatic and renal function. Gonadotropin titers are done weekly or more often, depending on the facilities available. This is an excellent index of the patient's response to therapy but not infallible in predicting the ultimate course of the cancer.

References

Acosta-Sison, H.: Chorioadenoma Destruens, Am. J. Obst. & Gynec. 80: 176, 1960.

Acosta-Sison, H.: Metastasis of Chorioepithelioma, Am. J. Obst. & Gynec. 75: 1149, 1958.

Barr, F. G., and Oktay, A.: Primary Ovarian Hydatidiform Mole, Am. J. Obst. & Gynec. 79: 1088, 1960.

Bateman, J. C., Carlton, H. N., and Thibeault, J. P.: Chemotherapy for Carcinoma of the Uterus, Obst. & Gynec. 15: 35, 1960.

Beecham, C., Peale, A., and Robbins, R.: Nitrogen Mustard and X-ray in the Treatment of Pulmonary Metastases From Choriocarcinoma, Am. J. Obst. & Gynec. 69: 3, 1955.

Berenblum, I.: Irritation and Carcinogenesis, Arch. Path. 38: 233, 1944.

Bergenstal, M., and others: Chemotherapy of Choriocarcinoma and Related Trophoblatic Tumors in Women, J. A. M. A. 168: 845, 1958.

Brown, W. E., Wood, C. D., and Smith, A. N.: Sodium Cyanide as a Cancer Chemotherapeutic Agent; Laboratory and Clinical Studies, Am. J. Obst. & Gynec. 80: 907, 1960.

Brunschwig, A.: Experiences With E-39 in the Treatment of Advanced Malignant Neoplasms, Cancer 11: 765, 1958.

Byron, R. L., and others: Left Brachial Arterial Catheterization for Chemotherapy in Advanced Intra-Abdominal Malignant Neoplasms, Surg., Gynec. & Obst. 112: 689, 1961.

Coonrad, E. V., and Rundles, R. W.: Mustard Chemotherapy in Ovarian Carcinoma, Ann. Int. Med. 50: 1449, 1959.

Creech, O. J., and others: Perfusion Treatment of Patients With Cancer, J. A. M. A. 171: 2069, 1959.

Cutis, J., Beer, C., and Noble, R.: Biological Properties of Vincaleukoblastine, an Alkaloid in Vinca Rosea Linn, With Reference to Its Antitumor Action, Cancer Res. 20: 1023, 1960.

De Roetth, H.: Chemical Characteristics and Varying Degrees of Malignancy in Tumors of the Human Ovary. I. Oxygen Consumption and Lactic Acid Production, Cancer Res. 17: 833, 1957.

Diamond, H. D.: The Chemotherapy of Lymphomas, New York J. Med. 61: 871, 1961.

Dunnebacke, T. H., and Zitcer, E. M.: Preparation and Cultivation of Primary Human Amnion Cells, Cancer Res. 17: 1043, 1957.

Edelman, S., Greenspan, E., and Baronofsky, I.: Isolation-Perfusion in Cancer Chemotherapy; Current Status and Preliminary Experiences, New York J. Med. 60: 2877, 1960.

Endicott, K. M.: Current Chemotherapy for Cancer, J. Nat. Cancer Inst. 19: 275, 1957.

Gellhorn, A.: A Critical Evaluation of the Current Status of Clinical Cancer Research, Cancer Res. 13: 205, 1953.

Gellhorn, A., and Jones, L.: Chemotherapy of Malignant Disease, Am. J. Med. 6: 188, 1949.

Goldin, A., and Mantel, N.: The Employment of Combinations of Drugs in the Chemotherapy of Neoplasia, Cancer Res. 17: 635, 1957.

Graham, J. B., and Graham, R. M.: The Effect of Vaccine on Cancer Patients, Surg., Gynec. & Obst. 109: 131, 1959.

Green, T. H., Jr.: Hemisulfur Mustard in the Palliation of Patients With Metastatic Ovarian Carcinoma, Obst. & Gynec. 13: 383, 1959.

Greenstein, J.: Biochemistry of Cancer, New York, 1954, Academic Press, Inc.

Haddow, A.: Mechanisms of Carcinogenesis in the Physiopathology of Cancer. In Homberger, F., and Fishman, W. (editors): The Physiopathology of Cancer, New York, 1953, Paul B. Hoeber, Inc.

Hartwell, J.: Survey of Compounds Which Have Been Tested for Carcinogenic Activity, United States Public Health Service, Publication No. 149, 1951.

Hitchcock, C., and others: Selective Intra-arterial Perfusion of Total Abdominal Viscera for Carcinoma, Surg., Gynec. & Obst. 111: 484, 1960.

Hitchings, G.: Present Status of Chemotherapy in Cancer, New York J. Med. 54: 2557, 1954.

Hueper, W.: Carcinogens and Carcinogenesis, Am. J. Med. 8: 355, 1950.

Humphrey, E. W., and Hitchcock, C. R.: Biological Effects of the Phosporamides in Patients With Advanced Cancer, Cancer 10: 231, 1957.

Hurley, J. D., and Hall, F. M.: Chemotherapy of Cancer, A. M. A. Arch. Surg. 80: 928, 1960.

Hurley, J., and others: Chemotherapy of Solid Carcinoma; Indications, Agents, and Results, J. A. M. A. 174: 1696, 1960.

Jackson, R. L.: Pure Malignancy of the Trophoblast Following Primary Abdominal Pregnancy, Am. J. Obst. & Gynec. 79: 1085, 1960.

Johnson, I. S., and others: Antitumor Principles Derived From Vinca Rosea Linn. I. Vincaleukoblastine and Leurosine, Cancer Res. 20: 1016, 1960.

Karnofsky, D.: Chemical Agents Used in the Treatment of Inoperable and Far Advanced Neoplastic Disease. In Bean, W. B. (editor): Monographs in Medicine, Series I, Baltimore, 1952, Williams & Wilkins Co., pp. 582-636.

Karnofsky, D.: In Dock, W., and Snapper, I. (editors): Advances in Internal Medicine, vol. 1, Chicago, 1950, Year Book Publishers, Inc.

Karnofsky, D.: The Bases for Cancer Chemotherapy, Stanford M. Bull. 6: 257, 1948.

Katsura, S., and others: Correlation Between Yoshida Sarcoma and Human Neoplastic Disease in Cancer Chemotherapy Studies, J. Nat. Cancer Inst. 23: 1, 1959.

King, G.: Differential Diagnosis and Therapy of Hydatidiform Mole and Chorioepithelioma, Proc. Roy. Soc. Med. 49: 381, 1956.

Kramer S. P., and Seligman, A. M.: The Distribution of Naphthylchloracetamidase With Implications for the Chemotherapy of Cancer, Cancer 14: 296, 1961.

Kramer, W. M., Eck, R. V., and Smith, R. R.: Prevention of Experimental Lung Metastases With Triethylenethiophosphoramide (ThioTEPA), Surg., Gynec. & Obst. 106: 427, 1958.

Larionov, L.: Peptides, Amides, and Esters of Chloroethylamino Derivatives of Amino Acids and of Phenylalkancarboxylic Acids; a New Class of Antitumor Compounds, Cancer Res. 21: 99, 1961.

Leighton, J.: Contributions of Tissue Culture Studies to an Understanding of the Biology of Cancer: A Review, Cancer Res. 17: 929, 1957.

Loeffler, R., Collins, V., and Hyman, G.: Comparative Effects of Total Body Radiation, Nitrogen Mustard and Triethylene Melamine on the Hematopoietic System of Terminal Cancer Patients, Science 118: 161, 1953.

Masterson, J. G., Calame, R. J., and Nelson, J. N.: A Clinical Study on the Use of Chlorambucil in the Treatment of Cancer of the Ovary, Am. J. Obst. & Gynec. 79: 1002, 1960.

Miller, B. J., and Kistenmacher, J. C.: Effects of P-Di-(2-Chloroethyl)-Aminophenylalanine on Malignant Tumors, J. A. M. A. 173: 98, 1960.

Modlin, R., and Morris, J.: The Effect of Certain Chemical and Physical Agents on the Radiation Sensitivity of Mouse Tumors, Cancer 14: 117, 1961.

Moore, G. E., Sandberg, A. A., and Watne, A. L.: Spread of Cancer Cells and Its Relationship to Chemotherapy, J. A. M. A. 172: 1729, 1960.

Moore, J. G., Brandkamp, W. W., and Burns, W. L.: Evaluation of Chemotherapy in Ovarian and Cervical Cancer by Tissue Culture Methods, Am. J. Obst. & Gynec. 77: 780, 1959.

Nadkarni, M. V., Trams, E. G., and Smith, P. K.: Preliminary Studies on the Distribution and Fate of TEM, TEPA, and Myleran in the Human, Cancer Res. 19: 713, 1959.

Peck, G., Mack, H., and Figge, F.: Cancer Detection and Therapy. III. Affinity of Lymphatic Tissue for Hematoporphyrins, Bull. School Med. Univ. Maryland 38: 124, 1953.

Perlson, S. G., and Whitsitt, R. E.: Adjuvant Therapy of Choriocarcinoma With Methotrexate, Obst. & Gynec. 15: 175, 1960.

Pietra, G., Rappaport, H., and Shubik, P.: The Effects of Carcinogenic Chemicals in Newborn Mice, Cancer 14: 308, 1961.

Pinkel, D.: The Use of Body Surface Area as a Criterion of Drug Dosage in Cancer Chemotherapy, Cancer Res. 18: 853, 1958.

Rassmussen-Taxdal, D., Ward, G., and Figge, F.: Fluorescence of Human Lymphatic and Cancer Tissue Following High Doses of Intravenous Hematoporphyrin, Cancer 8: 78, 1955.

Rath, H., and Enquist, L. F.: The Effect of Thio-TEPA on Wound Healing, A. M. A. Arch. Surg. 79: 812, 1959.

Reiner, I., and Dougherty, C.: Clinical and Pathologic Aspects of Hydatidiform Mole, Obst. & Gynec. 15: 735, 1960.

Rhoads, C.: Present Status of Chemotherapy in Cancer, New York J. Med. 54: 2557, 1954.

Rundles, R., and Barton, W.: Triethylenemelamine in Treatment of Neoplastic Disease, Blood 7: 483, 1952.

Russell, D., Jones, H., and Auerbach, S.: Choriocarcinoma; Report of a Case Showing Unusual Metastatic Behavior, Obst. & Gynec. 17: 84, 1961.

Salter, W.: Chemistry of Carcinogens, Occup. Med. 5: 441, 1948.

Salvaggio, A. T., Nigogosyam, G., and Mack, H. C.: Detection of Trophoblast in Cord Blood and Fetal Circulation, Am. J. Obst. & Gynec. 80: 1013, 1960.

Schell, R. F., and Hall, B. E.: Experience With Triethylene Melamine (TEM) and Triethylene Thiophosphoramide

(Thio TEPA) in Recurrent or Metastatic Solid Tumors, Surg., Gynec. & Obst. 106: 459, 1958.

Schulman, H.: Prerenal Azotemia and Hydatidiform Mole, Am. J. Obst. & Gynec. 80: 180, 1960.

Shanbrom, E., and others: Therapeutic Spectrum of Uracil-Mustard, a New Oral Antitumor Drug; With Special Reference to the Effects of Small Dosage in Lymphomas, Chronic Leukemias, and Ovarian Carcinomas, J. A. M. A. 174: 1702, 1960.

Shapiro, D. M., and Fugmann, R. A.: A Role for Chemotherapy as an Adjunct to Surgery, Cancer Res. 17: 1098, 1957.

Shimkin, M. B., and Moore, G. E.: Adjuvant Use of Chemotherapy in the Surgical Treatment of Cancer, J. A. M. A. 167: 1710, 1958.

Sholes, D. M.: Pelvic Perfusion With Nitrogen Mustard for Cancer: A Neurological Complication, Am. J. Obst. & Gynec. 80: 481, 1960.

Sokal, J. E., and Lessmann, E. M.: Effects of Cancer Chemotherapeutic Agents on the Human Fetus, J. A. M. A. 172: 1765, 1960.

Staley, C., and others: Treatment of Advanced Cancer With 5-Fluorouracil, Surg., Gynec. & Obst. 112: 185, 1961.

Stehlin, J. S., and others: The Leakage Factor in Regional Perfusion With Chemotherapeutic Agents, A. M. A. Arch. Surg. 80: 934, 1960.

Stevens, G. M., Thomas, S. F., and Wilbur, B. C.: Intraaortic Nitrogen Mustard for the Palliation of Advanced Pelvic Cancer, Radiology 75: 948, 1960.

Stirling, G. A.: An Unusual Case of Choriocarcinoma and a Consideration of the Vascular Lesion, J. Obst. & Gynaec. Brit. Emp. 67: 284, 1960.

Stock, C.: Experimental Cancer Chemotherapy, Advances Cancer Res. 2: 425, 1954.

Sullivan, R. D., Miller E., and Sikes, M. P.: Antimetabolite-Metabolite Cancer Chemotherapy, Cancer 12: 1248, 1959.

Swyer, G. L. M.: Oestrogen Therapeutics: Metabolic Considerations, J. Obst. & Gynaec. Brit. Emp. 66: 815, 1959.

Taylor, E. S., Isbell, N. P., and Dean, R. E.: An Experiment in the Use of Radioactive Gold for Cervical Cancer, Am. J. Obst. & Gynec. 80: 899, 1960.

Teller, M. N., and others: Transplantable Human Tumors in Experimental Chemotherapy, a Comparison With Animal Tumor Systems, Cancer Res. 20: 112, 1960.

Vaitkevicius, V., and others: Clinical Evaluation of Cancer Chemotherapy With 5-Fluorouracil, Cancer 14: 131, 1961.

Veterans Administration Adjuvant Cancer Chemotherapy Cooperative Group: Status of Adjuvant Cancer Chemotherapy; a Preliminary Report of Cooperative Studies in the Veterans Administration, A. M. A. Arch. Surg. 82: 466, 1961.

Warwick, O., Darte, J., and Brown, T.: Some Biological Effects of Vincaleukoblastine, and Alkaloid in Vinca Rosea Linn in Patients With Malignant Disease, Cancer Res. 20: 1032, 1960.

Watkins, E., and others: The Use of Intravascular Balloon Catheters for Isolation of the Pelvic Vascular Bed During Pump-Oxygenator Perfusion of Cancer Chemotherapeutic Agents, Surg., Gynec. & Obst. 111: 464, 1960.

Weisberger, A., Levine, B., and Storaasli, J.: Use of Nitrogen Mustard in Treatment of Serous Effusions of Neoplastic Origin, J. A. M. A. 159: 1704, 1955.

Wright, J.: Clinical Cancer Chemotherapy, New York J. Med. 61: 249, 1961.

Wright, J. C., and others: The Effect of Triethylenethiophosphoramide on Fifty Patients With Incurable Neoplastic Diseases, Cancer 10: 239, 1957.

Wynder, E.: Some Practical Aspects of Cancer Prevention, New England J. Med. 246: 492-503, 538-546, 573-582, 1952.

Zukoski, C. F., Lee, H. M., and Hume, D. M.: The Effect of 6-Mercaptopurine on Renal Homograft Survival in the Dog, Surg., Gynec. & Obst. 112: 707, 1961.

24 · Cancer of the Urethra, Vagina, Vulva, and Bartholin's Gland

CANCER OF THE URETHRA

Cancer of the female urethra is most often a squamous tumor arising in the terminal urethra. It spreads up to the internal meatus, penetrating to the submucosa of the vaginal wall rapidly, so that early lesions are rarely seen. I have excised the terminal urethra for a presumed caruncle that failed to respond to all conservative therapy and found an intraepithelial cancer in the specimen. This was confirmed by a quorum of gynecologic and urologic pathologists, and I regret that preoperative smears were not done for cytologic study. The symptoms are bleeding and dysuria. Diagnosis is established by the palpation of the tumor mass extending along the urethra or ulcerating into the vagina. Biopsy reveals the malignant nature of this rare lesion. Treatment has not been standardized. In view of the almost hopeless prognosis in the past and the early spread to the regional lymphatic stations, interstitial therapy by needles or a colloidal isotope followed by radical excision and groin dissection could be tried. An advanced lesion would necessitate an anterior exenteration and total vaginectomy with ureterointestinal or cutaneous anastomoses.

CANCER OF THE VAGINA

Primary cancer of the vagina is a rare but a highly lethal disease. The rich lymphatic drainage of the vagina and its vascularity make treatment difficult. The cancer is usually located on the posterior wall in the upper third of the vagina and is of the squamous cell type. Extension to the regional glands via the peri-rectal lymphatics occurs early as shown by histologic study of specimens removed from patients who have been subjected to surgery. The lesion can be irradiated with a gamma emitter placed in a dental mold to distribute the sources adequately. Deep roentgentherapy can be beamed at the lesion. The proximity of rectum and bladder, even in an early lesion, limits radiotherapy to palliation without undue risk of causing a fistula. Were one to see such a cancer and have modern facilities available, the lesion might be confined by irradiation by radioactive needles or threads, supplemented by interstitial radiation with a colloidal isotope emitting beta radiation. An exenteration operation with complete lymphadenectomy following the radiation could offer some chance of cure.

CARCINOMA OF THE VULVA AND BARTHOLIN'S GLAND
General Considerations

Carcinoma of the vulva and Bartholin's glands comprise about 3 per cent of all genital tract cancers in women. This would be less than 1 per cent of all malignancies afflicting women. It is a disease of later life, with the greater number of women presenting themselves with these cancers being between 60 and 70 years of age. Despite the accessibility of the lesion for early diagnosis, few patients are seen who have not neglected it or treated it for several months with salves. The saving grace in this disease is that it lends itself admirably to a block dissection—capably performed—that makes the gynecologist realize he must also be an anatomist.

Etiology and Pathologic Anatomy

Taussig, who made some of the major contributions to the understanding of this disease, has outlined some of the conditions found more commonly in patients who subsequently develop vulval cancer. About 50 per cent of squamous cell cancer is preceded by leukoplakia of the vulva. He found urethral caruncles, infections of Bartholin's glands, senile papillomas, syphilis, and other chronic infections about the vulva more common among patients with vulval cancer. The most common site is the labium majus. The primary site may be the labium minus, clitoris, perineum, and very rarely an adenocarcinoma develops in Bartholin's gland. The histologic type of vulval cancer influences the treatment, so the less common lesions, cancerous and precancerous, will be discussed separately.

Basal Cell Carcinoma

Compared with the face and neck, the appearance of a basal cell cancer of the vulva is a rarity. It is believed that basal cell cancers arise from the basal layer of the epidermis. The clinical appearance of these lesions is the same as seen elsewhere on the skin. Two types are distinguishable: the rodent ulcer (noduloulcerative type) and the flat epithelioma. The symptoms are minimal, and the patient may complain of only slight local irritation or pruritus. The diagnosis is confirmed by biopsy that is adequate enough for the pathologist to eliminate the possibility of a truly invasive squamous cell cancer. Since true metastatic spread of this disease does not occur, the treatment consists of a wide local excision with, perhaps, a selective lymphadenectomy to help the pathologist confirm the local nature of the malignancy.

Intraepithelial Carcinoma

Bowen, in 1912, described a precancerous lesion that is now generally recognized as a true intraepithelial carcinoma. Evidence has accumulated to confirm the fact that many true intraepithelial carcinomas progress to invasive cancer of the squamous or basal cell types. It is not possible to make a diagnosis from gross observation of the lesion. It is frequently found in conjunction with leukoplakia and may be suspected in an area of the vulva that shows a slight ulceration with surrounding erythema. Vulval pruritus is the common symptom. In the presence of leukoplakia, the treatment of choice is a simple vulvectomy. A wide local excision is indicated in young patients with small lesions in whom the vulva is preserved for cosmetic reasons.

Paget's Disease

Paget's disease of the vulva is a rare lesion that may represent a primary carcinoma or a secondary intraepithelial metastasis from an underlying adenocarcinoma of the sweat glands. Whether it is related to the hidradenoma of the vulva, which is more commonly seen, is not known. It is a true malignant disease with early metastatic spread and treatment is identical to that of squamous cell cancer of the vulva.

RADICAL GROIN DISSECTION
Surgical Anatomy

The surgical anatomy of radical groin dissection lends itself to discussion in four phases: (1) superficial lymphatics and anatomy of the saphenous vein, (2) femoral vessels and round ligament, (3) dissection of the deep lymphatics and external iliac, hypogastric, and common iliac vessels, and (4) resection of the vulva, which requires knowledge of the external genitalia. We deal, in this operation, with only the parietal lymphatics, those lying retroperitoneally. The visceral lymphatics, those accompanying large vessels to the pelvic organs, are not concerned except in the event of widespread metastatic disease.

Phase 1—Superficial Lymphatics and Anatomy of the Saphenous Vein

The superficial inguinal nodes lie just under the superficial fascia in Scarpa's triangle (Plate 60, *A*), vary from ten to twenty in number, and will be taken with the block dissection rather than being separately identified. The

PLATE 60

A

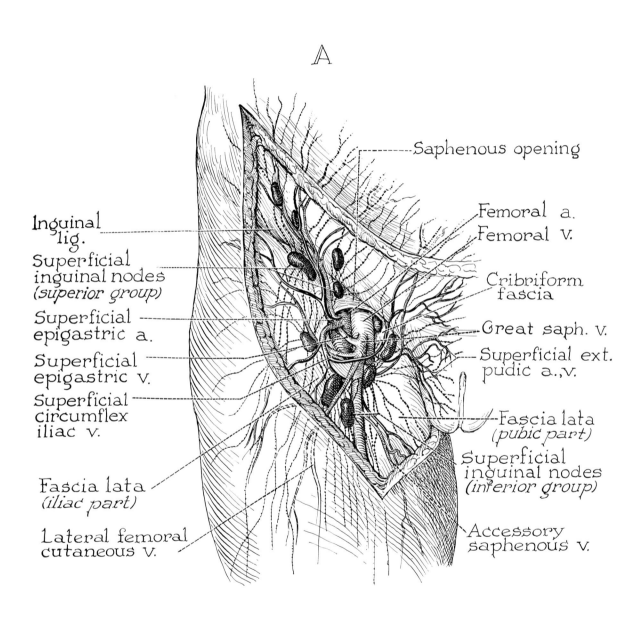

Saphenous opening

Femoral a.
Femoral v.

Cribriform
fascia

Great saph. v.

Superficial ext.
pudic a.,v.

Fascia lata
(pubic part)

Superficial
inguinal nodes
(inferior group)

Accessory
saphenous v.

Inguinal
lig.

Superficial
inguinal nodes
(superior group)

Superficial
epigastric a.

Superficial
epigastric v.

Superficial
circumflex
iliac v.

Fascia lata
(iliac part)

Lateral femoral
cutaneous v.

PLATE 60 (*Concluded*)

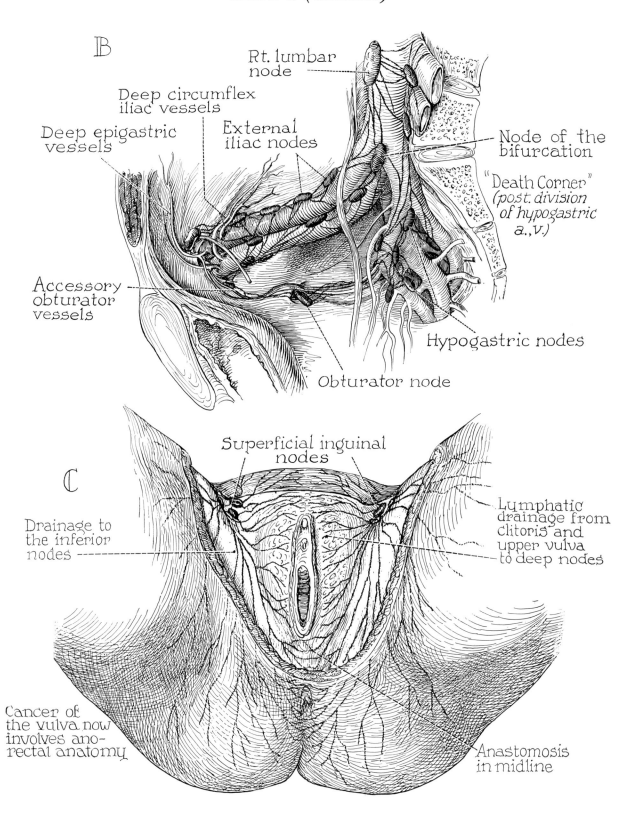

B

Rt. lumbar node

Deep circumflex iliac vessels

Deep epigastric vessels

External iliac nodes

Node of the bifurcation

"Death Corner" (*post. division of hypogastric a., v.*)

Accessory obturator vessels

Hypogastric nodes

Obturator node

C

Superficial inguinal nodes

Drainage to the inferior nodes

Lymphatic drainage from clitoris and upper vulva to deep nodes

Cancer of the vulva now involves anorectal anatomy

Anastomosis in midline

superficial inguinal nodes have been divided into a superior and inferior group by a horizontal line drawn through the middle of the fossa ovalis. This is arbitrary—an anatomist's prerogative—and contributes little to the understanding of the lymphatic drainage of the vulva. In general, the upper group drain the lower abdominal wall, mons pubis, and upper part of the buttocks. The lower group drain the clitoris, labia majora and minora, perineum, and parts of the lower extremity (Plate 60, C). Surgeons must appreciate that all drain into the deep inguinal lymphatics through the femoral canal. The node of Cloquet or Rosenmüller, a detailed description of which will be given later, thus becomes a sentinel node in diseases of the vulva. From the deep inguinal nodes the drainage is to the parietal lymphatics along the external iliac vessels, then to the common iliac nodes, and eventually to the para-aortic lymphatic systems (Plate 60, B). A cancer of the clitoris may metastasize directly to the deep nodes or even pass to the lower iliac nodes. A lesion deep in the vestibule has a poorer prognosis than one far out on the labia majora. The saphenous vein and its branches, superficial external pudic, superficial epigastric, and superficial circumflex iliac, are shown in Plate 60, A, in one of the more common arrangements.

Scarpa's triangle, in which a considerable part of the dissection will take place, has as its base the inguinal ligament. Its sides are formed by the sartorius laterally and the adductor longus medially. The fascia lata and its extensions require understanding in an extensive dissection such as this. In the thigh the fascia lata is divided into two portions: the lateral, or iliac, and the medial, or pubic. The saphenous opening (fossa ovalis) penetrates this fascia and is the outer opening of the femoral canal. The accessory saphenous vein is shown in Plate 60, A, and, when present, must be ligated during the dissection. The not uncommon inverted Y arrangement of the saphenous vein must be remembered, for this may lead to unnecessary bleeding during the saphenous ligation.

Phase 2—Femoral Vessels and Round Ligament

The femoral canal is about 2 cm. long and begins above at the femoral (crural) ring and ends at the fossa ovalis. Dissection of the fossa ovalis reveals the nerve, artery, vein, and canal in that sequence from the lateral side to the medial. The deep inguinal nodes, from one to three in number, lie in the canal medial to the vessels. The highest one is called the node of Cloquet or Rosenmüller. In this operation the inguinal ligament is not divided, since the femoral canal can be thoroughly cleaned out by attacking it from below in Phase 2 and from above in Phase 3. Plate 60, A, shows the detailed anatomy of the groin, but it must be remembered that the individual structures will not be identified in the operation.

The round ligament arises from the uterus, passes through the internal abdominal ring, and through the inguinal canal, and emerges from the subcutaneous ring to end in the labium majus. It brings with it the fascial coverings of the abdominal wall, but these may become very attenuated as the labium is reached. Small branches from the ovarian and deep epigastric vessels accompany the ligament. The ilioinguinal nerve and the external spermatic branch of the genitofemoral nerve pass through the inguinal canal. This operation requires the identification and section of the round ligament but no detailed dissection of it throughout its course or individual recognition of its accompanying fascial layers, canal of Nuck, nerves, veins, arteries, or lymphatics.

The surgical anatomy of inguinal and femoral hernias is concerned with this operation. Incision of the aponeurosis of the external oblique muscle, close to the inguinal ligament, from the anterior superior iliac spine to the pubic tubercle—extensive splitting of the internal oblique and transversalis muscles—opens the field for the retroperitoneal lymphadenectomy. The fascial extensions from the abdominal wall seen in the hernial sac contain the parietal lymphatics (Plate 60, B), with which this operation is much concerned.

Phase 3—Dissection of the Deep Lymphatics and External Iliac, Hypogastric, and Common Iliac Vessels

The external iliac artery is larger than the internal iliac (hypogastric) artery in the adult. It passes obliquely downward and outward along the inner border of the psoas muscle. The external iliac vein lies behind it in the upper part of its course but lower down is entirely to the medial side. The external iliac artery and vein are easily dislodged from their beds on the lateral wall over the iliopsoas muscle. The index finger is inserted between the muscle and the vessels and the muscle are drawn medially. This permits the removal of the lymphatics behind the vessels—they are parietal lymphatics and their removal is important. The artery and vein continue as the femoral vessels after passing under Poupart's ligament and entering the femoral canal. There are several muscular branches to the psoas muscle and neighboring lymph nodes which may require ligation. The two main branches are generally given off just above the femoral canal (Plate 60, B). The deep epigastric vessels pass along the medial margin of the internal abdominal ring and continue cephalad between the transversalis fascia and peritoneum. The vessels are crossed near their origin by the round ligament as it enters the internal or abdominal ring. An accessory obturator artery frequently arises from the deep epigastric artery. Both need to be ligated in order to perform a thorough dissection of the femoral canal. The deep circumflex iliac artery arises from the external iliac artery nearly opposite the epigastric artery. It passes outward behind Poupart's ligament to the region of the anterior superior spine of the ilium and gives off several muscular branches. This artery is ligated in the dissection.

The internal iliac or hypogastric artery arises at the bifurcation of the common iliac artery opposite the lumbosacral articulation. It descends into the pelvis, dividing into parietal and visceral branches, and terminates as the lateral umbilical ligament (obliterated hypogastric artery). The parietal branches are the iliolumbar, the lateral sacral, the obturator, the internal pudendal, and the gluteal vessels. Plate 60, B, shows the posterior divisions of the hypogastric artery and vein. They are short and thick in their intrapelvic portions, making clamping and ligation difficult, and frequently cause serious bleeding if lacerated inadvertently. The visceral branches are the umbilical, inferior vesical, middle hemorrhoidal, and uterine branches. It is not feasible in an extraperitoneal lymphadenectomy or otherwise to dissect out the course of each of these branches, especially the parietal vessels. One branch, the obturator, is readily cleaned of the surrounding lymphatic and fatty tissue along its course. It runs forward and downward a little below the brim of the pelvis, with the obturator nerve above and the vein below. It passes into the obturator canal and may have to be ligated to thoroughly clean the obturator membrane (Plate 60, B).

The lymph nodes are named from their arterial counterparts: common iliac, external iliac, and hypogastric. The obturator node is long and thin, embedded in fat, and quite constant. It can be palpated lying on the obturator membrane. Another node at the bifurcation of the common iliac artery, called the node of the bifurcation, is quite constant in location and should be specifically removed as an important prognostic node. The aortic nodes are large and lie lateral to the aorta, for which reason they are referred to as the para-aortic lymphatics.

Phase 4—Resection of the Vulva

The final phase of a radical groin dissection requires a complete vulvectomy. All of the structures of the vulva are removed down to the inferior fascia of the urogenital diaphragm. The detailed anatomy of the vulva is described in Chapter 16 (page 298).

Plate 60, C, illustrates some of the peculiarities of the lymphatic drainage of the vulva. The liberal anastomoses across the midline allow contralateral metastases in many cases. Carcinoma of Bartholin's gland may drain into the anorectal lymphatics. The clitoris may drain directly into the deep lymphatics.

RADICAL VULVECTOMY AND GROIN DISSECTION
Surgical Principles

A block dissection infers that the operator attacks the cancer from the periphery of healthy tissue without traversing any part of the malignant lesion. Thus one must start from the side opposite the cancer and proceed toward the lesion if healthy areas are not to be seeded with cancer cells—if seeding is a fact—during the operation. We must always enter some plane beyond the lesion and displace the tissues to be removed toward the center of the operative field. The complete removal of the primary lesion, together with its primary and secondary lymphatic stopping points, should be accomplished with the minimal amount of disturbance to adjacent structures. The temptation is always present to limit the block dissection and undermine large skin areas to close the skin edges. This completely defeats the only sound approach, poor as it is, we have to deal with vulval cancer.

The size of the primary lesion may modify the radicality of the primary incision. McKelvey, who knows a lot about this disease, modifies his incisions, depending on the size of the initial lesion and its position in the vulva. Since the percentage of positive nodes increases with the size of the primary lesion, as we have discussed earlier, the breadth of the incisions should be increased with the more advanced lesions. Lesions that may drain into the anorectal lymphatics (Plate 60, C), such as a cancer of the perineum or Bartholin's gland, may require an exenteration of the viscera to clear the lesion.

The combined operations most commonly associated with the names of Basset and Taussig have a major fault—they violate the principles of an en bloc dissection. Whether by stages or at one sitting, if the inguinal nodes must be removed, the intervening lymphatics, between inguinal and vulvar lymphatics, should not be left behind. It would be nice to believe that cancer cells restrain themselves to a primary growth in the vulva and then establish themselves in a secondary site in the super-ficial lymphatics, with no cells left in the lymphatics en route! Why leave a bridge of inoculated tissue between the primary lesion and its first metastatic station? Way and Marshall have made this clear to all who study pelvic cancer.

By indicating the structures left at the end of this dissection, one can better understand the steps of the procedure. At the end of the operation the field should show the following structures: the aponeurosis of the external oblique muscle, the internal oblique and transversalis muscles, the inguinal ligament, the femoral nerve, artery, and vein, the ligated ends of the greater saphenous vein, and the iliopsoas, pectineus, sartorius, adductor longus, and gracilis muscles.

By the same token, the following structures should be present in the gross en bloc dissection: a large segment of skin from the abdomen and groins, the vulva (labia majora, labia minora, clitoris, mons pubis, terminal portions of urethra and vagina, bulbocavernosi, ischiocavernosi, and other structures), the superficial and deep inguinal nodes, portions of the round ligaments, portions of the saphenous veins, and the lesion itself, together with the surrounding skin.

A saphenous ligation flush with the femoral vein is necessary in the course of this operation. This should be done early in the course of the procedure, and all the branches draining into the saphenous vein are ligated. The branches of the femoral nerve that are necessarily exposed are not cut, since the lymphadenectomy within the femoral canal can be done without severing these nerves.

It is amazing how the large denuded area of the vulva will granulate and close in. Full-thickness pinch grafts should be laid in cavities of healthy granulations to hasten the closure. Surgical principles are not violated in this operation, although the convalescent period may be lengthened. How foolish to attempt an approximation of the vulvar skin to the vaginal mucosa! This, almost invariably, pulls the urethra down and obliterates the posterior urethrovesical angle, with resultant incontinence. Urinary incontinence is then added to the management of a difficult malignancy.

The incisions for a radical vulvectomy open up the major lymphatic channels draining the lower extremities. Were it possible to individually identify and ligate these lymphatic vessels, the problem of postoperative seromas would be solved. The placing of sutures along the skin edges may interrupt some channels but also interrupts the blood supply. The question of early ambulation also arises. Certainly, movement of the lower extremity will increase the lymph flow, and this has been observed among patients who are ambulated early after a radical dissection. It is probably best to risk a lymph fistula and prolonged drainage of the wound than an extensive phlebitis with possible fatal embolic phenomena.

Steps of the Operation

1. Make the first skin incision on the side opposite the primary lesion (Plate 61, A). The horizontal incision is sweeping in its course and starts about 8 cm. above the anterior superior iliac spine and courses to the midline above the mons pubis. From the apex of this incision make a second vertical one through the skin and subcutaneous tela to a point about 6 cm. below and 6 cm. lateral to the femoral vessels as they are palpated through the fossa ovalis. From the end of this incision incise the skin and subcutaneous tissues upward and medially into the genitocrural fold of skin.

2. Adhering to the principles of a block dissection, grasp the upper end of the incision and deepen it down to the aponeurosis of the external oblique muscle. Always move the tissues from the periphery toward the cancer.

3. Continue the dissection, quickly cleaning everything off the fascia, over the inguinal ligament and onto the fascia lata of the upper thigh (Plate 61, B). Over the inguinal ligament the deep layer of the superficial fascia, as well as the deep fascia, is adherent and must be separated by sharp dissection. The superficial circumflex iliac artery and vein, the superficial epigastric artery and vein, and the superficial external pudic artery and vein may require repeated clamping and tying until they are clamped at their origin from the femoral vessels. Plate 61, B, shows the dissection advanced to expose the fossa ovalis and the next several steps of the operation.

4. Fibers of the iliohypogastric, ilioinguinal, external cutaneous, middle cutaneous, and crural branch of the genitofemoral nerve may be resected in the course of the operation. No attempt is made either to identify or spare them.

5. When a grossly suspicious node is found, identify its former bed by means of a brain clip (Plate 61, B) and place it in fixative with the container properly labeled as to its location. An x-ray later will show these clips in the former lymphatic bed.

6. Large tissue surfaces are exposed in this operation, and as the dissection is completed in an area, it is covered with warm, wet laparotomy pads.

7. Proceed with a high saphenous ligation, including all of the feeders. The main branches, the superficial circumflex iliac, the superficial epigastric, and the external pudic veins, are ligated. Their corresponding arteries are ligated as encountered. This clears the fossa ovalis of the more superficial part of the cribriform fascia and nodes. During this dissection the accessory saphenous and lateral femoral cutaneous veins may be resected and require ligation.

8. The base of Scarpa's triangle, bounded superiorly by the inguinal ligament, laterally by the sartorius muscle, and medially by the adductor longus muscle, is further cleaned of any lymphatic tissue. While all this seems remote from attacking the primary lesion, it must be done if surgery is to encompass the cancer and lend a promise of cure.

9. The second phase of this operation begins (Plate 61, C). Clean out the femoral canal of its lymphatics insofar as this can be done from below without unnecessary bleeding high in the canal out of reach. The lacunar (Gimbernat's) ligament may be cut for better exposure.

10. The deep inguinal nodes vary from one to three in number (are inconstant) and lie medial to the femoral vein. The lowest is situated below the junction of the saphenous and femoral veins and the middle at the entrance to the femoral canal. The largest is within the canal and is termed the node of Cloquet or Rosenmüller.

11. Plate 61, C, shows the dissection of the distal half of the femoral canal. The remainder of the canal will be cleaned out from above the inguinal ligament.

12. Continue the anatomic dissection above the inguinal ligament. Incise the aponeurosis of the

Text continued on p. 415.

PLATE 61

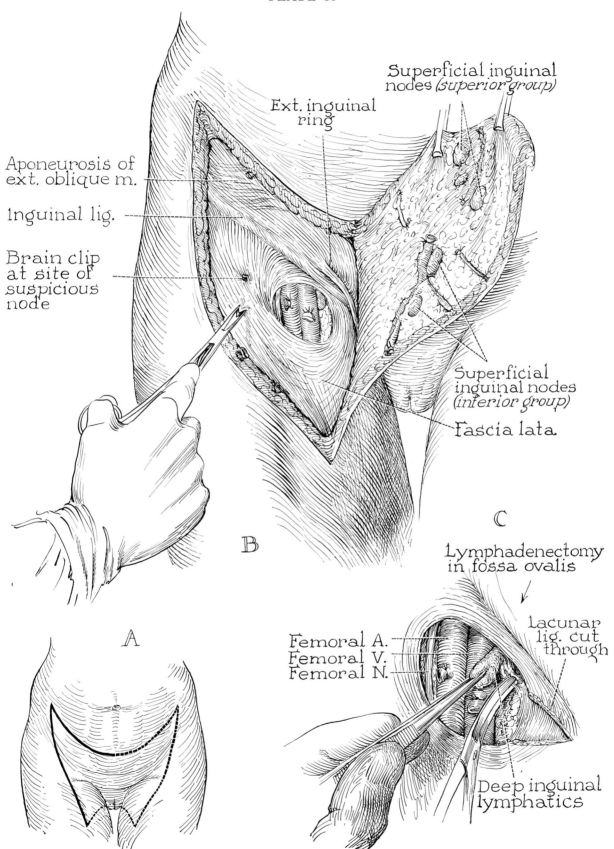

Ext. inguinal
ring

Superficial inguinal
nodes *(superior group)*

Aponeurosis of
ext. oblique m.

Inguinal lig.

Brain clip
at site of
suspicious
node

Superficial
inguinal nodes
(inferior group)

Fascia lata.

B

C

Lymphadenectomy
in fossa ovalis

A

Femoral A.
Femoral V.
Femoral N.

Lacunar
lig. cut
through

Deep inguinal
lymphatics

PLATE 61 (Continued)

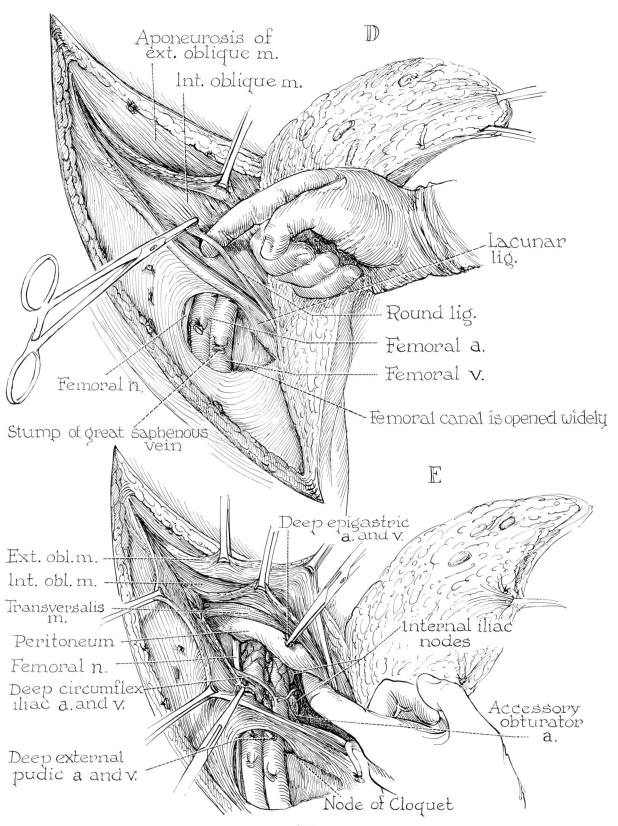

D

Aponeurosis of ext. oblique m.

Int. oblique m.

Lacunar lig.

Round lig.

Femoral a.

Femoral v.

Femoral n.

Femoral canal is opened widely

Stump of great saphenous vein

E

Deep epigastric a. and v.

Ext. obl. m.

Int. obl. m.

Transversalis m.

Peritoneum

Femoral n.

Deep circumflex iliac a. and v.

Internal iliac nodes

Accessory obturator a.

Deep external pudic a and v.

Node of Cloquet

PLATE 61 *(Continued)*

F

Psoas M.

Peritoneum

Iliacus M.

Femoral N.

Ext. iliac A. and V.

Ext. iliac lymphatics

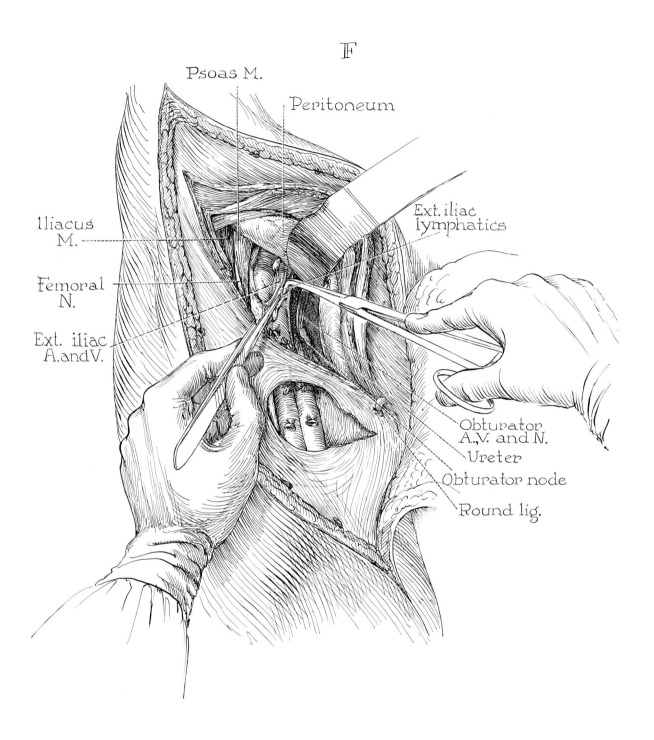

Obturator A., V. and N.

Ureter

Obturator node

Round lig.

PLATE 61 (Concluded)

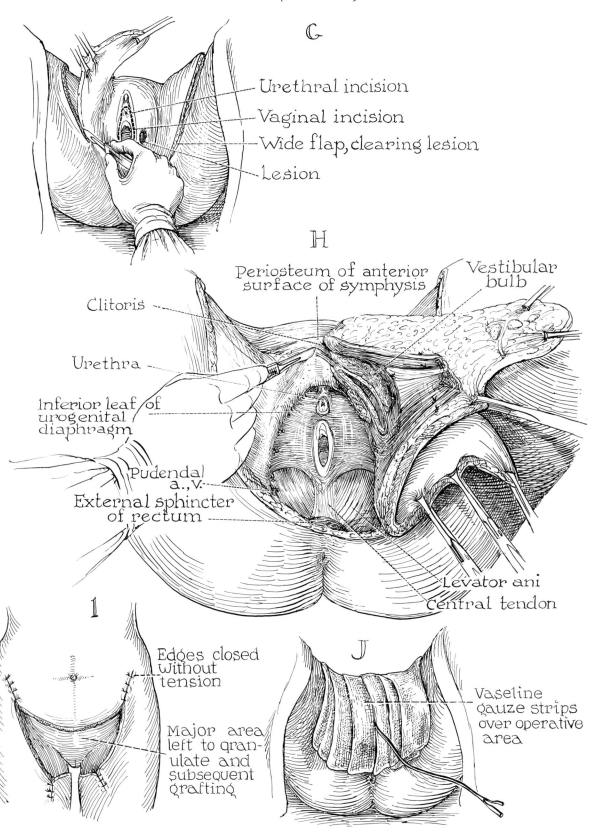

G

Urethral incision

Vaginal incision

Wide flap, clearing lesion

Lesion

H

Periosteum of anterior surface of symphysis

Vestibular bulb

Clitoris

Urethra

Inferior leaf of urogenital diaphragm

Pudendal a., v.

External sphincter of rectum

Levator ani

Central tendon

1

Edges closed without tension

Major area left to granulate and subsequent grafting

J

Vaseline gauze strips over operative area

414

external oblique muscle in the same manner as for a herniorrhaphy. Retract the flaps of the aponeurosis—below to the inguinal ligament and above to widely expose the round ligament and adjacent structures. Pull the round ligament out so it can be clamped well above the external abdominal ring (Plate 61, D).

13. Do not persist in isolating the round ligament when it is not obvious. Frequently it is so attenuated in the elderly patient as to make identification difficult. If easily identifiable, clamp, cut, tie, and draw it toward the midline; if not, open the internal oblique and transversalis muscles in the direction of their fibers.

14. The third phase, dissection of the deep lymphatics of the external iliac and hypogastric vessels, is begun. Push the peritoneum medially, off the iliopsoas muscle, and dissect the subperitoneal connective tissue (transversalis fascia) and the lymphatics and areolar tissue about the external iliac vessels and their attachments. Alternately, the use of angle clamps, Metzenbaum scissors, and small curved Halstead hemostats will facilitate the dissection (Plate 61, E).

15. The femoral nerve will be seen emerging from the lateral border of the psoas muscle and lying in the groove between the psoas and iliacus muscles. It enters the femoral canal lateral to the femoral vessels where the main branches go to the pectineus, sartorius, and quadriceps femoris. It should be carefully preserved in this dissection (Plate 61, E).

16. Three branches of the external iliac artery or the beginning of the femoral artery are encountered in cleaning out the femoral canal: the deep epigastric, deep circumflex iliac, and deep external pudic arteries. These, as well as their veins, are ligated in the course of the dissection (Plate 61, E). The node of Cloquet is removed from above if it was not possible to remove it from below.

17. Be alert for an accessory obturator artery! Troublesome bleeding may be encountered from this vessel when it arises from the deep epigastric or external iliac vessels. Particularly is this so if the accessory obturator artery or vein arches over medial to the femoral ring to reach the obturator foramen (Plate 61, E).

18. The parietal peritoneum is further dissected off the iliopsoas muscle and retracted medially. This will give you sufficient exposure to follow the external iliac vessels up to their origin from the common iliac. Again the principle of a block dissection, proceeding from the periphery toward

the primary lesion, can be adhered to. Continue the lymphadenectomy with sharp and blunt dissection from the common iliac vessels along the external iliac and hypogastric arteries and veins. Again let us not deceive ourselves that the branches of the hypogastric artery and vein, with their multiple variations and inaccessibility, can be clearly identified, completely isolated, and clearly denuded of lymphatic tissue except by tedious days in the dissecting room with a well-preserved corpse. The primary and secondary lymphatic stations are all parietal lymphatics, in the operable stage of the disease, so the dissection is entirely retroperitoneal.

19. Extend the dissection to the obturator foramen and clean out the obturator node and fatty tissue. This node is long and thin, and is readily palpable between the fingers. The obturator artery and vein may be sacrificed at random, but the obturator nerve should be preserved, since a clean dissection of the obturator fossa can be done without sacrificing it. The ureter will be drawn medially with the peritoneum and some retroperitoneal connective tissue. It need not be disturbed from its areolar and vascular bed in this operation. Plate 61, F, shows the structures involved in the depths of the pelvic lymphadenectomy. There remains, yet, the cleaning of the pelvic side wall behind the great vessels where some parietal nodes may be present.

20. Lift the external iliac artery and vein off the pelvic side wall and clean out the lymphatic and areolar tissue behind these vessels. This would be a rare metastatic station in this disease, but obvious nodes should be recognized and studied. This completes the deep lymphadenectomy and the abdominal phase of the operation on one side. Remember that the operation can be done in stages should the patient's condition suddenly deteriorate. There is usually a profuse drainage of serum after such a dissection, so tight closure is contraindicated. Some interrupted chromic sutures may be placed in the upper ends of the incisions into the external oblique aponeurosis if the field is reasonably dry. Hernia following this radical dissection is no problem and is unimportant insofar as the patient's survival is concerned.

21. The same dissection is now carried out on the side of the primary lesion. Suspicious nodes are tagged with brain clips, and those detached from the specimen are labeled and fixed separately for section and study. After this dissection the operation may likewise be stopped should the patient be in shock or, after consultation with the anesthetist, it is deemed inadvisable to continue with the vulval phase.

22. Plate 61, *G,* shows the skin incisions for the vulvectomy. Join these up with the abdominal and thigh incisions. The incisions should not be symmetrical, for the incision adjacent to the primary lesion should clear it by 5 cm. or more.

23. The incision within the vaginal orifice extends about the urethra, the terminal portion of which will be amputated. Here, again, the amount of the vagina and urethra that is excised depends on the location of the lesion. If the cancer originates on the labia minora or clitoris, greater clearance of the primary lesion is obtained by taking more of the distal vagina and urethra.

24. Working close to the periosteum of the symphysis, dissect the mons pubis cleanly from above downward toward the lesion. Proceed with the vulvectomy on the side opposite the lesion. Deepen the vulval incision, and clamp, cut, and tie the branches of the internal pudic (pudendal) artery and vein as they are encountered. Ligation of these branches may have to be done time and again at different stages of the dissection. They are the superficial perineal with its branches to the labia and bulbocavernosus and ischiocavernosus, the artery to the vestibular bulb and the superficial transverse perineal, both arising from the superficial perineal, and, finally, the terminal branches supplying the body, glans, and prepuce of the clitoris (Plate 61, *H*).

25. Incisions are now made encircling the urethra at the junction of its middle and outer thirds. Posteriorly, this incision is continued around the vagina so as to result in the eventual amputation of its lower one third or one fourth (Plate 61, *H*). Amputate the terminal portions of the urethra and vagina, taking them with the specimen as it is swept toward the lesion. The mons pubis, clitoris, frenulum, and prepuce of the clitoris, the crura of the clitoris, vestibular bulbs, bulbocavernosi, ischiocavernosi, transverse perineal muscles, Bartholin's and Skene's glands, plus all the other structures that make up the vulva and its fascial coverings, will be removed with the specimen.

26. Gradually bring the entire tissue mass toward the primary cancer, always avoiding incision near or pressure upon the lesion. Resect the remaining attachments and remove the block of tissue.

27. Do not be tempted to undermine the skin and close large portions of this wound. The upper edges of the abdominal incisions may lend themselves to partial closure without tension (Plate 61, *I*). Place an indwelling catheter in the bladder, and dress the wound with a layer of Vaseline gauze followed by a light pressure dressing (Plate 61, *J*). The latter will be replaced in a few days with a few thicknesses of gauze to permit exposure of the granulating surface.

28. As soon as healthy granulations appear, pinch grafts are done to expedite closure of the wound.

Postoperative Care

Because of the loss of lymph and the large area exposed, constant check must be made on the patient's electrolyte balance. An indwelling catheter is necessary for six to eight days, and the wound is cleaned by irrigations with normal saline solution after defecation. Grafting is begun as soon as healthy granulations appear. Penicillin, together with one of the wide-spectrum antibiotics, is continued for two weeks or more so that wound infection does not hinder the grafts or normal healing.

References

Abell, M. R., and Gosling, J. R. G.: Intraepithelial and Infiltrative Carcinoma of Vulva: Bowen's Type, Cancer 14: 318, 1961.

Arronet, G., Latour, J., and Tremblay, P.: Primary Carcinoma of the Vagina, Am. J. Obst. & Gynec. 79: 455, 1960.

Basset, A.: Traitment chirurgical operatoire de l'epithelioma primitif due clitoria, Rev. de chir. Paris 46: 546, 1952.

Berlin, H., and Winters, H. S.: Malignant Melanoma of the Vulva With Pregnancy, Obst. & Gynec. 15: 302, 1960.

Borja, M. N., and Graham, J. B.: Squamous Carcinoma of the Vulva, New York J. Med. 60: 398, 1960.

Bowen, J. T.: Precancerous Dermatoses; a Study of Two Cases of Chronic Atypical Epithelial Proliferation, J. Cutan. Dis. incl. Syph. 30: 241, 1912.

Brack, C. B., Merritt, R. I., and Dickson, R. J.: Primary Carcinoma of the Vagina, Obst. & Gynec. 12: 104, 1958.

Dahle, T.: Carcinoma of the Vulva and Subsequent Successful Pregnancy, Acta obst. et gynec. scandinav. 38: 448, 1959.

DeHaan, Q., and Johnson, C.: Adenocarcinoma of the Paraurethral Glands; Report of a Case, Am. J. Obst. & Gynec. 80: 1108, 1960.

Frank, L., and Miller, A.: Malignancy of the Vulva, Am. J. Surg. 53: 412, 1941.

Gemmell, A. A., and Haines, M.: Pregnancy Following Radical Vulvectomy for Carcinoma of the Vulva, J. Obst. & Gynaec. Brit. Emp. 67: 199, 1960.

Gosling, J. R. G., and others: Infiltrative Squamous Cell (Epidermoid) Carcinoma of Vulva, Cancer 14: 330, 1961.

Green, T., Ulfelder, H., and Meigs, J.: Epidermoid Carcinoma of the Vulva: An Analysis of 238 Cases; Part I. Etiology and Diagnosis, Am. J. Obst. & Gynec. 75: 834, 1958.

Kaufman, R., Boice, E., and Knight, W.: Paget's Disease of the Vulva, Am. J. Obst. & Gynec. 79: 451, 1960.

Kehrer, E.: Die Vulva und ihre Erkrankugen. In Veit, J.: Handbuch der Gynäkologie, ed. 3 (Stoekel, W., editor), Munich, 1929, J. F. Bergmann, vol. 5, pp. 1-592.

Knoblich, R.: Primary Adenocarcinoma of the Female

Urethra; a Review and Report of Three Cases, Am. J. Obst. & Gynec. **80**: 353, 1960.

Krantz, K. E.: Innervation of the Human Vulva and Vagina, Obst. & Gynec. **12**: 382, 1958.

Lang, W., Menduke, H., and Golub, L.: The Delay Period in Carcinoma of the Vagina; With Observations on Age Incidence and Survival Rate, Am. J. Obst. & Gynec. **80**: 341, 1960.

McAdams, A. J., Jr., and Kistner, R. W.: The Relationship of Chronic Vulvar Disease, Leucoplakia, and Carcinoma in Situ to Carcinoma of the Vulva, Cancer **11**: 740, 1958.

McKelvey, J.: Carcinoma of the Vulva, Obst. & Gynec. **5**: 452, 1955.

Marcus, S. L.: Primary Carcinoma of the Vagina, Obst. & Gynec. **15**: 673, 1960.

May, H. C.: Carcinoma in Situ of the Vagina Subsequent to Hysterectomy for Carcinoma in Situ of the Cervix, Am. J. Obst. & Gynec. **76**: 807, 1958.

Merrill, J. A., and Bender, W. T.: Primary Carcinoma of the Vagina, Obst. & Gynec. **11**: 3, 1958.

Monaco, A. P., Murphy, G. B., and Dowling, W.: Primary Cancer of the Female Urethra, Cancer **11**: 1215, 1958.

Paget, J.: On Disease of the Mammary Areola Preceding Cancer of the Mammary Gland, St. Barth. Hosp. Rep., Lond. **10**: 87, 1874.

Pelham, H., and Amreich, J.: Gynäkologische Operationslehre, Berlin, 1930, S. Karger.

Smith, F.: Primary Carcinoma of the Vagina, Am. J. Obst. & Gynec. **69**: 525, 1955.

Stoeckel, W.: Zur Therapie des Vulvakarzinoms, Zentralbl. Gynäk. **54**: 47, 1930.

Taussig, F.: Diseases of the Vulva, New York, 1923, D. Appleton & Co.

Taylor, G., and Nathanson, I.: Lymph Node Metastases: Incidence and Surgical Treatment in Enoplastic Disease, New York, 1942, Oxford University Press, pp. 314-323.

Tod, M.: Carcinoma of the Vulva. Radium Implantation Treatment of Carcinoma of the Vulva, Brit. J. Radiol. **22**: 508, 1949.

Way, S.: Malignant Disease of the Female Genital Tract, Philadelphia, 1951, The Blakiston Co., pp. 1-49.

417

25 · Cancer of the Cervix

General Considerations

Cancer of the cervix is the most common cancer of the female genital tract and second only to cancer of the breasts for all cancers afflicting women. The master radiotherapists in every generation have built their skill and knowledge in learning to distribute gamma emitters in the female pelvis. Roentgentherapy, with the advent of each new modality, seems to reach its zenith in attempts to deliver a cancerocidal dose to the female pelvic organs. Cancer of the cervix tends to remain confined to contiguous spread for a limited time in, perhaps, 80 per cent of the cases. It thus lends itself to radical excision that is undergoing a new trial in the present decade.

Etiology and Pathologic Anatomy

Predisposing causes to cervical cancer are parity, age, and race. Multipara have a higher incidence, as do non-Jewish women. The peak incidence is about 45 years of age. By this is meant that more women at the age of 45 years are eligible for the development of a cervical cancer than are those in other age groups presenting themselves for examination. There are more women in our population 45 years of age than there are 60 years of age. *The likelihood of a woman to develop this or other genital cancers increases with each year she lives.* Many other factors such as diet, chronic infection, age at marriage, venereal disease, and prolapse have been mentioned for lack of any other sound proposal.

Histologically, 95 per cent of the lesions are squamous carcinomas and 5 per cent are adenocarcinomas. The squamous carcinomas may be divided into several grades according to Broder's classification. Grade I is a well-differentiated tumor with keratinization, stratification, and epithelial pearl formation. Grade II is a spindle cell or transitional type in which the stratification is not as distinct. Grade III is more anaplastic and dedifferentiated, and the cell type of origin is often obscure. Grade IV is a medullary tumor; the cells are similiar to the basal cell layer of the normal cervical epithelium, and the tumor may contain long plugs of cells with central degeneration. Such a histologic grading is interesting in comparing the response to radiation of a series of tumors. With notable exceptions, there is correlation between the degree of dedifferentiation and the sensitivity of the tumor to radiation. The more anaplastic cancers are damaged more by electrons than are the less differentiated cell types. Of more immediate importance to the clinician, until we have newer modalities with which to attack this disease, is the lymphatic and contiguous spread of cervical cancer.

Lymphatic Spread

The lymphatic spread of cervical cancer is more important clinically than its spread by continuity, contiguity, or the vascular system. It is true metastatic spread—involvement of nodes distant and not continuous with the primary lesion—that frequently determines the prognosis. It is true metastatic spread that changes a clinically early cancer to a much more advanced condition when the nodes are studied by the pathologist after radical surgery. Most patients are seen after previous therapy by surgery or radiation has *disturbed the metastatic pattern* usually seen in the untreated disease. This, together with the changes caused by inflammation and destruction of lymphatic and venous drainage, will account for many unusual findings.

Studies of the lymphatic spread in surgical and autopsy material have the common weakness that the observations are not made on viable cells. The studies of Zeidman and Buss in the domestic rabbit have the weakness that inferences must be drawn that the same thing happens in human beings. When the pathologic histology of human nodes is compared with the above investigators' experimentally invaded rabbit nodes, one is convinced that there can be little difference between metastatic phenomena in human beings and rabbits. In their studies V_2 and Brown-Pearce carcinoma cells were injected into lymphatics below the popliteal nodes of rabbits. The popliteal nodes were removed one to three days later to see if cells could jump the subcapsular sinus and gain access to the efferent lymphatics immediately. They were shown to be trapped in the afferent subcapsular sinus. How long does a node remain a barrier? How soon do cells penetrate the parenchyma and finally gain access to the medullary sinus of the node? The rabbits were studied from one to forty-two days after injection of the viable cancer cells. The studies showed lymph nodes to be an effective barrier for about three weeks after emboli are first arrested in them. Then the node is seen to have large areas replaced and cancer cells in the medullary sinus. As with human metastatic disease, there are variations, and some of the rabbits showed distant metastatic spread that had to be hematogenous. *In general, the node is a good barrier, and it would appear that a thorough lymphadenectomy has sound surgical foundations.*

While the division of the lymphatic channels draining the cervix into multiple subgroups has limitations in its clinical application, we must still use any facts at our command. The frequent intercommunication and the presence of small anomalous groups of nodes do not permit consistent prediction of the direction of spread with any useful clinical accuracy. Henriksen divides the major lymphatic channels into three groups: an anterior channel, passing anterior to the ureter to link with the paracervical, external iliac, and obturator nodes; a posterior channel, behind the ureter, going to the hypogastric, obturator, external iliac, and sacral groups; and a sacral channel, passing along the perirectal connective tissue extensions to the lateral sacral nodes and presacral lymphatics. The course of the ureter determines this anatomic grouping. The uterine, middle, and superior vesical arteries are anterior to the ureter, and lymphatics along their courses follow tissue planes long ago described by Wertheim as the roof of the ureteral canal. Lymphatics coursing through the connective tissue of the hypogastric artery, and especially the middle hemorrhoidal branch, are posterior to the ureter and could be called a posterior channel. A sacral channel would be defined as those lymphatics that follow the perirectal connective tissue and thence along the branches of the superior hemorrhoidal artery up out of the pelvis. The predominance of positive nodes in the left side of the pelvis compared to the right side as found by several observers may bear some relationship to the presence of the pelvic colon and its descent from the left side of the abdomen to the middle and then downward to reach the rectum.

Consider the nodes themselves. Some generalities are known about the pelvic nodes: (1) The sacral nodes are very small and the hypogastric nodes slightly larger. The common iliac nodes are still larger, while the para-aortic nodes may be as large as any encountered. (2) The superficial and deep inguinal nodes drain into the external iliac chain after having received the lymphatic drainage from most of the lower extremity, with its frequent fungous infections of the toes, bruises, and other dermatologic conditions that often keep these nodes enlarged. (3) The deep inguinal glands may provide an index to the spread of carcinoma above the primary metastatic stations. (4) A frozen section may show cancer in the hilum of the node, and it must be presumed that cells have been dispatched to the next group of nodes. The surgeon is then

419

compelled to continue his dissection higher than contemplated and interdict the lymphatic channels, crude and inefficient as this may be, by radical surgery. (5) The size, shape, or consistency of a node is not indicative of the presence of invasion by cancer. (6) Nodes subjected to extensive irradiation and those out of the field have shown the same degree of hyalinization and fibrosis, so that present histologic techniques do not permit a positive distinction between an irradiated and a nonirradiated node. (7) The fibrohyaline capsule seen in some nodes after irradiation, like the trauma of surgery, possibly interrupts the metastatic flow of cancer cells from the primary bed. (8) The small intercalated node may harbor cancer cells or cause a retrograde extension of the cancer without the distinction of bearing any name corresponding to an artery that we use in describing the extension of this disease.

The distribution of nodes throughout the pelvis that are important in pelvic malignancies is shown in Plate 64, E to L, drawn during a radical hysterectomy. The names attached to many of the groups are confusing, since the nomenclature in England and on the Continent differs somewhat from that in the United States. Abroad, the obturator nodes are included with the hypogastric chain. In European literature the obturator nodes are lymphatics found at the exit of the obturator canal and not those that are intrapelvic and lie over the obturator fossa.

The involvement of nodes need not follow their anatomic nearness to the primary lesion. Secondary metastatic stations may be found to be involved without evidence of cancer in nodes close to the cervix. In the more common pattern of metastatic spread, small parametrial nodes can be demonstrated in the fixed specimen or in histologic sections of the parametrium. These would not be identified at operation, since an en bloc dissection is being done and the immediate paracervical tissues are widely circumscribed. According to some anatomists, the paracervical or ureteral nodes are located along the uterine artery where it crosses the ureter. These, if present and enlarged and firm, might be felt during the dissection of the ureter through the broad ligament. The obturator nodes lie in the obturator fossa over the obturator artery, vein, and nerve. These are frequently found as single, long nodes embedded in loose, fatty areolar tissue (Leveuf's node). The hypogastric nodes are small and vary from six to eight in number as they lie along the course and branches of the hypogastric artery and vein. The external iliac nodes lie along the course of the external iliac artery and vein and are more commonly found in the groove between the two. Some nodes may be found underneath the vessels, necessitating the detachment of these vessels from their beds on the psoas muscle to explore this region. Some anatomists have divided these nodes into superior, middle, and inferior chains, depending on whether they lie high up on the artery or lower and more medially on the vein. One quite consistent node (node of the bifurcation) is found in the groove between the hypogastric and external iliac veins. The sacral nodes lie along the course of the uterosacral thickenings, then on the sacrum until they reach the promontory, and then at the bifurcation of the aorta, where they drain into the para-aortic nodes.

The secondary metastatic stations in cancer of the uterus and upper vagina are the common iliac nodes, the inguinal nodes, and the para-aortic nodes. The common iliac nodes lie along the course of the common iliac vessels and drain into the para-aortic chain. In most instances nodes higher than the third or fourth lumbar vertebra will not be resected. The inguinal nodes are described thoroughly in Chapter 24, Cancer of the Urethra, Vagina, Vulva, and Bartholin's Gland (page 404).

The rectocervical and rectovaginal septa are more easily entered than is the vesicovaginal septum—this, of course, in the absence of extension to either side. The two branches of the superior hemorrhoidal artery are posterolateral in location. The point of origin of these branches depends to some extent on the formation of the mesosigmoid, and they make frequent anastomoses with the middle hemorrhoidal arteries. Because of this, the presacral lymphatics cannot be resected without ligation of many vessels and mobilization of the rectosigmoid.

Some generalizations regarding the frequency of the involvement of the various node groups can be determined by study of the statistics reported by Javert from lymphadenectomies in the operating room and by Henriksen from lymphadenectomies at autopsy. Their studies are in general agreement that spread to the hypogastric nodes, obturator nodes, and external iliac and common iliac nodes is statistically most common. Henriksen found many more ureteral nodes involved in his autopsy material than were discovered from the surgical specimens. This may be the result of the different sources. It is not possible to excise the pararectal lymphatics or the sacral nodes without a pelvic colectomy and excision of the rectum. Thus in only the autopsy material is involvement in the nodes behind the rectosigmoid reported. There is a marked discrepancy in the reported incidence of involvement of the ureteral nodes between the surgical and post-mortem material. The reason for this is not clear. Javert reasons that spread to more distant nodes—hypogastric, obturator, iliac—is relatively early and that retrograde involvement of the nodes immediate to the cervix, with edema and thickening of the parametrium, is the next step. Thus from the studies of these investigators, the surgeon resects fewer positive ureteral nodes at operation than are found at post-mortem examination, although the autopsy material represents more advanced cases. It seems more likely that the scarcity of positive ureteral nodes in autopsy specimens is because they have been eradicated by intense local therapy from an intracavitary gamma emitter which most of these patients would have had. Nodes farther from the cervix may not have received a destructive dose of radiation.

Everyone performing cancer surgery knows that the preoperative evaluation of the extent of the disease is frequently optimistic when the specimen is studied by the surgical pathologist. In our material at the New York Hospital and Cornell Medical Center the findings are very disturbing for carcinoma of the cervix. Many cases have to be upgraded after operation when positive nodes are found with a relatively early cervical lesion. In addition, when the complete cervix is available for study, some Stage O lesions are found to be true invasive cancer.

Direct Spread

The spread of cancer of the cervix by continuity follows tissue planes, nerves, and blood vessels. Thus, the usual spread is to the parametrium, but it is difficult to say whether this direct extension may not be dependent to some extent on the regional lymphatics. A normal, pliable parametrium does not exclude the presence of cancer, and a markedly indurated and retracted parametrium can be free of cancer. The cancer may spread to contiguous structures without a solid bridge of malignant tissue along the way. Here the lymphatics probably play a part with possible involvement of small, unnamed, intercalated nodes involved in the spread.

Symptoms and Diagnosis

The common symptom of cervical carcinoma is irregular vaginal bleeding. Not infrequently it is postcoital. Its character is different from the menstrual flow in that infection and sloughing in the advanced lesions cause it to be watery, brownish, and foul smelling. Unfortunately, symptoms can be entirely absent in the early lesions, except perhaps for a vaginal discharge, which many less fastidious women will tolerate for long periods before seeking relief. Pain is a late symptom, suggesting extension of the lesion or pelvic infection involving the parametrium. Rarely, the primary symptoms originate from an obstructive lesion of the urinary tract with pyelonephritis.

The steps in establishing the diagnosis of cancer of the cervix are divided into those performed in the office or clinic and those undertaken after hospitalization.

Office Procedures

1. Speculum examination
2. Bimanual examination
3. Cytologic examination
   Papanicolaou smears and scrapings
4. Phase-contrast microscopy
5. Colposcopy
6. Colpomicroscopy
7. Schiller's iodine test
8. Biopsy
   Punch method
   Ring biopsy

The speculum should be introduced with lukewarm water as a lubricant if cytologic studies are to be done. An obvious exophytic cancer or crater is grossly recognizable as malignant. Surface scrapings and a biopsy may thus complete the office diagnosis (Plate 62, *A* to *H*). With earlier lesions the inspection is not conclusive, and after a bimanual examination and routine smears and scrapings, further tests are done. Smears and scrapings should be repeated several times if inconclusive.

Wet-Staining Technique for Office Cytodiagnosis Screening

A rapid, polychrome, wet-staining technique provides an office cancer screening method that can be used by the gynecologist with basic training in cytodiagnosis. This wet technique causes less distortion of the cellular morphology than the complicated fixation and staining methods in common use. In fact, since the cells are suspended in the staining fluid, they roll around and can be viewed from several sides.

Red and blue-black Sheaffer Pen Company inks are used to make the stain. My own experience has been that the stain should be mixed just prior to the individual test. If large groups are to be screened, the solution is made in larger quantities. For an individual screening, the staining solution is made as follows:

Permanent blue-black ink, Sheaffer Pen Co.
   No. 232 _____ 4 drops
Permanent red ink, Sheaffer Pen Co. No.
   032 _____ 4 drops
Distilled water _____ 120 ml.

These proportions are different from those advocated by the original investigators of the method, but differences in the light sources and microscopes warrant changes in the formula to provide the clearest possible stain.

Smears of the desquamated cells in the posterior fornix, scrapings of the squamocolumnar junction with a tongue depressor, aspirations from the endocervical canal, and endometrial aspirations from the uterine cavity may be individually taken as indicated. Usually, one or two slides are sufficient. The slides are stained fifteen minutes, cover slips are placed over the areas of the smears, and then they are examined under medium power.

Papanicolaou would have been the first to recognize the usefulness of the wet technique and also the first to insist on a permanent record, should any suspicious cells be seen. This can be done by immersing the slide in equal parts of alcohol and ether after removing the cover slip. It is then fixed in the usual method and becomes a permanent record.

We have had limited experience with colposcopy, and phase-contrast microscopy and colpomicroscopy must be considered in the developmental stage. For practical purposes the Schiller's iodine test may suggest an abnormal area of epithelium. Whether from infection or cancer, or both, abnormal tissue does not stain as deeply as the normal epithelium. Gram's iodine is painted on the surface, and abnormal areas of epithelium remain whitish, whereas the normal, intact epithelium absorbs the dye. Ring biopsies may be taken with a knife or with one of several instruments, such as the Gusberg curette. The objective is to obtain the entire squamocolumnar junction (Plate 62, *L*). For this reason, biopsies requiring extensive excision of tissue (Plate 62, *I* to *N*) are best performed in the hospital and under anesthesia if necessary. Small or inadequate biopsies have no place in gynecology and only add to the pathologist's difficulties in deciding whether a lesion is truly invasive.

Technique of Diagnostic Procedures

1. Plate 62, *A,* shows the technique of taking a vaginal smear from the posterior fornix. In this

PLATE 62

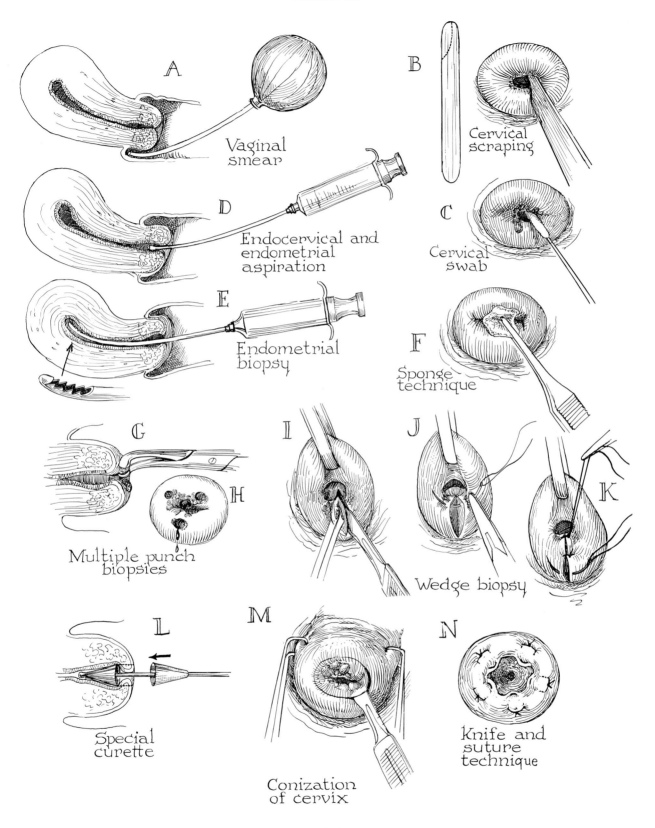

A — Vaginal smear

B — Cervical scraping

C — Cervical swab

D — Endocervical and endometrial aspiration

E — Endometrial biopsy

F — Sponge technique

G — Multiple punch biopsies

H

I, J, K — Wedge biopsy

L — Special curette

M — Conization of cervix

N — Knife and suture technique

location a composite picture of all of the exfoliation from the exocervix, the endocervix, and the endometrial cavity is pooled. It is the most valuable site from which exfoliated cells are obtained. No lubricant is used on the speculum in obtaining this smear. One or more spreads of the secretions in the posterior fornix are placed on the slide. An effort is made to make a thin spread that is instantly placed in a solution containing equal parts of 95 per cent alcohol and ether. Any delay in placing the smear in the solution voids the specimen.

2. Plate 62, B, shows a method of obtaining a scraping of the mucocutaneous junction of the cervix. Several devices have been made to accomplish this. A tongue depressor cut to fit the particular cervix in question makes an adequate device.

3. A method of obtaining exfoliated cells by the use of a simple swab is shown in Plate 62, C.

4. Plate 62, D, shows a method of aspirating the endocervical and endometrial cavities. Several devices can be used, but a malleable metal cannula attached to a 10 ml. syringe is adequate. This is molded to follow the contour of the uterine cavity to avoid perforation. The patency of the cervical canal is determined during this maneuver, since, if a stricture exists and the canal is closed, any exfoliation from the endometrial cavity or the cervix above the site of stricture is retained.

5. Plate 62, E, shows a method of endometrial biopsy with a serrated cannula attached to a 10 ml. syringe. Tissue is taken from representative areas of the uterine cavity unless this method of office curettage reveals grossly malignant tissue with the first few pieces aspirated.

6. Plate 62, F, illustrates a technique utilizing a special sponge. It is subsequently embedded in paraffin or other fixative and a permanent section cut.

7. The usual method of obtaining multiple punch biopsies from a suspicious cervix is shown in Plate 62, G and H. Four sites have been biopsied. There is no limitation on the amount of tissue or the number of areas that may be removed by this method. Bleeding from the biopsy sites is controlled by cautery or coagulants.

8. The method of taking a wedge biopsy, with subsequent suture and closure, is demonstrated in Plate 62, I to K. This is a useful technique when a carcinoma in situ has been found and the operator wishes to know whether there is an invasive cancer. An adequate sample of tissue is presented to the pathologist.

9. Plate 62, L, shows a method of obtaining the entire mucocutaneous junction by means of a special curette. The one pictured is that developed by Gusberg and the entire mucocutaneous junction can be excised by the surgeon.

10. The method of obtaining the mucocutaneous junction by means of the knife-and-suture technique is shown in Plate 62, M and N. This is the most satisfactory of all methods. All of the suspicious tissue is removed and presented in one piece to the pathologist for serial section to determine the invasiveness of the lesion. While any method that aims at obtaining the entire mucocutaneous junction can be done under local anesthesia as an office procedure, it is best performed in the hospital under general anesthesia, during which time other diagnostic procedures are performed.

Adjuncts in the Office Diagnosis of Cancer

Plate 63 shows some new and some old instruments that may aid the gynecologist in his office detection of cancer. Frequently, the cervix may be stenosed, and thin, delicate cannulae are needed to enter the uterine cavity for aspiration and endometrial biopsy (Plate 63, A and B). Plate 63, C, shows an endocervical speculum for visualization of the distal cervical canal. It is particularly useful when the cervix is everted and endocervical smears or scrapings are indicated. Since the endocervical canal is fractionally curetted during many diagnostic curettages, this instrument aids in the cytologic examination of this area of the cervix.

Plate 63, D and E, shows some thin instruments that permit the operator to explore and biopsy suspicious lesions within the endocervical canal. Almost always these causes of bleeding are benign, but with proper exposure the source of bleeding may be located and a hospital admission deferred or avoided while the office studies are being completed.

After Hospitalization

1. Routine history and physical examination
2. Medical studies as indicated
3. Routine blood count, urinalysis, and urine culture

PLATE 63

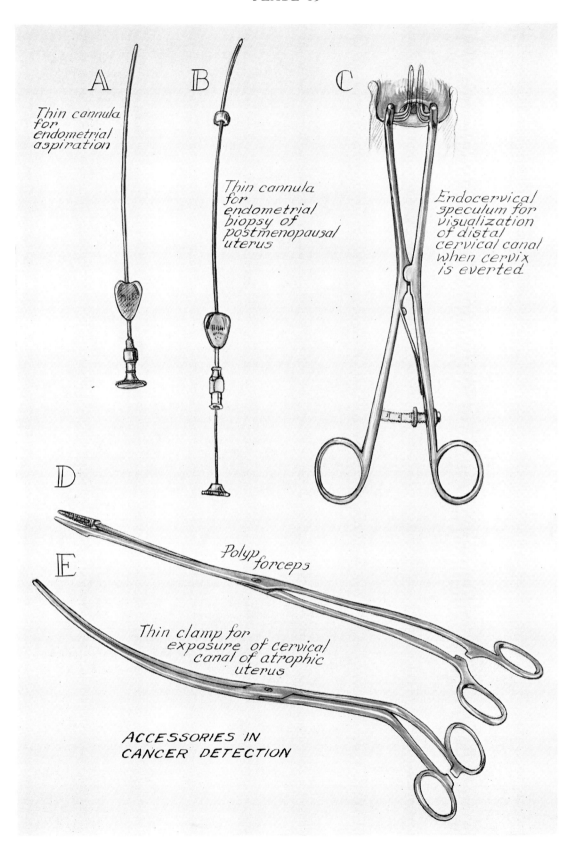

A — Thin cannula for endometrial aspiration

B — Thin cannula for endometrial biopsy of postmenopausal uterus

C — Endocervical speculum for visualization of distal cervical canal when cervix is everted

D — Polyp forceps

E — Thin clamp for exposure of cervical canal of atrophic uterus

ACCESSORIES IN CANCER DETECTION

4. Chest x-ray
5. Blood chemistry studies
6. Intravenous urography
7. Examination under anesthesia
8. Cystoscopy and other urinary tract studies
    Retrograde urography (as indicated)
    P.S.P. excretion tests (bilateral as indicated)
    Gemmell's maneuver
    Bladder biopsy (as indicated)
    Cytology of urinary sediment (as indicated)
    Differential urine cultures and microscopic examination after retrograde catheterization of the ureters
9. Proctosigmoidoscopy
10. Staging of lesion

After hospitalization with a positive diagnosis, we have established a routine in the Department of Obstetrics and Gynecology, The New York Hospital-Cornell Medical Center designed to determine the extent of the lesion and the ultimate plan of therapy. Routine history and physical examination are supplemented by any general medical studies deemed advisable. A blood count, urinalysis, and chest x-ray are done. Blood chemistries should include a BUN, NPN, sugar, K, and Na. Plasma proteins and CO_2 may be indicated. An intravenous urogram is made which may suggest further retrograde studies and kidney function tests. An examination under anesthesia is indispensable to determine, within the limitations of a bimanual examination, the status of the parametrium and paracolpium. Cystoscopic and proctoscopic examinations are often done at the same time. A careful note is dictated and written into the patient's record for future comparison. This should indicate the size of the lesion, a general description of its gross appearance, the depth and distensibility of the vagina, mobility of the cervix, size, shape, and mobility of the fundus, and a description of the adnexa. On combined rectovaginal examination the cardinal and uterosacral thickenings are individually described as to the existence of infiltration, thickening, and retraction. The distance of any suspected infiltration from the

pelvic side walls or actual fixation on one or both sides is essential to planning therapy.

For teaching and thoroughness, twenty-five steps in the inspection and palpation of a cervical lesion are suggested.

Twenty-Five Steps in Inspection and Palpation

An examination under anesthesia of a patient with malignant disease before and after instituting therapy has no substitute. Frequently your plan of treatment is modified by the findings not evident on examination with the patient awake. In our experience the additional information gained far outweighs the small risk of the anesthetic and saves the patient the psychic trauma of a prolonged and vigorous pelvic examination while awake. Listed below are twenty-five steps in the inspection and palpation of a cervical cancer. An examination under anesthesia can be just as informative in other pelvic malignancies.

1. Palpate the abdomen and note the presence of any masses, hernias, and scars. Note the thickness of the abdominal panniculus, edema of the mons or thighs, and any suggestion of ascites.

2. Palpate the superficial inguinal nodes above and below the inguinal ligament and over the fossa ovalis. The enlargement of these nodes usually represents the reaction to infection in advanced cases, with sloughing or involvement in the lower vagina and urethra.

3. The skin of the abdomen, back, and lateral aspect of the thighs is examined carefully for tanning, thickening, and telangiectasia in those patients previously irradiated.

4. With a dry speculum, repeat the vaginal and cervical smears or scrapings and any other method available to you for following the effects of therapy.

5. Inspect the vulva and lower vagina for visual evidence of extension. Turn the speculum sideways and inspect the urethra.

6. Inspect the upper vagina for visual evidence of extension, its location anteriorly or posteriorly, and the distance of such extension from the cervix.

7. Inspect the lesion on the cervix and note whether it tends to be ulcerative, endophytic, or exophytic. In the case of a crater or exophytic

lesion, note the dimensions in centimeters and record in your dictation. Note the amount of infection and slough.

8. Now observe the vaginal vault with particular reference to retraction of the lateral fornices and to which side, if any, the lesion seems to be drawn or extending. Note whether the lesion tends to extend anteriorly or posteriorly and to what degree it has obliterated the anterior and posterior fornices.

9. Estimate the volume of the upper third of the vagina and vaginal vault in the event of radiation by vaginal cone or radium and other radioactive sources. Note the distensibility and pliability of the vaginal vault by opening and closing the speculum.

10. Palpate the length of the urethra and anterior vaginal wall with special reference to thickening and induration. Note the distance that any thickening or suspicious areas extend from the cervix above and the external urethral meatus below. Compare with the cystoscopic tests for operability of cervical cancer.

11. Palpate the length of the posterior vaginal wall with special reference to thickening, induration, and pliability. Note the distance any suspicious areas extend from the cervix above and introitus below. Compare with the proctoscopic findings.

12. Palpate the cervix or lesion itself. Note its consistency—whether hard and unyielding or friable and prone to hemorrhage.

13. Study the mobility of the cervix in all directions. Note to which side of the pelvis it is drawn or has some limitation of motion. Note fixation to the bladder base and rectum.

14. Do a bimanual examination and note the size, shape, and position of the uterus. Observe its mobility and whether fixation by the cervical cancer or other intrapelvic disease is responsible for any limitation.

15. Follow any hardness or induration of the cervix into the lower uterine segment to study possible contiguous extension.

16. Palpate the adnexa for evidence of pelvic inflammatory disease, endometriosis, or other gynecologic lesion.

17. Do a combined rectovaginal examination and note any thickening or induration of the rectovaginal septum and any other intrinsic rectal lesion.

(If the vaginal examination suggested extension or retraction to one side or the other, start the next six steps on the opposite side. If not, start with the patient's right side.)

18. Palpate the right cardinal ligament for thickening and retraction. Note probable extent of the lesion from the cervix.

19. Palpate the right uterosacral ligament and note the extent of any thickening from the cervix.

20. Palpate the right pelvic side wall and note whether any direct extension is fixed to the obturator fascia. The pattern of spread is like a truncated pyramid, with the base on the pelvic side wall. A radiation shelf tends to be more broad, flat, and harder. If not fixed, estimate the distance in centimeters the lesion seems free of the pelvic side wall. Palpate the region of the obturator node.

21. Palpate the left cardinal ligament for the same observations.

22. Palpate the left uterosacral ligament for the same observations.

23. Palpate the left pelvic side wall for the same observations.

24. Do a combined rectovaginal-abdominal examination and estimate the mobility of the entire pelvic contents. In recurrent lesions study the feasibility of an exenteration of the pelvic mass.

25. Change gloves, reinsert the speculum, and take repeat biopsies. Control any bleeding by fulguration or compression.

Cystoscopic Tests for Operability of Cervical Cancer

Chart VII outlines some of the cystoscopic observations to be made in evaluating a cancer of the cervix. Designed to determine whether a lesion can be adequately removed by radical hysterectomy or whether an exenteration is necessary, the same observations provide much information of value in the event that radiotherapy is selected for treatment. These observations and tests are far from conclusive and are the subject of further study and investigation. At present, their value depends on the individual skill and experience of the cystoscopist who is treating cancer of the cervix or other genitourinary malignancies.

CHART VII

CYSTOSCOPIC TESTS FOR OPERABILITY OF CERVICAL CANCER

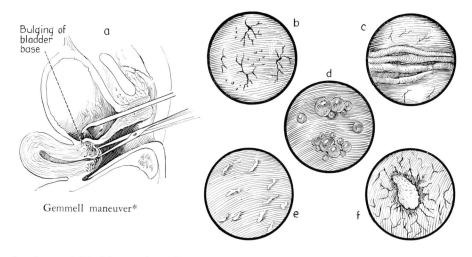

Bulging of bladder base

Gemmell maneuver*

1. Observe fundus and bladder neck and note capacity and sensation

----

----

2. Trigone and bladder base
   a. Bulging of floor

   ----

   b. Circulatory changes (dilatation vessels, telangiectasia, petechial hemorrhages)

   ----

   c. Transverse ridging

   ----

   d. Edema (diffuse, bullous)

   ----

   e. Pitting and retraction; superficial desquamation

   ----

   f. Ulceration

   ----

3. Gemmell maneuver*

   ----

*Gemmell maneuver. Place a volsellum on the cervix and remove the speculum. Proceed with cystoscopy. While watching the retrotrigonal area of the bladder base, make gentle traction on the volsellum. Note transverse ridging and whether it occurs immediately on traction. Indicates adherent bladder.

428

CHART VII (Continued)

CYSTOSCOPIC TESTS FOR OPERABILITY OF CERVICAL CANCER

Braasch bulbs of various sizes are passed to determine the site of constriction or compression

Biopsy sites in retrotrigonal area

A

B

If both ureters are involved studies are limited to one side at a time

Biopsy of superficially ulcerated area

4. Ureteral orifices (circulatory changes, irregular gaping, ulceration, nodules)

Right _____ Left _____

5. Meatoscopy* (fixation, retraction, movement on "strain")

Right _____ Left _____

6. Ureteral catheterization (easy passage, obstruction, angulation, where?)

_____

_____

7. Biopsies (location)

Right _____ Left _____

8. Remarks on operability

_____

_____

9. *Operative notes*
   a. Dissection of bladder base (stripped easily, gauze dissection, sharp dissection necessary, perforation, resection of bladder necessary)

   _____

   _____

   b. Dissection of right ureter   _____

   _____

   _____   _____

   c. Dissection of left ureter

   _____

   _____

Meatoscopy. While watching the ureteric orifice, have the patient strain down as if trying to void. Note movement of orifice. Normal orifice moves downward and outward promptly. Indicates fixation of ureters.

After a routine observation cystoscopy, attention is directed to the bladder base. The observations shown in Chart VII, *b* to *f*, suggest progressive degrees of invasion of the bladder wall by a cervical cancer or changes in the bladder base due to the cancer plus intracavitary radiation. The Gemmell maneuver is suggested for an adaptation of some observations of Professor Arthur Gemmell published in 1928 (Chart VII, *a*). The cystoscopist observes the bladder base for evidence of fixation between bladder, cervix, and vagina by manipulating the cervix in various directions. These observations promise to be valuable as more is learned by this method. As skill develops, it is possible to predict the difficulty that will be encountered in a radical dissection and, in some patients, whether surgery is feasible at all. The ureteral orifices are studies for evidence of fixation and compression. They are observed while the patient attempts to void, and their movement is compared with the normal. Catheters are passed to note the presence of strictures or extrinsic pressure and the location of ureteral involvement from the cervix (Chart VII, *A*). Biopsies are taken in the bladder base (Chart VII, *B*). These studies are then compared with the findings at operation if a radical dissection is done (Chart VII).

Proctosigmoidoscopy

Proctosigmoidoscopy is done following the cystoscopy. The rectal mucosa is inspected as high as possible, with particular reference to the area adjacent to the cervix. It is rare to find a lesion extending through the rectal mucosa except in the advanced cases. Positive findings or need for biopsy is more common after irradiation or radical surgery and in the presence of rectal symptoms. However, biopsy of any suspicious areas is done, since this modifies the staging and ultimate therapy in the event of tumor extension into the rectum.

With all this information available, the lesion is now staged according to the classification accepted by the American Medical Association and the World Health Organization. It should again be pointed out that a detailed description of the lesion, the ligaments and paracolpium, and the observations made on cystoscopy and proctosigmoidoscopy and the microscopic reports of biopsies of adjacent organs are more important than the stage, although the general usefulness of the classification is not denied.

Clinical Classification of Carcinoma of the Uterine Cervix

Stage O.—Carcinoma in situ, preinvasive carcinoma, intraepithelial carcinoma, and similiar conditions.

Stage I.—Carcinoma which is strictly confined to the cervix.

Stage II.—Carcinoma which extends beyond the cervix but has not reached the pelvic wall or which involves the vagina but not the lower third.

Stage III.—Carcinoma which has reached the pelvic wall or the lower third of the vagina.

Stage IV.—Carcinoma which involves the bladder or the rectum (or both) or has extended beyond the limits previously described.

Brunschwig's classification of cervical carcinoma has this in its favor—the type and adequacy of previous radiation therapy or inadequate surgery is appraised. The Memorial Hospital in New York, until recent years, received a great many patients with half-treated and advanced malignancies, as do most of our larger centers. Such institutions are still dumping grounds but get a gratifying share of new, untreated, and, at times, early lesions.

Surgical and Pathologic Classification of Carcinoma of the Uterine Cervix

Class O.—Carcinoma in situ, also known as preinvasive carcinoma, intraepithelial carcinoma, microcarcinoma.

Class A.—Carcinoma which is strictly confined to the cervix.

Class Ao.—After a positive biopsy of infiltrating carcinoma, no tumor found in the cervix in the surgical specimen.

Class B.—Carcinoma which extends from the cervix to involve the vagina, except the lower third; carcinoma which extends into the corpus; carcinoma which may involve the upper vagina and corpus; vaginal and/or uterine extension which may be by direct spread or be metastatic.

Class C.—Carcinoma which has involved paracervical and/or paravaginal tissue by direct extension or by lymphatic vessels, or in nodes within such tissues; vaginal metastases and/or direction extension into the lower third of the vagina.

Class D.—Lymph vessel and node involvement beyond paracervical and paravaginal regions—includes all lymphatic vessels and/or nodes in the true pelvis, except as described in Class C; metastasis to the ovary or tube.

Class E.—Carcinoma which has penetrated to the serosa, musculature, or mucosa of the bladder and/or of the colon or rectum.

Class F.—Carcinoma which involves the pelvic wall (fascia, muscle, bone, and/or sacral plexus).

Psychosomatic Considerations in Discussion of the Diagnosis With the Patient

The psychosomatic considerations in surgery of this type revolve around the nature of the disease and chances of cure, the resultant mutilation attendant upon the procedure, and finally the sexual function should the patient be in a sexually active age group or unmarried. In general, no matter how insistent the patient may be to "know the whole truth," there is a certain depressing reaction upon learning that she has cancer. This is true in even the most stoic individuals. Subterfuges are best substituted for an outright revelation of the nature of the illness. This is impractical in hospitals strictly devoted to neoplastic disease. Here the surgeon should emphasize the chances of cure and the new developments in therapy in order to maintain the patient's morale.

Treatment of malignant disease of the cervix aimed at cure rather than palliation is always radical, whether it be radiation or surgery. The extent of the operation, the postoperative course, and the possible complications should be judiciously presented to the patient, modified, of course, according to the individual temperament. It is a serious mistake to present the situation lightly to the patient. The shock of surgery or other forms of treatment may seriously depress a patient who is not given a reaonable explanation for each step in her management.

Treatment

Noninvasive cancer of the cervix is treated by amputation of the cervix or total hysterectomy. The ovaries need not be removed. Invasive cancer is treated by radiation or surgery alone and by a combination of these approaches. Radiation therapy has been outlined in Chapter 22 (page 385). Radical surgery alone may be employed in early lesions with about the same five-year survival as radiation. In Stage III and IV lesions therapy must be ultraradical to effect a cure. The operations will be described and are formidable procedures. Many combinations of radiation and surgery are under trial to improve the survival. At the present time in the Department of Obstetrics and Gynecology, The New York Hospital–Cornell Medical Center we are administering external roentgentherapy and two insertions of a gamma emitter and are subsequently performing a radical hysterectomy and pelvic lymphadenectomy. Gynecologists do not anticipate a marked increase in the survival of patients with cervical cancer until the basic cause is revealed by those engaged in fundamental research.

Special Situations in Treatment of Cancer of the Cervix
Cancer of the Cervical Stump

The present generation of gynecologists should be the last to be confronted with this problem in a country dedicated to and enlightened by preventive medicine. If devoted gynecologists could be relieved of the shackles and burden of treating cervical stumps, they might devote themselves to more pressing problems in the treatment of women. Cancer of the cervical stump is treated as if the uterus were

431

Text continued on p. 437.

CODE SHEET FOR GYNECOLOGICAL HISTORY

THE NEW YORK HOSPITAL

CODE NO. _____ NAME _____ PRIVATE ____ SEMI-PRIVATE ____ CLINIC ____ HISTORY NO. ____ DATE OF DISCHARGE ____

ADMISSION I (Col. 7)
0....Non-oper.
1....Oper.-peri & vag.
2....Oper.-abd.
3....Other oper.
4....Cystoscopic
5....For Study Only
6....
7....
8....
X....
△....Pavillon

ADMISSION II (Col. 8)
0....Private
1....Semi-Private
2....White
3....White (Jewish)
4....Black
5....Other Race
6....On Gyn. Before
7....On Obs. Before
8....On Gyn. Same Year
9....Single
X....Transfer
△....Pavillon

AGE (Cols. 9 & 10)

PARITY (Col. 11)

NUMBER ABORTIONS (Col. 12)

OBSTETRICAL HISTORY (Col. 13)
0....A. Nullipara
1.... Spont. Deliv.
2.... Oper. Deliv.
3.... Spont. & Oper. (vag.)
4.... Cesarean Sect.
5....B. Puerperia afebrile
6.... Puerperia febrile
7.... Puerperia unknown
C. Obst. Age (on adm.)
8.... Before puberty
9.... Child-bearing
X.... Post-Menopausal
△....

CONCURRENT CONDITIONS
MEDICAL I (Col. 14)
0....None
1....Rheum. Heart Dis.
2....Hypertensive H.D.
3....Arterioscler. H.D.
4....Coronary Art. Dis.
5....Quest. H.D.
6....Essent. Hypertension
7....Renal Disease
8....Pulm. T.B.-act.
9....Pulm. T.B.-Inact.
X....Pulm. T.B.-Quest.
△....Non-pulmonary TB

MEDICAL II (Col. 15)
0....Bronchiectasis
1....Bronch. Asthma
2....Pneumonia (pre-op)
3....U.R.I. (pre-op)
4....Diabetes
5....Anemia (pre-op)
6....Blood Dyscrasia
7....Endocrine Dyscrasia
8....Mental Dis. (pre-op)
9....Benign Tumors—Skin
X....Benign Tumors—Breast
△....Benign Tumors—Other (except Gyn)

MEDICAL III (Col. 16)
0....Lues c̄ lesions, STS+
1....Lues c̄ lesions, STS—
2....Lues s̄ lesions, STS+
3....Lues s̄ lesions, STS—
4....Lues Doubtful
5....Lues Unknown (No STS)
6....No lues
7....Gonorrhea
8....Stein-Leventhal Syndrome
9....
X....
△....

OTHER DISEASES (Col. 17)
0....None
1....Infect. & Parasitic
2....Malignancy (except gyn)
3....Nutrit. & Avitamin.
4....Poison & Intox.
5....Nerv. System & Sense
6....Circulatory
7....Respiratory
8....Digestive
9....Skin
X....Bone & Joint & Muscle
△....Other

GYNECOLOGICAL CONDITIONS
EXTERNAL GENITALIA I (Col. 18)
0....No disease
1....Hypertrophy Labia
2....Chancre
3....Ulcer (except Lues)
4....Anomaly
5....Absence Labia
6....Leukoplakia Vulvae
7....Kraurosis Vulvae
8....Pruritis
9....Condylomata
X....Lymphogranuloma
△....

EXTERNAL GENITALIA II (Col. 19)
0....Hypertrophy Clitoris
1....Disease Hymen (except imp.)
2....Imperforate Hymen
3....Bartholin Cyst
4....Bartholin Abscess
5....Carcinoma Vulva
6....Other Tumors Vulva
7....
8....
9....
X....
△....Other Dis. Vulva

VAGINA AND PERINEUM I (Col. 20)
0....Normal
1....Anomaly
2....Complete Lacer.
3....Cystocele
4....Rectocele
5....R.V.O.
6....Vaginitis
7....Stricture
8....Foreign Body
9....Cul-de-sac hernia (enterocele)
X....
△....

VAGINA AND PERINEUM II (Col. 21)
0....Inclusion Cyst
1....Gartner's Cyst
2....Carcinoma Vagina
3....Other Tumors
4....Fistula-Vesico-vag.
5....Fistula-Recto-vag.
6....Fistula Uretero-vag.
7....Fistula-Recto-peri.
8....C.T.C. doubtful
9....C.T.C. pos.
X....C.T.C. neg.
△....Other Dis.-Vag. & Peri.

CERVIX I (Col. 22)
0....No disease
1....Cystic
2....Hypertrophic
3....Lacerated
4....Anomaly
5....Stenosis
6....Descensus
7....Cervicitis, ac. (g.c.)
8....Cervicitis, ac. (other)
9....Cervicitis, chr.
X....Erosion
△....Endocervicitis

CERVIX II (Col. 23)
0....Leukoplakia
1....Squamous Metaplasia
2....Polyp
3....Myoma of Cervix
4....Adeno-carcinoma
5....Squamous Cell Ca (invasive)
6....Basal cell hyperactivity and question of Ca.
7....Intraepithelial Ca.
8....Hyperkeratosis
9....Sarcoma
X....Other Tumors
△....Other Diseases

UTERUS (CORPUS) I (Col. 24)
0....Normal
1....Anomaly
2....Prolapse
3....Retroversion
4....Anteflexion
5....Malposition—other
6....Hypoplasia
7....Chr. Endometritis
8....Hyperplasia Endomet.
9....Atrophic Endomet.
X....Pyometria
△....Foreign Body

UTERUS (CORPUS) II (Col. 25)
0....Submucous Myoma
1....Other Myoma
2....Adenomyosis
3....Adenomyoma
4....Endometrial Polypl
5....Endometriosis
6....Adenocarcinoma
7....Sarcoma
8....Adenoacanthoma
9....Carcinoma in Situ
X....Other Tumors
△....Other Dis. Uterus

TUBES I (Col. 26)
0....Normal
1....Anomaly
2....Hydrosalpinx
3....Pyosalpinx
4....Hematosalpinx
5....Acu. Salping.
6....Subacu. Salping.
7....Chr. Salping.
8....Salping. Isth. nod.
9....Tubo-Ovar. Absc.
X....T.B.
△....Endometriosis

TUBES II (Col. 27)
0....Carcinoma
1....Other Tumors
2....Previous removal (1 or 2)
3....Perisalpingitis
4....
△....Other Dis.

OVARY I (Col. 28)
0....Normal
1....Anomaly
2....Hypoplasia
3....Prolapse
4....Perioophoritis
5....Endometriosis (Not Cyst)
6....Follicular Cyst
7....Corpus Luteum Cyst
8....Simple Cyst
9....Endometrial Cyst
X....Para-Ovarian Cyst
△....Dermoid Cyst

OVARY II (Col. 29)
0....Corpus Hemorrhagicum
1....Serous Cystadenoma
2....Pseudomuc. Cystadenoma
3....Fibroma; Fibroadenoma
4....Carcinoma-Serous
5....Carcinoma-Pseudomuc.
6....Other malignant Tumors
7....Sarcoma
8....Other Benign Tumors
9....Cystic
X....Previous removal (one or both)
△....Other Dis. Ovary

MISCELLANEOUS DISORDERS (Col. 30)
0....None
1....Pelv. Cellulitis
2....Pelv. Abscess
3....Intraliga. Myoma
4....Intraliga. Cyst
5....Hermaphroditism
6....Pelv. Peritonitis
7....Extra-Genital Endometriosis
8....Other Pelvic Endometriosis
9....Previous Removal Uterus
X....Previous Amputation Cervix
△....Other Disorders

MENSES (Col. 31)
0....Normal
1....Ameno.
2....Dysmeno.
3....
4....Meno.
5....
6....Metro.
7....Dx.: Functional Bleeding
8....P-M Bleed
9....
X....Other Abnormal Menses
△....

MENOPAUSE (Col. 32)
0....Normal
1....After Radiation
2....After Surgery
3....Early (Under 35)
4....Not Reached

RECTAL DISEASES: (Col. 33)
0....None
1....Polyp
2....Stricture
3....Hemorrhoids
4....Prolapse
5....
6....Fistula-in-ano
7....Carcinoma (not gyn)
8....
9....
X....
△....Other Diseases

URINARY TRACT DISEASES

URETHRA I (Col. 34)
0....Normal
1....Anomaly
2....Absent
3....Incontinence
4....Urethrocele
5....Caruncle
6....Polyp
7....Stricture
8....Diverticulum
9....Carcinoma
X....Benign Tumors
△....Prev. Op. Incont.

URETHRA II (Col. 35)
0....Urethritis, ac. (g.c.)
1....Urethritis, ac. (other)
2....Urethritis, chr. (not g.c.)
3....Peri-urethral Absc.
4....Skene's Glands Dis.
△....Other Diseases

BLADDER (Col. 36)
0....Normal
1....Anomaly
2....Stone
3....Foreign Body
4....Cystitis, Acute
5....Cystitis, Chr.
6....Tumor, Benign
7....Tumor, Malig.
8....Retention (pre-op)
9....Endometriosis
X....Concurrent Urin. Tract Inf.
△....Other Diseases

URETER (Col. 37)
0....Normal
1....Stricture
2....Anomaly
3....Stone
4....Hydro-ureter
5....Ureteritis
6....Tumor
7....Surgical Injury
8....
9....
X....

KIDNEY I (Col. 38)
0....Normal
1....Lone Kidney
2....Other Congen.
3....Stone
4....Hematuria
5....Hydronephrosis
6....Pelvic Kidney
7....Pyelitis, acu.
8....Pyelitis, chr.
9....Pyelitis, T.B.
X....Chr. Nephr.
△....Pyelonephritis

KIDNEY II (Col. 39)
0....Tumor, benign
1....Tumor, malign.
△....Other Dis. Kidney

ABDOMINAL DISEASE I (Col. 40)
0....None
1....Hernia-Incis.
2....Hernia-Umbil.
3....Hernia-Inguin.
4....Hernia-Femor.
5....Ascites
6....Foreign Body
7....Appendicitis
8....Intestinal Obstr.
9....Paralytic Ileus
X....
△....

ABDOMINAL DISEASE II (Col. 41)
0....Gall Bladder Dis.
1....Diffuse Peritonitis
2....Adhesions
3....Perit. Incl. Cyst.
4....Previous Laparotomy
5....Previous Colostomy
6....
9....
X....
△....Other Dis.

OPERATIONS

VAGINAL & PERINEAL I (Col. 42)
0....None
1....Dilat. of Cervix
2....D & C
3....Tubal Insuffl.
4....Biopsy Cervix
5....Other Biopsy
6....Insert. Pessary
7....Insert. Radium
8....Cauteriz. Cervix
9....Remov. Condylomata
X....Bartholin's Excis.
△....Bartholin's.

VAGINAL & PERINEAL II (Col. 43)
0....Remov. Inclus. Cyst
1....Remov. Gartner's Cyst
2....Hymenotomy
3....Cervical Repair
4....Polypectomy
5....Amputat. Cervix
6....Vulvectomy
7....Perineorrhaphy
8....Ant. Colporrhaphy
9....Post. Colporrhaphy
X....Vag. Myomectomy
△....Repair Cul-de-Sac Hernia

VAGINAL & PERINEAL III (Col. 44)
0....Vag. Hysterect.
1....Vag. Hysterect. & Tu/Ov
2....Culdoscopy
3....Vaginectomy
4....Vaginoplasty (not A&P)
5....Colpotomy
6....Excision of Cervical Stump.
7....
8....
9....
X....
△....Other Vag. Oper.

ABDOMINAL 1 (Col. 45)
0....None
1....Tot. Hysterect.
2....Subtot. Hysterect.
3....Myomectomy
4....Suspension
5....Wertheim
6....Radica. Pelvic Eviscerectomy
7....
8....
9....
X....
△....Other Op.

ABDOMINAL II (Col. 46)
0....Salpingectomy-Unilat.
1....Salpingectomy-Bilat.
2....Oophorectomy-Unilat.
3....Oophorectomy-Bilat.
4....Resection of Ovary
5....Suspension of Ovary
6....Removal Para-Ovar. Cyst
7....Cauteriz. Endomet. Implants
8....Tubal Steriliz.
9....Salpingostomy
X....Pelvic Lymph Node Dissection
△....Other Abd. oper.

URINARY TRACT (Col. 47)
0....None
1....Plication Urethra
2....Supra-Pubic Susp. Ureth.
3....Repair Ves. Vag. Fist.
4....Repair Uretero-Vag. Fist.
5....Biopsy
6....Transplant. Ureters
7....Anastomosis Ureters
8....Cystectomy
9....Excision of Caruncle
X....
△....Other op.

RECTAL OPERATIONS (Col. 48)
0....None
1....Repair R-V Fistula
2....Hemorrhoidectomy
3....Polypectomy
4....
5....Removal Rectum
6....
7....
8....
9....
X....
△....Other Op.

OTHER OPERATIONS (Col. 49)
0....None
1....Explor. Lap-no removal
2....Explor. Lap-biopsy
3....Release of Adhes.
4....Appendectomy
5....Repair Hernia
6....I & D
7....Paracentesis
8....Second. Closure
9....Removal Perit. Cyst
X....Colostomy
△....Other Op.

NON-OPER. PROCEDURES (Col. 50)
0....None
1....Exam. under Anesth
2....Proctoscopy
3....Cystoscopy
4....Dilat. Ureters
5....
6....
7....
8....
9....
X....
△....Other

THERAPY (Col. 51)
0....Transfusions
1....X-ray
2....Radium
3....Sulfonamide
4....Penicillin
5....Streptomycin
6....Broad Spectrum Antibiotics
7....Other Antimicrobials
8....
9....
X....Transfusion reaction—mild
△....Transfusion reaction—severe

RADIATION THERAPY (Col. 52)
0....None
1....For Steriliz.
2....For Menopause
3....For CA Cervix
4....For CA Fundus
5....For CA Ovary
6....Other CA
7....Other Condit.
8....
9....
X....
△....

ANESTHESIA (Col. 53)
0....None
1....Local
2....Pudendal Block
3....N_2O-O_2
4....D-Tubocurarine
5....Ether
6....Cyclopropane
7....Spinal
8....Caudal
9....Basal Only
X....Pentothal
△....Other

POST-OPER. COMPLICATIONS I (Col. 54)
0....None
1....Febrile—Cause Unk.
2....Febrile-Pneumonia
3....Febrile-Urinary Infect.
4....Febrile-Thrombophleb.
5....Febrile-Infect. Oper. Sit
6....Febrile-Other Cause
7....Shock-Operative
8....Urinary Infect.-afebr.
9....Thrombophleb.-afebr.
X....
△....

POST-OPER. COMPLICATIONS II (Col. 55)
0....Pulm. Embolus.
1....Coronary Occlus.
2....Paralytic Ileus
3....Intestinal Obstruct.
4....Atelectasis
5....Wound Infection
6....Wound Disruption
7....Anemia
8....P-O Hemorrhage
9....Psychosis
X....Urinary Retention
△....Other

RESULT (Col. 56)
0....Well
1....Improved
2....Unchanged
3....Undetermined
4....Untreated
5....To Return
6....Died-Operation
7....Died-Gyn. Dis.
8....Died-Intercurrent
9....Autopsy
X....Transferred
△....Signed Release

YEAR OF DISCHARGE (Cols. 57 & 58)

INFERTILITY I (Col. 59)
0....None
1....1 year
2....2 years
3....3 years
4....4 years
5....Over 4 years
6....Sterility absolute
7....Male causes
8....Tubal occlusion
9....Cervical mucus

INFERTILITY II (Col. 60)
Anovulatory
0....(a) Pituitary dysfunction
1....(b) Ovarian dysfunction
2....Low metabolism
3....Malposition of uterus
4....Uterine tumors
5....Other tumors
6....Cause unknown
7....No statement

CODE SHEET FOR TUMOR REGISTRY 47124

NAME _____

TUMOR REG. NO. _____

FINAL TUMOR DIAGNOSIS _____

HISTORY NO. _____

DATE THIS REPORT _____

DATE POSITIVE Dx MADE _____

Underline all applicable categories in each column and fill in appropriate specific information.

HISTORY I (Col. :5)

Sex
0....Male
1....Female

Marital Status
2....Single
3....Married (Include divorced separated, widowed)

Race
4....White
5....Negro
6....Oriental

Hospital Status
7....In-patient, Pav.
8....In-patient, Pvt.
9....In-patient, S-Pvt.
X....Out-patient, NYH, OPD
△....Out-patient, VA clinic or pvt. M.D.

HISTORY II (Col. 16)

Service
0....Gen. Surgery
1....Obs.-Gyn.
2....Urology
3....Plastic
4....Neurosurg.
5....ENT
6....Eye
7....Pediatrics
8....General Medicine
9....Hematology
X....Dermatology
△....Other (Specify)

HISTORY III (Col. 17, 18)
Age (To nearest year at time of positive NYH tumor diagnosis)

HISTORY IV (Col. 19)
Other Neoplasms (Past or Present)
0....No other neoplasm
1....Other neoplasm

Type.....................
Date Dx. ....
Rx. ....
Result.....................
2....Unknown

Concurrent Condns.
3....Tbc
4....Diabetes
5....Cardiac disease (Specify)
6....Pregnancy
7....Premenopausal
8....Menopausal (to 8 years, after onset)
9....Postmenopausal
X....Endocrine disorder (Specify)
△....Other disease (Specify)

DIAGNOSIS I (Col. 24)
Basis of NYH Diagnosis
0....Autopsy
1....Surgical pathology
2....X-ray
3....Exfoliative cytology
4....Clinical only
5....Other (Specify)

HISTORY V (Col. 20)
Previous Diagnosis of this Neoplasm
0....No prev. Dx
1....Prev. Dx, histol
2....Prev. Dx, X-ray
3....Prev. Dx, cytol.
4....Prev. Dx, clinical only
5....Prev. Dx, method unknown
6....Unknown

HISTORY VI (Col. 21, 22)
Interval from Previous Dx to this Dx
(To nearest month, or year if greater than 8 years)

HISTORY VII (Col. 23)
Previous Treatment of This Neoplasm
0....No previous Rx
1....Prev. Rx, Surgery, curative
2....Prev. Rx, Surgery, palliative
3....Prev. Rx, Surgery, endocrine
4....Prev. Rx, Surgery, exploratory or diagnostic only

5....Prev. Rx, Radiation, X-Ray
6....Prev. Rx, Radiation, other (Specify)
7....Prev. Rx, endocrine
8....Prev. Rx, Chemotherapy (Specify)
9....Prev. Rx, other (Specify)
X....Unknown
(Specify for 1-9 above Name of Hosp. or M.D. who treated Pt.)
Address: ....

DIAGNOSIS II (Col. 25)
Extent
0....Localized
1....Regional, direct spread
2....Regional, lymph nodes
3....Remote metastasis, lymph nodes

4....Remote metastasis, abdominal and/or pelvic cavity.
5....Remote metastasis, thoracic cavity.
6....Remote metastasis, bones
7....Remote metastasis, CNS.
8....Remote metastasis, other (Specify)
9....Metastatic disease, primary site unknown or ablated
X....Unknown

DIAGNOSIS III (Col. 26)
Status at Time of Diagnosis
0....Asymptomatic
1....Ambulatory with symptoms related to neoplasm
2....Ambulatory with symptoms not related to neoplasm
3....Bedridden with symptoms related to neoplasm
4....Bedridden with symptoms not related to neoplasm
5....Moribund because of neoplasm
6....Moribund for condition not related to neoplasm
7....Dead

DIAGNOSIS IV (Col. 27)
Stage and Grade (where known)
0....Grade not given
1....Grade I
2....Grade II
3....Grade III
4....Grade IV
5....Stage not given
6....Stage I or A
7....Stage II or B
8....Stage III or C
9....Stage IV or D
X....Other grade and stage information (Specify).

DIAGNOSIS V (Col. 28, 29)
Interval Between Onset of Symptoms and NYH Dx
(To nearest month, or year if greater

than 8 years. If recurrent, use time of onset of recurrent symptoms)

TREATMENT I (Col. 30)
Type
0....Surgery, curative
1....Surgery, palliative
2....Surgery, endocrine
3....Surgery, diagnostic or exploratory only
4....Radiation, standard X-ray
5....Radiation, other
6....Endocrine
7....Chemotherapy
8....Other
9....No treatment

Details of Rx:
1. ....
2. ....

Rx Completed?
1. No....Yes....Date Completed

2. No....Yes....Date Completed

TREATMENT II (Col. 31)
Purpose
0....Curative
1....Palliative
2....Diagnostic only
3....Unknown

DISCHARGE CONDITION I (Col. 32)
Status of Patient
0....No clinical evidence of neoplasm
1....Clinical evidence of neoplasm
(Specify) ....

2....Alive and well
3....Ill, ambulatory, Sx related to Tumor

4....Ill, ambulatory, Sx not related to Tumor
5....Bedridden due to Tumor
6....Bedridden, but not due to Tumor
7....Dead (Specify whether due to Tumor or other cause)

8....No Autopsy
9....Autopsy performed

DISCHARGE CONDITION II (Col. 33)
Responsibility for Follow-up Care
0....Pvt. Physician (Specify)
Name: ....
Address: ....

1....Outside Hospital (Specify)
Name: ....
Address: ....

2....NYH Clinic (Specify)

3....Other (Specify)

4....Unknown or pt. refuses follow-up care

Follow-up treatment
5....No further specific Rx being continued
6....Radiation, X-ray
7....Radiation, other
8....Endocrine
9....Chemotherapy
X....Other
△....Unknown
(Specify for 6-X) Details of Rx:
....

Estimated date of completion:
....

Signed:.....................M.D.

CODE SHEET FOR TUMOR REGISTRY

THE NEW YORK HOSPITAL

FOR USE OF TUMOR REGISTRY. DO NOT UNDERLINE.

FOLLOW-UP DATA

STATUS I (Col. 34)

A. *Marital Status*

0....Single
1......Married (include divorced, separated, widowed)

B. *Type of Follow-up*

2....Pvt. Physician
3....Outside hospital
4....NYH clinic or in-patient
5....Other
6....Unknown or pt. refuses follow-up care
7....Lost to follow-up

STATUS II (Col. 35)

Service

0....Gen. Surgery
1....Obs.-Gyn.
2....Urology
3....Plastic
4....Neurosurg

5....ENT
6....Eye
7....Pediatrics
8....General Medicine
9....Hematology
X....Dermatology
△....Other (Specify in "Remarks")

TREATMENT I (Col. 36)

0....Radiation Std. X-ray
1....Radiation other
2....Endocrine
3....Chemo Rx
4....Surgery, curative
5....Surgery, palliative
6....Surgery, endocrine
7....Surgery, diagnostic only
8....Other
9....None
(Specify) ....

CONDITION (Col. 37)

A. *Status of Patient*

0....Alive and well
1......Ill, ambulatory, Sx related to Tumor
2......Ill, ambulatory, Sx not related to Tumor
3....Bedridden due to Tumor
4....Bedridden due to cause other than Tumor
5....Dead of Tumor
6....Dead of Other Cause

B. *Source of Information*

7....Outside Hospital or Private Physician
8....NYH Clinic or In-Patient
9....Information from Patient
△....Information from Visiting Nurse
X....Information from other source (Specify in "Remarks")

CONDITION II (Col. 38, 39)

Survival Time

(Months since first positive NYH Dx made or years if greater than 8 years)

CONDITION III (Col. 40)

A. *Status of Neoplasm*

0....No evidence neoplasm
1....Residual neoplasm, primary site
2....Residual neoplasm, regional
3....Residual neoplasm, remote metastases
4....Recurrent neoplasm, primary site
5....New metastases
6....Histological change, primary site (Specify in "Remarks")
7....New site(s), multicentric disease.

B. *Other Conditions*

8....New unrelated neoplasm (Specify. Give Tumor Reg. No.)
9....Non-neoplastic disease (Specify).

CONDITION IV (Col. 41)

Source of Information

0....Clinical exam alone
1....Clinical plus X-ray
2....Clinical plus Surg. Path
3....Clinical plus cytology
4....Other (Specify in "Remarks")

CONDITION V (Col. 42, 43)

Follow-up Time

(Months from first positive NYH Dx to last exam by M.D.)

DEATH INFORMATION I (Col. 44)

A. *Place of Death*

0....NYH
1....Other, hospital
2....Other, not hospital
3....Unknown (Specify for 1, 2 above and put date of death in "Remarks")

B. *Autopsy*

4....Yes
5....No
6....Unknown (Specify place of autopsy in "Remarks").

DEATH INFORMATION II (Col. 45)

Autopsy Diagnosis

0....No evidence this neoplasm
1....Local neoplasm
3....Neoplasm with remote metastasis
4....New Primary neoplasm
5....Histolog. change primary site without metas.
6....Histolog. change primary site with metas.
7....Unknown (For 3—6 give details in "Remarks")
8....Other major pathology (Specify in "Remarks")

READMISSIONS (Col. 46)

Date	34A	34B	35	36	37A	37B	38 39	40A	40B	41	42 43	44A	44B	45	46	Remarks

Follow-up sheet to be mailed to attending physicians

		CHECK ONE	CHECK ONE	CHECK ONE
PATIENT				
NYH History No.				
Diagnosis				
Discharge Date				
Tumor Reg. No.				
Date of our Last Info.				
1. No contact with patient since above date.		1. ( )	1. ( )	1. ( )
2. Patient contacted, not examined (Specify most recent date)		2. ( )	2. ( )	2. ( ) ....
3. Patient examined (Specify most recent date)		3. ( )	3. ( )	3. ( ) ....
Status of Patient	1. Well	1. ( )	1. ( )	1. ( )
	2. Ambulatory, ill of Neop.	2. ( )	2. ( )	2. ( )
	3. Ambulatory, ill of Other Cause	3. ( )	3. ( )	3. ( )
	4. Bedridden from Neop.	4. ( )	4. ( )	4. ( )
	5. Bedridden, other Cause	5. ( )	5. ( )	5. ( )
	6. Dead of Neop.	6. ( )	6. ( )	6. ( )
	7. Dead, other Cause	7. ( )	7. ( )	7. ( )
	a. Where	a.	a.	a. ....
	b. Date	b.	b.	b. ....
	c. Autopsy (Yes or No)	c.	c.	c. ....
Status of Neoplasm	1. No evidence of Neoplasm	1. ( )	1. ( )	1. ( )
	2. Evidence of residual Neoplasm not prev. eradicated (Specify Where)	2. ( )	2. ( )	2. ( ) ....
	3. Evidence of recurrent Neoplasm (Specify)	3. ( )	3. ( )	3. ( ) ....
	4. Evidence of new metastases (Specify)	4. ( )	4. ( )	4. ( ) ....
	5. Other changes (Specify)	5. ( )	5. ( )	5. ( ) ....
	6. New unrelated Neop. (Specify)	6. ( )	6. ( )	6. ( ) ....
	7. Serious non-neop. Disease (Specify)	7. ( )	7. ( )	7. ( ) ....
Since date of our last info.	Specific Diagnostic Procedures (Give Date and Results)	1. .... 2. .... 3.	1. .... 2. .... 3.	1. .... 2. .... 3. ....
	Specific Treatment (Give Date and Results)	1. .... 2. .... 3.	1. .... 2. .... 3.	1. .... 2. .... 3. ....

Signed .... M.D.

present, except that there are limitations to the use of intracavitary radiation. Radical surgery may be more difficult because of adhesions and the obliteration of the normal landmarks. Since the uterus has little to do with the surgical principles involved in a radical hysterectomy—except that it is removed—the technique of surgery is the same. The use of interstitial gamma emitters or colloidal beta emitters is ideal for this situation where intracavitary radiation is limited.

Cancer of the Cervix in Pregnancy

A small fraction of 1 per cent of patients with cancer of the cervix are found to be pregnant. This modifies the treatment considerably, depending on the duration of the pregnancy and, at times, religious factors dealing with the viability of the infant. In the first trimester the cancer is treated as if the conception did not exist, provided this is explained to and accepted by the parents. Radiation results in death of the embryo and spontaneous abortion. In the second trimester, if x-ray and radium are selected as the method of treatment, the uterus is evacuated by an abdominal hysterotomy. In the third trimester the gynecologist must weigh the fetal salvage against definitive treatment of the cancer in deciding on the proper course. Radical surgery in the presence of a pregnant uterus is feasible and the tissue planes are distinct. Blood loss is greater than in the nonpregnant patient. The patient should not be allowed to deliver vaginally not only because of the possibility of the spread of the lesion, but also because of the severe lacerations that may be sustained.

Code Sheet for Gynecologic History

For long-term study of factors relative to the development of pelvic malignancies some system of recording pertinent data about each gynecologic patient is needed. The code sheet for gynecologic history of The New York Hospital (pages 432 and 433) has proved adequate. A simple IBM punch-card machine and separator permit any investigator to assemble data with a minimum of time and effort.

Cancer Code The New York Hospital–Cornell Medical Center

For purposes of research and to satisfy the requirements of the American College of Surgeons, a Tumor Registry should be set up in every hospital to function in conjunction with the hospitals' record room. The Cancer Code of the New York Hospital–Cornell Medical Center (pages 434 and 435) has been used for over six years and found simple and satisfactory for this purpose.

Follow-up of Patients

The follow-up of patients is more important than the original coding since the latter information is already a matter of record in the patient's chart. A follow-up sheet (page 436) to be sent to doctors is useful in obtaining data. To keep the registry up to date, letters may also have to be sent to referring physicians not on a hospital's staff, to the patient, to other hospitals, and to relatives. This is facilitated by the use of form letters. The examples given on pages 438 and 439 will cover most of the correspondence required to obtain information.

Prognosis

The five-year survival of patients with carcinoma of the cervix follows a discouraging pattern despite efforts of the gynecologist to improve the result. This does not mean that the comprehensive care and comfort of the patient is not improving yearly. When the thousands of statistical reports enlarging the literature are sampled, about 80 per cent of patients with Stage I lesions are alive after five years (the others had positive nodes and actually have Stage IV cancer), about 40 per cent of those with Stage II cancer are alive, about 10 per cent of those with Stage III lesions are surviving with or without recurrence, and none with true Stage IV cancer have survived. The inaccuracies inherent in our system of staging the lesions must be considered in every statistical analysis of the results of therapy. Survivals after ultraradical surgery have yet to be appraised in terms of the patients who live when viable cancer is found in the specimen re-

Dear _____:

In the interests of following cases included in our Tumor Registry, we would appreciate current information as indicated on the patient(s) listed on the accompanying sheet.

We are grateful for your assistance in our maintenance of records so valuable for cancer research.

A self-addressed return envelope is enclosed for your convenience.

Sincerely yours,
Secretary, Tumor Registry

Enclosure

Dear _____:

We are interested in obtaining periodic follow-up medical information on people who have been treated at New York Hospital, in order to ensure that they are continuing to receive medical attention and in order to maintain records which are valuable for medical research. In accordance with this, we recently wrote to your physician, Dr. _____, inquiring about your present condition. He replied he has not seen you for some time.

We trust this means you are feeling fine and have had no further trouble. It is advisable, however, that you continue visits to a physician at least once a year.

Would you write a brief note on the back of this letter, telling us how you are and giving the name and address of your present doctor? We can then write him occasionally for reports on you. We will very much appreciate your cooperation in this matter. A self-addressed return envelope is enclosed.

Very truly yours,
Follow-up Secretary

Enclosure

Dear _____:

We are interested in obtaining periodic follow-up medical information on people who have been treated at New York Hospital, in order to ensure that they are continuing to receive medical attention and in order to maintain records which are valuable for medical research. Our records state that you are the _____ of _____ who was discharged from the New York Hospital on _____ and on whom we have been unable to obtain current information.

In a brief note on the back of this letter, would you please tell us what you know regarding this former patient's whereabouts and general condition and the name and address of his (her) present physician.

We appreciate very much your cooperation in this matter. A self-addressed return envelope is enclosed.

Very truly yours,
Follow-up Secretary

Enclosure

moved by block dissection. The over-all bulk of the surgical specimen precludes an unequivocal answer as to whether it contains cancer or not. Cytologic studies in prognosis have made progress.

Graham and Graham use observations on the normal, desquamated, cervical epithelium to determine the effectiveness of x-ray or radium. The effect on normal cells is qualitatively the same, and they can be more easily counted to measure the radiation effects. Four cellular changes take place: (1) vacuolization of the cytoplasm, (2) enlargement of the cells at least one and one third normal size, (3) enlargement, wrinkling, and disarrangement of the chromatin, and (4) increase in the number of nuclei in the cell. In this method, one hundred cells are counted consecutively and tabulated as normal or as falling in one of the four categories just given. A cell may show all four characteristics, so its category is determined by the predominant change. The

---

Dear _____:

    We have recently learned of the death of the patient listed below.

    In order that our follow-up may be complete on this patient, we would like to have the death information which appeared on the death certificate if one is available, or otherwise fill in the blanks at the bottom of this sheet and return it to us.

    We appreciate very much your assistance in our maintenance of records so valuable for cancer research. A self-addressed, return envelope is enclosed for your convenience.

                            Sincerely yours,
                            Secretary, Tumor Registry

Name:

Address:

Date of death:

Primary cause of death:

Contributory cause:

Autopsy?:

Name of attending physician:

Dear _____:

    We have recently learned of the death of patient _____ on _____ at _____.

    In order that our follow-up may be complete on this patient, we would like to have autopsy information. Would you kindly send us a summary of the autopsy report if one is available, or otherwise fill in the blanks at the bottom of this sheet and return it to us?

    We appreciate very much your assistance in our maintenance of records so valuable for cancer research. A self-addressed, stamped envelope is enclosed for your convenience.

                            Sincerely yours,
                            Secretary, Tumor Registry

Was neoplasm mentioned (specify):
Extent of neoplasm:
Other pathologic conditions:

most important change in studying the sensitivity of the lesion to radiation is vacuolization of the cytoplasm. If the first one hundred benign and malignant cells are counted, the percentage of malignant cells can be expressed. The observer then continues to count additional benign cells to make the necessary one hundred. A smear before treatment, one on the fourteenth day, and one upon conclusion of therapy suffice to predict sensitivity. With radium, a smear before insertion and one a week later allow a prediction of the effectiveness of the therapy. The cytologic end result would appear to be the same whether radium or medium, high, or supervoltage x-ray is used. If 75 per cent or more show radiation reaction (RR), the effect has been good. Less than 60 per cent is considered poor. Smears falling inbetween these percentages are not common, indicating that the cervical cancers either are or are not radiosensitive.

Graham and Goldie have studied the size of the cells to determine radiosensitivity. Both cornified and precornified cells enlarge during radiation. The size of the cells is accurately measured by an ocular micrometer or by a projection technique. The greater the number of cells showing swelling the more favorable the response. The peak effect of radium—at fourteen days—and the peak effect of radiation being summated shortly after the last treatment require that the smears should be counted at these times.

RADICAL PELVIC SURGERY
Surgical Anatomy of the Obturator Fascia, Obturator Membrane, Muscles and Related Vessels, Nerves, and Lymphatics Encountered in Radical Pelvic Surgery

The obturator internus originates from the pelvic surface of the pubic rami near the obturator foramen, from the pelvic surface of the ischium along a line from the foramen to the great sciatic notch, and from fibers inserting into the deep surface of the obturator fascia, the fibrous arch bounding the canal for obturator artery, vein, and nerve, and the upper aspect of the obturator membrane. It is a large, flat, triangular muscle and forms a tendon which, at the lesser sciatic notch, joins the combined tendon of the two gemelli, and all are inserted into the trochanteric (digital) fossa. This member of the powerful lateral rotators of the thigh is supplied by nerve fibers from the first and second sacral nerves. Besides the two gemelli, one of which arises on each side of the lessor sciatic notch, two additional lateral rotators belong to this group. The quadratus femoris passes from the tuber of the ischium to the femur behind the greater trochanter. The obturator externus arises from the outer surface of the bones bounding the ventral two thirds of the obturator foramen and inserts into the trochanteric fossa. The nerve supply of these muscles is from the lumbosacral plexus and branches of the obturator nerve. Again, the intrinsic diseases of these muscles are of no concern to the gynecologist, but, like the sacrospinous and sacrotuberous ligaments, they serve as landmarks or may be secondarily involved in pelvic disease. This is especially true in studying the extent of invasion and fixation of adjacent structures by cervical cancer. Radical surgery, knowledge of the pain distribution in malignant disease, and radiotherapy to the pelvic side walls focus our attention to the complex anatomy of the obturator region.

The obturator membrane is another structure in the anatomy of the female pelvis concerned with the attachment of the pelvic musculature and encountered in radical pelvic dissections. It is not connected with any pelvic joint, and its interlacement of fiber bundles closes the obturator foramen except in its uppermost part. Its margins are attached to the margin of the foramen except for the free borders of the obturator canal. This canal is bounded above by a rounded part of the margin of the foramen and below by the free edges of the membrane. The obturator vessels and nerves pass through the canal, and the obturator muscles arise from both its surfaces. The long, thin, and very constant obturator lymph node has its ventral extremity near the foramen but lies between the peritoneum and obturator membrane.

The obturator fascia covers the obturator internus and adjacent structures. It is attached to the body of the pubis, to the iliac portion of the arcuate line, along the ventral margin of the great sciatic notch, and to the sacro-sciatic ligament. There is a defect in this fascia at the obturator canal. Its extension beyond the pelvis forms the outer boundary of the ischiorectal fossa. The aponeurosis of origin of the iliococcygeus portion of the levator ani arises from a thickening of the obturator fascia. The surface of this aponeurosis has a thickening (arcus tendineus or the white line) from the ischial spine to the pelvic aspect of the body of the pubic bone. A complete dissection of the pelvis will involve large portions of this structure in determining the extent of the disease. As in other parts of the body, tissue condensations about major vessels and nerves are important landmarks to the surgeon. When the branches of the hypogastric arteries and veins are systematically dissected out and ligated to perform an authentically complete pelvic lymphadenectomy, large portions of the obturator fascia will be resected.

The obturator artery runs downward and forward just below the upper margin of the true pelvis. It passes through the upper part of the obturator canal with the obturator nerve above it and the obturator vein below. Muscular branches are given off to the surrounding muscles. Nutrient vesical and pubic branches can be seen before it divides, after emerging from the obturator canal, into its terminal branches to muscles about the head of the femur. The obturator nerve supplies the adductor muscles of the thigh together with branches to the skin and fascia of the medial aspect of the thigh. It can be identified by the pelvic surgeon in the substance of the psoas major muscle, where it is formed from three roots that lie in front of the femoral nerve. Its fibers are derived from the second, third, and fourth lumbar nerves. The nerve is first seen on the medial border of the psoas major,

behind the common iliac vessels, and on the lateral side of the ureter and hypogastric vessels. It passes foward below the pelvic brim in contact with the obturator artery to the obturator groove of the obturator foramen (canal), through which it reaches the thigh. The obturator lymph node—an important landmark in cervical cancer, whether treated by radical surgery or radiation—lies at the inner end of the obturator canal above the obturator vessels. It receives afferent lymphatic channels from the upper and medial parts of the thigh; its efferent lymphatic channels join the interiliac and common iliac chains of lymph nodes.

RADICAL HYSTERECTOMY AND PELVIC LYMPHADENECTOMY
Steps of the Operation

1. No. 6 ureteral catheters are inserted after the induction of anesthesia. While the use of these catheters is not recommended by some surgeons, I feel they facilitate the dissection of the ureters through the base of the broad ligament. Small catheters are atraumatic when the basic rules in handling the ureters—enumerated later—are observed. The presence or absence of evidence of vaginal extension either at the time of operation or before preoperative radiation therapy will suggest to the surgeon the advisability of circumcising the vagina well below the lesion prior to entering the abdomen. When it is felt that this will facilitate the abdominal operation or ensure adequate clearance of the lesion, the full thickness of the vaginal wall is incised and hemostasis secured along the wound edges. The vagina and rectum are separated for several centimeters cephalad to aid in identifying the level of incision as seen from the abdomen. The anterior and posterior walls are then sutured together, enclosing the cervix, as is done in the Schauta radical vaginal hysterectomy. The ease with which a guillotine incision of the vagina distal to the cervix (if decided upon) can be done will provide information as to the technical difficulties that may be encountered during the remainder of the operation. The adhesions, thickenings, and retractions caused by old endometriosis or inflammatory disease must be dissociated, if possible, from that caused by malignant disease. The solid, unyielding, retracted, and unpliable feel of cervical cancer extending in the parametrial connective tissue is soon recognized by the pelvic sur-

geon and more information is now available to determine the feasibility of adequately excising the lesion by a radical hysterectomy.

2. An interiliac incision with bisection of the recti muscles (see Chapter 33, page 565, for details) is preferred. This gives adequate exposure even in the very obese person with a deep funnel pelvis. The operation can be done through a right or left rectus incision or an extended midline incision. In any event, the surgeon must not handicap himself by inadequate exposure for this procedure.

3. The longest instruments available (some borrowed from the chest surgeon's set) and several vein retractors for handling of major vessels and the ureter are desirable. The illustrations were drawn to show a universal retractor in place. This versatile instrument is very satisfactory, particularly in conjunction with an interiliac incision.

4. Exploration of the abdomen is done with a systematic palpation of the abdominal and pelvic nodes. Special attention is paid to the aortic chain up to the renal pedicles. Metastatic disease beyond the pelvis will probably alter the decision to continue the operation.

5. Upon opening the peritoneum, the presence or absence of fluid is noted. The character of the fluid, if present, and the occurrence of blood or granules are observed. Fat necrosis from pancreatic disease appears as granules in the omentum or mesentery and should not be mistaken for metastatic disease. The cecum and appendix are first observed and then the ascending colon up to the hepatic flexure. The para-aortic nodes on the right side are felt several times during this maneuver. An enlarged and matted node should be removed and sent for frozen section. The liver edge and the round ligament are then exposed, and the surface is observed for metastatic tumor. Small fibroid nodules in the capsule of the liver are common and should not be mistaken for tumor. If doubt exists, the nodule, together with a representative area of liver, is excised and sent for frozen section. The substance of the liver is then felt for nodules within the parenchyma. The gall bladder is palpated for stones and thickening, and adhesions between it and the liver are noted. Differential diagnosis of abdominal conditions is difficult enough after pelvic surgery or radiation so that any information about the gall bladder that might clarify the cause of a surgical abdomen—days or years later—should be a matter of record. The pyloris, head of the pancreas, common duct, and pyloric end of the

stomach are then felt between the thumb and index finger by insertion of the latter into the foramen of Winslow.

6. The right kidney is felt, and its size and the firmness of its parenchyma are noted. The right ureter is palpated throughout its course, and its size, peristaltic response to stimulation, and the presence of anything causing extrinsic pressure are observed. After palpating the diaphragm, the splenic flexure of the colon and the spleen are explored. The size of the spleen, and its firmness, may vary from the normal because of the anesthetic or possibly as a result of infection associated with a malignancy in the pelvis. The left kidney is felt, but since the ureter on the left is cushioned by the root of the mesentery, its condition is difficult to ascertain without retroperitoneal exploration. During palpation of the descending colon to the pelvic brim the presence of any lesions in the bowel is noted and the left para-aortic nodes are felt as well as they can be through the mesentery. The small bowel is not always "run," but the terminal ileum should be inspected for the presence of a Meckel's diverticulum. The author has seen a Meckel's diverticulum adherent to the dome of an atrophic uterus that was perforated during a curettage for postmenopausal bleeding.

7. Convinced that the cancer is confined to the pelvis and with a negative report on any biopsies taken in the upper abdomen, the surgeon now does a meticulous palpation of the known glandular and connective tissue routes of metastatic spread in the pelvis. The glandular metastatic station first palpated is the bifurcation of the aorta. The common iliac vessels and the node of the bifurcation are observed on both sides. At the same time the ureter is palpated between the fingers as it crosses the pelvic brim. The external iliac vessels are then followed out to the femoral ring, and the presence of enlarged or matted nodes is decided. The surgeon should not hesitate to stop frequently and send nodes or biopsies for frozen section. The hypogastric vessels and the pararectal areas are then felt on both sides. Deeper in the pelvis the obturator fossae are felt and the characteristic long node and surrounding fat compared with the normal.

8. The uterus is then retracted either manually or by means of a tenaculum of some type and its mobility studied. The vesicouterine reflection of peritoneum is observed for thickening and adherency. With the uterus pulled to the left, the parametrial thickenings on the right are palpated

for extension, retraction, and fixation. An identical maneuver is done to determine the status on the left side. The uterus is then pulled forward and the uterosacral thickenings examined for infiltration, retraction, and extension of tumor or inflammatory reaction.

9. The appendix is now removed routinely. Even if the operation is not feasible and this fact is learned later, the appendix should not be left behind to confuse the diagnosis if intestinal complications develop. This is just as true if surgery is abandoned and radiation used, since the latter has its share of intestinal complications.

10. The next step determines whether the operation can be done without a subtotal cystectomy or other bladder surgery. The cystoscopic studies will have suggested the probability that the bladder can be dissected off the cervix and vagina but are not the final criteria. The right round ligament is grasped at the internal inguinal ring and is clamped, cut, and tied with a fixation ligature of medium silk or with 0 chromic catgut if you prefer. The vesicouterine fold of peritoneum is then opened from right to left across the uterus and as close to the bladder as possible (Plate 64, A). Frequently the ease with which the vesicouterine reflection of peritoneum can be incised will give an idea as to the ease of the subsequent dissection. Note in Plate 64, A, the pliability of the structure in this particular operation. No edema or thickening of the peritoneum was present, and the operative field showed the normal cleavage planes. The connective tissue extensions from the round ligament pass downward and inward toward the uterus. An artery and its veins frequently run in this connective tissue thickening —an arrangement so characteristic in the pelvis and abdomen. The connective tissue becomes more dense and converges just above the thickenings created by the uterine artery and its veins. The round ligament mesentery is another guide in this dissection and points the way to the uterine vessels and their connective tissue extensions. The fatty and areolar tissue of the posterior aspect of the lateral recess of the space of Retzius is exposed. A venous plexus (Santorini) ramifies throughout this space, and the vessels, being poorly supported, are easily ruptured. Bleeding should be controlled by a hot, tagged sponge for it is not worth the delay to attempt individual clamping and tying of these fragile veins.

11. A knife handle is then used to determine with what difficulty the bladder can be dissected free of the cervix and vagina (Plate 64, B). If the bladder base is rigidly fixed, firmly adherent, and devoid of any natural line of cleavage, it is improbable that an adequate dissection can be done without risk of leaving tumor or of obtaining multiple fistulas. Sharp dissection can be done to find the plane of cleavage between the vagina and bladder when the patient has been irradiated prior to the radical hysterectomy. As illustrated in Plate 64, B, the ease of dissection of the cervix and vagina from the bladder base may be the determining factor as to whether to continue the operation. Next, palpate the ureter close to the cervix with one index finger and strongly draw the entire uterus to the opposite side. The operator now learns how firmly the ureter may be attached to the paracervical connective tissue. The maneuver is repeated on the opposite side, with special attention to the side that seemed to have the most extension clinically. On the rectal side of the cervix the rectum is less intimately attached to the cervix and vagina at this level and rarely causes any technical difficulty. If the operation seems feasible, a warm, gauze sponge is tagged and left in the bed between the uterus and the bladder.

12. An incision is made in the peritoneum with dissecting scissors as shown in Plate 64, C. This extends from the resected distal end of the round ligament along the pelvic brim to the cecum. If the cecum is redundant and its peritoneal reflections extend over the common iliac vessels, it is mobilized and retracted cephalad as far as is necessary to expose the field of operation adequately. The appendiceal stump has been inverted, but the mesoappendix is ligated in a way that does not draw the cecum toward the ureter. The method of doing this will naturally depend on the developmental type of the appendix and its mesentery (Plate 64, C). The ileocecal vessels run in an extension of the mesentery of the small bowel. This is behind the ileocecal junction, so these vessels should be identified and preserved during the dissection. This incision is then continued above the pelvic brim along the infundibulopelvic pedicle. The ureter now comes into view on the retroperitoneal side, and the medial flap should be retracted toward the midline. The infundibulopelvic pedicle, together with the ovarian artery and veins, is clamped close to the ureter, cut, and doubly ligated (Plate 64, D). When the proximal end is retracted medially, the great vessels are visualized.

13. At this time the peritoneoareolar flap for the ureter is developed. The lateral peritoneal incision that was carried along the aorta medial to the cecum and ended with the ligation of the

443

Text continued on p. 455.

PLATE 64

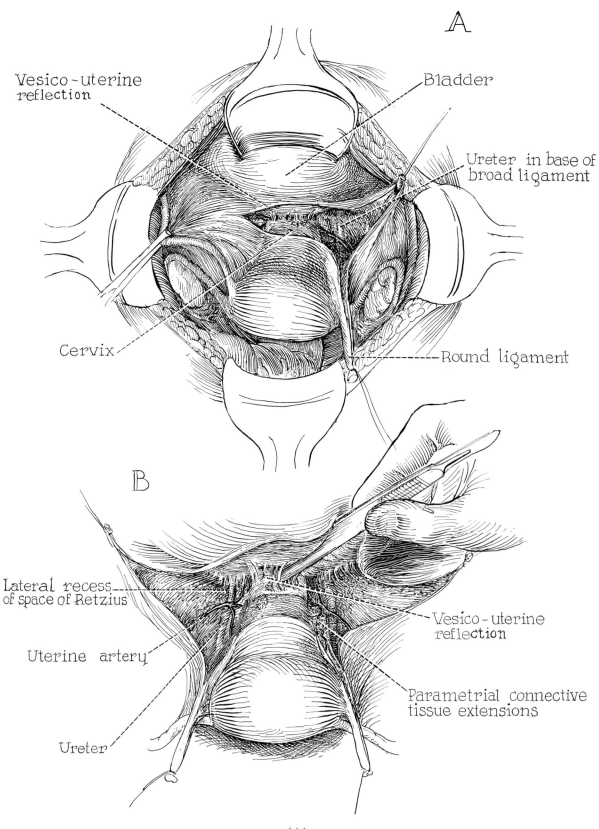

A

Vesico-uterine reflection

Bladder

Ureter in base of broad ligament

Cervix

Round ligament

B

Lateral recess of space of Retzius

Vesico-uterine reflection

Uterine artery

Parametrial connective tissue extensions

Ureter

444

PLATE 64 *(Continued)*

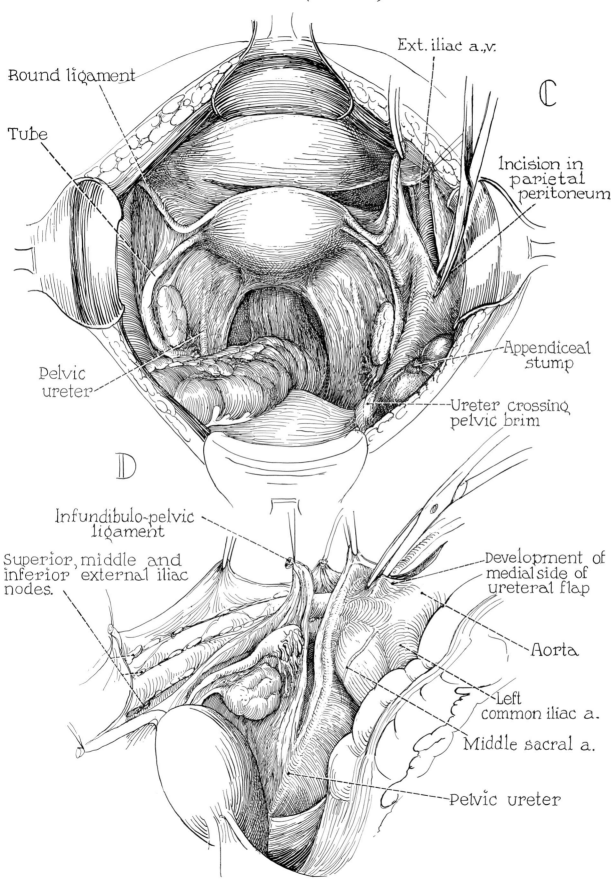

Round ligament

Tube

Ext. iliac a.,v.

C

Incision in
parietal
peritoneum

Appendiceal
stump

Pelvic
ureter

Ureter crossing
pelvic brim

D

Infundibulo-pelvic
ligament

Development of
medial side of
ureteral flap

Superior, middle and
inferior external iliac
nodes.

Aorta

Left
common iliac a.

Middle sacral a.

Pelvic ureter

PLATE 64 *(Continued)*

E

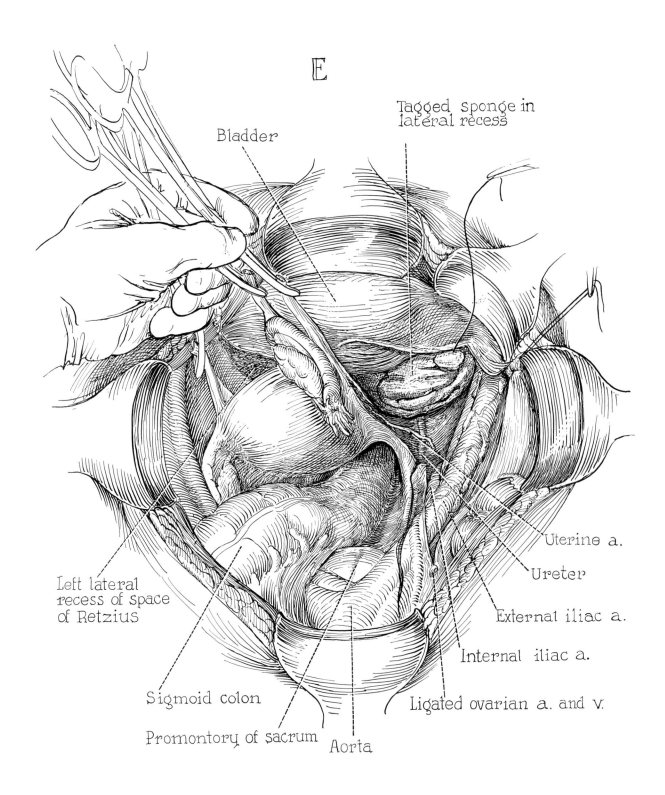

Tagged sponge in lateral recess

Bladder

Uterine a.

Ureter

External iliac a.

Internal iliac a.

Ligated ovarian a. and v.

Left lateral recess of space of Retzius

Sigmoid colon

Promontory of sacrum

Aorta

PLATE 64 *(Continued)*

F

External iliac lymphadenectomy

Node of the bifurcation

Deep epigastric a.

Accessory obturator a.

Obturator a.,v., and n.

Tagged sponge

Bladder

Ant. and post. divisions
of hypogastric artery

Uterine a.

Ureter retracted medially

Hypogastric nodes

Ureter entering connective
tissue at base of broad lig.

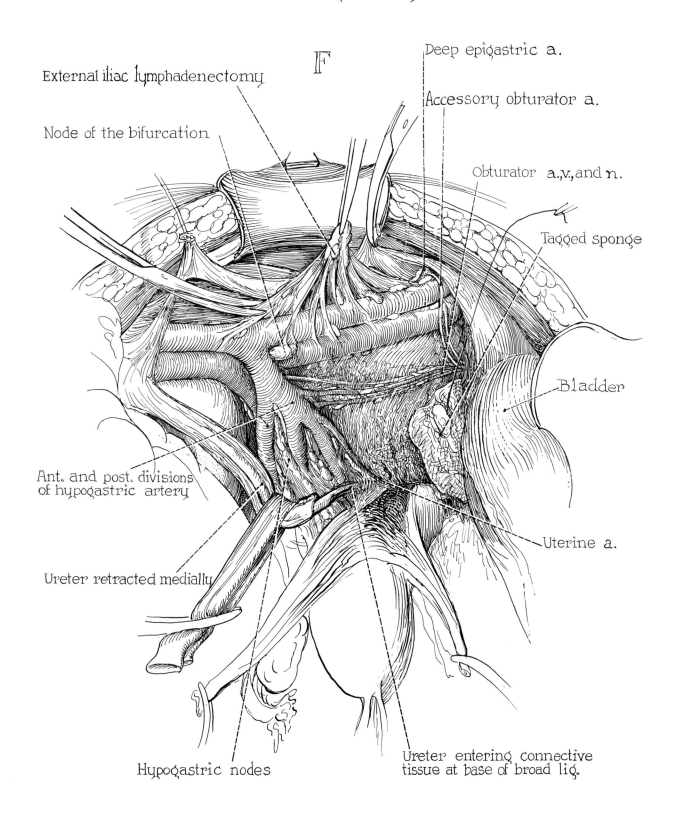

PLATE 64 (Continued)

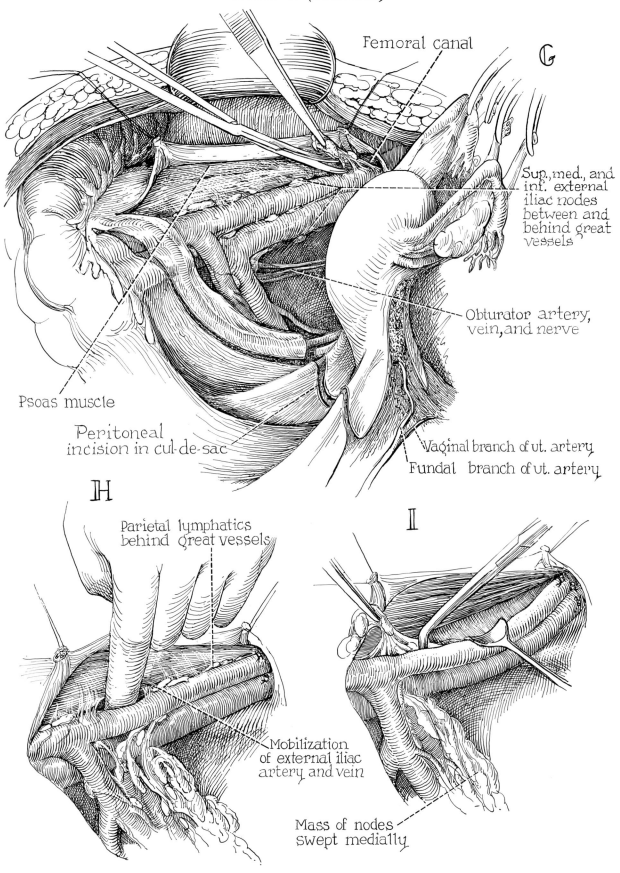

Femoral canal

G

Sup., med., and inf. external iliac nodes between and behind great vessels

Obturator artery, vein, and nerve

Psoas muscle

Peritoneal incision in cul-de-sac

Vaginal branch of ut. artery

Fundal branch of ut. artery

H

Parietal lymphatics behind great vessels

I

Mobilization of external iliac artery and vein

Mass of nodes swept medially

PLATE 64 (Continued)

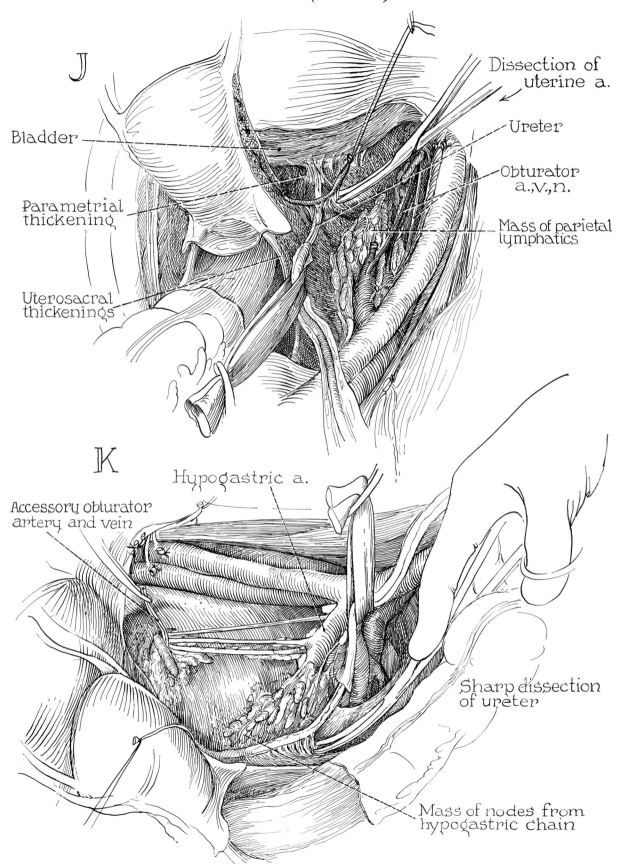

J

Bladder

Parametrial
thickening

Uterosacral
thickenings

Dissection of
uterine a.

Ureter

Obturator
a.,v.,n.

Mass of parietal
lymphatics

K

Accessory obturator
artery and vein

Hypogastric a.

Sharp dissection
of ureter

Mass of nodes from
hypogastric chain

PLATE 64 (Continued)

L

Deep epigastric and circumflex iliac vessels

Iliopsoas muscle

Ant. division of hypogastric artery

Post. division of hypogastric artery

Accessory obturator artery and vein

Obturator canal

Obturator nerve, artery, and vein

Dissection of obturator fossa and node

Mass of nodes and fatty areolar tissue from common and ext. iliac vessels

Hypogastric nodes

Uterine artery

M

Ureter drawn medially

N

Connective tissue of parametrium and paracolpium

Further stripping of ureter

Ureter handled by picking up sheath

PLATE 64 (Continued)

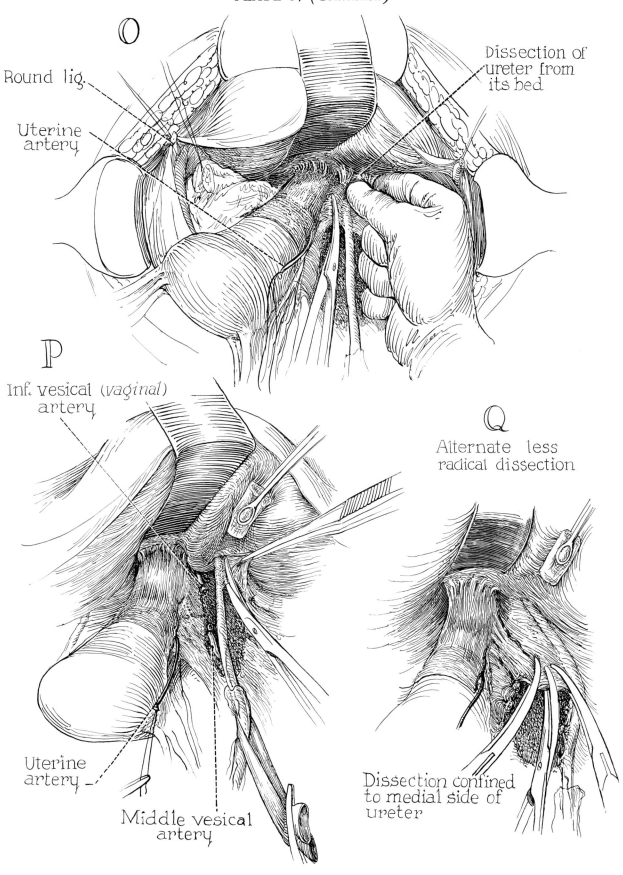

O

Round lig.

Uterine artery

Dissection of ureter from its bed

P

Inf. vesical (*vaginal*) artery

Uterine artery

Middle vesical artery

Q

Alternate less radical dissection

Dissection confined to medial side of ureter

PLATE 64 (Continued)

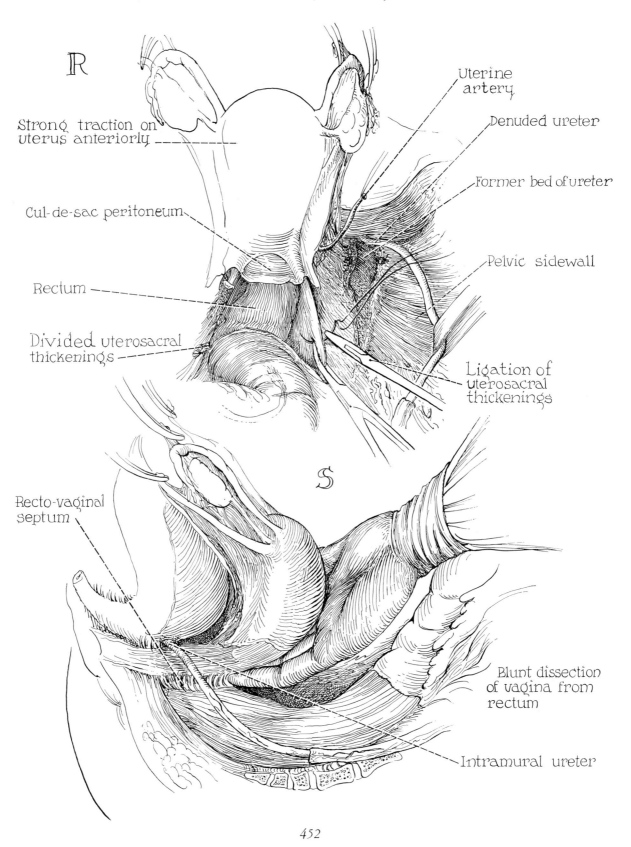

R

Strong traction on
uterus anteriorly

Cul-de-sac peritoneum

Rectum

Divided uterosacral
thickenings

Uterine
artery

Denuded ureter

Former bed of ureter

Pelvic sidewall

Ligation of
uterosacral
thickenings

S

Recto-vaginal
septum

Blunt dissection
of vagina from
rectum

Intramural ureter

PLATE 64 (Continued)

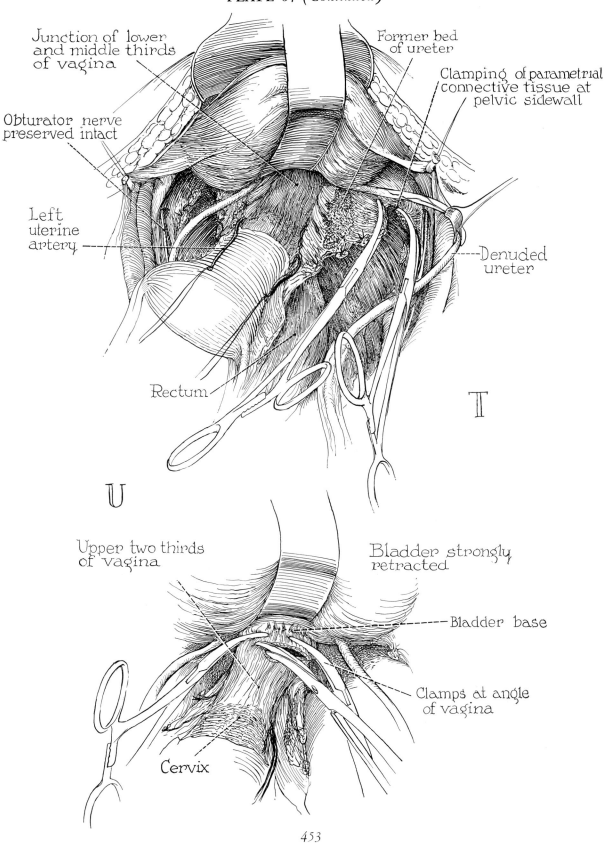

Junction of lower and middle thirds of vagina

Former bed of ureter

Clamping of parametrial connective tissue at pelvic sidewall

Obturator nerve preserved intact

Left uterine artery

Denuded ureter

Rectum

Ⅱ

Ⅰ

Ⅰ

Upper two thirds of vagina

Bladder strongly retracted

Bladder base

Clamps at angle of vagina

Cervix

453

PLATE 64 (Concluded)

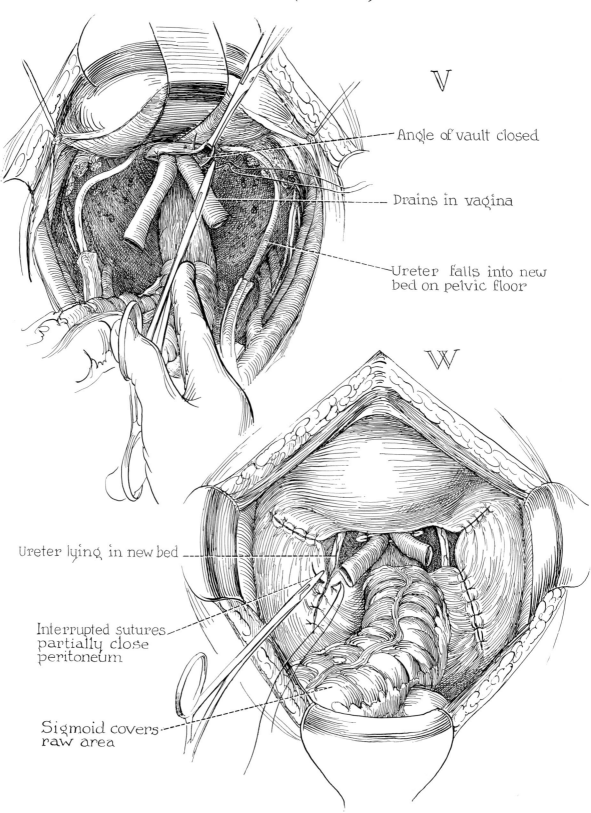

V

— Angle of vault closed

— Drains in vagina

— Ureter falls into new bed on pelvic floor

W

Ureter lying in new bed — — —

Interrupted sutures partially close peritoneum

Sigmoid covers raw area

ovarian vessels is carried down on the right side of the ureter. The peritoneum medial to the ureter is incised so as to make a flap about 3 cm. across (Plate 64, D). This is carried down the left side of the ureter about 5 to 6 cm. from the pelvic brim and then across the ureter to the lateral side of the flap. The medial end of this incision will later be carried down and across the rectum prior to ressection of the uterosacral ligaments (Plate 64, E). Care is exercised not to disturb the periureteral connective tissue between the peritoneum and ureter. At no time should the ureter be grasped by instruments indiscriminately. When necessary to clamp a small vessel in its sheath, a fine hemostat is used and a fine tie applied. The ureter is moved about in the operative field by means of small vein retractors and is carefully protected from the pressure of large retractors and other instruments used in the operative area. With the uterus drawn strongly to the left, some of the important landmarks of the operation are seen (Plate 64, E). The ureter is seen in the pelvis with the uterine artery coursing over it. The hypogastric artery (internal iliac artery) is seen dipping down into the pelvis. Note the lymphatics along the great vessels which are seen in their beds rather than coming away attached to the peritoneal flaps. The importance of good exposure, as demonstrated by Plate 64, E, will be more evident as the operation proceeds deeper in the pelvis.

14. A warm, gauze sponge, properly tagged, is now laid in the operative bed, and the same procedure up to this point is carried out on the left side. On this side the anatomy of the descending colon, sigmoid, and rectum modifies the technique. If the sigmoid mesentery is more caudad than average, the dissection is more limited unless the terminal branches of the inferior mesenteric artery, together with the sigmoid and descending colon, are displaced upward. The infundibulo-pelvic pedicle on this side is ligated high, after displacement of the bowel, and when the lateral flap is retracted, the vessels and ureter come into view.

15. The next few steps are shown from the left side to familiarize the surgeon with the appearance of the entire operative field during this block dissection (Plate 64, F). The left ureter is shown dissected out from above the pelvic brim to the base of the broad ligament. An adequate peritoneal sheath has been left for nourishment. It can be seen entering the connective tissue at the base of the broad ligament or so-called ureteric canal. As it is drawn medially, the anterior and

posterior divisions of the hypogastric artery and vein, together with the hypogastric chain of nodes, are visualized. As emphasized repeatedly in this operation, this is a dangerous area should these vessels be accidentally ruptured. This is especially true of the massive posterior muscular branches that dip between the nerve trunks of the lumbosacral plexus and above the upper border of the piriformis muscle. The obturator artery, vein, and nerve are seen as they course along the lateral wall of the pelvis to the obturator fossa. Injury to the artery or vein is unimportant, but the nerve is preserved if possible. The node dissection is now begun at a midpoint between the brim of the pelvis and the femoral canal. Forceps and dissecting scissors are alternately used with long angle clamps, and any bleeders are clamped and tied. It is not always possible or even desirable to keep the mass of nodes with the main specimen. They should be carefully labeled if detached. Note particularly in Plate 64, F, the node of the bifurcation that lies between the external iliac and hypogastric arteries. It should be carefully palpated for evidence of tumor, and if suspicious it should be sent for frozen section. The constancy of this node makes it an important landmark, and involvement with metastatic disease may represent the last metastatic station below the pelvic brim to which the cancer has spread.

16. The dissection proceeds distally along the external iliac vessels to the femoral canal, which is cleaned out (Plate 64, G). A variable artery with its companion vein, the accessory obturator, is frequently encountered in this dissection. Ligation of this accessory artery and vein will prevent troublesome bleeding later in the dissection when the obturator fossa is approached. The textbooks of anatomy describe these accessory obturator vessels as present in about one third of the dissections. Experience at the operating table during radical surgery and surgery on the lower one third of the ureter suggests that the absence of these vessels is more of an anomaly than their presence. The deep epigastric vessels may be cut, clamped, and tied if they interfere with the dissection or cause any bleeding. If an interiliac incision has been used, the deep epigastric vessels will have been ligated more cephalad already, and their subsequent ligation at their origin is of little importance. As the dissection of the femoral canal proceeds, the femoral nerve will be recognized lateral to the vein. The femoral nerve arises in the substance of the psoas major, from the back of the second, third, and fourth lumbar nerves and posterior to the obturator nerve. In

this dissection it will be recognized in the groove between the psoas and iliacus before entering the femoral canal. Since the deep inguinal nodes in the femoral canal occupy the areolar tissue medial to the nerve and vessels, there is little chance of traumatizing this important nerve, but it should be identified. The deep femoral node (Cloquet, Rosenmüller) is removed without difficulty. Some bleeding may be encountered from the superficial epigastric, superficial external pudic, and superficial circumflex iliac vessels when the more superficial part of the femoral canal is cleared of lymphatic and areolar tissue. Small nodes or intercalated nodes between and behind the great vessels are removed by the next maneuver. The node dissection is then carried proximally on the great vessels to clean all the tissue from the common iliac artery and veins well up on the aorta and vena cava. The individual groups of nodes are labeled and fixed separately for section as a prognostic aid. The lymphadenectomy and manipulation of the major vessels are the same as a periarterial sympathectomy. The large vessels will become smaller in diameter and will tend to undulate from the thorough dissection that is done.

17. In Plate 64, *H,* the technique of mobilizing the external iliac artery and vein is shown. This is done from the femoral canal to a point near the brim of the pelvis where a small branch to the ureter comes off the common iliac artery. This ureteral branch should be preserved, if possible, together with the flap of peritoneum and retroperitoneal connective tissue. The parietal lymphatics extend behind and between the external iliac vessels and are readily removed with the vessels lifted off the psoas. This is done by inserting the index finger between the belly of the muscle and the vessels and gently sweeping the vessels free (Plate 64, *H*). This technique is not as formidable a maneuver as would first be imagined. The vessels are lifted from their beds with comparative ease unless bound down by radiation or inflammatory reaction. As the bifurcation is reached, the operator proceeds with caution so as not to rupture any of the branches of the posterior division of the hypogastric artery or vein. The iliolumbar branch, which courses laterally from its origin, is identified and avoided. One or more vein retractors are then used to retract the vessels medially while the lymphatics behind and between the artery and vein are removed (Plate 64, *I*). Some of the muscular branches may be ruptured in this maneuver but are not difficult to ligate and control. It is rarely possible to keep these nodes together with the main mass being swept medially, so they are separately labeled for the pathologist. In any lymphadenectomy where a mass of nodes and fat become detached from the specimen—disallowing orientation and identification by the pathologist—a tag or marker of some kind should be placed for positive identification in the former bed of the node or nodes. The femoral nerve as it emerges between the iliacus and psoas may be exposed. It should be left undisturbed except where it is necessary to clean out the femoral canal of its fat and nodes. Pressure on the femoral nerve from retractors should be avoided by a liberal incision that permits lateral traction beyond the nerve.

18. A view of the right side of the pelvis is now used to show the dissection of the hypogastric chain of nodes and the removal of the contents of the obturator fossa (Plate 64, *J*). The common iliac artery and vein are now retracted laterally by a vein retractor while the ureter is gently drawn to the midline by a rubber dam. During the discussion of the surgical anatomy involved in this operation, the variability of the vessels arising from the hypogastric artery was emphasized. (See under Surgical Anatomy of the Pelvic Arteries and Veins, page 528.) Both veins and arteries of the parietal branches dip into muscle masses and through the greater and lesser sciatic foramina. The posterior division that gives rise to these branches may be very large and rather short. If the artery is accidentally severed or the vein ruptured in the node dissection, blood will well up in the pelvis in a most alarming manner. The nodes and areolar tissue along the hypogastric vessels are now removed. Long forceps and an angle clamp serve admirably in this dissection. The ureter, now beyond its peritoneal flap, is mobilized by gentle dissection until the uterine artery is seen to cross it to the uterus. A presacral neurectomy may be performed and the distal ends of the plexus used to help tease the lymphatics off the hypogastric vessels. The nerves, which lie over the vessels here, are stripped away with the lymphatics. The extent of the disease and palpation of the lymphatics along the hypogastric vessels may warrant their deliberate ligation and resection. This is a difficult step if each branch of the hypogastric artery and vein on both sides is dissected out and individually ligated and stripped of lymphatic and areolar tissue. An alternative is to ligate only the branches of the anterior division which is technically more simple. The steps in ligation of the hypogastric vessels and their branches are described under Hemorrhage From Hypogastric Vessels (page 527).

19. The uterine artery is now ligated close to its origin from the hypogastric artery (Plate 64, *J*). The tie on the distal end is left long. By gentle dissection the artery is drawn medial to the ureter, which is now seen entering the cardinal thickenings at the base of the broad ligament. The uterine veins may be two or more in number, and the ureter frequently courses through them. They are too fragile to retract by traction sutures like the artery and must be individually ligated. It is not possible to keep an absolutely dry field of operation at this point, but the bleeding should be adequately controlled so that the operator is not working blindly.

20. Plate 64, *K*, shows a continuation of the dissection of the pelvic ureter and hypogastric nodes. At this point the ureter is denuded of peritoneum, but as much areolar tissue of the periureteral sheath is preserved as possible. It is this tissue that must carry any blood supply for the terminal ureter—the site of postoperative fistulas. When the ureter has been dissected from its bed to the point where it enters the base of the broad ligament, it is then drawn laterally and the mass of hypogastric nodes swept under it toward the uterus if the nodes are attached to the specimen. Plate 64, *K*, shows the accessory obturator vessels—that seem to be present so frequently as to scarcely deserve the connotation of accessory—untied and held in a Kelly clamp. These vessels may be further encountered in the dissection of the obturator fossa. As indicated in the sketches, an assistant continually makes traction on the uterus in whatever direction will add to the exposure of the field and aid the surgeon in his dissection. The sequence of doing the steps of this operation on both sides may vary. In general, it is best to perform the steps alternately from side to side up to the node dissection of the hypogastric chain. This mobilizes the uterus considerably so that it can be retracted in whatever direction will aid the surgeon. From this point on, one side, usually the right, is dissected completely. This would be halfway or more down the vagina preparatory to the vaginectomy.

21. If there is considerable bleeding from surface bleeding points that defy individual ligation, a hot pack can be placed over the area. The operator then varies the sequence of the operation by proceeding with the opposite side. Usually by the time he is ready to return to the former field of operation the bleeding will have ceased. This is an important point to remember or much time will be wasted by attempting to operate in an obscured area.

22. The obturator artery, vein, and nerve are now seen entering the obturator fossa with its large elongated node and abundant areolar and fatty tissue (Plate 64, *L*). With the uterine artery removed from the field, the node dissection can continue further, with the ultimate cleaning out of the obturator fossa.

23. The terminal ureter is managed in two ways: The ureter may be completely dissected away from the cardinal thickenings or some connective tissue may be left attached to its lateral aspect. With the former technique the parametrium and its cardinal thickenings can then be resected adjacent to the pelvic side walls or parietal fascia. With the latter the resection of parametrium and its cardinal thickenings is limited to 2 to 3 cm. from the cervix. If the extent of the lesion was not evident before, the operator must decide at this point whether the more extensive operation is required to clear the lesion or whether the more simple modification will suffice.

24. The complete operation with free mobilization of the pelvic ureter from brim to bladder is first described (Plate 64, *M*). The uterus is drawn to the left and cephalad. A thin Deaver or malleable retractor is placed between bladder and vaginal wall in the plane established during the initial steps of the operation. The thumb and index finger now palpate the intraligamentary ureter (with or without a catheter) as it passes through the base of the broad ligament and over the angle of the vaginal vault and enters into the bladder.

25. The original Wertheim operation describes a ureteral canal with the ovarian vessels lying in the roof of the so-called canal. In this technique the index finger was passed in the canal, anterior to the ureter, and an aneurysm needle passed down to ligate the vessels and tissues in the roof of the ureteral canal. This was supposed to preserve the ureteral branch of the uterine artery. The relationship of the uterine artery to the ureter does not permit this assumption. If the parametrium is to be taken to the pelvic side wall—and the parametrium is only connective tissue extensions accompanying the vessels—the source of any blood supply has to be ligated in order to resect the parametrium. Two artificial spaces can be created by this technique of entering the areas above and below the connective tissue extensions, nerves, and lymphatics that accompany the uterine and superior vesical arteries. The artificial space caudad and somewhat anterior to this connective tissue (more commonly called cardinal or Mackenrodt's ligament) is referred to as the paravesical space (subvesical fossa), and lower down it is called the para-

vaginal space. The space cephalad and more posterior to the ligament is designated the pararectal space (subrectal fossa). With the parametrium drawn taut, the ureter is gently dissected out of its bed, and an attempt is made to leave a small amount of the periureteral sheath intact. Any traction should be made on the uterus or its ligamentous thickenings and never by pulling on the ureter (Plate 64, N). Clamps placed on bleeders should be set one notch and the ureter palpated between the fingers; if the ureter is free, the clamp can be set. The vaginal branch of the uterine artery may require repeated ligation.

26. After the angle of the vaginal vault is reached, the bladder base is further dissected off the vagina in a lateral direction. When the first part of the intramural ureter is recognized, great care should be exercised to prevent undue trauma in the area since the blood supply of the terminal ureter is essentially retrograde from the bladder (Plate 64, O). The dissection goes much easier from now on, and the operator must decide how much vagina to remove since it is a simple matter to remove all but the terminal few centimeters. Once the ureter is dissected out of the cardinal connective tissue thickenings and the natural vesicocervical and vesicovaginal lines of cleavage entered, the ureter is spared any further trauma (Plate 64, P). It is not necessary to dissect the trigone from the vaginal wall—that would have to be done by sharp dissection, for there is no natural line of cleavage —since a lesion not adequately cleared by a less extensive vaginectomy would not usually be cured by a simple radical hysterectomy. Bladder resection of some degree would probably be necessary. Plate 64, P, shows the ureter about to enter the bladder base. The bladder is retracted by sponge and forceps so that the intramural portion of the ureter is immediately recognized. To the left of the ureter is the inferior vesical artery—about the nomenclature of which there is some confusion. Some anatomists use the term synonymously with the vaginal artery. In operative dissections there are found branches from the hypogastric or middle hemorrhoidal arteries that pass to the upper vagina along the posterolateral wall. Realizing that many anatomic variations occur in the pelvis, it would still seem more accurate to assume that the inferior vesical and vaginal arteries are separate structures in most dissections.

27. With the modified and less radical operation, the dissection proceeds as shown in Plate 64, Q. Small bites of tissue are necessary with this modification of the operation. Large pedicles will result in kinking of the ureter. The ureter is

drawn laterally and its position in the base of the broad ligament ascertained. The parametrium is then clamped, cut, and tied with successive small bites immediately adjacent to the medial edge of the ureter. This continues until the angle of the vaginal vault is reached, whereupon the dissection is done exactly as if the ureter had been completely freed from its bed.

28. Attention is now directed toward the resection of the uterosacral ligament and the dissection of the rectum from the cervix and vagina. In Plate 64, R, the uterus has been drawn sharply forward, showing the reflection of the cul-de-sac peritoneum and the uterosacral thickenings. On the right side the uterine artery is seen retracted anteriorly, and the former bed of the ureter is visible. The denuded portion of the ureter is carefully retracted and protected at all times. Even though the critical phase of the operation—dissection of the ureter—is done, a carelessly placed retractor or inadvertent strong traction may still compromise the ureter with disastrous complications. The left uterosacral thickening has been ligated and cut close to the rectum. On the right side a suture is being placed prior to section of this ligament. A line of cleavage between vagina and rectum is readily found in the midline. This dissection should be started in the midline by knife and knife handle dissection until the operator is certain of the correct cleavage plane.

29. The posterior vaginal wall is longer than the anterior, so a correspondingly greater separation of vagina from rectum is done. This will normally carry the separation down to the level of the coccyx or beyond (Plate 64, S). This dissection is done by inserting the hand in the plane of cleavage already established and gently separating the vagina from the rectum. Do not be tempted to carry this too far laterally, or the rich anastomosis of vessels in the pararectum and paracolpium will be entered and unnecessary bleeding started. In Plate 64, S, the nearness of the denuded pelvic ureter and its intramural portion can be appreciated. The copious blood supply and rich anastomosis of the hemorrhoidal vessels relieve the surgeon of fear of rectal fistulas except under unusual circumstances.

30. Draw the right ureter out of the field and begin the resection of the parametrial connective tissue (Plate 64, T). Long Kelly clamps are used to ensure removal of all of the parametrium out to the pelvic side wall. Ligatures are placed on the tissue laterally. The medial part of the parametrium, together with the uterus, is ligated also, even though its blood supply has been interrupted

for the most part. Note in Plate 64, *T,* how far lateral to the former bed of the ureter it is possible to resect the parametrium and paracolpium. Most of the bleeding during this maneuver will come from that part of the paraproctium included in the clamps. The rectum has such a rich anastomosis, especially on the posterior and lateral aspects, that it is almost impossible to avoid some bleeding during the removal of the uterus and vagina. Progressive clamping of the parametrium, paracolpium, and paraproctium will eventually bring the dissection to the vaginal wall. In the operation illustrated the upper two thirds of the vagina were removed.

31. In the alternate less radical operation—insofar as the dissection of the ureter is less complete—the clamping of the parametrium will have been done as shown in Plate 64, *Q.* In this operation the ureter, with its lateral connective tissue attachments intact, is displaced to the side wall by vein retractors, and after it is lifted off the angle of the vaginal vault, the clamping of the paracolpium and paraproctium can proceed. Usually only the upper third of the vagina is removed in this technique, since it would be selected for early lesions strictly confined to the cervix.

32. Long Kelly clamps are now used to amputate the upper two thirds of the vagina that is to be included in the block dissection (Plate 64, *U*). As the vault is cut across, the angles are approximated with sutures of 00 chromic catgut since they can bleed slightly, although usually the extent of this operation results in considerable devitalization. Bleeding points on the cut edges of the vagina are ligated as necessary. The bladder is now strongly retracted, and hot packs are placed in the operative bed and are removed every few minutes to locate any uncontrolled bleeding points. Any areolar tissue that did not come with the specimen is excised until the entire field is clean and dry.

33. The ureters are now allowed to fall into their new beds on the pelvic floor. They should remain a reasonably good color, and a small amount of oozing along the denuded portions is a welcome thing to see. Two Penrose drains are now placed in the vaginal vault, with the intrapelvic ends straddling the rectum. Hemostasis should be complete enough to forego the placing of drains, but drains are left for a different reason. The opening of numerous lymphatic channels from the lower extremities will cause the collection of a large amount of lymph for several days, and a source of drainage for this is provided (Plate 64, *V*).

34. The bladder now falls naturally over the new vaginal vault, and its raw surface lies against that of the rectum. Several interrupted sutures are used to reperitonealize at the angles, but the extent of the operation leaves no choice except for the bladder and rectum to be adherent over the new vaginal vault. The reperitonealization does bring more of the peritoneum over the ureters, giving them a roof for their new bed (Plate 64, *W*).

35. The wound is then closed in the manner described in Chapter 33 (page 565), depending on the original incision selected. Silver wire stay sutures are recommended since postoperative distention is almost the rule.

Postoperative Care

Radical hysterectomy and pelvic lymphadenectomy is a formidable procedure and requires a team to execute the operation and take care of the patient postoperatively. Blood, as well as fluids and electrolytes, is replaced volume for volume. Parenteral therapy will be needed for several days. On the third postoperative day anticoagulants are given, since the incidence of thrombophlebitis from the pelvic dissection is high. Antibiotic therapy is continued with at least one agent that is effective against the enteric group of organisms. The urinary complications total 100 per cent. A radical hysterectomy, performed as described in this book, interrupts practically all the sympathetic and parasympathetic nerve fibers to the bladder with a resultant neurogenic bladder and urine retention. Function is restored in 4 to 6 weeks. From now on the patient should be in the hands of gynecologists with urologic training, since most other postoperative problems are minor compared with those in the urinary tract. (See Management of Electrolyte Abnormalities in Gynecologic Surgery, page 543.)

RADICAL VAGINAL HYSTERECTOMY
Indications and Surgical Principles

The art of performing a radical vaginal hysterectomy should not be lost even though the indications for its performance are limited at this time. Should research provide a method of controlling cancer of the lymph nodes of the parametrium and other metastatic stations in the pelvis by means of the injection of radio-active substance or other therapy, the indications for this operation would become more extended. The operation is indicated in an extremely obese patient who has been subjected to many laparotomies and has a radioresistant Stage I or early Stage II cancer of the cervix. Weighing the operative risk of an abdominal radical hysterectomy against the expectancy for positive lymph nodes among these patients with early carcinomas, a decision to do a radical vaginal hysterectomy might be made. One advantage of this operation is that it allows for a very wide extirpation of the paracolpium, paracervicum, parametrium, and the broad ligament with less technical difficulty than from above. It does not permit a pelvic lymphadenectomy, except for the nodes adjacent to the cervix and small intercalcated nodes that may be taken with the specimen.

Steps of the Operation

1. Ureteral catheters are inserted, and the patient is placed in the extreme lithotomy position. The instrument table should be equipped with four or more Jacobs clamps or some comparable type clamp for making strong traction upon the specimen. Long Deaver retractors, long needle holders, long Babcock type clamps, long angle clamps, and long Kelly clamps will facilitate the performance of the operation.

2. A left Schuchardt's incision is first made, provided the surgeon is right-handed. To do this a large Deaver retractor is placed in the vagina on the left side and strong traction made laterally. A posterior Sims retractor is placed on the right posterolateral wall and strong retraction made in this direction. The first incision is made from the point of insertion of the puborectalis, the thickening of which can be felt along the left lateral vaginal wall. This is continued through the skin and subcutaneous tissue and around the anus to the midline. The sphincters of the rectum are avoided by curving this incision outside the capsule of the external sphincter. The incision is further extended through the fat of the ischiorectal fossa and is carried up toward the cervix adjacent to the levator sling and the extensions of the obturator fascia. This may help the operator avoid the inferior and middle hemorrhoidal vessels and the arteries and veins of the vaginal

wall. The rich anastomosis of the vessels of the vagina prevents necrosis of any part of the vagina that will be left in this operation, so the ligation of large vessels is of no concern to the operator. The incision now permits displacement of the rectum and the vagina to the right, permitting adequate room for the surgeon to work. In carrying the incision up toward the cervix, it should be extended to the point at which the vagina will eventually be circumscribed.

3. Allis clamps are now placed in a circular fashion at about the junction of the upper and lower halves of the vagina. A circular incision is made through the full thickness of the vaginal wall, extending around to meet the upper end of the left Schuchardt's incision (Plate 65, A). The full thickness of the vaginal wall is then dissected in the vesicovaginal and rectovaginal septa upward toward the cervix. Posteriorly the reflection of the peritoneum of the cul-de-sac will soon be seen. It is incised and a deep retractor placed within the peritoneal cavity.

4. The bladder is now advanced to further free the vesicouterine reflection of the peritoneum to enter the peritoneal cavity anteriorly. The patient should now be put in a more extreme lithotomy position and either small laparotomy pads or tagged sponges used to pack off the bowel (Plate 65, B).

5. Plate 65, C, shows strong traction being made on the inverted vagina to the left and downward which outlines the right uterine artery and permits palpation of the ureter on this side. The right uterine artery and the ureter are both skeletonized so as to be positively identified prior to ligation of the uterine artery (Plate 65, C). If the patient is a nullipara or if there is minimal descensus at the start of this operation, part of the paracolpium and the paraproctium is clamped, cut, and ligated before the base of the broad ligaments is reached. This will permit enough descensus of the uterus to bring the uterine artery and the ureter into the field of operation.

6. The uterine artery is ligated both proximally and distally to the ureter (Plate 65, D). This may necessitate ligation of a small branch of the uterine artery to the ureter in this vicinity. Traction is made to the opposite quadrant while the same procedure is performed on the left side. The ureter is further dissected from its bed and is gently retracted laterally, with care being exercised not to compress the ureter against the descending rami of the pubis by means of the retractors.

Text continued on p. 465.

PLATE 65

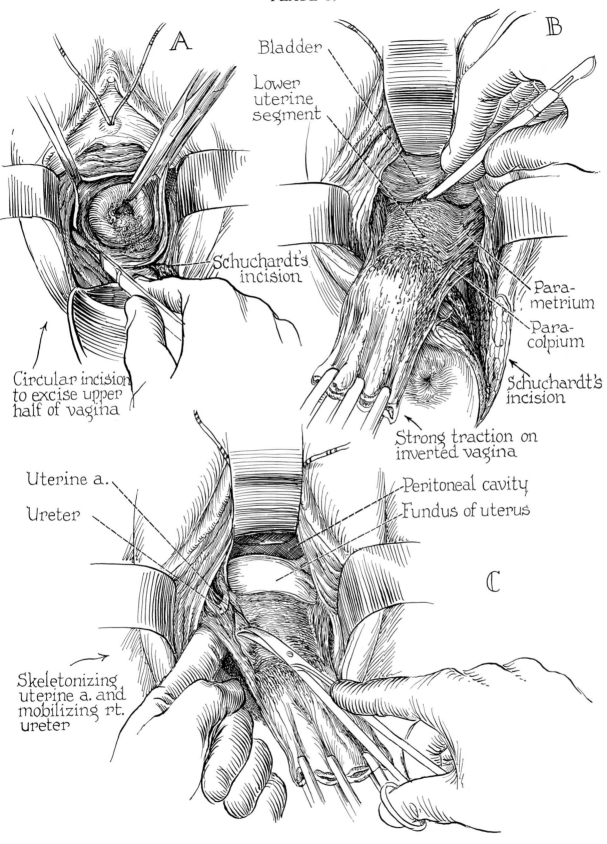

A

Bladder

Lower
uterine
segment

Schuchardt's
incision

Circular incision
to excise upper
half of vagina

B

Para-
metrium

Para-
colpium

Schuchardt's
incision

Strong traction on
inverted vagina

Uterine a.

Ureter

Peritoneal cavity

Fundus of uterus

C

Skeletonizing
uterine a. and
mobilizing rt.
ureter

PLATE 65 *(Continued)*

Uterine a.

D

Ligation of
distal stump
of uterine a.

Rt.
ureter

Wide resection of
paracolpium and
parametrium
after mobilization
and retraction of
the ureter

Omentum

Tube

Round lig.

Former bed
of ureter

Broad lig.

Parametrium

E

Ureter

PLATE 65 (Continued)

F

The fundus is readily delivered anteriorly after strong retraction of bladder and ureters

Infundibulopelvic pedicle

Retracted ureter

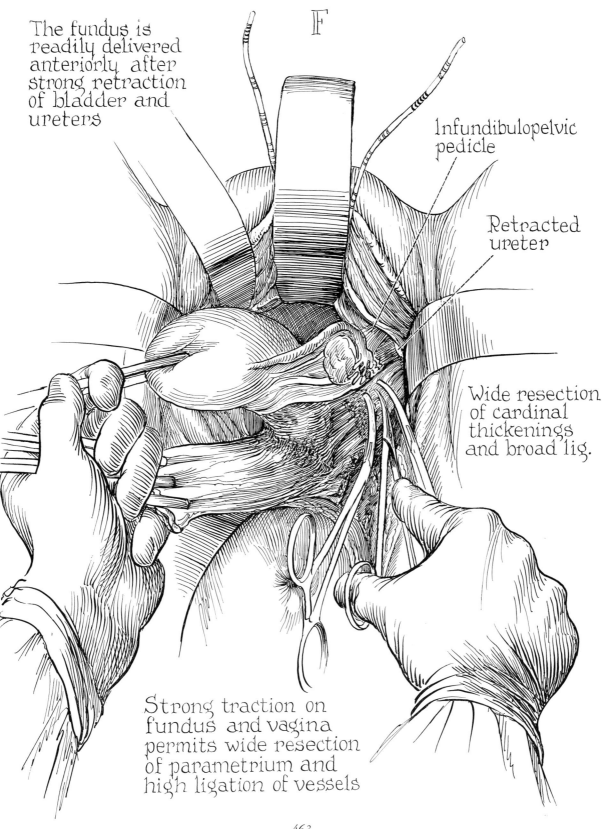

Wide resection of cardinal thickenings and broad lig.

Strong traction on fundus and vagina permits wide resection of parametrium and high ligation of vessels

PLATE 65 *(Concluded)*

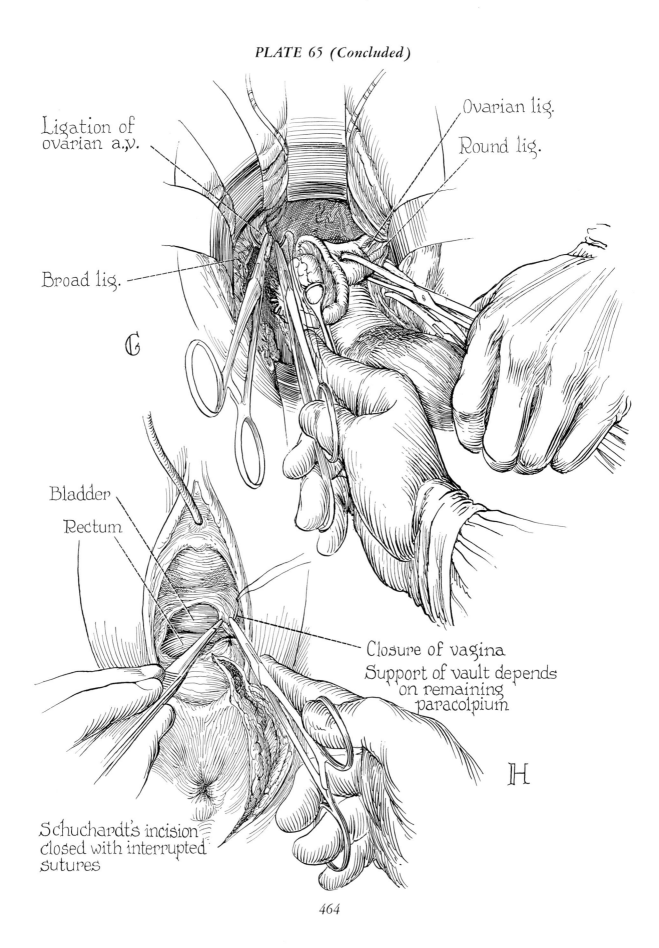

Ligation of
ovarian a.v.

Ovarian lig.

Round lig.

Broad lig.

C

Bladder

Rectum

Closure of vagina
Support of vault depends
on remaining
paracolpium

H

Schuchardt's incision
closed with interrupted
sutures

7. A wide resection of the paracolpium, paraproctium, and parametrium is done, with the structures resected flush with the pelvic wall (Plate 65, E). This resection is done on alternate sides so that as successive segments are resected the specimen can be brought nearer and nearer to the operator. The fundus of the uterus is delivered and a strong clamp used to draw it in the same direction as the inverted vagina (Plate 65, F). As the resection of the cardinal ligaments and broad ligaments is continued (Plate 65, F), the infundibulopelvic pedicle and the round ligament come into view. The degree of traction on the specimen is adjusted so as not to rupture these rather fragile connective tissue extensions, since retraction of the ovarian artery and vein leads to troublesome bleeding quite difficult to locate and control. The tubes and ovaries are removed in any operation for invasive cancer. In Plate 65, G, is shown the removal of the tube and ovary on the right side and ligation of the infundibulopelvic pedicle. The tube and ovary are grasped with an ovum forceps and drawn in the same direction as the specimen. The round ligament and then the ovarian artery and vein are successively clamped and ligated with transfixion sutures (Plate 65, G). The very strong traction on the specimen is released while the remaining attachments of the uterus are being resected.

8. After the retractors are removed, the bladder and rectum tend to fall together in areas that have been denuded of peritoneum. At times sufficient peritoneum can be mobilized to permit separate closure; however, in most instances the wall of the vagina is closed by interrupted sutures through the full thickness of the vaginal wall (Plate 65, H). Several small Penrose drains are left in the middle of the vaginal vault between the bladder and rectum to permit drainage of serum which is considerable due to the interruption of lymphatic channels. The paravaginal incision (Schuchardt's) is closed with interrupted sutures (Plate 65, H), eliminating any dead space in the deeper layers and in the ischiorectal fossa.

Postoperative Care

The postoperative care is essentially the same as that after a radical abdominal hysterectomy. An indwelling catheter is placed after the ureteral catheters are withdrawn. The drains are advanced a few centimeters after the first forty-eight hours and are removed entirely in a few days. For the management of electrolytes, general nutrition, and control of infection, see page 543.

ULTRARADICAL PELVIC SURGERY
Surgical Anatomy of the Iliofemoral Musculature and Their Arteries, Veins, and Nerves Encountered in Ultraradical Pelvic Surgery

Certain groups of muscles helping to make up the soft tissues of the pelvis are encountered in pelvic surgery. Their specific diseases are not the concern of the gynecologist. Their nerves and vessels are involved in several pelvic operations and create a need for the gynecologist to be familiar with these landmarks and structures.

The iliofemoral musculature is divided by the iliac blade into an anterior group (iliopsoas) supplied by nerves from the lumbar plexus and a posterior group (gluteal, piriformis, and tensor fascia lata) supplied by nerves from the sacral plexus. The fan-shaped iliacus and the fusiform psoas make up the iliopsoas. The former arises from the iliac fossa and the latter from the sides of the last thoracic and of the lumbar vertebrae. The two muscles insert by a common tendon into the lesser trochanter of the femur. The small, flat, fusiform psoas minor lies on the medial surface of the psoas major and extends from the twelfth thoracic vertebra to the iliopectineal eminence. A dense fascia covers these muscles from the iliac crest and iliolumbar ligament to the capsule of the hip joint, passing under the inguinal ligament, to which it is attached by some fibers. The course of a psoas abscess and its differential diagnosis from a femoral hernia is determined by the course of the fascia of these muscles down to their insertions (iliopectineal fascia). A psoas abscess descending below the inguinal ligament usually follows the lateral aspect of the femoral vessels. If the abscess ruptures through the fascial sheath or follows the profunda artery, it will pass beneath the adductor longus and point toward the medial aspect of the thigh. Examination of the back, signs of massive infection, and swelling below the fossa ovalis usually will clarify the diagnosis.

The iliopsoas muscle flexes the thigh at the hip together with weak action as a medial rotator and adductor. The action of the iliopsoas is of little interest to the gynecologist, but the relations of the muscle group to the female pelvic viscera and the landmarks the iliopsoas provides should be understood by anyone doing radical pelvic surgery. The iliopsoas fascia is covered by retroperitoneal connective tissue, in which the inferior vena cava runs to the right of the midline. As the inferior mesenteric artery and vein pass into the sigmoid meso-colon, they are anterior to the left iliopsoas and psoas minor. On both sides the ureter, ovarian artery and vein, and colic vessels are just anterior to these muscles with their overlying fascia. The external iliac artery lies medial to the psoas major in the pelvis. The femoral artery is medial to this muscle beyond the inguinal ligament. The iliacus in the region of the pelvis is covered by retro-peritoneal fat. The psoas crosses its medial margin with the femoral nerve, emerging be-tween to pass into the thigh through the femoral canal. These landmarks are impor-tant in radical dissections of the groin and pelvis.

The posterior group of the iliofemoral mus-culature contains a muscle that comprises a small segment of the pelvic floor and serves as a landmark in gynecologic surgery. The piriformis arises from the lateral part of the ventral surface of the second, third, and fourth sacral vertebrae, the posterior border of the great sciatic notch, and the deep surface of the sacrotuberous ligament. It inserts on the upper border of the greater trochanter. Its nerve supply is from the first or second sacral nerve, and it extends, adducts, and rotates the thigh laterally. The gynecologist encounters this muscle during radical pelvic surgery since the sacral plexus rests on its ventral surface and large parietal branches of the hypogastric ar-tery pass above and below its belly, going outward to supply the large iliolumbar and gluteal muscle masses. The iliolumbar artery runs upward and laterally beneath the common iliac artery, where it may be encountered during a lymphadenectomy. It passes up between the psoas and the vertebral column, dividing into branches supplying the iliacus, psoas, and quadratus lumborum. Out of the pelvis it represents no problems for the pelvic surgeon. The lateral sacral artery often has two branches. The superior passes downward and medially into the first anterior sacral foramina and out the first posterior sacral foramina, terminating by supplying the skin over the sacrum.

The superior gluteal artery is the largest branch of the hypogastric artery and is a short thick trunk which runs backward between the lumbosacral cord and first sacral nerve and passes out of the pelvis above the upper border of the piriformis muscle. It supplies muscular branches to the iliacus, piriformis, and ob-turator internus. This artery and vein are two of the most feared residents of "death corner" to be encountered in a pelvic lymphadenectomy or other retroperitoneal surgery in the area. If torn or cut, they will retract into the reaches of the sacral nerve and piriformis muscle. A liberal collateral circulation provides a serious hemorrhage from the distal end which is ex-ceedingly difficult to bring under control.

The inferior gluteal artery (sciatic) arises from the hypogastric artery and passes down to the lower part of the great sacrosciatic fora-men behind the internal pudic artery and rests on the sacral plexus of nerves and piriformis muscle. It leaves the pelvis through the sacro-sciatic foramen between the piriformis and coccygeus. It gives branches to the piriformis, coccygeus, and levator ani in the pelvis and muscular branches to the gluteus maximus in the buttock. Its course outside the pelvis does not concern us, but, like the superior gluteal artery, its accidental rupture causes a large hemorrhage, although technically it is easier to control.

The coccygeus is situated behind and parallel with the levator ani and together they complete the muscular pelvic diaphragm that supports the abdominal and pelvic viscera. The coccyg-eus is a triangular plane of muscular and tendinous fibers arising by its apex from the spine of the ischium and lesser sacrosciatic liga-ment and inserted by its base into the margin of the coccyx and lower sacrum. With the levator on one side and piriformis on the other, it closes the back part of the pelvic outlet. Its action is to pull the coccyx forward after it has been pressed backward by defecation or parturition. It is supplied with nerve fibers from the fourth and fifth sacral nerves.

Indications for Operation

Ultraradical operations are under study as a method of management of advanced pelvic malignancies. The degree of mutilation with ultraradical operations should not be disproportionate to the chance for cure. The surgeon should be guided by which course, simple palliation or ultraradical surgery, will give the patient the most comfort during the terminal phase of her illness if she is to inevitably succumb to the malignant disease. A colostomy and ureteral transplants are easier to manage than a sloughing, bleeding recurrent pelvic cancer with multiple fistulas.

TOTAL ABDOMINAL PELVIC EXENTERATION WITH CUTANEOUS URETEROSTOMIES
Steps of the Operation

1. The choice of incisions rests between a long left rectus or an interiliac approach. Cutaneous ureterostomies are easily placed and cared for with a rectus incision. An interiliac incision may traverse the site ideal for the ureterostomy. When the ureters are placed in the bowel, this is not so and the added advantage in exposure afforded by an interiliac incision may be made use of.

2. The abdomen is explored, with particular attention being given to the abdominal aorta and its lymphatics. Study of the pelvic lesion may reveal solid fixation of the lesion to the pelvic side walls or sacrum. If the operation cannot be done without leaving tumor, it is preferable to carry out some palliative procedure.

3. The small bowel and omentum are walled off with warm, moist packs. A moderate degree of Trendelenburg position is requested of the anesthetist.

4. The right round ligament is clamped, cut, and ligated flush with the internal inguinal ring. An incision is then made in the peritoneum lateral to the external iliac vessels and extending to the cecum, which is mobilized if it extends over the pelvic brim. The appendix is removed at this time. The peritoneal incision is then extended between the cecum and the ureter to the point

where the ureter is crossed by the ovarian artery and vein. Denudation of the parietal peritoneum below the brim of the pelvis is necessary for a complete and thorough lymphadenectomy. Subsequent exploration of patients subjected to this procedure shows the remarkable capacity of the peritoneum to regenerate over the entire surface. The operation to this point is essentially the same as a radical hysterectomy.

5. An incision is now made in the sigmoid mesentery preparatory to resection of the bowel. In Plate 66, A, is shown an operation in which a high resection of the bowel was done, and the colostomy site selected was just above and to the left of the umbilicus. When the ureters are transplanted into the colon, the resection is much lower in order to anchor the bowel near the promontory and to receive the right and left ureters without angulation or strangulation. The superior hemorrhoidal and sigmoidal arteries are ligated as encountered. The inferior mesenteric artery is preserved unless the nature of the lesion demands removal of most of the descending colon.

6. An incision is made in the peritoneum medial to the right ureter where it crosses the common iliac artery and dips over the brim of the pelvis. This is carried up to the ovarian vessels in order to leave a flap of peritoneum and subperitoneal connective tissue attached to the ureter for nourishment. A few centimeters of peritoneum can also be left below the pelvic brim. The pelvic ureter is now dissected out of its bed down to the point of entry into the base of the broad ligament. If tumor is suspected proximal to this, a shorter length of ureter is dissected out.

7. The ureter is cut and the distal end ligated. One should aim to keep as long a pelvic segment as possible. A No. 10 whistle-tip latex catheter is passed up to the kidney pelvis and the end passed out of the incision to minimize drainage of urine in the operative field. Handle the ureter gently and, if necessary to handle it with instruments, grasp only its outer areolar layer. It is especially vulnerable if compressed by retractors being changed about in the operative field.

8. The cecum and terminal ilium are now mobilized, and a retroperitoneal bed is formed for the ureter. This bed is created to avoid any kinking of the ureter as it curves gently toward the area of skin selected for the transplant. An area of skin, free of scar tissue, is selected about 8 cm. medial to and 4 cm. above the anterior superior spine. The tunnel under the cecum and parietal peritoneum of the abdominal wall is completed

467

Text continued on p. 476.

PLATE 66

A

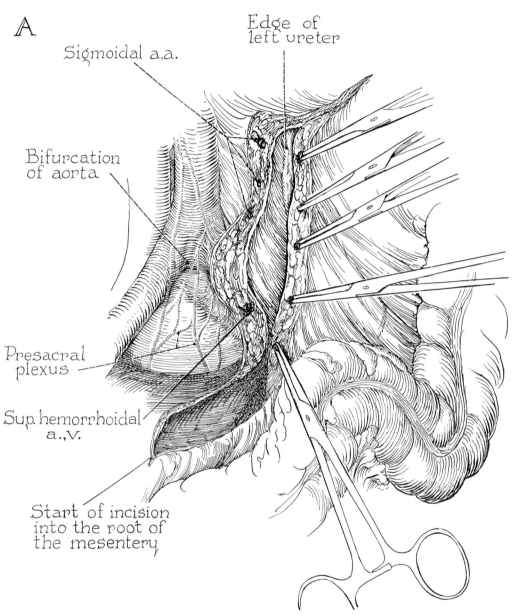

Edge of
left ureter

Sigmoidal a.a.

Bifurcation
of aorta

Presacral
plexus

Sup. hemorrhoidal
a., v.

Start of incision
into the root of
the mesentery

Incisions into root of mesentery for
high resection of descending colon,
sigmoid colon, and rectum

PLATE 66 (Continued)

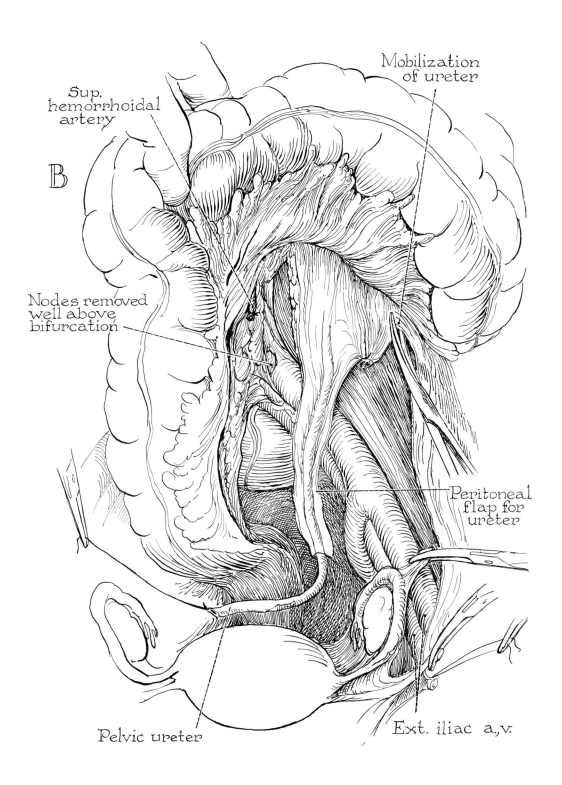

Sup.
hemorrhoidal
artery

B

Nodes removed
well above
bifurcation

Mobilization
of ureter

Peritoneal
flap for
ureter

Pelvic ureter

Ext. iliac a.v.

PLATE 66 *(Continued)*

Mesentery prepared
for colostomy

Lumbar
ureter

C

Division of
bowel by
actual cautery

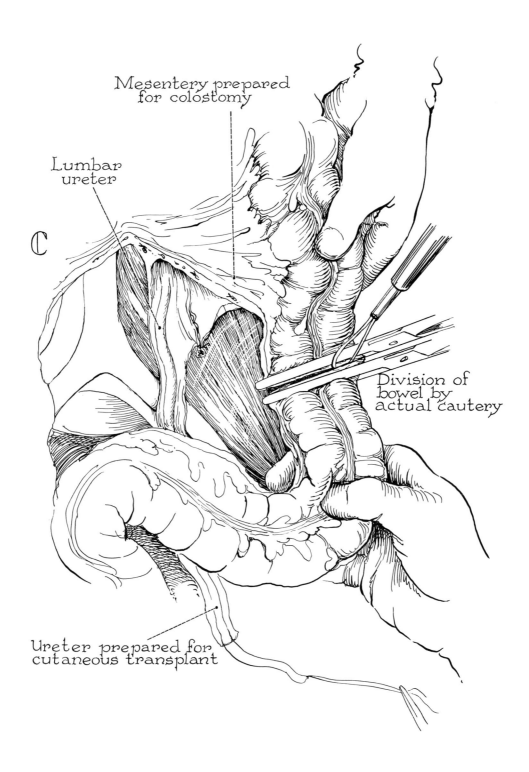

Ureter prepared for
cutaneous transplant

470

PLATE 66 (Continued)

D

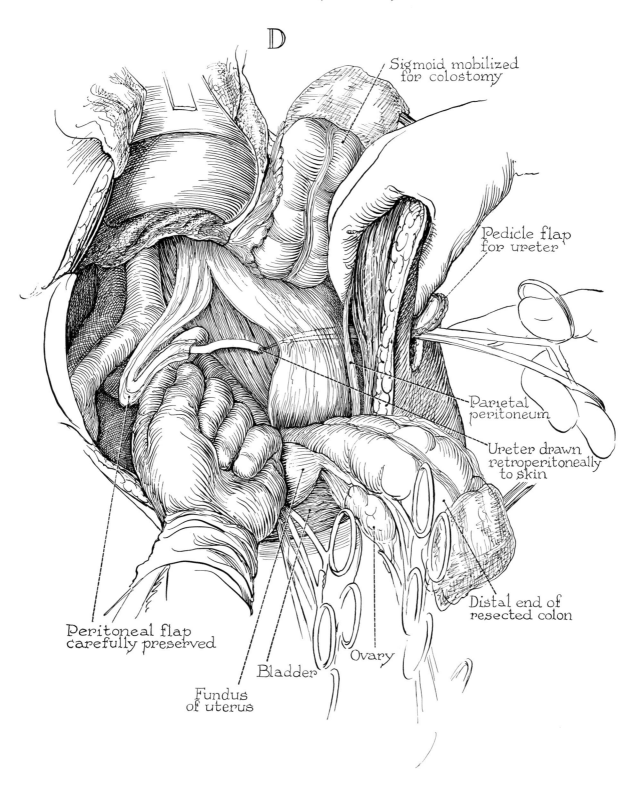

Sigmoid mobilized
for colostomy

Pedicle flap
for ureter

Parietal
peritoneum

Ureter drawn
retroperitoneally
to skin

Distal end of
resected colon

Peritoneal flap
carefully preserved

Bladder

Ovary

Fundus
of uterus

PLATE 66 (Continued)

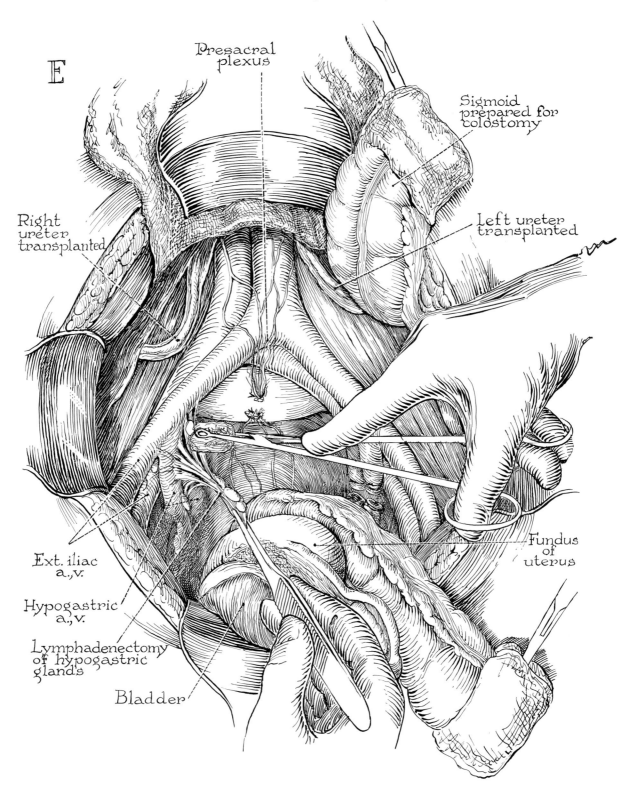

E

Presacral plexus

Sigmoid prepared for colostomy

Right ureter transplanted

Left ureter transplanted

Ext. iliac a.,v.

Fundus of uterus

Hypogastric a.,v.

Lymphadenectomy of hypogastric glands

Bladder

472

PLATE 66 (Continued)

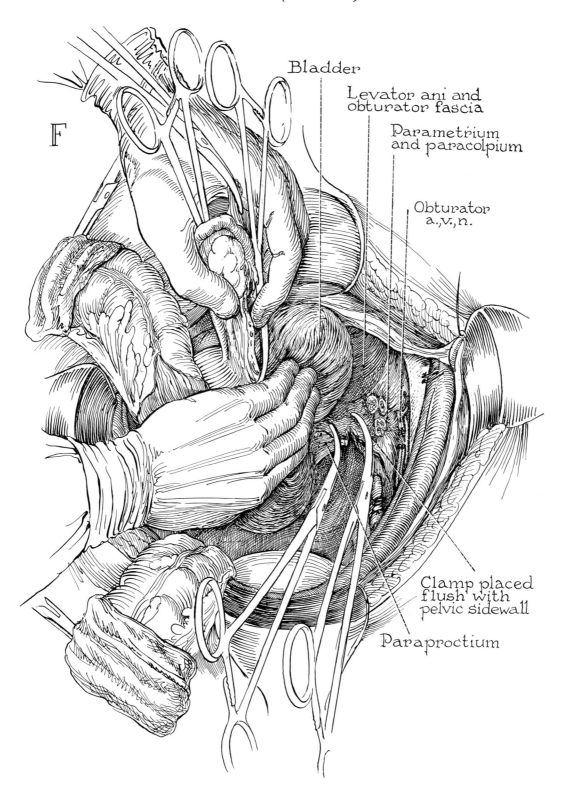

F

Bladder

Levator ani and
obturator fascia

Parametrium
and paracolpium

Obturator
a.,v.,n.

Clamp placed
flush with
pelvic sidewall

Paraproctium

PLATE 66 (Continued)

Mobilization of pelvic organs from
symphysis and antero-lateral walls
of pelvis

G

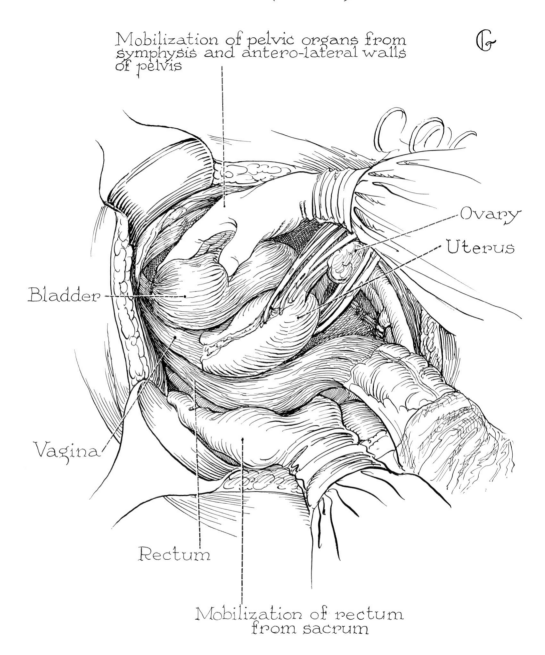

Ovary

Uterus

Bladder

Vagina

Rectum

Mobilization of rectum
from sacrum

474

PLATE 66 (Concluded)

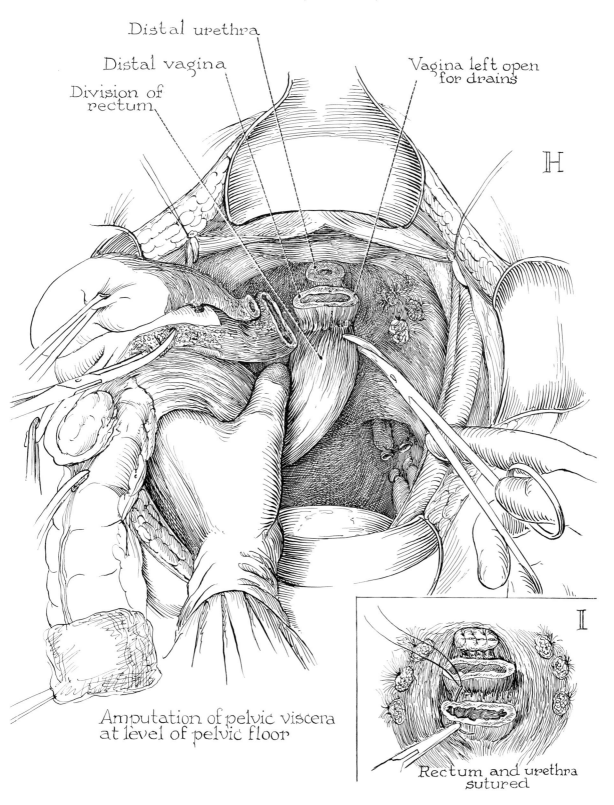

Distal urethra

Distal vagina

Division of rectum

Vagina left open for drains

H

Amputation of pelvic viscera at level of pelvic floor

I

Rectum and urethra sutured

to this point. The cutaneous ureterostomy is completed by the method illustrated under Cutaneous Ureterostomy: Treatment of the Terminal Ureter (page 263).

9. Preparation of the left ureter for cutaneous transplant is the next step. It is picked up as it dips over the brim of the pelvis, or lower down if the position of the ever-variable sigmoid mesocolon obscures it. The peritoneum is incised on each side of the ureter to form a peritoneal flap (Plate 66, *B*). The lateral incision in the left leaf of the sigmoid mesocolon is carried well up the lateral gutter. The incision medial to the ureter—to form the peritoneal flap—is carried up to a point above the site selected for the bowel resection. This keeps the ureter out of the way during the resection and subsequent cleaning of the area of areolar and lymphatic tissue. In contrast to a radical hysterectomy, in which bowel and bladder are left, the lymphadenectomy and the removal of the areolar tissue about the great vessels is not done segment by segment, since once the vital structures—ureters and large bowel—are prepared, the remainder of the operation can be done with dispatch and disregard for minor bleeding about the bladder and rectum. With the sigmoid mobilized as shown in Plate 66, *B*, the lymphatic and areolar tissue along the left side of the aorta is easily removed.

10. The mesenteric border of the bowel at the site selected for division is cleaned for a distance of about 10 cm., and any bleeding points are ligated. Long, straight Kocher clamps or other devices available or preferred by the surgeon are placed across the bowel, and the bowel is divided between clamps. The knife-phenol-alcohol technique or actual cautery (Plate 66, *C*) may be used. The actual cautery cannot be used if an inflammable anesthetic is being administered. The distal end of the bowel is inverted by placing several large mattress sutures over the clamp. The proximal end is covered with a warm, moist sponge and left in the upper part of the field, and its color is watched.

11. The remainder of the mesentery is incised, and any vessels encountered are ligated. The left colic and one or more sigmoidal arteries, if ligated during the resection of the remainder of the mesocolon, are tied off to preserve the continuity of the marginal arteries that provide the collateral circulation. Should the marginal artery adjacent to the colostomy stump fail to pulsate and the bowel discolor, a higher segment of the descending colon is mobilized until viable bowel is seen and the colostomy stump made there.

12. The left ureter, its lumbar segment having been well mobilized during the bowel division, is transplanted into the skin. Plate 66, *D,* shows the bowel resected and the left ureter being drawn to the skin. On the left side the distal part of the descending colon and the sigmoid have been mobilized so it is a simple matter to make a retroperitoneal channel for the ureter. A long Kelly clamp is passed from the skin just underneath the peritoneum of the flank and the traction suture on the end of the ureter grasped to draw it to the surface. It should reach the skin without tension, compression, or angulation.

13. We are continuing to do many of the time-consuming parts of this operation in preparation for the actual exenteration—the phase of the operation most likely to cause surgical shock. One may wonder when the site of the disease is to be attacked, but, with all the transplants done and the colostomy prepared, the removal of the pelvic organs may be speedily done. Then if the patient becomes surgically shocked, the abdomen can be quickly closed to help combat this complication.

14. Any remaining areolar and lymphatic tissue on the aorta and vena cava is removed by sharp and blunt dissection. The lymphadenectomy is continued along the external iliac vessels to the femoral canal, which is cleaned out. All tissue is dissected toward the midline—that is, toward the cancer in this operation. The parietal peritoneum is further incised from the round ligament over the bladder near the superior border of the symphysis. The bladder is then freed up laterally to expose the obturator fossa, which is now cleaned of its long node and connective tissue. This is left attached to the bladder. (Plate 66, *E.*)

15. A similiar dissection is done on the left side. A sweep of the hand will now detach the bladder from its fragile attachments to the posterior border of the symphysis and adjacent descending rami of the pubis.

16. Return now to the region of the bifurcation of the right iliac vessels. The node of the bifurcation (constant in location), together with the adjacent areolar and lymphatic tissue, is removed. This dissection is carried down over the pelvic brim, dissecting out the hypogastric nodes. The utmost caution is used when the region of the posterior (muscular) division of the hypogastric artery is reached. The hypogastric artery and vein are now ligated and resected distal to the posterior division. This area is known as "death corner," and positive control of the major vessels in the area can avert massive hemorrhage. Plate

66, *E*, shows the hypogastric lymphadenectomy on the right side. In this particular operation the hypogastric vessels were ligated on the left side at the time of this sketch. The thoroughness of the dissection is facilitated by resecting the presacral plexus and removing this with the retroperitoneal connective tissue and lymphatics. In practice, the remainder of the operation can be done in less time than the pelvic dissection of a radical hysterectomy, since the ureters are out of the field and the other structures—rectum and bladder—are to be removed.

17. The rectosigmoid is now separated from the sacrum. The superior hemorrhoidal vessels may require successive ligation. Later, the paired middle hemorrhoidal vessels are encountered when the pelvic viscera are about to be removed.

18. The longest Kelly clamps available, the longest needle holders, and considerable fortitude are now worth while. Anteriorly, the umbilical artery and its branches to the bladder, together with their parietal connective tissue extensions, are successively clamped, and suture ligatures are used for hemostasis. The uterine arteries and parametrium are likewise clamped, cut, and tied close to the pelvic side wall. This technique is done alternately on each side as the exenteration proceeds. No pretense is made that the hypogastric artery and vein with all its parietal and visceral branches can be systematically dissected out and denuded of lymphatics. (Plate 66, *F*.)

19. The middle hemorrhoidal artery with its connective tissue extensions is often referred to as the suspensory ligament of the rectum or paraproctium. This is clamped in successive bites close to the pelvic side wall until the levator ani is reached (Plate 66, *F*).

20. The right hand is then introduced between the symphysis and bladder, while the left hand is placed between the rectum and the sacrum (Plate 66, *G*). By blunt dissection the remaining attachments are released. It is not feasible to stop for minor bleeding at this time but better to perform this shocking phase of the operation as expeditiously as possible. Particularly if the patient has had radiation therapy, the rectum and bladder in the region of the cervix may be adherent to the levator ani and extensions of the obturator fascia. Segments of the levator ani may be resected with the pelvic contents. Posteriorly, the piriformis and coccygeus form the pelvic floor with the branches of the large lumbosacral plexus. Damage

to these muscles is unimportant, but the large trunks of the lumbosacral plexus should be spared any trauma consistent with a clean dissection of the pelvis.

21. The urethra, vagina, and ampulla of the rectum are now cut across and the specimen delivered (Plate 66, *H*). Multiple hot laparotomy pads are placed in the pelvic cavity for a few minutes while you and your assistants make ready to clamp the major bleeding points. Should the extension of the lesion necessitate a vaginal phase and vulvectomy to complete the procedure, the mobilization need not be so extensive at this time since it can be done with greater ease from below.

22. The pelvic cavity is now inspected, and all bleeding points are ligated. When the field is dry, several interrupted sutures of 0 chromic catgut are used to close the rectum and urethra (Plate 66, *I*). A 5-yard, 2-inch plain gauze pack is placed in the pelvis and the end delivered through the vagina.

23. The stump for the colostomy is now drawn out of the upper end of the incision and the intra-abdominal part of the colon studied to see where it tends to lie. The mesentery is then sutured to the parietal peritoneum or other structures—psoas or underside of the internal oblique—to obliterate any holes where small bowel may enter and become strangulated.

24. The upper end of the incision is now prepared for the permanent colostomy by suturing the peritoneum to the anterior sheath of the rectus. No attempt is made to reperitonealize the field of operation since large segments of the parietal peritoneum were removed.

25. The wound is closed in layers together with interrupted sutures of No. 32 steel wire. Wet saline dressings are bunched around the ureterostomies, followed by a sealed dressing with a catheter included for instillation of saline solution to keep them moist. The rectus incision is dressed depending on whether the colostomy is left open with an indwelling rectal tube or left with a clamp attached. If open, the rest of the wound should be sealed as well as can be.

Postoperative Care

The postoperative care of cutaneous ureterostomies is discussed on page 265; postoperative care of the colostomy, page 597; fluid and electrolyte management, page 543.

Total Pelvic Exenteration With Ureterointestinal Anastomoses and Wet Colostomy
Steps of the Operation

1. A greater length of the sigmoid colon is left in preparation for the ureteral transplants than one selects for the cutaneous transplant operation. The inferior mesenteric artery and left colic artery are carefully preserved. The arrangement of the sigmoidal arteries may warrant saving the most proximal of these.

2. Study the anatomy of the colon and fit it over the brim of the pelvis near the midline. Decide where it can be anchored in order to receive the right ureter without angulation. Note how much additional bowel is needed beyond the transplants to bring the colostomy out below and to the left of the umbilicus.

3. Outline the usual V-shaped area on the mesocolon extending from the root of the mesentery to points about 4 cm. proximal and distal to the point selected for resection. Denude the mesenteric border of the colon and resect the V-shaped area of mesocolon. The superior hemorrhoidal artery and vein and one or all of the sigmoidal arteries and veins may have to be clamped and ligated, depending on the extent of the lesion.

4. Straight Kocher clamps are placed across the bowel, which is divided either by the knife-phenol-alcohol technique or by the actual cautery. The distal end is inverted by mattress sutures placed over the clamp and returned to the pelvis. The colostomy stump and adjacent bowel are observed for viability while holding them in the position they will subsequently occupy.

5. The ureters are further mobilized with an adequate flap of peritoneum to retain some of their blood supply. The arrangement of the terminal peritoneal flap will depend on the technique selected for the ureterointestinal anastomosis. Dehiscence of the anastomosis postoperatively is a major surgical problem that frequently causes the death of the patient. Tension on the line of suture can be avoided by careful study of the length of the colon and the subsequent fixation of the descending colon and sigmoid colon leading to the skin surface as is described in the next step. The implantation of the ureter into the bowel is a success if the mucosa of the ureter unites with the mucosa of the bowel. The myriad of methods of ureterointestinal anastomosis result in stricture or abnormal reflux regardless of the ingenuity of

the surgeon; but if the method used allows, by chance, the mucosal surfaces to unite, a successful transplant is the result. The method selected in each situation has varied from the simple technique of pushing the ureter into a hole in the bowel to elaborate techniques of devising channels, flaps, tunnels, variously shaped funnels, and other operations that are equally unsuccessful if a band of scar tissue forms about the anastomosis and causes a surgical urinary obstruction. With annoying consistency, techniques that employ a mucosa-to-mucosa approximation which permit a constant reflux of urine from the bowel present the surgeon with the problem of a recurrent pyelonephritis that soon becomes resistant to all therapy.

6. The ureters are now brought alongside the bowel to sites they tend to go naturally. They are implanted into the bowel by the method illustrated under Ureterointestinal Anastomosis in Chapter 12. The variation in the length of the sigmoid mesentery among patients is the deciding factor in selecting the point of implantation of the ureters and resection of the bowel. The shorter the mesocolon, the more distal the resection in order to bring the bowel to the skin with the ureters implanted without tension. You can err on the other side. The mesocolon and sigmoid mesentery can be exceptionally long, and when the ureters are transplanted at the pelvic brim, they may flow into a cloaca that is difficult to empty from the abdominal stoma. Each patient must be studied to decide the site of colostomy and ureteral anastomosis that will give the best functional and cosmetic result.

7. The colon is not anchored to the parietal peritoneum until the abdomen is to be closed. It is then anchored by interrupted sutures to adjacent structures to close any pockets and fix it firmly in the region of the ureteral transplants. Now, simply pack off the bowel with warm, moist packs and take care to keep instruments—heavy retractors especially—away from the area.

8. The operation then proceeds as previously described for a total pelvic exenteration with or without a vulvectomy with delivery of the pelvic organs from below.

Postoperative Care

The postoperative care of ureterointestinal anastomoses is discussed on page 259; fluid and electrolyte management, page 543; postoperative care of the colostomy, page 597.

Total Pelvic Exenteration With Vulvectomy
Steps of the Operation

1. During the abdominal phase the viscera are left within the pelvis after the dissection has been completed to the point where the three major organs—bladder, vagina, and rectum—are about to be amputated. Bleeding points at or near the pelvic aperture, hard to ligate from above, are controlled by packs that are subsequently removed from below.

2. The entire vulva is excised, using an incision as shown in Plate 67, *A*. Begin anteriorly by cutting down through the subcutaneous tela and fat of the mons pubis until the pubic bone is exposed. Continue the dissection close to the anterior surface of the pubic rami and symphysis, excising the clitoris, base of the labia majora, base of the labia minora with the frenulum and prepuce of the clitoris, insertions of the ischiocavernosi and bulbocavernosi, and veins of the vestibular bulbs. The index finger of the left hand is inserted between the urethra and the inferior border of the symphysis. The laparotomy pad left anteriorly can now be palpated.

3. The remnants of the urogenital diaphragm are cut and any bleeding points ligated. Laterally the anterior edges of the levator muscles are seen (Plate 67, *B*). These muscles are clamped, cut, and tied by successive bites so that any vessels in the muscle body do not retract and cause annoying bleeding.

4. At times it makes things easier to deliver the bladder, uterus, and colon at this time (Plate 67, *C*). If this interferes with the dissection posteriorly, the pelvic organs are left within the pelvis until later.

5. The vulva is displaced to the right, and the incision around the rectum is continued deeper through the ischiorectal fossa (Plate 67, *C*). The perineal and inferior hemorrhoidal branches of the internal pudendal artery and vein are clamped and ligated. Cut the anococcygeal raphe and extend the dissection close to the sacrum to meet the point of mobilization from above. The laparotomy pad left between the sacrum and the rectum can now be removed.

6. At this point the pelvic contents are easily delivered and the exenteration accomplished by severing the remaining connections on the right.

7. All bleeding points are controlled. A large sheet of rubber dam is put in the cavity, and six or more yards of 2-inch packing are introduced behind this (Plate 67, *D*). The upper and lower ends of the wound are approximated with interrupted sutures of 0 chromic catgut where they tend to fall together (Plate 67, *D*). It is possible in some patients to close the perineal wound with several drains at the posterior extremity of the incision. This permits the small bowel to fall into the depths of the pelvis and become adherent there. The rubber sheet and packing method of terminating this procedure tends to have the small bowel become adherent at a higher level. This may be of some advantage in avoiding intestinal obstruction. Preventing the small bowel and cecum from descending into the depths of the pelvic cavity may save some indirect traction on the ureters and colostomy which should pass to their cutaneous ostia without angulation. The longer period required for the wound to granulate in as compared with a primary closure with drainage is little handicap to the patient who must be in the hospital or convalescent home for six to eight weeks after this formidable procedure.

Postoperative Care

Strict attention is given to fluid balance, electrolytes, general nutrition, and bowel function. (See Fluid and Electrolyte Management After Radical Surgery or Postoperative Complications in Pelvic Surgery, page 543.) The packing is loosened in forty-eight hours, and a few feet of it are removed. Opening of the lymphatics draining the lower extremities pours a great deal of lymph into the pelvis that will drain from the wound. On the third and fourth postoperative days the remaining packing is removed. By the fifth day the rubber sheet can be teased away from the wound and bowel after irrigation with warm saline solution. The cavity itself is then irrigated one or more times daily to remove serum and debris. Granulations readily form. Areas not forming healthy granulations are débrided as indicated, and the wound is managed as any incision healing by secondary intention.

Anterior Pelvic Exenteration
Indications and Surgical Principles

An anterior pelvic exenteration is indicated when a malignancy of the cervix has extended into the base of the bladder, leaving the rectum free. All examinations and proctoscopy must

PLATE 67

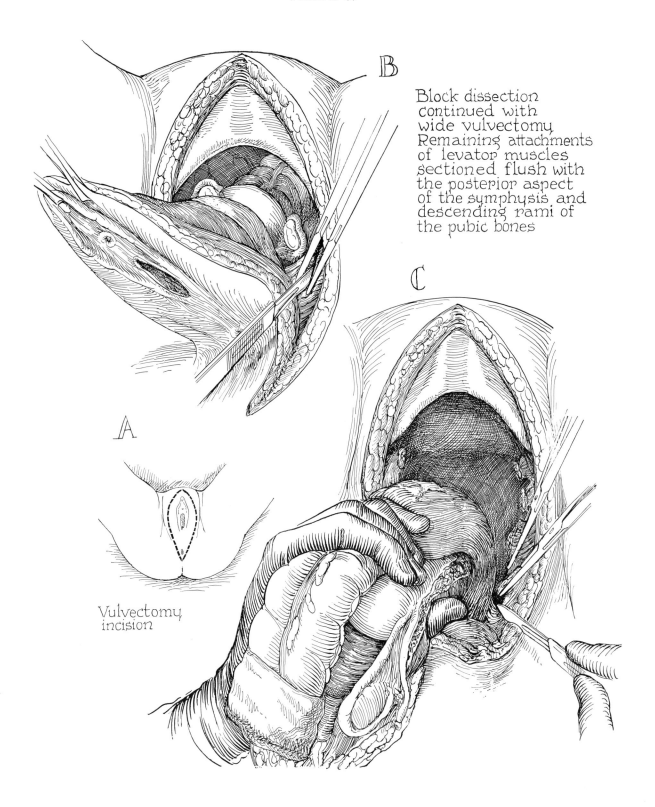

Block dissection continued with wide vulvectomy. Remaining attachments of levator muscles sectioned flush with the posterior aspect of the symphysis and descending rami of the pubic bones

Vulvectomy incision

PLATE 67 (*Concluded*)

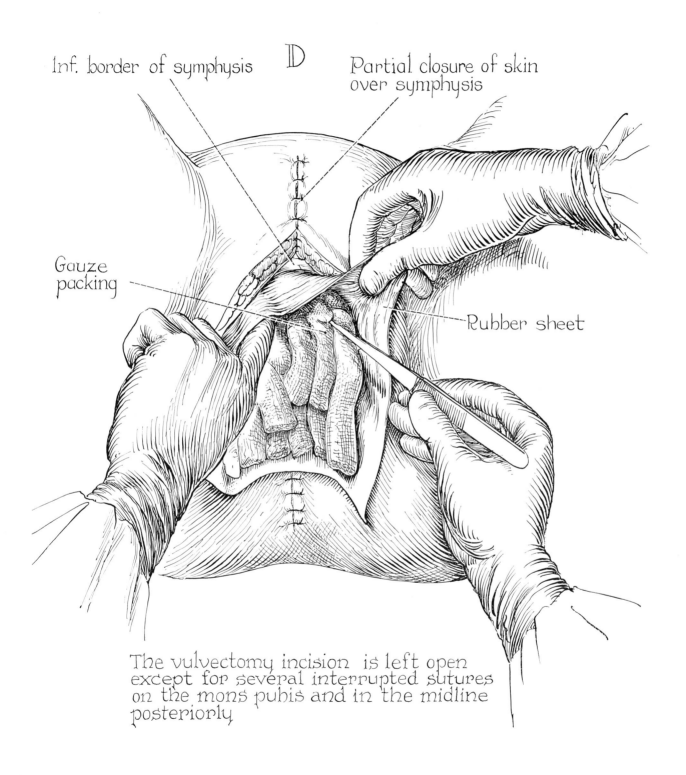

Inf. border of symphysis

D

Partial closure of skin over symphysis

Gauze packing

Rubber sheet

The vulvectomy incision is left open except for several interrupted sutures on the mons pubis and in the midline posteriorly show no evidence of extension to the presacral lymphatics. The operation may also be indicated when a fistulous tract exists between the vagina and bladder, particularly when it is large and follows both radiation and surgery. It may be impossible to ascertain whether the fistula is on the basis of the radiation and surgery or these factors combined with a recurrence of the malignancy. An anterior pelvic exenteration is frequently indicated in cancer of the urethra or a primary cancer of the vagina that involves the anterior vaginal wall. The operation is most frequently done for a primary cancer of the bladder, particularly if it has extended to the uterus or the anterior vaginal wall. If the lesion extends only a relatively short distance down the vagina, the entire operation can be done from the abdomen. If the lower one third of the vagina is involved, a vulval phase of the operation is necessary to complete the block dissection.

Preoperative Preparation and Anesthesia

In addition to the nutritional and psychotherapeutic measures taken to prepare the patient for a major procedure, the bowel is prepared, since exploration of the pelvis may reveal that a total exenteration is necessary. General anesthesia is most commonly employed. If an anesthetist is available who is experienced with hypotensive anesthesia, it is recommended that such anesthesia be used since it has been found to conserve a considerable amount of the blood loss experienced in this operation. Preoperative urinary antiseptics are given.

Steps of the Operation

1. Any lower abdominal incision that is extensive enough to give adequate exposure will suffice for this operation. A long left rectus or paramedian incision is preferable if it is anticipated that the ureters have to be transplanted to the skin. A long lower midline incision that can be extended upward with excision of the umbilicus is adequate. Should it be found necessary to perform a total pelvic exenteration with a colostomy, the colostomy can be placed at the site of the former umbilicus. A transverse interiliac incision gives excellent exposure. It is not quite so satisfactory when the ureters have to be transplanted to the skin or a colostomy performed.

2. The pelvis is explored following the steps suggested under Radical Hysterectomy and Pelvic Lymphadenectomy. Any suspicious nodes or tissue is sent to the laboratory for frozen section, for this information may necessitate a modification of the operation that had been planned.

3. The operation proceeds as a radical hysterectomy until the mobilization of the right ureter is completed. The ureter is dissected down to the base of the broad ligament and transected at this point, provided it appears to be free of tumor. If there is any suspicion that the ureter may be involved in the malignant process proximal to this point, the ureter is transected several centimeters above the suspicious area of involvement (Plate 68, A). An adequate peritoneal flap is developed in the mobilization of the ureter that provides blood supply whether it is transplanted either to the skin or into the bowel (Plate 68, A).

4. A suture is placed on the distal ureter to control bleeding at the point of transection and prevent reflux of urine in the field of operation. The proximal end of the ureter is tagged with a suture and drawn out of the field of operation and protected by moist gauze (Plate 68, B). The hypogastric artery and vein are ligated beyond the posterior division (Plate 68, B). Great care is exercised not to rupture the fragile veins comprising the posterior division. Subsequent bleeding is difficult to control.

5. A similar procedure is carried out on the left side. With the bladder and uterus drawn sharply anteriorly, the peritoneum of the cul-de-sac is incised close to the rectum, and the uterosacral ligaments are clamped, cut, and tied. The line of cleavage between the vagina and the rectum is developed laterally to the parametrium and paracolpium. These connective tissue thickenings carry vessels and nerves to the uterus and vagina.

6. After ligation of the left hypogastric artery and vein, the dissection of the lymphatic tissue about the great vessels is completed by sweeping the mass of tissue toward the uterus.

7. The bladder is detached from the symphysis by blunt and sharp dissection. Many vessels in the space of Retzius will cause some oozing. These should be clamped and ligated close to the periosteum (Plate 68, C). This process is continued until the urethra is mobilized and can be felt penetrating the urogenital diaphragm (Plate 68, C). Meanwhile the anterolateral aspect of the bladder

Text continued on p. 487.

PLATE 68

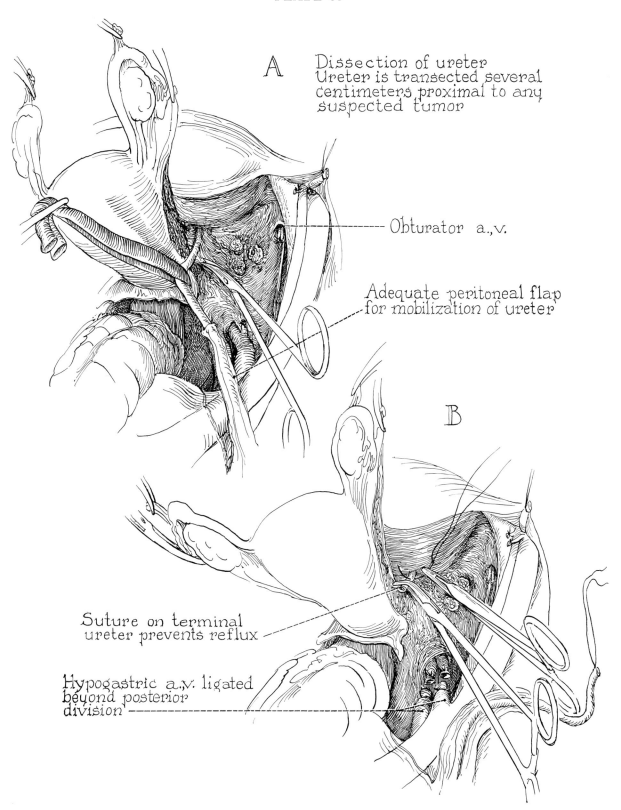

A Dissection of ureter
Ureter is transected several
centimeters proximal to any
suspected tumor

Obturator a.,v.

Adequate peritoneal flap
for mobilization of ureter

B

Suture on terminal
ureter prevents reflux

Hypogastric a.,v. ligated
beyond posterior
division

PLATE 68 (Continued)

𝕮

Bladder detached
from symphysis

Urethra
mobilized

Strong
traction

Vessels in space of Retzius
clamped and ligated close
to periosteum

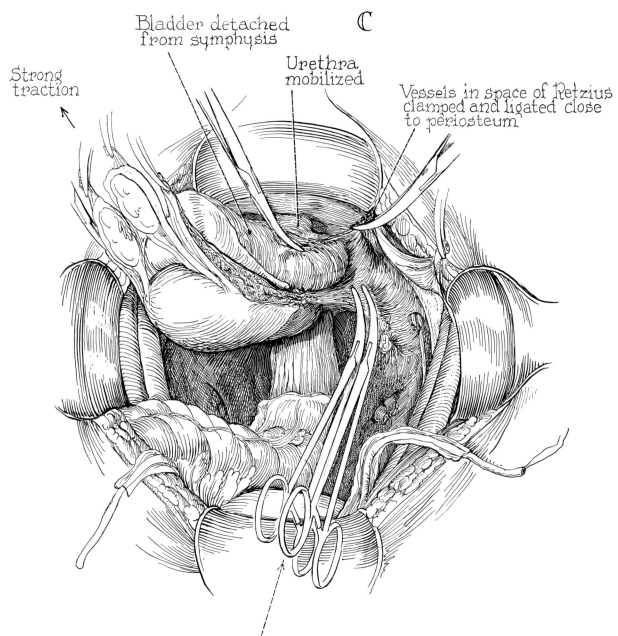

Successive clamping of parametrium and
paravesicum to mobilize uterus and bladder

PLATE 68 (Continued)

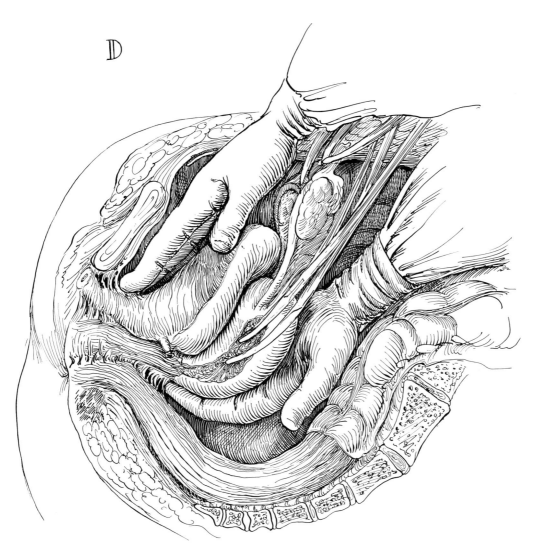

D

Mobilization of bladder and uterus by
blunt dissection in space of Retzius
and rectovaginal septum

PLATE 68 (Concluded)

E

Resection of vagina at
level of pelvic floor

Stump of urethra

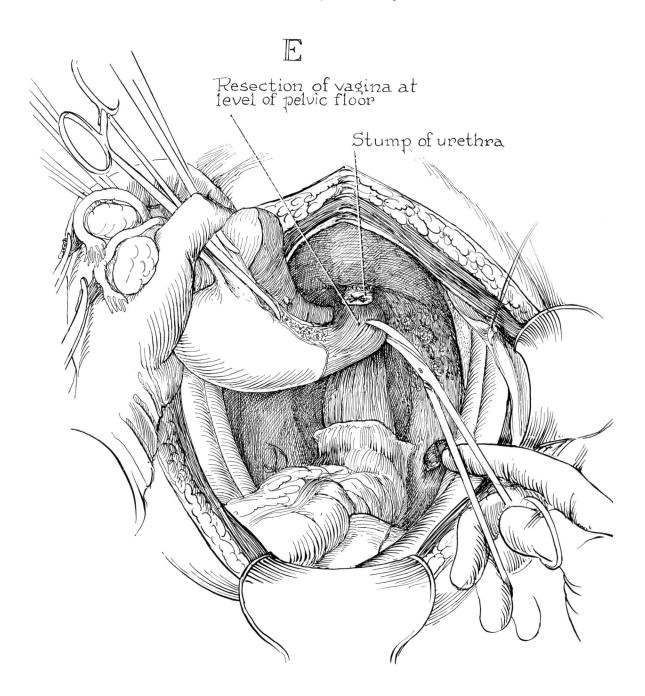

Resection of urethra and vagina for
removal as a block dissection without
vaginal stage

has been mobilized down to the levator ani and the extensions of the obturator fascia upon that muscle. An identical procedure is done on the left side. This completes the mobilization of the bladder except for connective tissue extensions that accompany the middle and inferior vesical arteries which will be clamped when the uterus and vagina are mobilized and dissected from the rectum.

8. The dissection is continued, successively clamping, cutting, and ligating the upper portion of the parametrium and paravesicum (Plate 68, C). No attempt is made to isolate and individually ligate vessels in this procedure. During the dissection the middle and inferior vesical arteries and veins are clamped, cut, and tied.

9. One hand of the operator is placed in the rectovaginal septum and the other between the bladder and symphysis. With blunt dissection, the bladder and uterus are further mobilized and the level of the lesion palpated. Plate 68, D, shows the position of the hands during this part of the dissection. The operator palpates the structures to be sure that the dissection is adequately clearing the area of the malignancy (Plate 68, D).

10. If it has been decided, both from the pelvic examination and from palpation of the lesion during the abdominal phase of the operation, that the lesion can be cleared without a vulvectomy, the urethra and vagina are resected at the level of the pelvic floor (Plate 68, E). The stump of the urethra is closed with a figure-of-eight suture, bleeding points on the vaginal cuff are ligated, and the pelvis is inspected for any active bleeding. Several Penrose drains are placed through the middle portion of the vaginal cuff down into the remains of the vagina. Should there be a generalized oozing in the field of operation, a 2-inch, 5-yard pack can be placed in the pelvic cavity and the lower end pushed out through the remains of the vagina.

11. In the description of a total pelvic exenteration the transplantation of the ureters either into the bowel or the skin was accomplished in the early and less shocking phase of the operation. However, in this procedure, since it might be determined at almost any stage of the operation that it was necessary to remove the rectum, the disposition of the ureters is best left until after the removal of the specimen. The operator then decides whether he wishes the ureters to be placed in the bowel or whether cutaneous ureterostomies are preferable. The ureters are transplanted, usually into the bowel, by the technique described

under Ureterointestinal Anastomosis (page 256). The abdomen is closed without drainage.

Postoperative Care

The drains left through the vagina should be withdrawn a few centimeters each day as long as there is considerable drainage and accumulation of serum and lymph. If a large pack has been placed in the pelvis, this is removed in forty-eight hours. Light Pentothal anesthesia may be induced for this procedure. In addition to the usual postoperative care after major pelvic surgery, all of the electrolyte studies required in the management of patients with ureterointestinal transplants are done. (See Fluid and Electrolyte Management After Radical Surgery or Postoperative Complications in Pelvic Surgery, page 543.)

Anterior Pelvic Exenteration—
Vulval Phase
Steps of the Operation

1. In Plate 69, A, is shown the incision for a vulvectomy in the event that a vaginal phase is necessary to complete the anterior pelvic exenteration. This incision completely circumscribes the labia majora and labia minora and takes with it all the structures down to the periosteum of the symphysis, including the clitoris, the crura of the clitoris, all of the vagina, and urethra. Posteriorly the incision should be just above the level of the sphincters of the rectum so that these are not impaired during the course of the operation. This is particularly important in the event that the ureters are transplanted into the bowel and the lower rectum must serve as a reservoir for the diverted urine.

2. The dissection starts on the mons pubis and is carried down through the subcutaneous tissue and fascia until the periosteum of the symphysis is reached (Plate 69, B). Those portions of the levator ani and the visceral extensions of the parietal connective tissue that have not been clamped, cut, and tied from above are now resected. During the course of this dissection strong traction should be made posteriorly that will permit the clamping of all the tissues flush with the pelvic side wall.

3. Posteriorly the ischiorectal fossa is entered on both sides and the rectum separated from the vagina until the level of the dissection done from above is reached. The entire specimen, together

PLATE 69

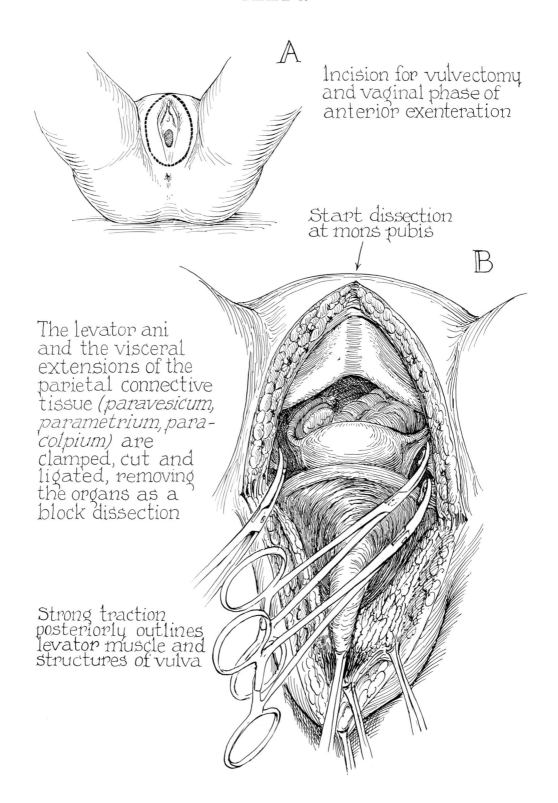

A

Incision for vulvectomy and vaginal phase of anterior exenteration

Start dissection at mons pubis

B

The levator ani and the visceral extensions of the parietal connective tissue *(paravesicum, parametrium, paracolpium)* are clamped, cut and ligated, removing the organs as a block dissection

Strong traction posteriorly outlines levator muscle and structures of vulva with all of the lymphatic tissue mobilized from above, is lifted out of the pelvis. The field of operation is inspected for any bleeding points and partial closure of the wound attempted. This is done by interrupted sutures of 0 chromic catgut, approximating the skin beginning at the anterior edge of the wound. Extensive undermining of the wound in order to effect a more complete closure is inadvisable, since this may possibly serve to disseminate malignant cells and unnecessarily open up tissue planes.

4. When as much of the wound as will close without tension has been sutured, both anteriorly and posteriorly, drains are placed in the most dependent portion of the wound. It is usually not necessary to insert a large sheet of rubber dam to hold back the bowel as is necessary in a total pelvic exenteration. However, should the small bowel tend to prolapse into the lower portions of the wound, this can be done. The packing is left in place for several days until the small bowel becomes adherent in the upper pelvis.

Postoperative Care

The postoperative care is the same as if the operation were done entirely from above, with the addition of the management of the vulval wound. The drains are withdrawn a few centimeters each day and may be removed completely about the fourth or fifth day. It may be necessary to irrigate the wound to aid in the formation of healthy granulations, but complete closure can be expected in the course of several weeks.

References

Ackerman, L. V., and del Regato, J. A.: Cancer: Diagnosis, Treatment and Prognosis, ed. 4, St. Louis, 1963, The C. V. Mosby Co.

Amreich, J.: Zur Anatomie und Technik der Erweiterten Vaginalen Carcinomoperation, Arch. Gynäk. 122: 497, 1924.

Amreich, J.: Lymph Node Involvement in Carcinoma of the Cervix Treated by Surgery and Irradiation, (Das Lymphknotenproblem bei Operation und Bestrahlung des Kollumkarzinoms), Wien. med. Wchnschr. 107: 6, 1957.

Antoine, T.: La colpomicroscopia, Rev. port. obst. ginec. e cir. 5: 379, 1952.

Arnas, N., and Foix, A.: Treatment of Carcinoma of the Cervical Stump (Tratamiento del carcinoma del munon cervical), Obst. y ginec. latino-am. 16: 161, 1958.

Arneson, A. N., and Quimby, E. H.: Distribution of Roentgen Radiation Within the Average Female Pelvis for Different Physical Factors of Irradiation, Radiology 25: 182, 1935.

Atlee, H. B., and Tupper, C.: The Vaginoabdominal Approach in Radical Pelvic Surgery, Am. J. Obst. & Gynec. 73: 141, 1957.

Ayre, J. E.: Cancer Cytology of the Uterus, New York, 1951, Grune & Stratton.

Bacon, H. E., and McCrea, L. E.: Abdominoperineal Proctosigmoidectomy for Rectal Cancer. The Management of Associated Vesical Dysfunction, J. A. M. A. 134: 523, 1947.

Baker, W. S.: Further Experience With Parametrial Radiogold as an Adjunct to Radium Therapy in Treatment of Pelvic Lymph Nodes in Cancer of the Cervix, Am. J. Obst. & Gynec. 81: 797, 1961.

Ball, T.: Carcinoma of the Cervix. In Forkner, C.: Practitioners' Conferences, vol. 5, Jan. 15, 1957, New York, Appleton-Century-Crofts, Inc., p. 103.

Barbieri, G.: Squamous Metaplasia, Atypical Hyperplasia, and Carcinoma in Situ of the Cervix Uteri (Metaplasia squamosa, iperplasia atipica e carcinoma "in situ" della cervice uterina), Lav. Ist. anat. e istol. pat. 18: 51, 1958.

Betson, J. R., and Golden, M. L.: Cancer and Pregnancy, Am. J. Obst. & Gynec. 81: 718, 1961.

Bonney, V.: Hunterian Lecture on Surgical Treatment of Carcinoma of the Cervix, Lancet 1: 277, 1930.

Breitner, J.: A Unified Approach to the Classification of Carcinoma of the Genital Tract (Vorschlag zur Vereinheitlichung der Stadieneinteilung bei den Genitalkarzinomen), Geburtsh. u. Frauenh. 18: 499, 1958.

Broders, A. C.: Carcinoma, Grading and Practical Application, Arch. Path. 2: 376, 1926.

Brunschwig, A.: Complete Excision of Pelvic Viscera for Advanced Carcinoma, Cancer 1: 177, 1948.

Brunschwig, A, and Daniel, W.: The Surgical Treatment of Cancer of the Cervix Uteri, Am. J. Obst. & Gynec. 75: 875, 1958.

Bruntsch, K. H.: The Value of Microscopic Examination of the Parametrium of Surgically Removed Specimens of Cervical Carcinomas for the Determination of the Degree of Infiltration, (Die Wertung der histologischen Untersuchung der Parametrien beim operierten Kollumkarzinom im Hinblick auf die Festsellung des Ausbreitungsgrades), Geburtsh. u. Frauenh. 17: 518, 1957.

Burns, B. C., Everett, H. S., and Brack, C. B.: Value of Urologic Study in the Management of Carcinoma of the Cervix, Am. J. Obst. & Gynec. 80: 997, 1960.

Cahill, J. J., and Zeit, P. R.: Intra-arterial Infusions of Pelvic Tumors With Amethopterin, Am. J. Obst. & Gynec. 81: 970, 1961.

Carter, B., and others: The Follow-up of Patients With Cancer of the Cervix Treated by Radical Hysterectomy and Radical Pelvic Lymphadenectomy, Am. J. Obst. & Gynec. 76: 1094, 1958.

Cherry, C., and Fraser, W.: The Influence of Focal Size on Local Radiocurability of Tumors of the Uterine Cervix, Cancer 13: 951, 1960.

Christopherson, W., and Parker, J.: A Critical Study of Cervical Biopsies Including Serial Sectioning, Cancer 14: 213, 1961.

Cole, W. H., and others: The Dissemination of Cancer Cells, Bull. New York Acad. Med. 34: 163, 1958.

Courtney, W. B., and others: Field Trial of the Cytoanalyzer: 1,184 Specimens Analyzed, J. Nat. Cancer Inst. 24: 1167, 1960.

Courtney, W. B., and others: Modified Drop Technique: Preparation of Smears for Automatic, Electronic Scanning, J. Nat. Cancer Inst. 25: 703, 1960.

Crisp, W. E., Davis, C. E., and Snow, D. L.: Preservation of Vaginal Function Following Radical Pelvic Surgery, A. M. A. Arch. Surg. 81: 632, 1960.

Cullen, T. S.: Cancer of the Uterus, Philadelphia, 1909, W. B. Saunders Co.

Dahle, T.: Combined Radiologic-Surgical Treatment of Carcinoma of the Cervix, Surg., Gynec. & Obst. 109: 600, 1959.

Dearing, R.: A Study of the Renal Tract in Carcinoma of the Cervix, J. Obst. & Gynaec. Brit. Emp. 60: 165, 1953.

De Girolami, E.: The So-Called Perinuclear Halo, Obst. & Gynec. 17: 175, 1961.

Delario, A. J.: Roentgen, Radium and Radioisotope Therapy, Philadelphia, 1953, Lea & Febiger.

Diddle, A. W., and Kinlaw, S.: Cervical Carcinoma: Radical Hysterectomy and Pelvic Lymphadenectomy, Am. J. Obst. & Gynec. 81: 792, 1961.

D' Incerti Bonini, L.: Fluorescent Microscopy in the Cytological Diagnosis of Carcinoma of the Uterus (La microscopia a fluorescenza per la citodiagnosi del carcinoma utero), An. obst. e ginec. 77: 929, 1955.

Douglas, R. G., and Sweeney, W. J.: Exenteration Operations in the Treatment of Advanced Pelvic Cancer, Am. J. Obst. & Gynec. 73: 1169, 1957.

Eckert, C.: Extended Operations for the Treatment of Cancer; Present Status of Controversial Extended Radical Surgical Procedures, A. M. A. Arch. Surg. 82: 562, 1961.

Eichner, E., Goldberg, I., and Bove, E. R.: In Vivo Studies With Direct Sky Blue of the Lymphatic Drainage of the Internal Genitals of Women, Am. J. Obst. & Gynec. 67: 1277, 1954.

Eichner, E., Mallin, L. P., and Angell, M. L.: Further Experiences With Direct Sky Blue in the in Vivo Study of Gynecic Lymphatics, Am. J. Obst. & Gynec. 69: 1019, 1955.

Elevitch, F., and Brunson, J.: Rapid Identification of Malignant Cells in Vaginal Smears by Cytoplasmic Fluorescense, Surg., Gynec. & Obst. 112: 3, 1961.

Engler, H. S., and McInnes, G. F.: Experiences With Iliac Artery and Vein Resection in Radical Pelvic Surgery, Cancer 11: 48, 1958.

Estrada, W. J., and others: Cytology: An Evaluation and Follow-up of 25,000 Genital Smears, Am. J. Obst. & Gynec. 77: 175, 1959.

Fluhmann, C. F., and Dickmann, Z.: The Basic Pattern of the Glandular Structures of the Cervix Uteri, Obst. & Gynec. 11: 543, 1958.

Foraker, A. G., and Reagan, J. W.: Nuclear Mass and Allied Phenomena in Normal Exocervical Mucosa, Squamous Metaplasia, Atypical Hyperplasia, Intra-Epithelial Carcinoma, and Invasive Squamous Cell Carcinoma of the Uterine Cervix, Cancer 12: 894, 1959.

Frick, H. C., and others: Surgical and Radiological Treatment of Cancer of the Cervix in 397 Cases, Surg., Gynec. & Obst. 107: 457, 1958.

Friedell, G. H., and Graham, J. B.: Regional Lymp Node Involvement in Small Carcinoma of the Cervix, Surg., Gynec. & Obst. 108: 513, 1959.

Garret, R.: Extrauterine Tumor Cells in Vaginal and Cervical Smears, Obst. & Gynec. 14: 21, 1959.

Gemmell, A.: Cystoscopy in Carcinoma of the Cervix, J. Obst. & Gynaec. Brit. Emp. 35: 465, 1928.

Graham, R. M.: Effect of Radiation on Vaginal Cells in Cervical Carcinoma. I. Description of Cellular Changes. II. The Prognostic Significance, Surg., Gynec. & Obst. 84: 153, 1947.

Graham, R. M.: Cytologic Prognosis in Cancer of the Cervix, Am. J. Obst. & Gynec. 79: 700, 1960.

Graham, R. M., and Goldie, K. R.: Prognosis in Irradiated Cancer of the Cervix by Measurement of Cell Size in the Vaginal Smear, Cancer 8: 71, 1955.

Graham, R. M., and Graham, J. B.: Cytological Prognosis in Cancer of the Uterine Cervix Treated Radiologically, Cancer 8: 59, 1955.

Gray, M. J., Gusberg, S. B., and Guttman, R.: Pelvic Lymp Node Dissection Following Radiotherapy, Am. J. Obst. & Gynec. 76: 629, 1958.

Gray, M. J., Taylor, H., and Planti, A.: The Lymphocyst: A Complication of Pelvic Lymp Node Dissections, Am. J. Obst. & Gynec. 75: 1059, 1958.

Gross, S. J., and Danziger, S.: Histochemical Techniques Applied to the Study of Benign and Malignant Squamous Epithelium of the Cervix Uteri, Am. J. Obst. & Gynec. 73: 94, 1957.

Henriksen, E.: Distribution of Metastases in Stage I Carcinoma of the Cervix; a Study of 66 Autopsied Cases, Am. J. Obst. & Gynec. 80: 919, 1960.

Henriksen, E.: The Lymphatic Spread of Carcinoma of the Cervix and of the Body of the Uterus, Am. J. Obst. & Gynec. 58: 924, 1949.

Hinselmann, H.: Gesteigert atypisches Epithel oder "Oberflächenkarzinom"? Ztschr. Geburtsh. u. Gynäk. 138: 153, 1953.

Holzaepfel, J. H., and Ezell, H. E.: Carcinoma of the Cervix, Western J. Surg., Obst. & Gynec. 68: 378, 1960.

Javert, C. T.: Pathogenesis of Endometriosis Based on Endometrial Homeoplasia, Direct Extension, Exfoliation and Implantation, Lymphatic and Hematogenous Metastasis (Including Five Case Reports of Endometrial Tissue in Pelvic Lymph Nodes), Cancer 2: 399, 1949.

Javert, C. T.: The Spread of Benign and Malignant Endometrium in the Lymphatic System, With a Note on Coexisting Vascular Involvement, Am. J. Obst. & Gynec. 64: 780, 1952.

Javert, C. T., and Hofammann, K.: Observations on the Surgical Pathology, Selective Lymphadenectomy and Classification of Endometrial Adenocarcinoma, Cancer 5: 485, 1952.

Jones, H., and others: Cellular Changes in Vaginal and Buccal Smears After Radiation: An Index of the Radiocurability of Carcinoma of the Cervix, Am. J. Obst. & Gynec. 78: 1083, 1959.

Jones, W. N., and Osband, R.: Cancer of the Cervix in Pregnancy, South. M. J. 53: 199, 1960.

Kaplan, L., and others: Acridine Orange Fluorochrome in the Study of Normal and Malignant Epithelium of the Uterine Cervix, Am. J. Obst. & Gynec. 80: 1063, 1960.

Kaufman, R. H., Topek, N. H., and Wall, J.: Late Irradiation Changes in Vaginal Cytology, Am. J. Obst. & Gynec. 81: 859, 1961.

Kelly, J. W. M., Friedell, G. H., and Sommers, S. C.: A Pathological Study in 55 Autopsies After Radical Surgery for Cancer of the Cervix, Surg., Gynec. & Obst. 110: 423, 1960.

Kickham, C.: Urologic Problems in Carcinoma of the Cervix, Surg., Gynec. & Obst. 112: 27, 1961.

Kickham, C. J. E.: Urologic Pitfalls in the Management of Carcinoma of the Cervix, J. Urol. 80: 229, 1958.

Koss, L. G., and Wolinska, W. H.: Trichomonas Vaginalis Cervicitis and Its Relationship to Cervical Cancer, Cancer 12: 1171, 1959.

Kottmeier, H. L.: Carcinoma of the Female Genitalia, Baltimore, 1953, The Williams and Wilkins Co.

Kottmeier, H. L.: Carcinoma of the Cervix, Acta obst. et gynec. scandinav. 38: 522, 1959.

Krieger, J. S., and McCormack, L. J.: The Indications for Conservative Therapy for Intraepithelial Carcinoma of the Uterine Cervix, Am. J. Obst. & Gynec. 76: 312, 1958.

Lang, W. R.: Colposcopy—Neglected Method of Cervical Evaluation, J. A. M. A. 166: 893, 1958.

Lash, A.: Management of Carcinoma of the Cervix in Pregnancy, Obst. & Gynec. 17: 41, 1961.

Lock, F. R., Greiss, F. C., and Blake, D. D.: Stage I Carcinoma of the Uterine Cervix; Comparison of Results With Variations in Treatment, Am. J. Obst. & Gynec. 80: 984, 1960.

McCall, M. L.: The Radical Vaginal Operative Approach in the Treatment of Carcinoma of the Cervix, Am. J. Obst. & Gynec. 78: 712, 1959.

McDuff, H. C., Jr., Carney, W. L., and Waterman, G. W.: Cancer of the Cervix and Pregnancy, Obst. & Gynec. 8: 196, 1956.

McDuff, H. C., Martin, R. E., and Waterman, G. W.: Accidentally Encountered Cervical Cancer, Am. J. Obst. & Gynec. 71: 407, 1956.

McDuff, H. C., Waterman, G. W., and Martin, R. E.: The Use of Surgery in the Total Management of Cancer, Ann. Surg. 139: 420, 1954.

Mackenzie, L. L.: The Cytology of Early Squamous-Cell Carcinoma of the Cervix, Am. J. Obst. & Gynec. 69: 629, 1955.

490

Martzloff, K. H.: Carcinoma of the Cervix Uteri; Its Operative Prognosis. A Clinical and Pathological Study to Ascertain the Prognosis Following Operation for Extirpation of the Malignant Process, Bull. Johns Hopkins Hosp. **40**: 160, 1927.

Masin, M., and Masin, F.: Cresyl Violet Staining in Exfoliative Gynecologic Cytology, Obst. & Gynec. **15**: 702, 1960.

Maliphant, R. G.: Variations in the Malignancy of Cancers of the Uterine Cervix, J. Obst. & Gynaec. Brit. Emp. **67**: 420, 1960.

Meigs, J. V.: The Wertheim Operation for Carcinoma of the Cervix, Am. J. Obst. & Gynec. **49**: 542, 1945.

Mitra, S.: Radikale vaginal Hysterektomie und extraperitoneal Lymphadenektomie bei Zervix-krebs, Zentralbl. Gynäk. **73**: 574, 1951.

Mitra, S.: Extraperitoneal Lymphadenectomy and Radical Vaginal Hysterectomy For Cancer of the Cervix (Mitra Technique), Am. J. Obst. & Gynec. **78**: 191, 1959.

Moorhead, P. S., and Hsu, T. C.: Cytologic Studies of HeLa, a Strain of Human Cervical Carcinoma. III. Durations and Characteristics of the Mitotic Phases, J. Nat. Cancer Inst. **16**: 1047, 1956.

Munnell, E. W., and Bonney, W. A.: Critical Points of Failure in the Therapy of Cancer of the Cervix; a Study of 250 Recurrences, Am. J. Obst. & Gynec. **81**: 521, 1961.

Navratil, E.: Zur Technik der vaginalen Radikaloperation des Carcinoma colli uteri, Arch. f. Gynäk. **178**: 57, 1949.

Navratil, E.: Die Entwicklungstendenz der operativen Behandlung des Collumkarzinoms, Bull. schweiz. Akad. med. Wissensch. **6**: 376, 1950.

Navratil, E., and others: Simultaneous Colposcopy and Cytology Used in Screening for Carcinoma of the Cervix, Am. J. Obst. & Gynec. **75**: 1292, 1958.

Nyberg, R., Tornber, B., and Westin, B.: Colposcopy and Shiller's Iodine Test as an Aid in the Diagnosis of Malignant and Premalignant Lesions of the Squamous Epithelium of the Cervix Uteri, Acta obst. et gynec. scandinav. **39**: 540, 1960.

Ober, K. G.: The Uterine Cervix at Different Age Periods; the Significance of Changes in Its Appearance in Cancer Diagnosis and the Question of So-Called Portio Erosion (Cervix Uteri und Lebensalter; die Bedeutung der Formwandlungen der Zervix fuer die Krebsdiagnostik und die Frage der sogenannten Portioerosion), Deutch. med. Wnschr. **83**: 1661, 1958.

Papanicolaou, G. N., and Traut, H. F.: Diagnosis of Uterine Cancer by Vaginal Smear, New York, 1943, The Commonwealth Fund.

Parsons, L., Cesare, F., and Friedell, G. H.: Primary Surgical Treatment of Invasive Cancer of the Cervix, Surg., Gynec. & Obst. **109**: 279, 1959.

Peham, H.: Operative Gynecology, Philadelphia, 1934, J. B. Lippincott Co.

Peham, H., and Amreich, I.: Gynakologische Operationslehre, Berlin, 1930, S. Karger, p. 237.

Pereyra, A. J.: The Relationship of Sexual Activity to Cervical Cancer; Cancer of the Cervix in a Prison Population, Obst. & Gynec. **17**: 154, 1961.

Poirier, P.: Lymphatiques des organes genitaux de la femme, Paris, 1890, Lecrosnier & Babe.

Pruitt, J. C., and others: Spray Technique for Preparation of Cytologic Specimens for Automatic Scanning Machines, J. Nat. Cancer Inst. **22**: 1105, 1959.

Przybora, L. A., and Plutowa, A.: Histological Topography of Carcinoma in Situ of the Cervix Uteri, Cancer **12**: 263, 1959.

Randerrath, E., and Hieronymi, G.: The Question of the So-Called Surface Carcinoma of the Portio Uteri (Zur Frage des sog. Oberflaechenkarzinoms der Portio Uteri), Munchen. med. Wchnschr. **98**: 1269, 1956.

Rastgeldi, S., and Turanli, I.: Concentration of Malignant Cells From Vaginal Washings by Means of a New Type of Centrifuge, Acta obst. et gynec. scandinav. **37**: 393, 1958.

Read, C. D.: The Role of Surgery in the Treatment of Carcinoma of the Cervix, Edinburgh M. J. **55**: 675, 1948.

Richardson, H. L., and Thiersch, J. B.: A Study of the Anatomical Distribution of Residual Carcinoma of the Cervix, Cancer **12**: 10, 1959.

Riva, H. L., Hefner, J. D., and Kawasaki, D. M.: Carcinoma in Situ of the Cervix; a Review of 156 Cases, Obst. & Gynec. **17**: 525, 1961.

Rotkin, I.: Studies on the Inheritance of Cancer of the Human Uterine Cervix, Cancer **14**: 179, 1961.

Sagiroglu, N.: The Nature of the "Perinuclear Halo": Further Clinical, Cytological, and Pathological Studies, Am. J. Obst. & Gynec. **77**: 159, 1959.

Salzer, R.: Colposcopy—an Aid in the Detection of Early Cancer and Precancerous Conditions of the Cervix, Obst. & Gynec. **13**: 451, 1959.

Sandifer, M. G., and Pritchett, N. L.: Psychologic Reactions Causing a Delay in Treatment of Cancer of the Cervix, Obst. & Gynec. **11**: 82, 1958.

Schauta, F.: Die Operation des Gebarmutterkrebses mittels des Schuchardt'schen Paravaginalschnittes, Monatschr. Geburtsh. u. Gynäk. **15**: 133, 1902.

Schauta, F.: Die Berechtigung der vaginalen Totalexstirpation bie Gebarmutterkrebs, Monatschr. Geburtsh. u. Gynäk. **19**: 475, 1904.

Schauta, F.: Die erweiterte vaginale Totalextirpation des Uterus bei Kollumcarzinom, Wien. and Leipzig, 1908, J. Safar.

Scheffey, L. C., and Thudium, W. J.: End-Results in the Treatment of Carcinoma of the Cervix With Radium, Am. J. Obst. & Gynec. **22**: 247, 1931.

Schiller, W., Daro, A. F., Gollin, H. A., and Primiano, N. P.: Small Preulcerative Invasive Carcinoma of the Cervix: the Spray Carcinoma, Am. J. Obst. & Gynec. **65**: 1088, 1953.

Schjott-Rivers, E., and Istre, B S: Pre-Operative Irradiation in Carcinoma of the Uterine Cervix, Acta obst et gynec. scandinav. **38**: 681, 1959.

Schmitt, A.: Colposcopy Detection of Atypical and Cancerous Lesions of the Cervix, Obst. & Gynec. **13**: 665, 1959.

Schmitz, H.: The Relation of the Degree of the Histological Malignancy to the Prognosis and Treatment of Carcinoma of the Uterine Cervix, Radiology **9**: 322, 1927.

Schmitz, H. E., and others: The Technique of Synchronous (Two Team) Abdominoperineal Pelvic Exenteration, Surg., Gynec. & Obst. **108**: 351, 1959.

Schmitz, H. E., Isaacs, J. H., and Fetherston, W. C.: The Value of Routine Cytologic Smears in Pregnancy, Am. J. Obst. & Gynec. **79**: 910, 1960.

Senior, H. D.: An Interpretation of the Recorded Arterial Anomalies of the Human Pelvis and Thigh, Am. J. Anat. **36**: 1, 1925-1926.

Sotto, L. S., Graham, J. B., and Pickren, J. W.: Postmortem Findings in Cancer of the Cervix; an Analysis of 108 Autopsies in the Past Five Years, Am. J. Obst. & Gynec. **80**: 791, 1960.

Stander, R. W., and others: The Intravenous Pyelogram and Carcinoma of the Cervix, Obst. & Gynec. **17**: 26, 1961.

Stern, E., and Dixon, W.: Cancer of the Cervix—a Biometric Approach to Etiology, Cancer **14**: 153, 1961.

Stoeckel, W.: Zur Technic der vaginalen Radikaloperation beim Kollumkarzinom, Zentralbl. Gynäk. **55**: 53, 1931.

Studdiford, W. E., and Hecht, E. L.: A Dual Purpose Cannula for the Cytologic Method, Am. J. Obst. & Gynec. **67**: 206, 1954.

Sussman, W.: Detection of Gynecologic Cancer by Fluorescence Microscopy, Obst. & Gynec. **13**: 273, 1959.

Symmonds, R., and Pratt, J.: Prevention of Fistulas and Lymphocysts in Radical Hysterectomy; Preliminary Report of a New Technic, Obst. & Gynec. **17**: 57, 1961.

Takeuchi, A., and McKay, D. G.: The Area of the Cervix Involved by the Carcinoma in Situ and Anaplasia (Atypical Hyperplasia), Obst. & Gynec. **15**: 134, 1960.

Taussig, F. J.: Iliac Lymphadenectomy for Group II Cancer of the Cervix: Technique and Five-year Results in 175 Cases, Am. J. Obst. & Gynec. 45: 733, 1943.

Taylor, R. S., Carroll, B. E., and Lloyd, J. W.: Mortality Among Women in Three Catholic Religious Orders With Special Reference to Cancer, Cancer 12: 1207, 1959.

Thornton, N., Fox, C. H., and Smith, D. E.: The Relationship of the Squamocolumnar Junction and the Endocervical Glands to the Site of Origin of Carcinoma of the Cervix, Am. J. Obst. & Gynec. 78: 1060, 1959.

Thornton, W. N., Jr., Waters, L. N., Pearce, L. S., Wilson, L. A., Jr., and Nokes, J. M.: Carcinoma in Situ; Value of Cold-Knife Cone Biopsy, Obst. & Gynec. 3: 587, 1954.

Tietze, K.: A Tampon Smear Method in Cytological Diagnosis (Ueber eine Tamponausstrichmethode in der zytologischen Diagnostik) Geburtsh. u. Frauenh. 18: 746, 1958.

Tolles, W. E., Horvath, W. J., and Bostrom, R. C.: A Study of the Quantitative Characterists of Exfoliated Cells From the Female Genital Tract. II. Suitability of Quantitative Cytological Measurements for Automatic Prescening, Cancer 14: 455, 1961.

Toplin, I.: A Tissue Culture Cytotoxicity Test for Large-Scale Cancer Chemotherapy Screening, Cancer Res. 19: 959, 1959.

Tornberg, B., Westin, B., and Norlander, A.: Fluorescence Microscopy and Acridin—Orange Staining in the Cytological Diagnosis of Atypical Changes in Cervical Epithelium, Acta obst. et gynec. scandinav. 39: 517, 1960.

Tucker, J. L., and Talley, R. W.: Prolonged Intra-arterial Chemotherapy for Inoperable Cancer: A Technique, Cancer 14: 493, 1961.

Twombly, G. H., and Taylor, H. C., Jr.: The Treatment of Cancer of the Cervix Uteri; a Comparison of Radiation Therapy and Radical Surgery, Am. J. Roentgenol. 71: 501, 1954.

Uhlenhuth, E., Day, E. C., Smith, R. D., and Middleton, E. B.: The Visceral Endopelvic Fascia and the Hypogastric Sheath, Surg., Gynec. & Obst. 86: 9, 1948.

Van Bouwdijk Bastiaanse, M. A.: Treatment of Cancer of the Cervix Uteri, Am. J. Obst. & Gynec. 72: 100, 1956.

Varga, A.: Cytological Cancer Screening: A Simple, Rapid Staining Procedure Applicable to Office Use, Obst. & Gynec. 15: 9, 1960.

Von Bertalanffy, L., Masin, M., and Masin, F.: A New and Rapid Method for Diagnosis of Vaginal and Cervical Cancer by Fluorescence Microscopy, Cancer 11: 873, 1958.

Walther, H. E.: Untersuchungen über Krebsmetastasen, Ztschr. Krebsforsch. 46: 313, 1937.

Watson, E. M., Herger, C. C., and Sauer, H. R.: Irradiation Reactions in the Bladder: Their Occurrence and Clinical Course Following the Use of X-ray and Radium in the Treatment of Female Pelvic Disease, J. Urol. 57: 1038, 1947.

Welch, J. S., Pratt, J. H., and Symmonds, R. E.: The Wertheim Hysterectomy for Squamous Cell Carcinoma of the Uterine Cervix; Thirty Years' Experience at the Mayo Clinic, Am. J. Obst. & Gynec. 81: 978, 1961.

Wertheim, E.: Bericht über die von der erweiterten Uteruskrebsoperation zu erwartenden Dauererfolge, Wien. klin. Wchnschr. 17: 783, 1904.

Wertheim, E.: A Discussion on the Diagnosis and Treatment of Cancer of the Uterus, Brit. M. J. 2: 689, 1905.

Wertheim, E.: The Extended Abdominal Operation for Carcinoma Uteri (Translated by Hermann Grad), Am. J. Obst. & Gynec. 66: 169, 1912.

Wheatley, R., and Foraker, A.: Protein Characterization in Normal and Abnormal Cervical Squamous Mucosa—"pH Signature," Am. J. Obst. & Gynec. 80: 1074, 1960.

Wied, G. L.: Stereophotocolpography; a Method for Centralized Screening for Cervical Carcinoma, Am. J. Obst. & Gynec. 71: 1301, 1956.

Winter, G. F.: Recent Experiences With Carcinoma in Situ (Neue klinische Erfahrungen beim Oberflaechenkarzinom), Geburtsh. u. Frauenh. 18: 484, 1958.

Woodruff, J. D.: Epithelial Changes Preceding Spinal-Cell Carcinoma of the Cervix Uteri, Am. J. Obst. & Gynec. 77: 977, 1959.

Zeidman, I., and Buss, J. M.: Experimental Studies on the Spread of Cancer in the Lymphatic System. I. Effectiveness of the Lymph Node as a Barrier to the Passage of Embolic Tumor Cells, Cancer Research 14: 403, 1954.

26 · Cancer of the Fundus, Tube, and Ovary

CARCINOMA OF THE BODY OF THE UTERUS
General Considerations

Carcinoma of the body of the uterus occurs less frequently than carcinoma of the cervix. Several statistical studies in the New York Metropolitan area show a ratio of 1:3. Most of the patients presenting themselves with this disease are between the ages of 55 and 60 years. When such statistics are correctly interpreted in terms of cases per thousand per age group, the longer a woman lives, the greater are her chances of developing this cancer or, in fact, any other cancer exclusive of those peculiar to children. The disease seems to have a predilection for the short, heavy-boned, obese type of woman, particularly one with high blood pressure and diabetes. When diabetes is not present, studies in progress seem to indicate a statistically higher percentage of abnormal glucose tolerance curves among women developing carcinoma of the corpus.

Etiology and Pathologic Anatomy

Carcinoma of the body of the uterus is practically always an adenocarcinoma. Ewing's classification is still adequate for the majority of the histologic types.

1. Malignant adenoma is the most frequent histologic type, showing greatly enlarged and elongated glands which are beginning to show a back-to-back arrangement. Histologically the cells show anaplastic changes.

2. Papillary adenocarcinoma is a more advanced dedifferentiation, with many areas of papillary formation, although these may be interspersed among adenomatous areas.

3. The alveolar type of histologic picture shows solid masses of cells that may be seen infiltrating the stroma of the endometrium, blood, and lymph vessels.

4. Adenoacanthoma is a histologic type in which squamous cells form a prominent element among areas of an adenocarcinoma.

The neoplasms may be classified on the basis of the degree of dedifferentiation from the normal cells. As with Broder's classification of squamous cell carcinomas, these tumors can be graded into four groups. In this grading, Grade I would show a minimum amount of dedifferentiation of the cells, progressing through the remaining grades to Grade IV, which shows the most highly malignant cells, the greater number of mitotic figures, a high degree of anaplasia and dedifferentiation. When a large series of tumors are graded in this manner, the survival of the patient roughly parallels the degree of histologic malignancy, although many other clinical factors and the method of treatment alter the prognosis.

Symptoms and Diagnosis

The common symptom is postmenopausal bleeding. Before the menopause there is a history of abnormal menstrual bleeding or intermenstrual bleeding. There may be some abdominal discomfort due to the passage of clots, but persistent pain signifies that the disease has spread beyond the uterus and is involving peritoneal surfaces. The disease may occlude the cervical canal and give rise to a pyometra or hematopyometra, in which event the patient has pain, fever, a tender, enlarged uterus, an elevated white count, and other signs and symptoms of an abscess. On physical examination, enlargement of the uterus, in the absence of incidental fibroids, is a grave prognostic sign. In advanced cases a friable mass of tissue may protrude from the cervix, or the lesion may have already extended along the submucosal lymphatics of the vagina. The diagnosis is confirmed by endometrial aspiration smears and curettage. The percentage of positive smears and the difficulty of interpretation of endometrial smears, as compared with cervical smears, make this test less reliable. The gross appearance of the tissue removed at curettage may be indistinguishable from a hyperplastic endometrium, and the final diagnosis rests on histologic examination. If a pyometra is encountered during the course of the curettage, drainage is established and the actual curetting of the endometrial cavity deferred for a week or more until the infection subsides. The cavity can then be curetted with less danger of perforation or extension of the infection.

Indications and Surgical Principles

A considerable difference of opinion exists as to the efficacy of preoperative and postoperative radium or x-ray in addition to the surgical management of carcinoma of the body of the uterus. The exponents of preoperative radiation insist that such intracavitary radium reduces the size of the lesion in addition to closing lymphatic channels into which tumor cells may be inadvertently displaced during subsequent surgery. This would presume that it were possible to classify the extent of the disease prior to removing the specimen. It also neglects to account for the lymphatic spread of endometrial carcinoma. This factor has been somewhat discounted in the past, while emphasis has been placed on extension of the disease to the vagina, cervix, tubes, and ovaries. Studies of the lymph node involvement in fundal cancer by Hendriksen suggest the necessity of dissection of the inguinal nodes, as well as the obturator, hypogastric, and iliac nodes. Therefore, in a classification such as that suggested by Finn, each stage would have to be determined after an operation, including a pelvic lymphadenectomy with removal of the deep inguinal nodes. Essentially his classification is as follows: Stage I, lesion confined to endometrium; Stage II, myometrium involved; Stage III, extension beyond myometrium but limited to reproductive organs; Stage IV, involvement of other pelvic organs or pelvic lymph nodes, including the bladder and rectum; and Stage V, distant metastasis outside of the pelvis. The classification therefore has its greatest usefulness in determining the prognosis in an individual patient and comparing the methods of therapy in various centers.

Since the question of preoperative radiation has not been settled, what bears closer scrutiny is, first, the advisability of waiting four to six weeks after radiation to perform surgery and, second, the extent of the operation that is ultimately done. Should the time between the insertion of preoperative radiation and surgery in carcinoma of the fundus be shortened to a few weeks or a few days? The extension of cancer would seem to be a constant process, with the lymphatics containing the malignant cells for a matter of weeks. The radiation effects insofar as the alteration of one individual cancer cell—when radium or similar massive dose agent is used—should occur within a short time after therapy. One might then question the advisability of waiting any length of time and performing the surgery within a few days of the radiation. Cancers require radical operation, with attention to the primary and secondary metastatic stations. Why, then, should a simple total hysterectomy be considered an adequate procedure for cancer of the fundus? In what way is it different from other cancers that need a wide excision?

Corscaden, an inveterate teacher and investigator, has repeatedly pointed out the inadequacy of a single tandem applicator in preoperative radiation of the uterus for fundal cancer. The size and distortion of the uterine cavity should govern the selection of an applicator to be used. If one is sure that the cavity is small and undistorted, a single tandem could conceivably deliver an adequate dose, decrease the local necrosis, and not have a rapid fall-off. An irregular cavity distorted

494

by fibroids is best handled by multiple applicators, ten or more. As many as possible are packed into the fundus and cornua of the uterus, while several are arranged in the lower segment (see Chapter 22, page 387). Doses are then calculated from these sources by use of the Quimby tables, but even here it is difficult to ensure that 6,000 gamma roentgens or more are delivered to points several centimeters from the source.

In summary, preoperative radium reduces the size of the uterus and makes it more firm and less susceptible to fracture during hysterectomy. It reduces the number of viable cancer cells that may be spilled in the operative field. Whether cells so spilled in the operative field can survive and cause recurrent cancer has yet to be proved. Whether the reduction of the size of the uterus, with its attendant simplification of the operation, is important to the cancer surgeon is dubious. That a uterus fibrosed by radium is easier to handle than a soft, friable, easily traumatized organ cannot be denied. But are we not concerning ourselves with an organ unessential to life—containing a cancer —when the patient may die of cancer due to involvement of vital structures or lymphatics removed from the primary site that are not influenced by local radiation treatment to the nonessential organ. Is the waiting period between radiotherapy and surgery justified in view of the possibility that lymphatic spread of this disease may be progressing in spite of the radiation? What good can come of a surgical specimen showing dramatic radiation results in the uterus when the common iliac nodes contain viable cancer? Perhaps the answer lies in using all the means at our command to intercept metastatic cancer cells—x-ray, radioactive compounds, radium, radical surgery—until the basic sciences discover a chemical or some other cure for each of the types of cancer. At The New York Hospital–Cornell Medical Center we have adapted for the present time a policy of an immediate, modified, radical surgical attack upon the disease with the subsequent use of other modalities if the malignancy has spread beyond the confines of the uterus.

Surgical Treatment

A modified radical hysterectomy and pelvic lymphadenectomy are performed. In this operation the ureter is permitted to remain attached to the parametrial tissue of the pelvic side wall. The rationale for this procedure is that the lymphatics involved in endometrial carcinoma tend to be in the higher groups of nodes, although retrograde involvement of the deep inguinal nodes is not denied. The deep inguinal nodes are therefore removed from the femoral canal because of the finding of involvement of these nodes in both post-mortem and surgical specimens. Involvement of the vagina is found to be through the submucosal lymphatics, so the upper third or more of the vagina is resected. The lymphadenectomy is carried beyond the pelvis in the aortic nodes as long as enlarged nodes that may represent the last metastatic station of the disease are encountered. If the disease has spread beyond the uterus and into the lymphatics, postoperative deep x-ray therapy is given and recurrent cancer treated by radical excision or palliative therapy. Whether resection of the upper third of the vagina is more efficacious in preventing vault recurrences than a simple hysterectomy with the subsequent placement of gamma sources in the vaginal vault is not known. The proximity of the bladder and rectum to the vaginal vault after removal of the cervix limits the dose that can be delivered to this area. Undoubtedly the newer modalities for delivering deep x-ray therapy will be placed within the uterine cavity and into the parametrium prior to hysterectomy for endometrial carcinoma so that the effects upon the adjacent lymphatics and the adnexa can be studied (see Radiation and Isotope Methodology in Gynecologic Cancer, page 387, and Plate 58, page 386).

SARCOMA OF THE UTERUS
General Considerations

A true appraisal of the incidence of sarcoma of the uterus has been confused by the inclusion of sarcomas with the endometrial cancers in some series of patients, while in others they are grouped with sarcomatous changes in fibro-myomas. The criteria for malignancy in a fibroid require clinical as well as histologic confirmation. Many cellular myomas that may be considered to have undergone sarcomatous change do not fulfill all of the requirements of a malignancy in that metastatic spread by blood vessels, lymphatics, or the invasion of adjacent tissue cannot be established.

Etiology and Pathologic Anatomy

The etiology of sarcoma of the uterus from the stroma of the endometrium results in several cell types. There is an endometrial sarcoma composed of cells resembling the source in that they are long, spindle cells with deeply staining nuclei. They satisfy all of the criteria of anaplastic cells. A rare group of tumors appear to arise from mixed mesenchymal elements and are composed of various mesoblastic elements, including cartilage and muscle. Another group of tumors show malignant connective tissue together with an adenocarcinoma of the endometrium and are called carcinosarcomas. The tumors that represent a malignant change in a fibroid are leiomyosarcomas. A fraction of 1 per cent of fibroids undergo malignant degeneration when the strict criteria of malignancy, invasion and metastatic spread, are applied.

Symptoms and Diagnosis

There are no specific symptoms indicating a sarcoma of the uterus. The symptoms common to many lesions—bleeding, vaginal discharge, or development of pyometra—are sometimes found. Pain is a late symptom and indicates widespread dissemination of the disease. The diagnosis of a sarcoma of the endometrium is made on histologic examination of the tissue, since grossly there is nothing to distinguish this disease from an adenocarcinoma of the endometrium. Occasionally distinct pulmonary metastasis, incidentally discovered during a chest examination and x-ray, together with some symptoms pointing to the uterus, will permit the diagnosis without histologic examination. The diagnosis of a leiomyosarcoma of the uterus is frequently incidental to other find-ings. A rapid increase in the size of an otherwise stationary fibroid tumor may suggest sarcomatous degeneration.

Indications and Surgical Principles

Definitive therapy in the form of surgery is undertaken as soon as the diagnosis is either suspected or confirmed. The prognosis in sarcoma of the uterus is so poor that most longtime survivals have been achieved when an early lesion has been incidentally removed during a hysterectomy for other reasons. The prognosis in sarcoma of the uterus has been studied by Novak by means of the number of mitotic figures in the histologic sections. Where there are more than twenty mitotic figures per high-power field, the prognosis is poor. This is a generalization that has some clinical usefulness. Sarcomas of the uterus that arise in a submucous myoma either do not have a definite capsule or are less likely to remain confined within the capsule of the tumor. A sarcoma arising within a fibroid that is subserous or is some distance from the fundus proper presents a more favorable situation. The question may arise in a young woman desiring children as to whether the uterus, tubes, and ovaries can be left in the event that a sarcoma is diagnosed in one of the specimens from a myomectomy. Patients have refused hysterectomy under these circumstances and subsequently conceived and carried to term without incident. In patients desiring a child, it is probably worth the risk to leave the genital organs in the event of a histologic leiomyosarcoma found well confined within the capsule of an intramural or subserous fibroid. While such a tumor may fulfill the requirements of anaplasia, as stated before, it may not fulfill all the requirements of invasion and metastatic growth to unequivocally classify it as a malignant disease.

Treatment

Irradiation by any of the conventional means employed have had no effect upon the progress of sarcoma of the uterus. Surgical treatment by simple total hysterectomy and bilateral salpingo-oophorectomy has been equally discouraging, with few survivals over a two-year period. No extensive experience with ultraradical surgery has been reported. An incidental histologic leiomyosarcoma found in a subserous or intramural fibroid is a different problem. One may not remove the uterus if the patient is adamant in retaining the organ for the purposes of childbearing. There have been some isolated instances of survival beyond two years with known extension beyond the uterus from a true endometrial sarcoma that was treated with triethylene melamine (TEM). One cannot be sure that the patient would have survived the same length of time without therapy. A discussion of chemotherapy in gynecologic cancer is given in Chapter 23 (page 398).

CANCER OF THE FALLOPIAN TUBE
General Considerations

Cancer of the Fallopian tube is a rare disease constituting only a fraction of 1 per cent of all gynecologic cancers. The Fallopian tube is not as accessible to the study of cyclic changes as is the endometrium or cervical epithelium. The common origin from the Müllerian duct suggests that the tube should be the site of more cancers. Extensive study of advanced undifferentiated pelvic cancers, reputedly of ovarian or uterine origin, might reveal that the incidence of tubal cancer is higher than believed.

Etiology and Pathologic Anatomy

Cancers of the Fallopian tube are almost always adenocarcinomas and vary from a strictly adenomatous pattern to solid medullary types in histologic appearance. The degree of dedifferentiation parallels that of endometrial adenocarcinomas, but the tumor is so rare that prognosis on the basis of histologic change has not been evaluated.

Symptoms and Diagnosis

There are no characteristic symptoms, and the diagnosis is made after study of the gross and microscopic appearance. As in the case of an endometrial cancer, the tube may exfoliate cells into the vagina that are recognized by cytologists. This has been a rather infrequent observation. Bleeding and vaginal discharge are the common symptoms, and pain appears after the disease has become advanced. On physical examination the lesion may be palpated immediately adjacent to the uterus, so that a diagnosis of ovarian cancer with adhesions to tube and the adjacent portions of the uterus and broad ligament is made. A hysterosalpingogram might suggest the disease, but this would certainly be an accidental finding. Gynecologists experienced in abdominal palpation frequently suspect the disease when a unilateral mass is adherent, and the size of the mass suggests that it is probably not a rapidly growing ovarian cancer. Most frequently these small masses are found to be metastatic disease from an endometrial cancer rather than a primary cancer of the Fallopian tube.

Treatment

The number of patients treated by any one individual is so limited that a standard method of treatment cannot be recommended. In the few cases in which x-ray therapy has been employed either preoperatively or postoperatively, there has been little indication that the patient survived any longer than she would have without therapy. Were one fortunate enough to make such a diagnosis preoperatively or at the operating table, it would seem that a modified radical operation with complete lymphadenectomy, particularly of the preaortic nodes above the pelvic brim, would give the best chance of interrupting the distant metastatic stations of this disease and improve the duration of survival.

CARCINOMA OF THE OVARY
General Considerations

The palliative therapy of carcinoma of the ovary is improving, but the over-all cure rate is unchanged. The symptoms of this disease appear after the chance of cure is remote. An opportunity exists to improve the early diagnosis by repeated examinations of patients with ovarian enlargements. The use of an exploratory colpotomy and culdoscopy to visualize the tumor directly is helpful. Rapidly enlarging tumors require definitive steps to establish a diagnosis and institute therapy, and this is done with a sense of urgency.

Etiology and Pathologic Anatomy

Approximately 70 per cent of the malignant tumors of the ovary are serous cystadenocarcinomas. Pseudomucinous cystadenocarcinomas make up another 12 to 14 per cent. The tumors of mesenchymal origin, such as the granulosa cell tumor, account for approximately 8 to 10 per cent. The remainder of the malignant tumors are malignant dysgerminomas, arrhenoblastomas, or tumors, the cell structure of which does not permit classification.

Symptoms and Diagnosis

Pain, postmenopausal bleeding, ascites, cachexia, and edema of the extremities are late manifestations of carcinoma of the ovary. The early carcinomas of the ovary seldom produce any symptoms, and it is only by the careful examination and observation of the gynecologist that these tumors are diagnosed preoperatively. Many of the early carcinomas are histologic diagnoses. There is nothing characteristic of an early malignant tumor that differentiates it from a benign lesion on bimanual examination. The rapid enlargement of a tumor, together with a nodular feeling, is an indication of possible malignant change. In the advanced cases, nodules are palpated in the cul-de-sac, which also bulges from ascitic fluid. A large ovarian cyst may simulate ascites. To decide between ascites and a large ovarian cyst, the tumor and abdomen are palpated, percussed, and auscultated first with the patient lying flat and then in a pronounced Trendelenburg position. Gravitation of the ascitic fluid changes the physical signs significantly and suggests the nature of the abdominal enlargement. A paracentesis is performed and the fluid studied either by section of the centrifuged sediment or by smears. In isolated instances the diagnosis of a malignant tumor with ascites has been made on vaginal smear. This technique has not as yet attained any degree of reliability as compared with the cytologic diagnosis of cancer of the cervix.

Treatment

An extended total hysterectomy is done with removal of both appendages and an adequate cuff of the vagina. Enlarged lymph nodes following the major vessels in the pelvis and the aorta are removed for prognosis. In the advanced cases, the omentum and other peritoneal structures, as well as bowel, may be involved with tumor masses. If feasible and if the patient's condition permits, all of the large masses, in addition to the entire omentum, are resected. Statistically, patients receiving postoperative radiation, even when the lesion appears to be confined within the capsule of the tumor, have not shown a higher survival rate than those in the nonirradiated group. These studies do not include postoperative irradiation with supervoltage therapy or the equivalent irradiation from a cobalt bomb. Whether radioactive gold should be administered as a prophylactic measure in a lesion that is confined to the capsule has yet to be studied. Certainly if there are ascites and minute implants on the parietal and visceral peritoneum, the omentum should be removed. At the time of operation, polyethylene tubes or rubber catheters can be left in the abdomen until a shipment of radioactive gold is received. Little improvement can be expected from intraperitoneal therapy either with radioactive gold or nitrogen mustard if there are large, malignant deposits that cannot be surgically removed. Distant extra-abdominal metastatic disease is given palliative therapy only. A discussion of intraperitoneal therapy in ovarian cancer is found in Chapter 22 (page 389) and Chapter 23 (page 399).

OMENTECTOMY FOR ABDOMINAL CARCINOMATOSIS
Surgical Anatomy of the Omentum

The greater omentum consists of a double sheet of peritoneum folded on itself so that it consists of four layers (Plate 70, *A*). The two layers descending from the greater curvature of the stomach pass in front of the small

PLATE 70

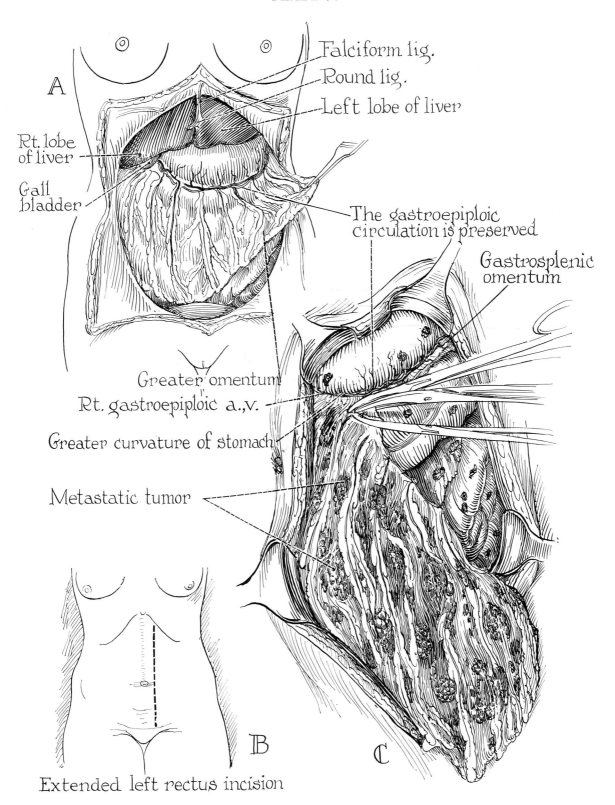

A

Falciform lig.

Round lig.

Left lobe of liver

Rt. lobe of liver

Gall bladder

The gastroepiploic circulation is preserved

Gastrosplenic omentum

Greater omentum

Rt. gastroepiploic a.,v.

Greater curvature of stomach

Metastatic tumor

Extended left rectus incision

B

C

499

bowel, often as low down as the true pelvis. The layers turn on themselves and ascend to the transverse colon, where they split and enclose that part of the large bowel. In the adult the layers are inseparably blended together and contain varying amounts of fat, depending on the obesity of the person. The left border of the greater omentum is continuous with the gastrosplenic omentum; its right border extends only as far as the duodenum (Plate 70, C). The anastomosis between the right and left gastroepiploic arteries is between the two anterior layers, and these vessels should be avoided when the omentum is resected (Plate 70, A and C).

Indications for Operation

The most common indication for resection of the omentum in gynecologic surgery is the removal of an omental "cake" in abdominal carcinomatosis of ovarian origin. This may be done as a palliative procedure for the patient's comfort or preparatory to the use of intraperitoneal gold to control ascites. The omentum may be large without the infiltration of malignant disease and present a problem of exposure to the surgeon. The short, stocky, obese female always poses a problem in exposure of the pelvic organs. Frequently, the distance from the costal margins to the pelvic brim is so short that it is difficult both to expose the pelvis and to pack the fat-laden bowel and copious omentum in the upper abdomen where there just is not enough room. The bowel should be laid outside the abdomen and covered with warm pads—it will suffer no harm and take less abuse than when forceful attempts are made to pack it where it cannot go.

Partial resection of the omentum may be done for a variety of reasons. Omental torsion has been reported in the pregnant as well as the nonpregnant patient. This condition is more common in sections of the right side, which is longer than the left half of the omentum. Displacement by the pregnant uterus, distortion by adhesions, hyperperistalsis, and strenuous physical exercise have all been indicted as etiologic factors. Sections of omentum are

frequently removed when releasing adhesions.

The omentum may become adherent over large areas of the anterior abdominal parietal peritoneum. It is often advisable to perform the operation deliberately through an incision in the structure rather than to attempt to dissect it free. Large areas within the abdomen may be denuded of peritoneum, which will regenerate. This "in situ peritonealization" after its wide denudation either from its visceral or parietal coverings is difficult to explain in terms of the ordinary epithelization that will eventually cover large skin areas. It would appear that it arises from cells in other tissues, probably the retroperitoneal connective tissues, that have the potential to develop into this remarkable membrane. A rent in the omentum should be closed in such a way as to prevent the bowel from finding its way through some small aperture, with subsequent strangulation. The omentum frequently forms part or all of the contents of a hernial sac. This is almost invariably true of an umbilical or midline incisional hernia. It should be remembered that this can also be a blessing with some hernias where there is a contraindication to surgery. The omentum may act as a convenient plug to prevent herniation of the bowel into the sac, with the possibility of strangulation. Pelvic tumors of ovarian or uterine origin, deprived of their blood supply by a narrow or twisted pedicle, may become parasitic on the omentum and avoid degeneration or gangrene.

The omentum may interfere with a paracentesis if it is adherent to the anterior wall and has formed multiple locules within the abdomen. The injection of radioactive colloids under these circumstances has considerable hazards should a necrotizing dose be delivered to a segment of bowel because of puddling of the isotope. The counting chamber will locate such areas during the first survey of the abdomen and alert the gynecologist to the possible complications.

Steps of the Operation

1. If the preoperative diagnosis is clear, the best incision to employ, not only to perform the pri-

mary surgery in the pelvis, but also in anticipation of a total resection of the omentum, is a left rectus incision. When it is decided that the omentum must be removed, the left rectus incision can be extended, if necessary, up to the costal margin (Plate 70, *B*). This allows adequate exposure for the resection of an omental cake that may have attained large proportions.

2. The surgeon begins on the left side by identifying the reflection of the peritoneum that forms the gastrosplenic omentum and the other landmarks shown in Plate 70, *A* and *B*. The spleen and the tail of the pancreas are identified and palpated frequently so that these structures are not inadvertently injured or torn.

3. Kelly clamps are placed just caudad to the gastroepiploic circulation along the greater curvature of the stomach (Plate 70, *C*). Relatively small bites of tissue are taken. The resection proceeds and vessels are tied off periodically to free the field of multiple clamps.

4. The operation is done as expeditiously as possible, since removal of this amount of tissue—grossly enlarged and edematous by virtue of the metastatic deposits contained—is a shocking procedure. The resection is continued from left to right until the region of the foramen of Winslow is reached. This marks the reflection of the anterior leaf of the peritoneum that passes over the pyloric end of the stomach and to the underside of the liver. The surgeon attempts to avoid cutting through solid masses of malignant tissue wherever this is possible. The stomach and the antimesenteric edge of the transverse colon are then inspected for any bleeding and for any areas that may have been denuded. Appropriate repair is made to any surface, and bleeding points are ligated.

References

Aaro, L. A., and Dockerty, M. B.: Leiomyosarcoma of the Uterus, Am. J. Obst. & Gynec. 77: 1187, 1959.

Addington, E., and Betts, R.: Immediate Hysterectomy Following Irradiation for Carcinoma of the Uterine Fundus; a Preliminary Report, Am. J. Roentgenol. 69: 442, 1953.

Anderson, H., and others: Primary Carcinoma of the Fallopian Tube, Obst. & Gynec. 3: 89, 1954.

Andrews, W. C., and Andrews, M. C.: Stein-Leventhal Syndrome With Associated Adenocarcinoma of the Endometrium; Report of a Case in a 22-Year-Old Woman, Am. J. Obst. & Gynec. 80: 632, 1960.

Arneson, A., Standbro, W., and Nolan, J.: The Use of Multiple Sources of Radium Within the Uterus in the Treatment of Endometrial Cancer, Am. J. Obst. & Gynec. 55: 64, 1948.

Ball, T. L., and Javert, C. T.: Fertility and Dysgerminoma Ovarii, J. Clin. Endocrinol. 8: 694, 1948.

Beecham, C. T.: Primary Surgical Treatment of Endometrial Carcinoma, Obst. & Gynec. 10: 230, 1957.

Blaikley, J., and others: Classification and Clinical Staging of Carcinoma of the Uterus; a Proposal for Modification of the Existing International Definitions, Am. J. Obst. & Gynec. 75: 1286, 1958.

Borell, U., Nilsson, O., and Westman, A.: The Cyclical Changes Occurring in the Epithelium Lining the Endometrial Glands, Acta obst. et gynec. scandinav. 38: 364, 1959.

Bromberg, Y. M.: Estrogen-Induced Uterine Cancer, Obst. & Gynec. 14: 221, 1959.

Brunschwig, A., and Murphy, A.: The Rationale for Radical Panhysterectomy and Pelvic Node Excision in Carcinoma of the Corpus Uteri, Am. J. Obst. & Gynec. 68: 1482, 1954.

Bunker, M. L.: The Terminal Findings in Endometrial Carcinoma, Am. J. Obst. & Gynec. 77: 530, 1959.

Cassidy, R. E., Hansford, D. P., and Crawley, R. J.: Random Inguinal Node Biopsy and Peritoneal Fluid Study in Ovarian Cancer, Am. J. Obst. & Gynec. 74: 616, 1957.

Colman, H. I., and Rosenthal, A. H.: Carcinoma Developing in Areas of Adenomyosis, Obst. & Gynec. 14: 342, 1959.

Copenhaver, E.: Atypical Endometrial Hyperplasia, Obst. & Gynec. 13: 264, 1959.

Corscaden, J.: Gynecologic Cancer, New York, 1951, Thos. Nelson & Sons.

Damon, A.: Host Factors in Cancer of the Breast and Uterine Cervix and Corpus, J. Nat. Cancer Inst. 24: 483, 1960.

Doko, F.: Histological Study of Recurrence in Adenocarcinoma of the Corpus Uteri, Am. J. Obst. & Gynec. 78: 180, 1959.

Eichner, E., and Bove, E. R.: In Vivo Studies on the Lymphatic Drainage of the Human Ovary, Obst. & Gynec. 3: 287, 1954.

Farrar, H., and Bryan, R.: Equilateral Distribution of Ovarian Tumors, Am. J. Obst. & Gynec. 80: 1085, 1960.

Faulkner, J. B.: Primary Carcinoma in a Diverticulum of the Female Urethra, J. Urol. 82: 337, 1959.

Garnet, J. D.: Constitutional Stigmas Associated With Endometrial Carcinoma, Am. J. Obst. & Gynec. 76: 11, 1958.

Gribb, J. J.: Hysteroscopy: An Aid in Gynecologic Diagnosis, Obst. & Gynec. 15: 593, 1960.

Gusberg, S. B., and Hall, R. E.: Precursors of Corpus Cancer. III. The Appearance of Cancer of the Endometrium in Estrogenically Conditioned Patients, Obst. & Gynec. 17: 397, 1961.

Hayden, G., and Potter, E.: Primary Carcinoma of the Fallopian Tube, Am. J. Obst. & Gynec. 79: 24, 1960.

Henriksen, E.: The Lymphatic Spread of Carcinoma of the Cervix and of the Body of the Uterus: A Study of 420 Necropsies, Am. J. Obst. & Gynec. 58: 924, 1949.

Hubbard, T.: The Effect of Adrenalectomy on Adenocarcinoma of the Uterus, Cancer 13: 1032, 1960.

Javert, C.: The Spread of Benign and Malignant Endometrium in the Lymphatic System With a Note on Co-Existing Vascular Involvement, Am. J. Obst. & Gynec. 64: 780, 1952.

Javert, C.: Prognosis of Endometrial Cancer, Obst. & Gynec. 12: 556, 1958.

Johansson, H.: Clinical Aspects of Metastatic Ovarian Cancer of Extragenital Origin, Acta obst. et gynec. scandinav. 39: 681, 1960.

Johnson, R. V., and Roddick, J. W.: Incidence of Adenomyosis in Patients With Endometrial Adenocarcinoma; a Study of 100 Patients, Am. J. Obst. & Gynec. 81: 268, 1961.

Kottmeier, H.: Carcinoma of the Female Genitalia, Baltimore, 1953, Williams & Wilkins Co.

Kottmeier, H.: Carcinoma of the Corpus Uteri: Diagnosis and Therapy, Am. J. Obst. & Gynec. 78: 1127, 1959.

Kottmeier, H. L.: Carcinoma of the Corpus Uteri, Am. J. Obst. & Gynec. 78: 1127, 1959.

Latour, J., and Davis, B.: A Critical Assessment of the Value of X-Ray Therapy in Primary Ovarian Carcinoma, Am. J. Obst. & Gynec. 74: 968, 1957.

Lefevre, H.: Node Dissection in Cancer of the Endometrium, Surg., Gynec. & Obst. 102: 649, 1956.

Liu, W.: Correlation Between Vaginal Cytology and Endometrial Histology, Am. J. Obst. & Gynec. 80: 321, 1960.

Lombardo, F. A., and Wood, H. T.: Primary Adenocarcinoma of the Uterine Tube; Report of 6 Cases, Obst. & Gynec. 17: 611, 1961.

McCall, M. L.: The Causes and Significance of Delay in the Management of Adenocarcinoma of the Endometrium; a Review of 683 Proved Cases From the Philadelphia Pelvic Cancer Committee, South. M. J. 50: 17, 1957.

Mc Clure, J. H., and Mengert, W. F.: Experiences With Intra-abdominal Nitrogen Mustard; a Report on 11 Women With Pelvic Malignancy, Am. J. Obst. & Gynec. 77: 676, 1959.

Madden, J. L., and others: The Pathogenesis of Ascites and a Consideration of Its Treatment, Surg., Gynec. & Obst. 99: 385, 1954.

Melander, E., Kullander, S., and Melander, Y.: Chromosome Analysis of a Human Ovarian Cystocarcinoma in the Ascites Form, J. Nat. Cancer Inst. 16: 1067, 1956.

Montgomery, J. B., and others: End Results in Adenocarcinoma of the Endometrium Managed by Preoperative Irradiation, Am. J. Obst. & Gynec. 80: 972, 1960.

Novak, E. R., and Woodruff, J. D.: Postirradiation Malignancies of the Pelvic Organs, Am. J. Obst. & Gynec. 77: 667, 1959.

Parsons, L., and Cesare, F.: Wertheim Hysterectomy in the Treatment of Endometrial Carcinoma, Surg., Gynec. & Obst. 108: 582, 1959.

Roddick, J. W., Jr., and Greene, R. R.: Relation of Ovarian Stromal Hyperplasia to Endometrial Carcinoma, Am. J. Obst. & Gynec. 73: 843, 1957.

Rosenblum, J. M., and Hendricks, C. H.: Estrogenated Vaginal Epithelium; Relationship to the Development of Carcinoma of the Endometrium, Obst. & Gynec. 3: 535, 1954.

Rutledge, F. N., Tan, S. K., and Fletcher, G. H.: Vaginal Metastases From Adenocarcinoma of the Corpus Uteri, Am. J. Obst. & Gynec. 75: 167, 1958.

Scheffey, L., and others: Further Experience in Management and Treatment of Carcinoma of the Fundus of the Uterus, With Five Year End Results in 75 Patients, Am. J. Obst. & Gynec. 46:786, 1943.

Schwartz, A. E., and Brunschwig, A.: Radical Panhysterectomy and Pelvic Node Excision for Carcinoma of the Corpus Uteri, Surg., Gynec. & Obst. 105: 675, 1957.

Sherman, A. I., and Woolf, R. B.: An Endocrine Basis for Endometrial Carcinoma, Obst. & Gynec. 77: 233, 1959.

Swerdlow, M.: Mesothelioma of the Pelvic Peritoneum Resembling Papillary Cystadenocarcinoma of the Ovary, Am. J. Obst. & Gynec. 77: 197, 1959.

Taylor, H., Jr., and Becker, W.: Carcinoma of the Corpus Uteri: End-Results of Treatment in 531 Cases From 1926-1940, Surg., Gynec. & Obst. 84: 129, 1947.

Turner, J. C., ReMine, W. H., and Dockerty, M. B.: A Clinicopathologic Study of 172 Patients With Primary Carcinoma of the Ovary, Surg., Gynec. & Obst. 109: 198, 1959.

Vander, J. B.: The Association of Diabetes Mellitus and Carcinoma of the Endometrium, Obst. & Gynec. 77: 243, 1959.

Waterman, G., Raphael, S., and Moskowsky, W.: Carcinoma of the Uterine Corpus, Am. J. Obst. & Gynec. 64: 1073, 1952.

Way, S.: Vaginal Metastases of Carcinoma of the Body of the Uterus, J. Obst. & Gynaec. Brit. Emp. 58: 558, 1951.

Wetterdal, P.: The Value of Surgery in the Treatment of Carcinoma of the Corpus Uteri, Acta obst. et gynec. scandinav. 38: 717, 1959.

27 · Control of Pain and Comprehensive Care in Gynecologic Cancer

General Considerations

Intractable pain from the spread of residual pelvic cancer is a difficult problem associated with incurable and terminal disease. Pain resulting from the extension of such residual pelvic cancer to the fascia, muscles, ligaments, periosteum, and contiguous structures is poorly localized. Nerve fibers synapse into common paths in the spinal cord, so the sensation of deep pain is diffuse rather than discrete. The pain is projected to all areas of the cord receiving fibers from the general area of invasion of the cancer. Seldom can the stimulus causing deep pain in the pelvis be localized to one cord segment. Pain arising in the parietal structures of the pelvis as well as the viscera may be referred to the back as well as to the extremities. No dependable relationship between the severity of pain and the degree of extension of the cancer exists. The pain threshold is extremely variable among individuals and makes the evaluation of the problem more complex. The gynecologist approaches this problem with orderly thinking. He must first decide whether or not he can gain control over the disease responsible for the pain. If it is not possible to control the disease, he must then decide whether radiation therapy, hormonal therapy, chemical therapy, or other palliative agents may relieve the pain without necessarily interrupting the progress of the disease. The choice of agents to control either the sensation of the pain or the patient's recognition of the stimuli as painful are considered. The surgeon prognosticates the duration of life and decides whether some of the more complex attacks upon the sensation of pain are justified. The method he selects to modify the pain and manage the patient falls into several approaches. It is realized that one or more methods may be used in combination and modified to the individual requirements of the cancer patient.

Analgesics and Combined Therapy With Tranquilizing Drugs

Large doses of chlorpromazine (Thorazine) may relieve the distress of pain, although not the sensibility of pain. In addition to its antiemetic action, this drug appears to potentiate the action of several analgesic drugs. Mephenesin, 0.25 Gm., combined with glutamic acid hydrochloride, 0.30 Gm., for better absorption, relaxes skeletal muscle and is practical, safe, and clinically useful. A total dose of mephenesin of 1 to 3 Gm., orally, may be given in twenty-four hours. In the early cases of residual cancer the nonaddicting drugs, such as aspirin, phenacetin, and antipyrine, are combined with a tranquilizing agent for a moderate analgesic effect. Signs of toxicity to these drugs after prolonged administration may result in anorexia, secondary anemia, changes in the mucous membranes, jaundice, and various skin reactions. The dosage and the combinations used are varied before resorting to the addicting drugs. The administration and dosage are adjusted to the individual patient. The analgesic drugs are given on a regular schedule around the clock; at the same time, a tranquilizing agent is introduced in the therapy. The tranquilizing drugs are started in small doses and are increased as the tolerance to these drugs manifests itself. Thorazine may be added to the analgesic drugs. Begin with 10 mg. every six hours and gradually increase the dose up to 25 mg. Where immediate control of symptoms is desirable without waiting for the results of oral therapy, an initial dose of 25 mg. can be given by deep intramuscular injection and continued on an eight-hour schedule, with gradual replacement by oral administration. Thorazine solution must be injected deep in the intramuscular tissues of the buttock, well diluted in physiologic saline solution. The area of injection should be massaged to reduce local irritation. The analgesics may be combined with a tranquilizing agent such as meprobamate, commonly known as Miltown, Equanil, etc. This preparation is given together with the analgesic drugs in the dosage of 400 mg. every six hours; the dose is increased in large and obese patients by giving 400 mg. every four hours. The withdrawal of the tranquilizing drugs is not a problem to the gynecologist dealing with terminal cancer. Withdrawal of drug therapy used in emotional states is a different problem, and the physician must estimate the psychologic weakness and dependency of each patient on the drug and determine how to cut down the dosage or withdraw therapy entirely without a relapse.

Narcotics and Combined Therapy With Tranquilizing or Potentiating Drugs

The control of chronic pain by the use of analgesics and combined therapy with the tranquilizing or potentiating drugs is limited. Extension of the disease to involve more nerve roots and an increase in the intensity of the pain by invasion of bone and surrounding structures soon necessitate the use of addicting drugs. The tolerance to addicting drugs and the need for increasingly larger doses must be appreciated. Routine orders for a certain dosage schedule should not be left and continued over an extended period of time. Daily re-evaluation of the patient's requirements and the substitution of combinations with other drugs and other measures prolong the usefulness of the

narcotics in managing the chronic pain of cancer. It must be appreciated that each narcotic has an optimum dose where the maximum relief of pain is achieved. These critical doses for the commonly used addicting drugs are as follows: codeine, 65 mg.; meperidine hydrochloride (Demerol), 150 mg., and morphine sulfate, 30 mg. Above these doses the resultant analgesic effect of the drugs is not appreciably increased, whereas the side effects become bothersome. Until tolerance develops, the surgeon uses the smallest amount of a mild addicting drug that gives relief. He progresses to the more powerful narcotics when the previous agent fails to control the patient's pain.

When narcotics are indicated, codeine phosphate 65 mg. by mouth together with a tranquilizing agent, such as meprobamate 200 mg. can be given on a four- to six-hour schedule. The dosage of meprobamate can be increased up to 400 mg. if it seems to potentiate the effect of the codeine. Drug therapy is supplemented with simple nursing procedures, such as hot or cold applications to the affected area. Combinations of a narcotic and a barbiturate are useful.

When the less potent narcotics fail to give relief, Demerol in a dosage of 50 to 150 mg. orally and morphine sulfate in a dosage of 10 to 30 mg. hypodermically are prescribed. These potent narcotics can be combined with a tranquilizing or potentiating drug and regulated to the individual patient. Chlorpromazine (Thorazine) is a useful supplementary agent, particularly when nausea and vomiting are present, either as a result of advanced cancer or from the administration of the narcotic. Chlorpromazine can be given on an increasing dosage schedule up to 25 mg. orally every four hours. For more immediate control of nausea and vomiting, the drug can be given intramuscularly in dosages as high as 50 mg. every four hours during an acute episode. Dihydromorphinone (Dilaudid) is somewhat more effective orally than morphine and is given in a 2 to 3 mg. dose. The subcutaneous dose is 2 mg. Its action is of shorter duration than morphine but is more potent. 6-Methyldihydromorphinone

504

(Metopon) is given orally in a 3 mg. capsule and has approximately the same analgesic effect as morphine. Methadone is a synthetic, morphinelike agent. It is given in the usual dose of 10 mg. orally and in smaller amounts subcutaneously or intramuscularly. Its depressive toxic effects are similar to those of morphine, with the same undesirable effects such as vertigo, nausea, and vomiting. Levorphan (Levo-Dromoran) is an extremely potent opiate given on a weight basis, with a subcutaneous injection of 2 mg. producing an analgesic effect equal to approximately 10 mg. of morphine. It has a longer action, but it is a respiratory depressant the same as morphine. Alphaprodine (Nisentil) is another synthetic opiate that is less potent than morphine on a weight basis. It seems to be equally effective orally or by any parenteral route. A subcutaneous dose of 20 mg. will produce approximately the same relief of pain as 10 mg. of morphine. Larger doses of alphaprodine are possible—up to 40 or 60 mg.—without the marked respiratory depression following the administration of most agents.

With the skillful use of these drugs, much of the patient's discomfort can be controlled. At the same time other measures of palliation are instituted.

Nerve Block and Neurosurgery for Control of Intractable Pain in Pelvic Cancer

With the exception of the ovaries, the female genital organs are situated in the midline. Cancer arising from the vulva, vagina, cervix, or fundus of the uterus involves organs with a bilateral innervation, and the pain emanating from the dissemination of these cancers may be referred to both sides. In addition, the malignancies arising in the female genital organs are in close proximity to the lumbosacral plexus, which contains the nerve supply to both lower extremities. The use of nerve blocks to interrupt pathways to the female genital organs may interfere with the nerve supply of the lower extremities. Nerve blocks may be attempted, but, when pain is uncontrolled by every other means, a surgical interruption of

the pain pathways in the spinal cord or higher up in the central nervous system is indicated.

Pain referred to surface areas in the pelvis unfortunately does not develop uniformly and seldom in any pattern that permits local injection of trigger points or surface treatment to a trigger area. Invasion of the myofascial layers of the skeletal muscles within the pelvis undoubtedly causes pain like skeletal muscle pain elsewhere. However, it is difficult to localize such pain and to inject a specific area. The involvement of the bladder and rectum provokes pain and further complicates the interruption of the nerve pathways. Pressure on the external iliac artery and vein can cause a disturbance of the blood supply to the extremity, with resultant pain that is difficult to control. Involvement of the periosteum and bony pelvis gives pain that is poorly localized and may be referred to distant sites. After having explored a pelvic malignancy in which the extent of the disease does not permit an exenteration type operation, resection of certain nerve groups that may afford some relief may be done. Extension of the malignancy to the pelvic side wall causes irritation of the obturator nerve from fibrosis or infection. An obturator neurectomy is a simple procedure and may relieve discomfort along the distribution of the sensory fibers. A presacral neurectomy reduces midline pain. The uterosacral ligaments and the infundibulopelvic ligaments may be resected, with the interruption of some nerve fibers.

A lumbar, paravertebral, or sympathetic block may help some patients. Pain emanating from the cervix or vagina and involving the rectum and nerve routes in the hollow of the sacrum may be affected little by this procedure. It is worth a trial, however, and any obstetrician and gynecologist familiar with the technique of paravertebral block in labor and delivery may employ such a procedure with a local anesthetic. After achieving an effective lumbar block, indicated by warmth in the corresponding leg, a solution of absolute alcohol or 6 per cent phenol can be considered for a prolonged effect on the sensory fibers involved. Surgical interruption of the sensory channels in the cord or

505

a surgical leukotomy may be advisable if there is a life expectancy of three months or more. However, if the patient is in the terminal stage of illness, extensive neurosurgical procedures are contraindicated. In these patients one may consider the intrathecal injection of alcohol, the injection of phenol in glycerin as a 6 per cent solution, or the injection of other destructive agents that may produce a permanent anesthesia. Many of these patients may already be without bladder or rectal control and be bedridden. They may have had an exenteration, and a colostomy or ureterointestinal or ureterocutaneous transplants will have eliminated the necessity for any sphincter control.

The effects on the lower extremities need only be considered. Again, the distribution of the pain of pelvic origin determines the site of injection. Pain along the distribution of the obturator and femoral nerves in the groin and lower extremities requires intrathecal injection as high as the twelfth dorsal or first lumbar interspaces. Pain along the distribution of the sciatic nerve requires injection in the second or third lumbar interspace, with the solution permitted to flow caudad to interrupt other sensory channels. Deep sacral pain requires the injection in the fifth lumbar or first sacral interspace, and the solution is allowed to gravitate so as to have an effect upon the lower sacral nerve roots.

Cordotomy provides excellent relief of pain in pelvic cancer, since it can be done below the upper thoracic segments of the cord and be performed bilaterally. The spinothalamic tracts are interrupted by a tractotomy in the upper thoracic segments or cervical cord, where they are most constant in position and more certain to give a high level of analgesia. The complications of bladder and rectal sphincter disturbances, paresthesia and analgesia of the legs, and hypotension may be reduced by doing the operation in two stages. Occasionally the pain is completely unilateral so the opposite side of the cord above the white commissure need only be interrupted. More often the development of pain on the other side indicates that a bilateral operation has to be done.

The employment of unilateral frontal leukotomy or bilateral medial frontal quadrant section in patients in the terminal stage must be reevaluated in view of the possible chemical leukotomy that may be induced by large doses of the tranquilizing and potentiating drugs. The employment of hypophysectomy in the treatment of advanced gynecologic cancer involves hormonal palliation, although it is a neurologic procedure. The hormonal and chemical palliation of pelvic cancer is discussed in Chapter 21 (page 378) and Chapter 23 (page 398).

Palliative Surgery and Radiation in Gynecologic Cancer

Palliative surgery in the treatment of female genital cancer involves a primary attack upon the site of the lesion or the use of surgery to remove recurrent or persistent malignant disease in or about the primary site. The most common cancer of the female genital organs is that of the cervix. Since this tends to remain largely localized in approximately 40 per cent of patients without presenting extrapelvic metastatic lesions, a block dissection, including the removal of the rectum and bladder, has produced an occasional cure and reduced the pain and suffering of many patients. My feelings and indications for the various exenteration procedures has been expressed before and are determined solely on the patient's comfort and possibility of cure of the disease. Exenterations are mutilating procedures, and unless they promise the patient a reasonable survival without pain and other inconveniences, the operations are not indicated. If the patient is faced with a life complicated by multiple fistulas of the bladder and rectum, plus a sloughing, bleeding lesion in the pelvis, the terminal period is probably more comfortable with a colostomy and some type of ureteral transplants that are, at least, manageable. Excision of recurrent lesions in the vagina or vulva may make the patient more comfortable during her terminal illness and relieve distressing pain, discharge, and odor.

Palliative radiation of malignancies within

the pelvis, even with the use of supervoltage sources, seldom makes the patient's terminal illness more tolerable. Recurrent cancer is a misnomer when applied to the same site— residual cancer with subsequent spread is what is meant. Since the patient has usually been subjected to all of the mechanical, chemical, and radiologic means to obstruct the spread of malignant cells, the use of further radiation is seldom indicated. The employment of radioactive isotopes, as well as other isotopes under investigation, to reduce the ascites associated with abdominal carcinomatosis is discussed in Chapter 22 (page 391).

Comprehensive Care for the Cancer Patient

Cornell University Medical College has instituted a comprehensive care and training program designed to make the student more familiar with the relationship of a person to his environment and the modification of this relationship that takes place during serious illness. The principles of such care that heretofore have been learned after years of private practice or after apprenticeship to an older physician are essential in the management of the cancer patient who must be returned to her home environment. Training in the management of a colostomy or diversion of the urinary stream, management of the skin or other areas that have been radiated, and the restoration of normal nutrition can be taught to some extent in the hospital with its enormous facilities. An entirely different situation exists when the patient must be returned to her home environment and cared for by some member of the family without medical training. Many patients develop an abnormal dependence upon the hospital and physicians if a comprehensive plan for home care is not developed before the patient is discharged.

The rehabilitation of the cancer patient starts immediately after definitive therapy and depends, to some extent, upon the agencies available in the community that may supplement her care by her family. In some communities the church or some charitable organization may be the only institution available to support the patient. In other communities extensive health facilities are available, including emergency doctor call services, dressings, hormones, practical nurse services, blood transfusions, transportation to and from the hospital for revisits, services of medical students studying courses in comprehensive family care, and many other special facilities that can be integrated to support the patient during a long-term illness. Arrangements for comprehensive care are started in the hospital so the patient realizes that many agencies and individuals, in addition to her family, will give her support and share the burden of her illness. This sharing of the patient's dependency by a variety of people and organizations will foster new strength within many individuals, relieve anxiety, and prevent invalidism and deterioration of the patient who becomes insecure.

References

David, N., Semler, H., and Burgner, P.: Control of Chronic Pain by DL-Alpha Acetylmethadol, J. A. M. A. 161: 599, 1956.

Dripps, R. D., Millar, R. A., and Kneale, D. H.: A Comparison of Anileridine, Morphine, and Meperidine in Man, Surg., Gynec. & Obst. 103: 322, 1957.

Goldfarb, A. F., and Stone, M. L.: A Total Care Program for Advanced Pelvic Malignancy, Am. J. Obst. & Gynec. 77: 206, 1959.

Guerriero, W., and Stuart, J.: Pelvic Pain of Gynecic or Other Origin, Am. J. Obst. & Gynec. 67: 1265, 1954.

Hay, R. C., Yonezawa, T., and Derrick, W. S.: Control of Intractable Pain in Advanced Cancer by Subarachnoid Alcohol Block, J. A. M. A. 169: 1315, 1959.

Luft, R., and Olivecrona, H.: Hypophysectomy in the Management of Neoplastic Disease; the Ludwig Kast Lecture, Bull. New York Acad. Med. 33: 5, 1957.

Lundy, J. S.: Available New Drugs for Systemic Control of Previously Difficult Pain Problems, J. A. M. A. 163: 1455, 1957.

Miller, N. F.: Terminal Care for the Gynecologic Cancer Patient (After Office Hours), Obst. & Gynec. 4: 470, 1954.

Nolan, R., and Peyton, W.: Cordotomy for Relief of Pain in Incurable Squamous-cell Carcinoma of the Cervix Uteri, Am. J. Obst. & Gynec. 71: 790, 1956.

Pearson, O., Ray, B., Harrold, C., West, C., MacLean, J., and Lipsett, M.: Hypophysectomy in Treatment of Advanced Cancer, J. A. M. A. 161: 17, 1956.

Perese, D.: How to Manage Pain in Malignant Disease, J. A. M. A. 175: 75, 1961.

Raven, R.: Rehabilitation of Patients After Treatment for Cancer, Brit. J. Phys. Med. 18: 35, 1955.

Roberts, E.: A New Approach to Nighttime Sedation, Am. J. M. Sc. 227: 609, 1954.

Sadove, M., and others: Chlorpromazine and Narcotics in the Management of Pain of Malignant Lesions, J. A. M. A. 65: 626, 1954.

Schiffrin, M. J. (editor): The Management of Pain in Cancer, Chicago, 1956, Year Book Publishers, Inc.

Schulman, C.: Home Care of Cancer Patients, J. A. M. A. 173: 1530, 1960.

Selling, L.: A Clinical Study of Miltown, a New Tranquilizing Agent, J. Clin. & Exper. Psychopath. 17: 7, 1956.

Smith, R.: Environmental Support in Long-Term Illness, J. A. M. A. 161: 836, 1956.

Sutherland, A. M.: Psychologic Barriers to Rehabilitation of Cancer Patients, Postgrad. Med. 17: 523, 1955.

Sutherland, A. M.: The Psychological Impact of Postoperative Cancer, Bull. New York Acad. Med. 33: 428, 1957.

Turnbull, F.: The Nature of Pain in the Late Stages of Cancer, Surg., Gynec. & Obst. 110: 665, 1960.

28 · Penetrating, Straddle, Coital, and Foreign Body Injuries

PENETRATING AND STRADDLE WOUNDS OF THE BLADDER, VAGINA, VULVA, AND RECTUM
Etiology and Pathologic Anatomy

Wounds of the vulva and perineum are rare because of the protection afforded the area. Excluding trauma caused by abortions, coitus, and parturition, the most common cause of penetrating wounds is impalement upon some sharp object. In young children injuries occur as a result of climbing fences or falling on rakes or garden tools or various toys. Lacerations and hematomas have been reported after kicks to the labia or falling in the bathtub.

Classification of Vaginal Injuries

I. Trauma to the vagina during infancy and childhood
   A. Foreign bodies (safety pins, crayons, pencils, coins, glass rods, toys, or parts of toys, etc.)
   B. Impalement injuries (fences, toys, bicycles, trees, garden tools, etc.)
   C. Rape lacerations
   D. Masturbation injuries
II. Injuries of the vagina from accidents, missiles, sexual aberrations, and foreign bodies after surgery
   A. Automobile injuries and straddle wounds
   B. Gunshot, war, missiles, and other objects
   C. Neglected pessaries
   D. Forceful coitus and rape

E. Sexual aberrations and masturbation injuries
F. Sexual excesses in prostitutes
G. Foreign bodies (needles, sponges, instruments, etc.)
III. Chemical injuries of the vagina
   A. Allergic reactions to bases for vaginal creams
   B. Irritative, infective pastes, solutions, or tablets to induce abortion or as emergency substitutes for standard contraception
      1. Permanganate, cresol, Lysol, other chemicals, and strong oxidizing agents
IV. Radiation injuries of the vagina
   A. Classification as to the source
      1. Deep roentgen ray injuries (super, high, medium, or low voltage)
         (a) External radiation reactions
         (b) Vaginal cone injuries
         (c) Perineal port reactions
      2. Gamma ray injuries (radium, radon, cobalt[60], iridium[192])
         (a) Intracavitary sources
         (b) Interstitial sources
         (c) Vaginal colpostats
      3. Isotope injuries (radioactive gold[198])
         (a) Interstitial radiation
         (b) Secondary to intraperitoneal isotope therapy
   B. Classification as to nature of injury
      1. Early injuries
         (a) Acute radiation vaginitis, partially reversible (usually with concomitant reactions in the bladder and rectum)
         (b) Early, progressive, irreversible, radiation injuries (usually associated

with advanced or persistant cancer of or involving the vagina)

2. Late injuries
   (a) Slowly progressive, late changes, without fistula formation (occlusion of vessels, ischemia, telangiectasia, contracture, loss of pliability or complete vaginal closure)
   (b) Progressive late changes with fistulas (ulceration of bladder and rectum with inevitable fistula formation)

V. Surgical injuries of the vagina
   A. Vault dehiscence after simple total hysterectomy
   B. Vault dehiscence after radical abdominal or radical vaginal hysterectomy
   C. Vaginal, bladder, and rectal injuries from constricting sutures

VI. Abortion wounds of the vagina
   A. Self-inflicted
      1. Radio-opaque objects
         (a) Crochet hooks, hat pins, hair pins, bobby pins, metal syringe tips, umbrella ribs, metal catheters, brass and iron wires, metal knitting needles, etc.
      2. Not radio-opaque
         (a) Rubber catheters, woven urethral catheters, knitting needles, slippery elm bark, rubber or wood penholders, pencils, glass catheters, glass drinking tubes, celluloid or plastic bobby pins, earpiece of shell rim glasses, cocktail stirrers, douche and enema nozzles, feathers, stalks of diverse plants, etc.
   B. Inflicted by abortionist
      1. Instrumental
         (a) Curettes, packing forceps, ovum forceps, needles, tenaculi, etc.
      2. Injected solutions
         (a) Iodine, mercurochrome, various oils, etc.

Symptoms and Diagnosis

The symptoms depend on the extent of the lesion and whether or not there is copious bleeding. Lesions of the bladder have the characteristic symptom of the escape of large amount of urine into the peritoneal cavity or retroperitoneally. Involvement of the rectum is marked by the escape of gas and fecal material. The diagnosis is made by inspection and by determining the course of the wound. The perineum, by definition, is a lozenge-shaped area that includes all of the structures of the pelvic outlet. It is bounded anteriorly by the inferior pubic rami and the arcuate ligament of the pubis, laterally by the ischium and the ischial tuberosities, and posteriorly by the coccyx and sacrotuberous ligaments. The wound may occupy only one portion of this area, or it may involve several sites. It may be confined to the urogenital region anteriorly, with lacerations of the vulva, urethra and bladder. The wound may primarily involve the anus or the anus and the ischiorectal fossa. Deeper and more severe wounds penetrate the pelvis and peritoneal cavity. Proctosigmoidoscopy, cystoscopy, catheterization of the ureters, urinalysis, and cultures are done to confirm the extent of the lesion.

Surgical Principles and Treatment

In the urogenital region, lacerations of the urethra are repaired in layers with 0000 atraumatic catgut. If necessary, a vaginal or suprapubic cystostomy is done to divert the urinary stream. Wounds extending into the anal region are repaired to reapproximate and restore the function of the sphincters. Drainage of the perianal space is indicated. For severe lacerations about the rectum and rectal sphincters a temporary colostomy is indicated. Wounds lateral to the anus that involve the ischiorectal region are débrided, cleaned, and repaired and require drainage. Lacerations of the vagina are repaired in layers with careful attention to hemostasis. A large hematoma can form in the paracolpium and extend into the pelvis between the sheaths of the broad ligament. If it is not clear whether the wound has penetrated into the pelvic cavity, the abdomen is explored. If the wound has not extended through the pelvic peritoneum, the retroperitoneal portion of the rectosigmoid may still be investigated by incision of the lateral and medial reflections of the peritoneum. Foreign bodies or fragments of the object that was responsible are removed. Extensive injuries to the bladder and ureters may have to be approached from the abdominal aspect. Wounds of the vagina are observed closely during the healing process since contractures of the vagina or cervix influence the function of menstruation and childbearing. Dilators are used to maintain the normal contour and pliability of the vagina.

VULVOVAGINAL INJURIES DUE TO COITUS
Etiology and Pathologic Anatomy

Vaginal injuries during coitus have been attributed to excessive sexual excitement, disproportion between the size of the male and female organs, abnormal positions of the uterus, spasm of the muscles of the pelvic floor, scars from previous vaginal surgery, senile changes in the vaginal vault, and a long abstinence from coitus and intercourse during the puerperium. Since vulvovaginal injuries resulting from rape are seldom the subject of case reports in the literature, it is not known how many such lacerations occur in proportion to those from the causes listed above. A state of virginity is not important in the etiology of these injuries, excluding, of course, the simple laceration of the hymen that may take place during the first sexual experience. Serious lacerations have been reported in prostitutes after many consecutive sexual acts in a short period. The injuries most frequently involve longitudinal lacerations of the posterior vaginal vault, since the posterior fornix of the vagina is the area that must accommodate the penis in the sexual act. Less frequently the lesions involve the vulva, the rectum, the anterior vaginal wall or the bladder.

Symptoms and Diagnosis

The patient may experience moderately severe sudden pain during intercourse, followed by vaginal bleeding. If the hemorrhage is profuse, shock ensues, with the patient showing the characteristic symptoms. Smaller lacerations are painful and are not infrequently seen in newlyweds; bleeding may be minimal and the only symptom pain on intercourse.

Treatment and Surgical Principles

Treatment consists of combating shock if the bleeding is severe, with subsequent suture of the laceration. The bladder and rectum are carefully investigated for injuries. Abstinence from intercourse and subsequent instruction of both husband and wife will usually suffice in the management of the small superficial lacerations. The severe lacerations require surgery and antibiotic therapy to prevent infection and undesirable sequelae.

FOREIGN BODIES LEFT IN THE PELVIS
General Considerations

Sponges, laparotomy pads, needles, and instruments will continue to be accidentally left in the chest, abdomen, and pelvis despite every known precaution and method of accounting for all objects in the operating room. The method of marking sponges with a radiopaque wire and tagging other objects that are not visualized on x-ray may not reduce the number of these accidents, but it will facilitate the diagnosis and localization after the patient shows the signs and symptoms of the presence of a foreign body. When in doubt, the surgeon should immediately begin all diagnostic procedures that will confirm or disprove the presence of a foreign body. These tests include x-rays of various types, studies to determine the presence or absence of obstructive symptoms to the bowel, and the probing of sinuses and wounds that fail to heal in the expected length of time. The medicolegal aspects of such an accident are far reaching, and many lawsuits can be avoided if the surgeon uses good judgment. The laws and outcome of lawsuits in the different states vary widely, and it is difficult to make generalizations. Some obvious rules to be followed that are applicable anywhere, since they represent the best medical ethics, are as follows: (1) The patient, or closest relative if the patient is too ill, is notified as soon as the complication is diagnosed. (2) The circumstances and reasons why this might have occurred are explained. (3) The steps that the surgeon intends to take to correct the condition are outlined to the patient or relative. (4) One or more consultants are obtained to confirm the steps the surgeon takes and to use their special skills to meet the situation. (5) The appropriate hospital authorities and the surgeon's insurance carrier are notified. (6) All possible preparations and tests are performed so the patient is in the best possible condition for reoperation. Careful and accurate notes indicating everything that is done and the time it is done are recorded. With this honest and straightforward approach, many patients accept the complication without animosity toward the surgeon. The surgeon can do much by his attentiveness and thoroughness to overcome the depressive features that occur to a patient requiring further surgery for foreign body complications.

Gynecologic surgeons are able to remove accessible foreign bodies through a posterior colpotomy. This may avoid a laparotomy if the patient has had an abdominal operation. There is little to lose by attempting removal by the vaginal approach. After a total hysterectomy the vault can be reopened from below, with the possibility that the foreign body may be retrieved. Serious bleeding may have occurred during the primary operation in which the foreign body was inadvertently left behind. Since the operative area where the object is likely to be found was a source of bleeding during the primary operation, adequate measures for blood replacement are made available. These accidents are regrettable, but their effect, both immediately and subsequently, should the patient demand compensation through the courts, can be minimized by attention to every detail of good surgical practice and avoidance of the temptation to conceal the facts that are easily brought out by even the simplest investigation.

PENETRATING WOUNDS OF THE PREGNANT UTERUS AND FETUS
General Considerations

The presence of the pregnant uterus modifies the type of injury that is sustained from objects penetrating the abdominal wall and perineum. The pregnant uterus affords protection to the other viscera and displaces the abdominal and pelvic contents to somewhat different locations, depending on the duration of the pregnancy. Many pregnant women were injured by bullets, shrapnel, and other objects capable of inflicting a penetrating wound during the last two conflicts, where attacks upon military targets in the vicinity of large cities were commonplace. It is expected that many more such accidents would happen in any future conflict, since it would not be possible, at least in the early stages of an attack, to single out pregnant women for evacuation.

Etiology and Pathologic Anatomy

In civilian accidents the most common penetrating object is an accidentally discharged bullet. The accidents occurring during the bombing of large cities place secondary objects in motion by the explosion. The change in the position of the peritoneal reflections of the bladder, uterus, and bowel in the various months of pregnancy is the most important factor in determining the type of injury. The protection given to other abdominal organs by the pregnant uterus and fetus varies with the duration of pregnancy, and organs that are ordinarily vulnerable to penetrating wounds of the abdomen are less so in the presence of a term pregnancy. Plate 71 shows some of the common wounds that may occur with the fetus at term. The bowel is crowded into the upper abdomen at this time, and a penetrating wound entering above the fundus might be expected to penetrate several loops of bowel. Perforations of the bowel, whether in the presence of a pregnancy or not, tend to occur in multiples of two. This fact should be remembered in exploring the abdomen after accidents, since fragments passing through a segment of bowel have a wound of entrance and a wound of exit. The fragment may pass through the bowel and the uterine wall to lodge in the placenta. This may cause a premature separation of the placenta, with concealed bleeding. The fragment may enter the

PLATE 71

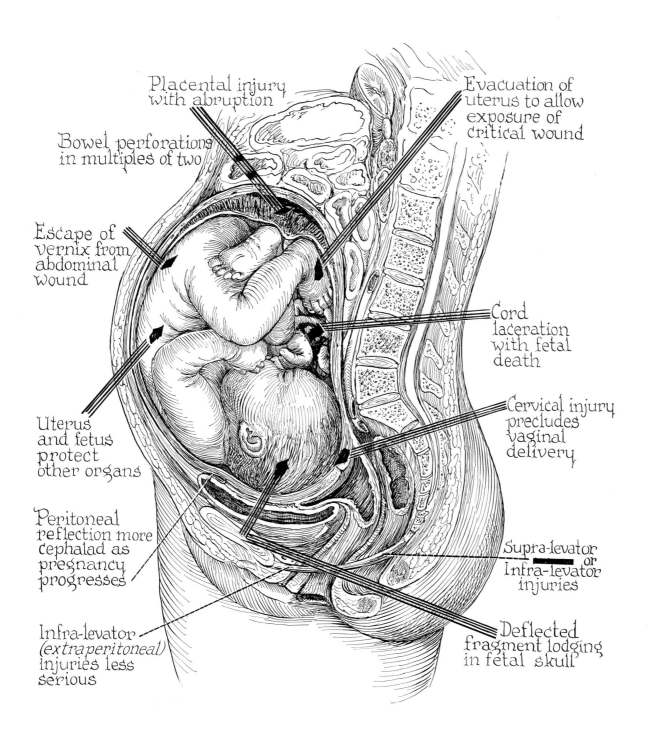

Placental injury
with abruption

Bowel perforations
in multiples of two

Escape of
vernix from
abdominal
wound

Uterus
and fetus
protect
other organs

Peritoneal
reflection more
cephalad as
pregnancy
progresses

Infra-levator
(extraperitoneal)
injuries less
serious

Evacuation of
uterus to allow
exposure of
critical wound

Cord
laceration
with fetal
death

Cervical injury
precludes
vaginal
delivery

Supra-levator
or
Infra-levator
injuries

Deflected
fragment lodging
in fetal skull

uterus and cause a laceration of the cord, with death of the fetus. The deflection of fragments from bony structures within the pelvis, with the creation of secondary fragments of bone, causes many bizarre wounds. Wounds from missiles in which the entrance is in the perineum are less serious if they are below the levator muscle (Plate 71). The possible course of these missiles is determined to decide whether supralevator or infralevator injuries or a combination of both have occurred. Lacerations of the cervix and vagina occur and may preclude vaginal delivery. There is almost an unlimited combination of wounds that may occur in addition to those injuries sustained by the fetus. In assessing the probable damage, the surgeon constantly keeps in mind the change in the peritoneal reflection and the position of the fetus, placenta, and abdominal and pelvic viscera at the various weeks of pregnancy. Despite the apparent vulnerability of the fetus and pregnant mother to such penetrating wounds, the number of case reports is relatively small and the survival rate is reasonably good. There are no statistical studies available to suggest the number of casualties that may be anticipated among pregnant women during a mass attack. They have undoubtedly occurred in considerable numbers, but seldom, under wartime conditions, does the physician stop to analyze the individual factors resulting from the pregnancy that may have influenced the type of wounds observed.

Symptoms and Diagnosis

The wounds of entrance and exit are noted on all parts of the chest, abdomen, and perineum. The wound of entrance is usually smaller than the wound of exit and may be further identified by threads of cloth or grease from the object along the edges of the entrance hole. Amniotic fluid, as well as vernix, may escape from the abdominal wound, and this confirms a perforation of the uterine wall. The passage of meconium in the abdominal wound suggests severe injury, with death of the fetus or severe injuries to the fetus itself. If x-ray facilities are available, the fetus and placental site are studied to locate objects or bullets that may have lodged in either the fetus or placenta. Fragments of shrapnel and other objects have been passed in the lochia after penetrating wounds of the pregnant uterus and subsequent delivery. Injuries to other organs in conjunction with the pregnant uterus may not show the characteristic signs and symptoms seen in the nonpregnant state due to their displacement and the added confusing factors resulting from injury to the pregnant uterus or fetus. Many injuries are not diagnosed until the uterus is emptied and an exploratory laparotomy performed.

Surgical Principles

The surgical principles in dealing with penetrating wounds during pregnancy are discussed under four headings: (1) abdominal injuries involving the pregnant uterus with the fetus alive and viable, (2) abdominal injury not affecting the pregnant uterus with the fetus alive and viable, (3) abdominal injuries that have a favorable prognosis but with a fetus that is premature or not viable, and (4) abdominal or perineal injuries with no involvement of the uterus itself in which labor is either in progress or imminent. There are many other possible situations, each of which must be evaluated individually. If the fetus is alive and viable, the abdominal injuries are repaired, usually after evacuation of the uterus by cesarean section. The obstetrician decides at this time whether a Porro section or a section hysterectomy should be done, depending on the extent of the damage to the uterus. The judgment of the obstetrician in this decision will be the result of his many years of experience and skill in determining the future capabilities of the uterus and the possible complications that would result from its retention. Injuries that do not affect the uterus, in which the fetus is alive and viable, are managed by evacuating the uterus to facilitate the repair of other organs. In exceptional cases the pregnant uterus is removed to manage wounds in the pelvis in which the presence of the recently evacuated uterus causes technical difficulties. The presence of a premature fetus and an abdominal injury with a favorable prognosis again requires the skill and judgment of the obstetrician to decide whether or not the pregnancy can be allowed to continue or whether the uterus must be evacuated and the fetus lost. Many factors will enter into the final decision, but, if it appears that the patient is going into premature labor, the most conservative course would be to evacuate the uterus at the time of abdominal surgery. If study of the abdominal wounds and uterus indicates that the prognosis is just as favorable with the uterus remaining, the uterus is left and measures are taken to prevent premature labor. Subsequently the patient can be expected to deliver vaginally provided there are no injuries to the perineum or vagina that would contraindicate this method of delivery. The problem of managing abdominal injuries while labor is in progress requires the nicety of judgment as to the mode of delivery. Abdominal hemorrhage or perforation of the bowel or other vital organs cannot wait the termination of labor and a vaginal delivery. A cesarean section is done and uterine contractions are stopped by a general anesthetic, regardless of the cervical dilatation. If delivery is imminent, one might be faced with the problem of delivering the infant vaginally and immediately proceeding with a laparotomy for multiple abdominal injuries that may not have seriously affected the uterus.

Prognosis

Some of the factors influencing the outcome of the patient with a perforating wound of the abdomen in the presence of a pregnant uterus are as follows: the greater the number of perforations and the greater the length of time between injury and treatment, the higher the mortality; the further the pregnancy is advanced, and therefore occupying more space, the greater is the chance of uterine injury. The contractility of the uterine musculature, however, permits severe lacerations without exsanguinating the patient. Experience in labor

with a previously myomectomized uterus has taught us that the organ need seldom be sacrificed for any lacerations caused by perforating objects. The age of the patient is a consideration. Older gravidas do not tolerate abdominal wounds as well as younger patients because of arteriosclerotic changes in the vessel walls that prevent vasoconstriction. The location of wounds in the abdominal viscera is an important factor. A tear in the left colon, with the escape of formed fecal material, does not produce the dramatic symptoms of a lacerated stomach, with the escape of a large quantity of gastric contents. It likewise does not produce symptoms as soon as lesions of the small bowel, with pouring of liquid contents into the peritoneal cavity. Lack of symptoms due to the escape of formed fecal material may delay surgery, and time is a factor in the ultimate prognosis. In reviewing many of these injuries, one cannot help but be impressed with the remarkably safe locale the fetus occupies in utero, compared with the rest of us on the outside.

RUPTURE OF THE PREGNANT UTERUS BY EXTERNAL VIOLENCE

Rupture of the pregnant uterus by external violence, such as automobile accidents, falls, and crushing injuries from other accidents, is quite uncommon despite the large number of pregnant women exposed to these possibilities. The patients usually show a laceration or contusion of the abdominal wall. The signs of primary shock, loss of fetal heartbeat, and a tetanic contraction of the uterus indicate an intra-abdominal and uterine catastrophe. Examination of the abdomen reveals the tender uterus and suggestive signs of intra-abdominal hemorrhage. The pulse rate continues to rise, while the blood pressure falls, and immediate preparations must be made to combat shock and prepare the patient for operation. Treatment consists of a laparotomy, with the decision as to the preservation of the uterus being made by the obstetrician for each individual case. The fetus is frequently lost, and the placenta and fetus may be found free in the abdominal cavity. After expulsion of the fetus into the peritoneal cavity, the uterus contracts down around the point of rupture and serious hemorrhage is less likely to occur. The obstetrician decides whether the uterus can be preserved as a functional organ. If so, the rent in the uterus is repaired in layers, and systematic examination of all of the pelvic and abdominal viscera is done to exclude injury to any other organs.

References

Armstrong, C. L., and Andreson, P. S.: Metallic Intrauterine Foreign Body in Term Pregnancy, Am. J. Obst. & Gynec. **78**: 442, 1959.

Beattie, J., and Daly, R.: Gunshot Wound of the Pregnant Uterus, Am. J. Obst. & Gynec. **80**: 772, 1960.

Belkap, R.: Gunshot Wound of the Pregnant Uterus, J. Maine M. A. **30**: 13, 1939.

Black, B.: Surgical Treatment With Recovery in a Case of Perineo-Abdominal Shotgun Wounds From Close Range With Multiple Injuries to Viscera, S. Clin. North America **24**: 952, 1944.

Bowles, H.: Laceration of Vaginal Vault at Coitus, Proc. Staff Meet. Clin., Honolulu **8**: 35, 1942.

Carciotto, S.: Vulvovaginal Laceration Due to Coitus in a Woman Who Remained a Virgin, Rassegna d'ostet. e ginec. **49**: 96, 1940.

Conger, S., and Paternite, C.: Massive Intra-Abdominal Hemorrhage From Utero-Ovarian Vein Rupture Following Delivery, Am. J. Obst. & Gynec. **67**: 426, 1954.

Cushman, G., and Kilgore, A.: The Syndrome of Mesenteric or Subperitoneal Hemorrhage (Abdominal Apoplexy), Ann. Surg. **114**: 672, 1941.

Echerling, B.: Obstetrical Approach to Abdominal War Wounds Late in Pregnancy, J. Obst. & Gynaec. Brit. Emp. **57**: 747, 1950.

Elias, M.: Rupture of the Pregnant Uterus by External Violence, Lancet **2**: 253, 1950.

Flamrich, E.: Gunshot Wounds of the Pregnant Uterus, Zentralbl. Gynäk. **65**: 25, 1941.

Fowler, R.: Gunshot Wounds of the Pregnant Uterus, New York J. Med. **11**: 525-527, 1911.

Giuffrida, F.: A Singular Genital Lesion From Coitus, Clin. ostet. **42**: 123, 1940.

Goodman, J.: Management of Diabetes Mellitus During Keto-Acidosis, Acute Infection, and Surgery, J. A. M. A. **159**: 831, 1955.

Gourlay, N.: Accidental Rupture of the Female Urethra, J. Obst. & Gynaec. Brit. Emp. **67**: 991, 1960.

Griswold, R., and Collier, H.: Perineal, Anal and Rectal Injuries in Civilian Practice, S. Clin. North America **35**: 1431, 1955.

Helsper, J.: Nonperforating Wounds of the Abdomen, Am. J. Surg. **90**: 580, 1955.

Hinrichs, F.: Vaginal Injuries, Monatsschr. Geburtsh. u. Gynäk. **94**: 240, 1933.

Hodgkinson, C., and Christensen, R.: Hemorrhage From Ruptured Utero-Ovarian Veins During Pregnancy, Am. J. Obst. & Gynec. **59**: 112, 1950.

Holters, O., and Daversa, B.: Bullet Wound of a Gravid Uterus With Intestinal Perforation, Am. J. Obst. & Gynec. **56**: 985-86, 1948.

Holzapfel, K.: Closure of the Vulva Due to a Burn, Monatsschr. Geburtsh. u. Gynäk. **97**: 89, 1934.

Hudock, J., Dupayne, N., and McGeary, J.: Traumatic Vulvar Hematomas, Am. J. Obst. & Gynec. **70**: 1064, 1955.

Jacobus, W.: Gunshot Wound of the Gravid Uterus, Am. J. Obst. & Gynec. **63**: 687, 1952.

Jurishica, A., and Gutglass, M.: Bleeding From Utero-Ovarian Vessels, Obst. & Gynec. **6**: 315, 1955.

Kobak, A., and Hurwitz, C.: Gunshot Wounds of the Pregnant Uterus, Obst. & Gynec. **4**: 383, 1954.

Lorimer, W. S., Jr.: Nonpenetrating Wounds of the Abdomen, Texas J. Med. **55**: 160, 1959.

Marsh, R., Coxe, J., and Ross, W.: Factors Involving Wound Dehiscence, J. A. M. A. **155**: 1197, 1954.

Motta, M., and Vianna, G.: Bullet Wound in a Pregnant Uterus, Rev. de gynec. e d'obst. **23**: 319, 1929.

Pasman, F., and Lovazzano, G.: Traumatic Injury of the Vagina Due to Coitus. Fatal Sepsis, Rev. Assoc. méd. argent. **53**: 59, 1939.

Placintianu, G., and Turcanu, G.: Bullet Wound in a Pregnant Uterus at Term, Spitalul **48**: 224, 1928.

Prestini, O., and Sardi, J.: Traumatic Incised Vulvoperineal Wounds, Boll. d. Soc. d'ostet. e ginec. **15**: 523, 1936.

Russo, S.: A Rare Case of Vulvovaginal Injury From Coitus, Clin. ostet. **35**: 741, 1933.

Savlov, E.: The Healing of the Disrupted and Resutured Wound, Surgery **36**: 362, 1954.

Shuey, P. B.: Spontaneous Rupture of a Uteroovarian Vein During a Normal Spontaneous Delivery, Am. J. Obst. & Gynec. **80**: 764, 1960.

Siler, V.: Trauma to the Perineum, Anus, Rectum and Colon, Am. J. Surg. **80**: 652, 1950.

Souter, R. J. de N.: Penetrating Gunshot Wound of a Pregnant Uterus, M. J. Australia **2**: 111, 1947.

Zondek, B.: Shrapnel Shot Through the Placenta, Lancet **1**: 674, 1947.

29 · The Obstetrician and Gynecologist in Civilian Defense

General Considerations

The present civilian defense plans are based on the principle that civilian defense is a responsibility of civilians and their governments. While the possibilities of an atomic war seem remote, I do not feel that any surgical text should be published that does not devote some space to forecasting an educated guess as to what is expected of a particular specialist. Despite the initiative and excellent work done by the Armed Forces in outlining the problems of civilian defense, it is a tragic fact that very little information has filtered down to civilian medical personnel. For this reason alone some general principles of civilian defense are included in this text. The complete evacuation of pregnant patients, at least from areas of obvious military targets, would not be feasible in the initial phase of a major conflict. The demands on all physicians, surgeons, and related personnel would be so great that only those patients expected to live and contribute to the war effort would be singled out for specific and definitive care. It is probable that only two thirds or less of the available medical personnel, and this includes anyone who has even the most elementary medical training, would survive. The hard fact in such a disaster—and this is appreciated by very few physicians—is that priority of medical care would have to go to those who can survive and be effective in continuing the National effort. Those who need medical attention the most would have to be disregarded. This is contrary to our usual medical thinking, but, if the nation is to survive, all our medical resources would have to be expended on those who would receive immediate benefit.

The generation of casualties in the hundreds of thousands results in a mass casualty situation in which the number of doctors and other medical personnel surviving, in relation to the number of wounded, would result in a situation in which the physician would simply decide who is to be treated and who is not to be treated. Initially, physicians could not stop sorting patients to render specific treatment to a few. All medical personnel would be immediately upgraded, and most of the immediate treatment would not be done by physicians.

Effects and Injuries From Nuclear Weapons

The atomic bomb differs from a conventional explosion in several particulars: (1) The explosive force released from an atomic explosion is much greater than that produced by any other type of bomb. (2) In addition to releasing intense heat and light, an atomic explosion releases highly penetrating invisible radiations that are destructive to living organisms. (3) Ionizing radiations that remain after the explosion are capable of producing harmful effects long after the initial explosion.

It has been customary to consider effects of nuclear weapons in terms of the nominal weapon of 20 kt., that is, roughly equivalent to the explosion of 20,000 tons of TNT. Weapons of much greater magnitude are designed. Nuclear weapons produce injuries by one or a combination of the following three effects: (1) blast, (2) thermal, and (3) ion-

PROBABLE EARLY EFFECTS OF ACUTE RADIATION DOSES OVER WHOLE BODY*

ACUTE DOSE (IN ROENTGENS)	PROBABLE EFFECT
0-25	No obvious injury
25-50	Possible blood changes but no serious injury
50-100	Blood cell changes, some injury, no disability
100-200	Injury, possible disability
200-400	Injury and disability certain, death possible
400	Fatal to 50 %
600 or more	Usually fatal

*From Department of Defense and Atomic Energy Commission: The Effects of Atomic Weapons, Washington, D. C., December, 1950.

izing radiation. Blast injuries occur from the primary shock wave of the explosion and from the secondary effects of flying debris. The latter, indirect blast injuries, are more of a problem than the direct blast injuries, particularly in the densely populated areas. Burns are of two types: (1) flash burns resulting directly from the intense heat released by the explosion and (2) flame burns resulting from the many fires that would be started by the heat and collapsing buildings. Radiation injuries are caused by the penetrating ionizing radiations emitted by the bomb and its by-products. Radiation sickness resulting from whole body radiation results in the acute radiation syndrome. This should be differentiated from radiation injury to certain parts of the body exposed to intense radiation and leading to local tissue damage. The severity of symptoms is dependent on the amount of radiation absorbed and is summarized in the accompanying table.

General Principles of Medical Care

"The mission of the medical service is to provide the maximum contribution to the success of the military effort through conservation of manpower. Successful accomplishment of the medical mission can be obtained by adherence to the following basic principles:

"a. Realization of Sound Professional Sorting by—

"(1) Prompt return to duty of patients with minor injuries, who are or easily can be rendered effective.

"(2) Establishment of a system of treatment priorities for the injured such that—

"(a) Early priority is given to those injured who are most likely to respond to the treatment available at the time and place.

"(b) Only the most expedient therapeutic procedures sufficient to meet immediate medical requirements will be performed.

"(c) Excepting urgent life-saving procedures, nothing will be done which decreases the patient's ability to care for himself.

"b. Economical Utilization of Medical Assets by—

"(1) Maximum conservation of medical effort, in that trained medical individuals are not assigned to first aid, rescue, transportation, or non-technical labor functions.

"(2) Rigorous conservation of essential supplies.

"c. Planning and Training for Medical Management of Mass Casualties in Nuclear Warfare, in Which—

"(1) Preparation is based on knowledge of nuclear weapons effects and sound medical practices.

"(2) Training is practical rather than theoretical."*

Medical Sorting and Treatment

In the early stages of a disaster, sorting becomes a key to the effective management of large numbers of casualties. The patients are grouped according to type and seriousness of injury and their likelihood of survival before any priority of treatment can be established. Insofar as treatment is concerned, four categories have been established, examples of which follow:

"1. *Minimal treatment:* In this group are effective individuals who can be returned to duty with minor injuries such as small lacerations and contusions, simple fractures of small bones, particularly of an upper extremity, and second degree burns of less than 10 per cent of the body surface, not including incapacitating burns of the hands or face. Also included in this group are noneffective individuals who require holding facility care for their daily needs, such as persons with second degree burns of

*From the Departments of the Army, the Navy, and the Air Force: Early Medical Management of Mass Casualties in Nuclear Warfare, Washington, D. C., TB MED 246, NAVMED P-5046, AFP 160-2-4, October, 1955.

TIME AFTER EXPOSURE	LETHAL DOSE (600 r OR MORE)	MEDIAN LETHAL DOSE (400 r)	MODERATE DOSES (300-400 r)
First week	Nausea and vomiting after 1-2 hours	Nausea and vomiting after 1-2 hours	No definite symptoms
	Short or no latent period	No definite symptoms	
Second week	Diarrhea Vomiting Inflammation of mouth and throat Fever Rapid emaciation Death (Mortality probably 100 %)	Beginning epilation	
Third week		Loss of appetite and general malaise Fever	Possible symptoms epilation Loss of appetite and general malaise
Fourth week		Severe inflammation of mouth and throat	Sore throat Pallor Petechiae Diarrhea
		Pallor Petechiae, diarrhea, and nosebleeds Rapid emaciation Death (Mortality probably 50 %)	Moderate emaciation (Recovery likely unless complicated by poor previous health or superimposed injuries or infections)

*From Department of Defense and Atomic Energy Commission: The Effects of Atomic Weapons, Washington, D. C., December, 1950.

the face interfering with sight and/or eating, incapacitating burns of both hands, disabling fractures of minor bones, or moderate neuropsychiatric disorders.

"2. *Immediate treatment:* This group includes patients with hemorrhage from an easily accessible site, extensive lacerations, rapidly correctable mechanical respiratory defects, severe crushing injuries of the extremities, open fractures of major bones, and incomplete amputations.

"3. *Delayed treatment:* This group includes patients with critical injuries to the respiratory or central nervous systems, significant penetrating abdominal wounds, multiple severe injuries, and severe burns of large areas of the body surface (40 per cent and above)."*

―――――

*From the Departments of the Army, the Navy, and the Air Force: Early Medical Management of Mass Casualties in Nuclear Warfare, Washington, D. C., TB MED 246, NAVMED P-5046, AFP 160-2-4, October, 1955.

Special Obstetric Problems

At the present time there is no plan for the special evacuation of pregnant women, and it is unlikely that this would be feasible in an attack without warning. For planning purposes it may be assumed that with a birth rate of approximately 2,400 per 100,000 of population, there would be approximately 200 births a month. It is probable that women at the scene of disaster would have to be delivered by someone other than a physician. Obstetricians would have to carry on their primary function of sorting casualties. Emergency maternity facilities could possibly be set up sometime after the disaster where ante-partum and postpartum services could be established. After the Hiroshima bomb explosion, approximately

27 per cent of the surviving pregnant women within two miles of the explosion aborted or had premature deliveries. For purposes of planning, it is estimated that about 10 per cent of the pregnant women in the area between two and three miles from ground zero will abort. They may suffer other injuries without aborting. The problem of prophylactic abortion for women who are exposed to significant radiation and survive the attack is difficult. Many women spontaneously abort during any serious disaster. The relationship between the dosage of radiation the patient receives and the probability of abnormality is difficult because the amount of radiation the patient received would have to be estimated after careful study and observation. In addition, one would be faced with the problem of the amount of radiation received by the fetus and what the effects of such radiation would be upon the newborn infant radiated after the infant was viable. The problem is so staggering without even probing the possible ramifications that it defies the imagination.

References

Artz, C.: Treatment of Burns. In: Management of Mass Casualties, Army Medical Service Graduate School, No. 553, March, 1955.

Brav, E.: The Treatment of Fractures. In: Management of Mass Casualties, Army Medical Service Graduate School, No. 552, March, 1955.

Dearing, W. P.: National Medical Preparedness, J. A. M. A. 169: 354, 1959.

Department of Defense and Atomic Energy Commission: The Effects of Atomic Weapons, Washington, D. C., December, 1950.

Departmens of the Army, the Navy, and the Air Force. Early Medical Management of Mass Casualties in Nuclear Warfare, Washington, D. C., TB MED 246, NAVMED P-5046, AFP 160-2-4, October, 1955.

Garb, S.: The Physician in Civil Defense. Survival in a Thermonuclear War; II. The Effects of Hydrogen Bombs, New York J. Med. 60: 2579, 1960.

Garb, S.: The Physician in Civil Defense. Survival in a Thermonuclear War; IV. Basic Principles of Protection From Hydrogen Bombs, New York J. Med. 60: 1897, 1960.

Garb, S.: The Physician in Civil Defense. Survival in a Thermonuclear War; V. Types of Shelters, New York J. Med. 60: 3129, 1960.

Garb, S.: The Physician in Civil Defense. Survival in a Thermonuclear War; VI. Providing Safe Ventilation, New York J. Med. 60: 3292, 1960.

Garb, S.: The Physician in Civil Defense. Survival in a Thermonuclear War; VII. Comparison of Different Shelters, New York J. Med. 60: 3457, 1960.

Garb, S.: The Physician in Civil Defense. Survival in a Thermonuclear War; VIII. Basic Dietary Supplies and Equipment for Shelters, New York J. Med. 60: 3666, 1960.

Garb, S.: The Physician in Civil Defense. Survival in a Thermonuclear War; IX. Hope for the City Dweller, New York J. Med. 60: 3863, 1960.

Garb, S.: The Physician in Civil Defense. Survival in a Thermonuclear War; XII. Final Considerations, New York J. Med. 61: 297, 1961.

Gundersen, G.: The Profession's Civil Defense Responsibilities, J. A. M. A. 169: 380, 1959.

Hansen, C. L.: Radiological Warfare, J. A. M. A. 175: 9, 1961.

Health Services and Special Weapons Defense, Federal Civil Defense Publication AG-11-1, Washington, D. C., December, 1950.

Hingson, R. A.: Resuscitation Techniques, J. A. M. A. 169: 384, 1959.

Hoegh, L. A.: The Federal Civil Defense Program— OCDM, J. A. M. A. 169: 351, 1959.

Hughes, C.: Débridement. In: Management of Mass Casualties, Army Medical Service Graduate School, No. 557, March, 1955.

Hungate, C. P.: The American Medical Association Civil Defense Program, J. A. M. A. 169: 349, 1959.

Larson, D. L., and others: The Use of Modified Exposure in the Management of Burn Wounds, Surg., Gynec. & Obst. 112: 577, 1961.

Lindquist, P. A.: Chemical and Biological Warfare, J. A. M. A. 169: 357, 1959.

McCarthy, E.: Para-Medical Role of Nursing in the Medical Care of Atomic Casualties. In: Management of Mass Casualties, Army Medical Service Graduate School, No. 551, March, 1955.

McNally, N.: Anesthesia and Analgesia in the Management of Mass Casualties. In: Management of Mass Casualties, Army Medical Service Graduate School, No. 556, March, 1955.

National Academy of Sciences: The Biological Effects of Atomic Radiation, Washington, 1956, National Academy of Science–National Research Council.

Schade, F. F.: California CPX–Medical and Welfare Services, J. A. M. A. 169: 358, 1959.

Shaeffer, J. R.: Rationale and Principles of Planning for Disaster, Surg., Gynec. & Obst. 108: 488, 1959.

Upton, A. C., and others: Some Delayed Effects of Atom-Bomb Radiations in Mice, Cancer Res. 20: 1, 1960.

Warren, S., and Bowers, J.: The Acute Radiation Syndrome in Man, Ann. Int. Med. 32: 207, 1950.

30 · Thrombophlebitis and Phlebothrombosis, Wound Dehiscence, Postoperative Hemorrhage, Accidental Injuries to the Ureter, and Management of Electrolyte Abnormalities in Gynecologic Surgery

Surgical Anatomy of the Pelvic Arteries and Veins

There are basic differences in the arrangement of the pelvic veins when compared with their respective arteries. The studies of Farabeuf and Kownatski have shown the important variations that influence surgery in the pelvis. Study of the pelvic venous system reveals how impossible it is to perform a complete lymphadenectomy of the parietal nodes about the hypogastric vessels. The veins arise from venous plexuses about their respective organs and anastomose freely. The veins surrounding an artery may be double or triple, and this variation may be found up to the common iliac vein. The superior vesical arteries and the obliterated umbilical arteries have no venous counterparts. Recall that the left ovarian vein empties into the renal vein, while the right drains into the inferior vena cava.

Some generalizations regarding the pelvic veins can be made despite their various formations. They are closer to the pelvic wall and more intimately bound to the parietal connective tissue than are the arteries. When double or triple, they tend to surround the artery but always tend to lie toward the pelvic wall. The arteries run internal, anterior, and superior to the veins, and parietal branches of the hypogastric artery pass through forks formed by the junction of the veins to form the hypogastric vein. Kownatski's dissections frequently showed the superior vesical, uterine, and in-

ferior vesical arteries arising from a patent segment of the umbilical artery, which has no corresponding vein. Venous drainage from the areas supplied by these arteries is by union of the vesical, uterine, vaginal, and obturator veins into a common trunk (middle iliac vein) that empties into the external iliac vein. At times, the pudendal, gluteal, and sacral veins unite in a common trunk (internal iliac vein) that empties into the external iliac vein. These radical variations from the usual pattern make pelvic surgery interesting but not hazardous if recognized.

The venous plexuses of the pelvis are named according to the organ or region they drain. A free anastomosis exists between the plexuses, so that one will merge imperceptibly into the adjacent plexus. The anatomic names do not, therefore, describe a sharply delineated structure. The plexus of Santorini is formed from the junction of the dorsal vein of the clitoris, veins from the anterior surface of the bladder and urethra, and from anastomotic channels from adjacent bone or obturator veins. The vesicovaginal plexus drains the middle and lower vagina and the adjacent base and superior surface of the bladder. The uterovaginal plexus receives blood from the upper vagina, cervix, and uterus. The uterine portion of this plexus lies between the layers of the broad ligament. The pampiniform plexus surrounds the ovarian arteries and ramifies in the connective tissue extensions accompanying these vessels (infundibulopelvic ligament). The hemorrhoidal plexus extends the length of the rectum. The proximal segment of the rectum drains by several veins into the inferior mesenteric vein and portal system. The middle part of the rectum is drained by the middle hemorrhoidal veins into the hypogastric veins. The veins draining the terminal few centimeters of the rectum, together with the anus, form the inferior hemorrhoidal plexus that empties into the internal pudendal veins. The anterior sacral plexus lies in the hollow of the sacrum and forms the middle and lateral sacral veins.

Surgical Principles in Operations Involving the Pelvic Arteries and Veins

Some surgical principles applicable to many pelvic operations may be formulated from a study of the pelvic anatomy. Few will argue that the anatomy of the pelvis is not difficult and complex and, as a corollary of this, requires constant review and study by the gynecologist. The rich blood supply permits ligation of many large vessels without necrosis of the organs. It is almost impossible to cause ischemia of the posterior vaginal wall without amputating the organ. Denudation of the external iliac artery or its ligation may seriously impair the lower limb, although collateral channels through the hypogastric artery may maintain the circulation. The hypogastric artery, in contrast, may be ligated without fear for the pelvic organs, even though they have been irradiated both by x-ray and radium. The major veins, including the vena cava, may be ligated without complications in most instances. The uterus will survive after ligation of both uterine arteries. Interruption of both ovarian arteries does not affect either ovaries or uterus. Observations on the uterus after ligation of all four vessels have not been studied. The visceral extensions of the parietal connective tissue that surround the arteries and veins provide a more secure pedicle than does individual isolation and ligation of the vessels. Particularly is this true of the thin-walled pelvic veins.

Clearing of the abdominal portion of the femoral canal may involve bleeding from the deep epigastric, deep external pudic, deep circumflex iliac, and, if present, the accessory obturator arteries and veins. Ligation of any or all of these branches is without incident to the patient. Experience with bleeding from vessels within the femoral canal indicates that the best way to control them is by systematic ligation of the bleeding points one at a time, since multiple clamps in so small a space hinder the surgeon.

THROMBOPHLEBITIS AND PHLEBOTHROMBOSIS
Etiology and Pathologic Anatomy

Thrombophlebitis is more common after pelvic surgery because of renewed interest in radical operations for pelvic malignancies. Trauma to the pelvic veins, infection, stasis, and damage to the surrounding tissues cause the disease process that subsequently extends to involve the deep veins of the leg. The ascending type of disease is also seen, with the initial lesion in the veins of the calf. A phlebothrombosis, with no clinical evidence of infection, is seen, and this is more frequently followed by pulmonary emboli.

Symptoms and Diagnosis

The patient is usually running a septic course and complains of more than the usual amount of pain in the lower abdomen and one or both legs. Often the wound is healing slowly or the vaginal vault, either left open or reopened for drainage or diagnostic reasons, drains more serum or purulent material than anticipated even after radical surgery. Subsequently one or both legs show calf tenderness exaggerated on extension (Homans' sign). The legs become swollen and edematous. Tenderness to palpation is noted over the femoral ring.

Treatment

The leg or legs are elevated and continuous hot packs applied. Blood is drawn for prothrombin level determination before anti-coagulant therapy is started and each morning thereafter while the process is acute. Chemotherapy and wide-spectrum antibiotics are continued, since in the thrombophlebitis encountered by the gynecologist there is pelvic infection and the ever-present threat or presence of a urinary tract infection. The patient is given combined Tromexan-Dicumarol therapy as follows: Tromexan, 1,500 mg., and Dicumarol, 300 mg. The following day Tromexan, 750 mg., and Dicumarol, 150 mg., are given. The morning prothrombin level may show a change as reported later in the day. On the third or fourth day the Tromexan can be discontinued and the patient maintained on Dicumarol. The daily dose is adjusted to keep the prothrombin level about 30 per cent of normal, depending on the laboratory facilities available and the method used. After the acute process is controlled, the patient is fitted with elastic stockings and gradually mobilized. Repeated pulmonary emboli may necessitate ligation of one or both common iliac veins.

DEHISCENCE OF AN ABDOMINAL INCISION
Etiology and Pathologic Anatomy

A wound dehiscence occurs most commonly on or about the eighth postoperative day. The incidence of this complication is probably less than 1 per cent of all abdominal surgery despite many of the adverse conditions under which incisions are expected to heal. The exact mechanism by which this occurs is not understood, but it is probable that the essential factors for wound healing in the patient's general nutrition are lacking. In examining the edges of dehisced wounds, one is impressed with the appearance of all layers of tissue. There do not appear to be any solid bridges of fibroblastic union throughout the length of the wound. Other factors, such as the rough handling of tissues, the indiscreet use of heavy suture material, and the failure to remove devitalized tissue in the operative field, are contributory. Sutures that are tied too tight strangulate rather than approximate the edges of a wound and eventually cut through the tissues in which they are placed. Infection, obesity, allergy to catgut, vitamin C deficiency, excessive coughing, vomiting, and distention have all been sug-

gested as contributory causes, but many patients whose postoperative courses are complicated by these factors have a wound that heals without incident. Dehiscence of a wound without intestinal obstruction does not have a high mortality rate. When, however, obstruction as well as a wound disruption is present, the mortality rate may be as high as 25 per cent. The incidence of this complication is exceedingly rare in the hands of any surgeon who pays strict attention to the patient's preoperative nutritional requirements, judiciously uses antibiotics preoperatively and postoperatively as indicated, and performs his operations with a delicate technique that avoids the development of seromas and hematomas in the wound.

Symptoms and Diagnosis

Patients frequently present an unfavorable postoperative course with a low-grade fever and signs of abdominal distention. They do not appear to be doing well and frequently express apprehension concerning their recovery. Some eviscerations occur without any warning, but in most instances a serosanguineous fluid may be reported on the dressing or the patient may complain of more than the usual amount of pain in and about the operative area. Auscultation over the incision, which may appear to be healing normally insofar as the union of the skin edges is concerned, may suggest that the bowel is very close to the surface. A lateral x-ray at this time shows that a knuckle of bowel which has escaped from the abdominal cavity is lying just beneath the skin, and the patient shows the signs of an early intestinal obstruction. More often than not, the wound simply gives way throughout its entire length, with a large amount of the small bowel and omentum bulging through the wound or laying on the adjacent abdomen.

Preoperative Care and Anesthesia

The dehiscence of an abdominal wound is a surgical emergency and rarely leaves more than an hour to ready the patient for secondary closure. One thousand milliliters or more of whole blood is made available before the patient is taken to the operating room. If the patient has eaten within three hours, a stomach tube is passed and the contents aspirated before anesthesia. A gastric suction tube is passed before anesthesia even though the vomiting occasioned by the introduction of the tube may cause the expulsion of more bowel. If there is any evidence or suggestion of intestinal obstruction, the patient is intubated under local anesthesia before the induction of a general anesthetic. There is no stomach tube or other means available that could possibly prevent aspiration of the stomach contents occasioned by the reverse peristalsis that takes place when the bowel is replaced or manipulated during surgery for obstruction. Spinal anesthesia has definite advantages in these patients provided they are not in shock. When the infusion is started, blood is drawn for blood chemistry studies, with special reference to the total proteins, albumin, and globulin.

Steps of the Operation

1. Plate 72, A, shows the dehiscence of a lower midline incision that is typical of this complication. The wound is separated throughout its length and loops of small bowel and omentum emerge. The area of the incision has been draped, and the remnants of the original suture material are being removed.

2. The abdomen is gently explored for obstruction of the bowel. Assured that no obstruction exists, the operator replaces the bowel and omentum within the abdomen. The wound is closed with through-and-through sutures of large-caliber silver wire that are subsequently tied after being threaded through a piece of small rubber tubing (Plate 72, B). The silver wire sutures are placed about an inch apart, and, as each one is tied, a finger is inserted within the abdomen and the intra-abdominal portion of the wire bent to conform to the curvature of the parietal peritoneum in the area.

3. Interrupted black silk sutures are used to approximate the skin between the through-and-through silver wire sutures (Plate 72, B).

Postoperative Care

The maintenance of the patient's nutrition is the most important factor in healing by secondary intention. Studies of the patient's electrolytes and serum proteins are done daily for several days postoperatively, with appropriate replacement as needed. If serum albumin is available, several units are given to the patient, particularly if the serum albumin is borderline or low. Gastric suction is continued until bowel sounds reappear and the patient is able to retain liquids by mouth. No laboratory-supervised replacement of electrolytes, proteins, and the other essential substances in metabolism and kidney function can take the place of the body's natural handling of these substances. In the absence of nausea and distention, the patient is encouraged to eat as soon as possible and to take adequate fluids by mouth. If progress is satisfactory, a tap-water enema may be given on the third postoperative day, and mild catharsis may be sufficient thereafter. The interrupted black silk sutures are removed on the seventh postoperative day. In the event that the wound heals satisfactorily, the silver wire stay sutures may be removed on or about the twelfth day. The antibiotics selected during the postoperative period should include a urinary antiseptic to prevent a urinary tract infection from complicating the patient's recovery.

WOUND DEHISCENCE OF THE VAGINAL VAULT
Etiology and Pathologic Anatomy

Healing of the vaginal vault after a total abdominal hysterectomy or vaginal hysterectomy is dependent on the same factors as the healing of wounds elsewhere. The vaginal vault can be left open after these procedures, with the insertion of drains, and will usually close without incident provided that the patient's general condition permits of good wound healing and the operation has been performed with due respect for the gentle handling of tissues. A dehiscence of the vaginal vault is accompanied by bleeding from the edges of the incision, or a hematoma or seroma may have formed between the peritoneum and the vaginal wall. This subsequently drains into the vagina. Plate 72, C, shows some of the directions that a hematoma may dissect after dis-

PLATE 72

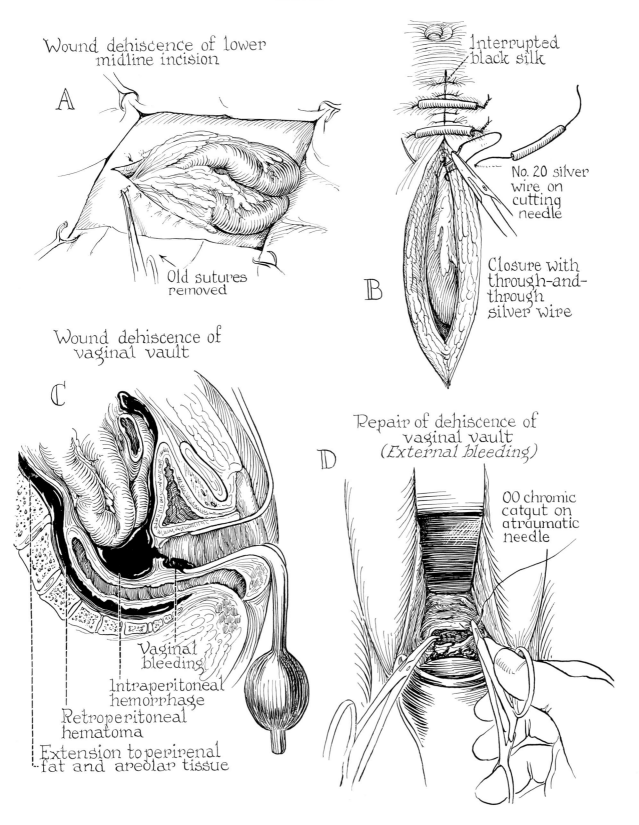

A

Wound dehiscence of lower midline incision

Old sutures removed

B

Interrupted black silk

No. 20 silver wire on cutting needle

Closure with through-and-through silver wire

C

Wound dehiscence of vaginal vault

Vaginal bleeding

Intraperitoneal hemorrhage

Retroperitoneal hematoma

Extension to perirenal fat and areolar tissue

D

Repair of dehiscence of vaginal vault
(External bleeding)

00 chromic catgut on atraumatic needle

ruption of the vaginal vault with bleeding. The most common and simple form of this complication is separation of the vaginal cuff, with external bleeding. The more extensive and serious hemorrhages from the vaginal vault occur intraperitoneally and dissect into the retroperitoneal tissues and broad ligament. The hematoma may extend to the perirenal fat and areolar tissue.

VAGINAL REPAIR OF DEHISCENCE OF THE VAGINAL VAULT WITH EXTERNAL BLEEDING
Steps of the Operation

1. The vault of the vagina is exposed, and if the bleeding is coming from a single isolated vessel, this vessel may be clamped and tied without anesthesia. If the remaining edges of the vaginal vault are reasonably healthy and there is no further bleeding, this will usually suffice to correct the complication.

2. If there is oozing from several areas of the vaginal vault, it is probably better to obtain hemostasis under anesthesia. Several sutures can be placed to close the vault and control the bleeding. Since the tissue is usually very friable, sutures of 00 chromic catgut on atraumatic needles are used to resuture the vault (Plate 72, D).

3. Active bleeding from the angles of the vault suggests that the vaginal branch of the uterine artery may be the source. Since there is such free anastomosis of the vaginal vessels on the lateral wall, sutures are placed not only to control the exact point of bleeding, but also a centimeter above and below the vessel. Recurrent bleeding from such a site is usually the result of failure to place hemostatic sutures in healthy tissue above and below a bleeding artery. A single suture placed on the bleeding point frequently sloughs in a few days, with recurrence of the bleeding and further retraction of the vessel. This makes each subsequent attempt at control more difficult. When the control of hemorrhage in the angles of the vaginal vault is more than just the simple ligation of a minor bleeding area, ureteral catheters are inserted. The sutures are immediately adjacent to the terminal and intramural ureter in this area. The control of bleeding in the angle of the vaginal vault may become a major complication if the ureter is accidentally injured.

Postoperative Care

The surgeon should review the patient's general nutritional condition with regard to protein replacement. Blood loss is replaced and the patient kept on adequate antibiotic therapy, including urinary antiseptics. The patient is mobilized on the day after operation, since there is little reason to believe that movement is a factor in wound dehiscence of the vaginal vault any more than in an abdominal wound.

RETROVAGINAL BLEEDING AFTER TOTAL HYSTERECTOMY
Etiology and Pathologic Anatomy

Retrovaginal bleeding after total hysterectomy represents a more serious type of bleeding due to blood loss from the flaps of the vaginal wall. The latter, like any cuff of tissue separated from its normal attachments, may necrose and slough, with considerable bleeding. Compartmented retrovaginal hemorrhage behind the vault is usually from a larger artery. This is commonly the vaginal branch of the uterine artery or the uterine artery itself. A hemorrhage just as serious can result from a total vaginal hysterectomy, although this is less likely to be concealed. Bleeding of a major vessel after a vaginal procedure more often is manifested by massive vaginal bleeding.

Symptoms and Diagnosis

The patient shows signs of shock out of proportion to the external blood loss if a large retroperitoneal and retrovaginal hematoma is filling. On vaginal examination the flaps are fragile and may be oozing. Close inspection suggests a higher and more inaccessible source of the major hemorrhage. On rectovaginal examination the mass of clotted blood is felt filling the pelvis and may extend up out of the true pelvis.

Preoperative Care and Anesthesia

Blood is replaced unit for unit, and several additional units of blood are available for the operation and during the crucial moments of locating and ligating the source of hemorrhage.

A general anesthesia, using gas, oxygen, and ether or cyclopropane, is preferable.

Surgical Principles

The ureters are catheterized prior to exploration, although the bladder base may be so edematous and distorted as to make this a time-consuming and difficult procedure. Direct catheterization at the brim of the pelvis may be easier in the presence of a massive hematoma, with edema and brawniness of the peritoneum. The primary pitfalls and finally the awakening of sound surgical judgment in the management of this complication follow a familiar pattern and fall into three phases: (1) the packing phase, (2) the suturing phase, and (3) the correct phase. During the first phase, packs—plain or saturated with various coagulants—are hopefully stuffed into the vault in the hope that they may control the bleeding by pressure, although they seldom could reach within several centimeters of the offending vessel. In the second phase, sutures—usually figure-of-eight—are profligately placed through the necrotic flaps of the vault. Since these necrotic flaps are not the source of the serious bleeding, and closure of the vault only helps a retroperitoneal hematoma to expand further, the seriousness of the hemorrhage is further concealed and the patient placed in added jeopardy. In the third phase the bleeding is systematically located and stopped by adherence to sound surgical principles and technique. The bleeding is controlled at the source after a primary ligation of the major vessels supplying the area. The operator can work in a less obscured field to locate the unligated vessel and also avoid injuring other vital structures during the critical moments of the operation.

Technique of the Operation

Exploration of the pelvis is first done to determine the approximate location of the bleeding vessel. This vessel may be obscured by the peritoneal reaction and clots in the operative field. If the specific vessel cannot be readily identified and clamped without grasping large portions of the adjacent tissue, a hot pack is placed over the source of the bleeding, and the hypogastric artery and vein on the side of the bleeding are ligated (Plate 73, A and B). This considerably reduces the amount of blood obscuring the operative field. The uterine artery is then identified at its origin from the hypogastric artery, the ureter is located and retracted out of the field of operation, and the uterine artery or its vaginal branch is clamped and secured without damaging adjacent tissue. The control of hemorrhage from the hypogastric vessels themselves, whether from injury or from damage during radical pelvic surgery, will be discussed separately, since it represents one of the more technically difficult surgical problems the gynecologist encounters.

Postoperative Care

If a catheter was introduced from the pelvic brim, this is left to splint the ureter for eight days and is removed under cystoscopic observation. The management of the drains, parenteral fluids, blood replacement, and electrolytes are discussed on page 543.

HEMORRHAGE FROM HYPOGASTRIC VESSELS
Etiology and Pathologic Anatomy

The hypogastric artery and vein are most frequently injured during the course of radical pelvic surgery. There is less danger of uncontrolled hemorrhage if these vessels are systematically clamped and ligated during the course of the hypogastric lymphadenectomy. If the indication for surgery does not require as complete and radical a dissection as this, the rupture of one of the deeper vessels while the remaining branches remain intact may present a major disaster, and patients have been lost at the operating table when every means of control of hemorrhage from these vessels has been exhausted. The hypogastric artery and vein may be injured from perforating wounds of the uterus or from accidental wounds to the pelvis. Unless such injuries are quickly recognized, the patient is exsanguinated, particularly if the perforation of the uterus and vessels has occurred during pregnancy.

527

Symptoms and Diagnosis

The amount of blood that can well up from an injury to the hypogastric artery, vein, or one of the major branches is alarming. The general area from which hemorrhage from a major arterial or venous trunk arises is readily recognized, but the location of the exact point of the laceration of the vessel can be exceedingly difficult. Rupture of these vessels from injury or perforation of the uterus is suspected if the patient goes into severe shock, with evidence of intra-abdominal or retroperitoneal hemorrhage.

Surgical Anatomy and Principles

The branches of the hypogastric vessels pass between the trunks of the lumbosacral plexus and also between the muscle bundles of origin of the coccygeus and piriformis. Their retraction between these structures presents the greatest difficulty. It is the short length before it disappears behind muscles, nerves, and ligaments that makes control of bleeding from the posterior division technically difficult. The iliolumbar artery at first passes dorsally and cephalad and then medially behind the obturator nerve to supply the iliacus. The lateral sacral artery passes medially and then caudally, with branches dipping into the sacral foramina, and also anastomoses with the middle sacral artery from the aorta. The superior gluteal artery passes dorsally and medially between the fifth lumbar and first sacral nerve roots. It leaves the pelvis through the suprapiriform part of the sciatic notch to reach the gluteal muscles. The inferior gluteal artery leaves the pelvis between the second and third sacral nerve trunks and through the infrapiriform part of the sciatic notch to reach the gluteus maximus. Again its intrapelvic course is short. The intrapelvic segment of the internal pudendal artery is not so short as the previous vessels. It leaves the pelvis on the upper edge of the sacrospinous ligament, external to the ischial spine, and enters Alcock's canal. Its perineal course is described in Chapter 16 (page 301) as it applies to surgery of the vulva, lower vagina, and rectum.

A systematic approach to control bleeding results in less blood and time lost than if clamps are blindly placed in what may well be considered the bloody angle of the pelvis. The hypogastric artery is first clamped, cut, and ligated close to the common iliac artery. The distal end is retracted to reveal points of rupture or defects in the posterior division. If the site of bleeding is still obscured, the hypogastric vein is clamped, cut, and ligated beyond the origin of the posterior division. The bleeding should be considerably diminished now, aiding in ligation of the bleeding point. If this fails, the hypogastric vein is also ligated proximal to the posterior division of the vein. The bleeding artery may have retracted behind the pyramidalis or lumbosacral plexus and must be dissected out to clamp and ligate it securely.

I have been unable to find any reports on the ligation of these vessels from an approach through the buttocks. The incisions to reach these vessels have been described in surgical anatomy texts, and as a possible means of controlling bleeding after pelvic surgery, this surgical approach merits more consideration. The ligation of the branches of the hypogastric vessels from the gluteal aspect might be a last resort measure when every means of controlling hemorrhage from the pelvic approach has been unsuccessful.

Preoperative Care and Anesthesia

Preoperative care and anesthesia are already decided since the patient is under some type of anesthesia when most of the accidents occur. Several units of blood are typed and cross-matched for the patient. Ligation of the bleeding vessel or vessels may be a prolonged procedure so blood loss is replaced immediately.

Steps of the Operation

1. In Plate 73, *A,* is illustrated an injury to the inferior gluteal artery, one of the major branches of the anterior division of the hypogastric artery.

2. The hypogastric artery and vein have been clamped at their origin from the common iliac (Plate 73, *A*). Long angle clamps are excellent in this situation, and vein retractors should be used to expose the major vessels.

***PLATE* 73**

CONTROL OF HEMORRHAGE FROM HYPOGASTRIC VESSELS

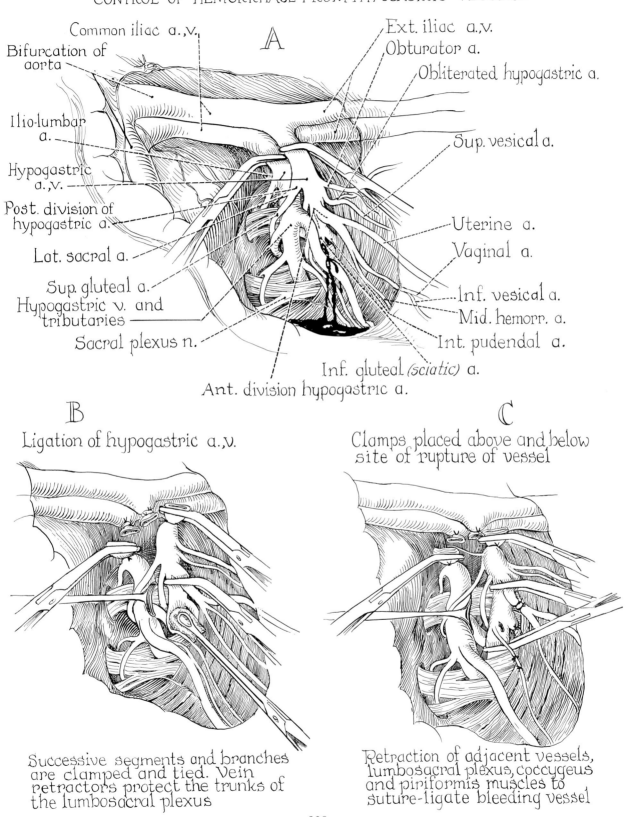

A

Common iliac a.,v.

Bifurcation of aorta

Ilio-lumbar a.

Hypogastric a.,v.

Post. division of hypogastric a.

Lat. sacral a.

Sup. gluteal a.
Hypogastric v. and tributaries

Sacral plexus n.

Ext. iliac a.,v.
Obturator a.
Obliterated hypogastric a.

Sup. vesical a.

Uterine a.
Vaginal a.

Inf. vesical a.
Mid. hemorr. a.
Int. pudendal a.

Inf. gluteal *(sciatic)* a.
Ant. division hypogastric a.

B

Ligation of hypogastric a.,v.

Successive segments and branches are clamped and tied. Vein retractors protect the trunks of the lumbosacral plexus

C

Clamps placed above and below site of rupture of vessel

Retraction of adjacent vessels, lumbosacral plexus, coccygeus and piriformis muscles to suture-ligate bleeding vessel

529

3. An aneurysm needle is passed first under the artery and a ligature of medium silk used to tie the vessel. A suture ligature of medium silk is placed distal to the first tie. An identical procedure is done with the hypogastric vein. The distal ends of the two major vessels are then tied and held by angle clamps (Plate 73, *B*). Gentle traction on the vessels will help to identify branches in the immediate field of operation.

4. A sponge stick is used to keep pressure over an area of active bleeding while successive segments and branches of the hypogastric artery are clamped, cut, and tied (Plate 73, *B*). This systematic approach to the lacerated vessel is preferable to blind clamping in the vicinity of the bleeding. The vessels are fragile, and if the clamp slips or tears, it only means that the laceration is extended deeper and deeper between the trunks of the lumbosacral plexus and the muscles of the pelvic floor.

5. In Plate 73, *B,* is shown an angle clamp placed over the anterior division of the hypogastric artery. The uterine artery, as well as other branches in the vicinity, can now be ligated. There is great variability in the arrangement of the hypogastric vessels, and this is considered during the systematic approach to the actual bleeding point.

6. An angle clamp is placed below the point of laceration of the vessel, while the more proximal portion of the hypogastric trunk is used to make gentle traction (Plate 73, *C*). With the bleeding controlled, the field may be cleared of blood and the specific structures identified. Nerves and muscle bundles are retracted from the specific branch that was injured, and the injured vessel is ligated with medium silk. Caution is observed to tie the vessels so as just to occlude the lumen and not to cut through these fragile vessels.

Bleeding From Posterior Division of the Hypogastric Vein

Since the hypogastric vein lies behind the artery, the latter will usually have to be ligated and retracted before a rent in the vein can be visualized. As in the control of arterial bleeding, intact vessels may have to be sacrificed for the purpose of exposure. The walls of the hypogastric veins are quite fragile, and, once successful in clamping the bleeding point, the operator should refrain from making traction on the clamp until a ligature is placed.

Postoperative Care

The measured or estimated volume of blood loss is replaced either on the operating table or in the immediate postoperative period. The patient's intake and output are observed for signs of urinary retention. Other details of postoperative care will depend on the reason for the primary operation.

TRANSGLUTEAL APPROACH TO THE DEEP BRANCHES OF THE HYPOGASTRIC ARTERY AND VEINS AND THE LUMBOSACRAL PLEXUS
Introduction

Rarely, in pelvic surgery by the general surgeon, gynecologist, or urologist, branches or the main vessels that exit from the pelvis through the greater sciatic notch are lost through retraction and produce bleeding difficult to control. The main branches are the superior gluteal, inferior gluteal, and the pudendal arteries and veins. Because the extravasation is limited by certain peculiarities of the superficial and deep fascia covering the huge muscle masses of the buttocks, an enormous hemorrhage pointing through the greater sacrosciatic foramen has gone unrecognized and patients have been lost. It is a most unusual complication but with the recent advances in all types of surgery involving the pelvis, an approach to control of hemorrhage from the buttocks should be described. Re-entry of the abdomen for the second or third time to control such bleeding, in the rare instances this complication occurs, provides the surgeon with a formidable operation through edematous, friable, unidentifiable, necrosed tissues where each movement or attempt at isolation and dissection of a structure simply adds to the blood loss. An approach from the buttock, posterior through the gluteal muscles, may provide a last-resort operation to control such hemorrhage.

Etiology

Probably the most common cause of hemorrhage from these vessels is pelvic trauma sustained during crushing wounds of the pelvis.

Since few could be expected to survive an injury accompanied by rupture of major vessels of the hypogastric chain and since such an injury would likely involve intra-abdominal or pelvic organs, control of such bleeding from the buttock is unlikely. The vessels may be ruptured during an abdominoperineal resection and retract so that ligation of the vessels is difficult. Retroperitoneal tumors frequently involve major vessels and nerves, and the same holds for those growths about the hypogastric vessels and the lumbosacral plexus. Radical pelvic surgery whether it involves the genitourinary system or rectosigmoid exposes major arterial and venous trunks in the pelvis to damage. Perforation of the uterus during dilatation and curettage, especially for purposes of abortion, has produced a share of the injuries reported to these vessels. The vessels are directly exposed and must be avoided during a superior hypogastric and pelvic splanchnic sympathectomy.

Surgical Anatomy

The skin of the buttock is coarse, thick, and partially fixed in the region of several bony landmarks. It does not slide over the underlying structures as freely as in most parts of the body. The superficial fascia is a deep, loose layer filled with large quantities of fat. Thus, trauma to vessels in this fascia may result in large effusions of blood or abscesses assuming large size. In contrast, as will be emphasized later, effusions or abscesses beneath the deep fascia take on an entirely different character.

The gluteal fascia or deep fascia of the buttock is continuous with the fascia lata. It is attached to the anal fascia near the coccyx, to the sacrum, to the sacrosciatic (sacrotuberous) ligament, and to the crest of the ilium (Plate 74, A). At the anterior border of the gluteus maximus, the deep fascia splits into two layers to envelope the muscle on both its superficial and deep surfaces. The nature of this deep fascia permits effusions or abscesses from the pelvis to escape through the exit foramina of the great vessels and nerves and extend down the leg underneath the deep fascia of the thigh since they are continuous.

The gluteus maximus is the largest muscle of the body and the most superficial of the buttock (Plate 74, A). It arises from the posterior fourth of the crest of the ilium, from the lumbar aponeurosis at its attachment to the crest of the ilium; from the posterior surfaces of the fourth and fifth sacral vertebrae, and from the great sacrotuberous (sacrosciatic) ligament. The fibers pass obliquely downward, lateralward, and forward. The anterior two thirds of the gluteus maximus is inserted into the deep fascia of the lateral surface of the thigh, the iliotibial band; the posterior and distal third is inserted into the gluteal ridge (gluteal tuberosity), the rough line of the femur leading from the greater trochanter to the linea aspera, between the vastus externus and adductor magnus. Its nerve supply comes from the inferior gluteal nerve and branches of the small sciatic nerve (posterior cutaneous nerve of the thigh). Details of its bursa, action, and variations are orthopedic considerations of the muscle relationship to the vessels with which the pelvic surgeon might be concerned are important.

The thick, long, inferior border of the gluteus maximus bounds the ischiorectal fossa and extends obliquely across the back of the thigh over the flexor muscles. The sciatic vessels and nerves pass beneath its inferior border, later to be pointed out as a landmark for the ligation of these vessels. When the gluteus maximus is reflected laterally from its origin, the gluteus medius muscle, the piriformis muscle, and the sacrotuberous ligament are among the major structures exposed. This also unveils the great sciatic nerve, the small sciatic nerve (posterior femoral cutaneus), the inferior gluteal artery, vein, and nerve, and the internal pudental artery, vein and nerve. All these structures pass beneath the inferior border of the piriformis muscle into and out of the subgluteal triangle. The latter landmark has the following boundaries. Laterally it is bounded by the line of insertion of the gluteus maximus to the femur and by the greater trochanter, and the medial boundary or base of the triangle is formed by the sacrotuberous ligament, part of the tuber ischii, and the long head of the biceps femoris muscle. The superior boundary is formed by the lower edge of the piriformis muscle. The apex of the triangle points laterally. These landmarks are important in the posterior approach to the control of bleeding from the inferior gluteal or internal pudendal vessels.

The gluteus medius muscle arises from the dorsum of the ileum between the posterior curved line and the crest above and the anterior curved line below, from the anterior four-fifths of the lateral lip of the crest, and from the fascia covering the muscle. The fibers converge to form a strong tendon that is inserted into the oblique line on the lateral surface of the greater trochanter. It is supplied by the superior gluteal nerve. When the muscle is reflected downward from its point of origin, the superior gluteal artery and vein and the superior gluteal nerve are exposed, emerging from the pelvis just above the superior border of the piriformis muscle.

The gluteus minimus muscle arises from the dorsum of the ilium between the anterior and inferior curved lines as far back as the greater sciatic notch. Its fibers converge into a flattened tendon to insert into a depression upon the anterior part of the greater trochanter. It is supplied by the superior gluteal nerve.

Indications for Operation and Surgical Principles

Since the operations are done as a desperate measure to control hemorrhage or rarely to drain a pelvic abscess pointing into the subgluteal triangle, the deep landmarks will be obscured. Thus the superficial landmarks are all-important in the locations of the vessels and the placing of the skin incisions directly over the vessels.

The superior gluteal artery and vein are pinpointed as follows (Plate 74, A). A line is drawn from the posterior superior spine of the ilium to the greater trochanter of the femur. The thigh should be rotated medialward. The junction of the medial (iliac) fourth of this line with the adjacent fourth of the line is directly over the vessels. Since the vessels are

emerging from the sacrosciatic notch in a downward and lateral course, the incision is started a few centimeters above the junction described above and carried down along the line toward the greater trochanter for 8 to 10 cm. or further to ensure adequate exposure.

The inferior gluteal artery and vein may be located within a few centimeters by the use of the following external landmarks (Plate 74, A). A line is drawn from the posterior superior iliac spine to the lateral side of the ischial tuberosity. This line is divided into thirds. The junction of the upper or superior (iliac) third of this line with the middle third will be directly over the inferior gluteal artery and its venae comitantes. Since the vessels are directed laterally and caudad, the incision should start 2 to 3 cm. cephalad to the vessels and continue along the line described for 6 to 8 cm. toward the tuberosity. This will give adequate exposure, even considering the thickness of the superficial fascia and the large muscle masses of the buttocks.

The pudendal artery and its venae comitantes lie under the following external landmarks (Plate 74, A). The same line drawn for the inferior gluteal vessels is utilized; namely, a line drawn from the posterior superior iliac spine to the lateral side of the ischial tuberosity. The pudendal artery and veins lie a few centimeters cephalad to the junction of the middle and distal thirds (toward the posterior superior iliac spine). The incision starts a few centimeters above this point and extends along the original line for 6 to 8 cm. At their lowermost point they will be seen re-entering the pelvis through the lesser sacrosciatic foramen. Although it is possible that a posterior approach to these vessels would be indicated without involvement of the other larger muscular branches, their location is important to avoid confusion with the gluteal vessels more commonly the cause of hemorrhage or in the path of a pelvic abscess.

Preoperative Care and Anesthesia

Blood, fluid, and electrolyte replacement are effected, weighing postponement of surgery against the amount of active bleeding. Most often it will be necessary to proceed with the patient in a critical condition.

Local anesthesia could be used but has two drawbacks that one might foresee. First, there is a large mass of tissue to be infiltrated until one dissects deep into the buttocks and relatively insensitive muscular tissue. Second, in the event that one of the vessels suspected as the primary site of hemorrhage is not found to be the source, time will be lost in infiltrating another site. General anesthesia need not be deep and is probably the method of choice although the limited number of times this approach has ever been used would not dictate any choice of an agent.

The patient must be intubated, preferably before induction, but certainly soon after induction since this type of surgical complication would frequently be associated with a paralytic ileus and abdominal distention. Since the patient is placed in the prone position for surgery, it is mandatory at this time.

TRANSGLUTEAL LIGATION OF THE SUPERIOR GLUTEAL ARTERY AND VEINS
Steps of the Operation

1. After intubation, the patient is placed in the prone position, and the thigh of the affected side rotated medialward.

2. A length of suture material is stretched between the posterior superior iliac spine and the greater trochanter of the femur.

3. The junction of the medial (iliac) fourth of this line and the adjacent fourth is marked (Plate 74, A).

4. An incision is made, starting a few centimeters above this point and extending toward the greater trochanter of the femur for an additional 6 to 8 cm.

5. The superficial fascia and fat are incised in the same direction as the skin incision, and all bleeding points ligated.

6. With the skin and superficial fascia widely retracted, the superficial layer of the deep (gluteal) fascia is exposed. Since many septa from this fascia pass deep into the gluteus maximus, distinct incision of this fascia before separating the muscle bundles of the gluteus maximus is not usually possible.

7. The muscle bundles run slightly more cephalo-caudad than the skin incision, and the incision and separation through the muscle are done in the direction of its fibers.

8. The vessels will be seen emerging over the superior borders of the piriformis muscle (Plate 74, B). They are clamped, cut, and doubly ligated, and the proximal ends of the ligatures left long. If the vessels are not obscured by bleeding, an aneurysm needle may be passed under them, and the ligation effected by this technique to avoid the use of clamps in an area containing major nerve trunks.

9. The inferior edge of the coccygeus muscle and the superior border of the piriformis muscle are retracted, and the vessels traced into the pelvis through the greater sciatic foramen. The source of the hemorrhage from the vessel or vessels may be proximal to their point of exit from the pelvis (Plate 74, B).

10. Blind clamping of the vessels should be avoided because of their intimate relationship with major nerves to the buttocks and legs. However, even this refinement may have to be discarded if the operation is a life-saving measure and the field grossly distorted by blood, clots, and local tissue reaction.

11. After control of the bleeding is achieved, the major nerves in the area are inspected, and any ligatures that may have involved them are replaced after deligation.

12. If infection is present with the hemorrhage, there is no question about draining the wound. Even without infection a small drain is left for twenty-four hours since the walls of the vessels are fragile from local tissue reaction and the unpleasant possibility of sloughing of the vessel wall and recurring hemorrhage may occur.

TRANSGLUTEAL LIGATION OF THE INFERIOR GLUTEAL ARTERY AND VEINS
Steps of the Operation

1. After intubation the patient is placed in the prone position, and the thigh on the side of the ligation rotated medialward.

2. A length of suture material is used to mark a line extending from the posterior superior iliac spine to the lateral surface of the tuber ischii.

3. The junction of the upper (medial, superior) third of this line and the middle third is marked.

4. A skin incision starting a few centimeters above this point is carried for a distance of 6 to 8 cm.

PLATE 74

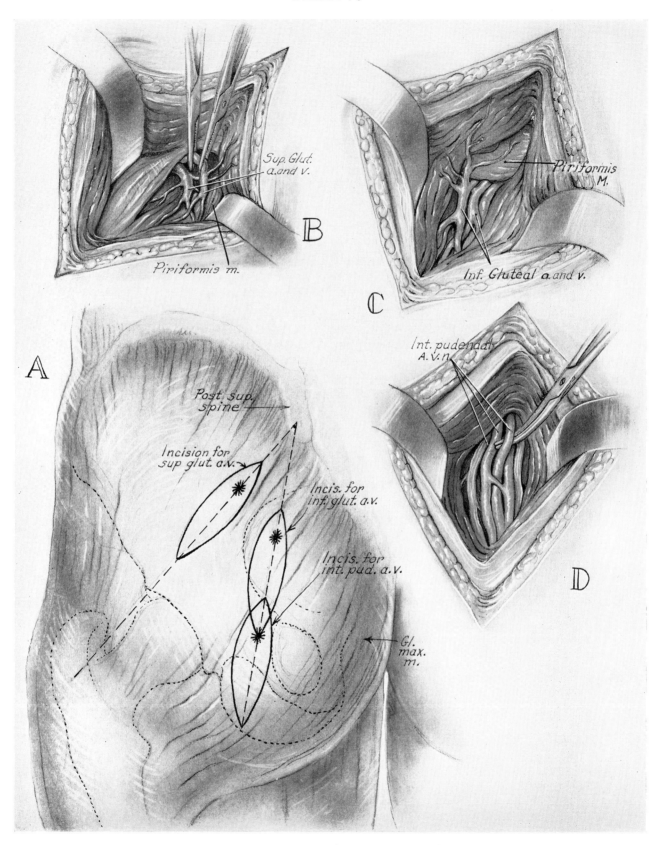

toward the lateral aspect of the ischial tuberosity along the line previously outlined (Plate 74, *A*).

5. The incision is carried down through the subcutaneous tela and superficial fascia. The superficial layer of the deep fascia over the gluteus maximus is identified.

6. The gluteus maximus is incised or split by blunt dissection in the direction of its fibers. Since the superficial layer of the deep fascia sends many septa into the muscle, this fascia is split with the muscle without any attempt to proceed at this point layer by layer (Plate 74, *C*).

7. The inferior glutea artery and its venae comitantes will be seen emerging under the inferior border of the piriformis muscle to enter the subgluteal triangle (Plate 74, *C*).

8. The vessels are clamped, cut, and doubly ligated. An aneurysm needle can be used to avoid the use of clamps if the field of the operation is not obscured so as to make this refinement impossible.

9. The ligatures on the proximal ends of the ligated vessels are left long for gentle traction in following the vessels into the pelvis to ensure that the vessels have not been ligated distal to the point of fracture and hemorrhage of the vessel wall.

10. The great sciatic nerve and the small sciatic (posterior cutaneous nerve of the thigh) lie just lateral to the vessels. They are inspected for any trauma since the ligation may have had to be done in the presence of a large hematoma and local tissue reaction that obscures the normal landmarks.

11. The wound is drained in the presence of infection or a great deal of serum or old blood coming from the pelvic cavity.

TRANSGLUTEAL LIGATION OF THE PUDENDAL ARTERY AND VEINS
Steps of the Operation

1. After intubation the patient is placed in the prone position, and the thigh on the side of the ligation rotated medialward.

2. A length of suture material is used to mark a line extending from the posterior superior iliac spine to the lateral surface of the tuber ischii.

3. The junction of the medial and lateral (tuber ischial) thirds of the above described line is marked. Two to three centimeters toward the posterior iliac spine will orient the surgeon directly over the pudendal vessels.

4. A skin incision is made, starting a few centimeters above this point and continuing along the line of orientation toward the tuber ischii for a distance of 6 to 8 cm. (Plate 74, *A*).

5. The skin incision is carried down through the superficial fascia and fat until the superficial fibers of the deep fascia and the muscle bundles of the gluteus maximus are identified.

6. The gluteus maximus and the extensions of the superficial layer of the deep fascia between its muscle bundles are incised or separated by blunt dissection in the direction of its fibers.

7. Caudad and somewhat lateral to the inferior gluteal vessels, the internal pudendal artery and veins are seen. Just medial to the vessels the great sacrosciatic ligament can be palpated (Plate 74, *D*). The vessels emerge from the pelvis under the inferior edge of the piriformis muscle.

8. The vessels are clamped, cut, and doubly ligated, and the proximal ligature left long for traction. An aneurysm needle and ligatures may be substituted for the clamp technique, depending on the surgeon's ability to clearly visualize the vessels.

9. The inferior border of the piriformis muscle is retracted, and the vessels followed higher in their course from the pelvic cavity to ensure that the bleeding has been adequately controlled (Plate 74, *D*).

10. Again, the major nerve trunks in the operative area–the pudendal nerve, the inferior gluteal nerve, and the greater sciatic nerve–are inspected for injury.

11. The decision to drain the wound will usually be in the affirmative since local tissue reaction or infection will necessitate drainage even if the surgeon is convinced that his ligatures on what are frequently friable vessels are secure.

Postoperative Care

Insofar as the gynecologist is concerned, these operations are desperate measures to control hemorrhage or an unusual approach to the drainage of a pelvic abscess pointing in the subgluteal triangle. Primary tumors, fractures of the pelvis, or orthopedic indications would allow, in most instances, more time for contemplation. Therefore, all the measures out-

535

lined (Chapter 30, page 543) for management of fluids, electrolyte balance, blood replacement, and the critically ill surgical patient are applicable.

The drains are advanced 4 to 6 cm. each day. The weight of the patient and thickness of the buttock determines the depth to which they may have been placed. Immediately after operation in the recovery room, patients are placed on the opposite side to avoid pressure or traction on the gluteal muscles that could disturb the operative area.

Antibiotic therapy is administered specifically if there is infection and the organism is known. Since drainage of the wounds is almost inevitable, prophylactic therapy is given even in the absence of obvious infection.

HEMORRHAGE FROM THE OVARIAN ARTERIES OR VEINS
Etiology and Pathologic Anatomy

Postoperative bleeding from the ovarian artery or vein occurs as a result of the ligatures or suture ligatures cutting through the vessel. The ovarian arteries and veins, like the superior mesenteric and celiac axis and their branches, are surrounded by thin, areolar, fibroelastic tissue. If the ligatures strangulate the vessel wall, rather than simply obliterate the lumen, the sutures cut through the vessels. Bleeding is divided into intra-abdominal and retroperitoneal types. Retroperitoneal bleeding is the more serious, since large amounts of blood are lost without the warning symptoms and series of events that occur with intra-abdominal bleeding.

Symptoms and Diagnosis

Massive bleeding into the abdominal cavity results in severe pain from local irritation and the rapid development of shock. Abdominal distention ensues, and a paralytic ileus follows. Retroperitoneal bleeding causes the same symptoms if it is extensive, but it is marked by periods of regression and exacerbation as the bleeding intermittently starts and stops. A retroperitoneal hematoma may rupture into the peritoneal cavity, with acute abdominal symptoms.

Surgical Principles and Treatment

The ovarian arteries and veins tend to retract with the infundibulopelvic pedicle to a position above the pelvic brim. They are frequently found, when bleeding and retracted, at the point where they cross the ureter. If time permits, intravenous and retrograde pyelograms are done to note the position of the ureters and the displacement of the kidneys. Before the abdomen is re-entered, the ureters are catheterized, particulary if the diagnosis is that of a retroperitoneal hemorrhage rather than bleeding into the abdominal cavity. The abdomen is reopened, the old clots are evacuated, and the bleeding sources are ligated.

Postoperative Care

The blood is replaced volume for volume during the course of the operation. The patient's intake and output are carefully observed, for there exists the possibility of renal shutdown in those patients who have suffered a massive hemorrhage. Appropriate antibiotic and other supportive therapy is given.

BLADDER INJURIES
Etiology and Pathologic Anatomy

Injuries of the bladder concerning the gynecologist result from the surgical scalpel and obstetric forceps almost exclusively. A contusion of the bladder results in submucosal hemorrhage and edema and is seen following many deliveries, pelvic operations, or urologic instrumentation. Rupture may be extraperitoneal or intraperitoneal. In the former, urine escapes only into the perivesical tissues, while in the latter the peritoneal cavity is involved. Rupture of the adjacent pelvic vessels will distort the contour of the bladder, which often appears pear-shaped in the cystogram and is referred to as a "teardrop bladder."

Symptoms and Diagnosis

The peritoneum can withstand small amounts of sterile urine, but large quantities or the presence of infected urine results in peritonitis. When urine permeates undrained soft tissue, suppuration, necrosis, and sloughing follow. Thus, the classical symptoms of shock, low abdominal pain, and desire to void without being able to do so or with gross hematuria are followed by symptoms arising from the toxic effects of the urine. An intravenous pyelogram is done as soon as the patient's systolic blood pressure is 90 or more. Kidney function is thus ascertained. A retrograde cystogram is done with 150 ml. of 10 per cent methiodal (Skiodan) sodium. Anteroposterior and oblique films are taken. What is more important is that they are repeated with the bladder empty. A small rupture may be obscured when the bladder is filled with dye. Cystoscopy rarely will contribute much to the diagnosis, and the instrumentation may be harmful at this time. Observations on the effect of the urine on the peritoneum during pelvic eviscerations indicate that it is benign in small, uninfected quantities.

Surgical Anatomy

See under Surgical Anatomy of the Female Bladder (page 180).

Preoperative Care and Anesthesia

Shock is combated before undertaking surgery, and urinary antiseptics are administered. General anesthesia is preferable.

Treatment and Surgical Principles

Extraperitoneal ruptures are treated by suprapubic cystotomy and drainage by suprapubic tube. Penrose drains are placed in the perivesical tissues. Intraperitoneal rupture requires a suprapubic cystotomy with drainage. Urine is suctioned from the peritoneal cavity and the peritoneum closed. These recommendations do not apply to perforations of the bladder incident to pelvic surgery. Unless there is damage of the bladder from radiation or a tumor complicating the problem, the wound heals promptly.

Postoperative Care

The indwelling catheter (suprapubic or urethral) is connected to straight drainage for ten days. Urinary antiseptics are continued for seven to ten days after removal of the catheter.

URETERAL INJURIES
General Considerations

Urologists may damage the female genital organs during general urologic surgery. Injuries the urologist may cause to the female genital tract, however, do not compromise vital organs. The gynecologist, by contrast, operates intimately with the urinary tract, where damage may be fatal. A female urologist may be defined as a well-trained regional surgeon and gynecologist who possesses adequate knowledge of the urinary tract so that he not only may skillfully manage the most radical surgery or radiotherapy in the pelvis, but also is capable of managing coincident lower urinary tract complications. Less important, but habitually seen in practice, are the benign conditions of the bladder neck and urethra where a gynecologic cause is responsible for urinary symptoms. The incidence of ureteral injury will not be known until surgeons are as enthusiastic about reporting primary injuries as they are about reporting new surgical techniques in the cure of such sequelae.

Etiology and Pathologic Anatomy

Injuries to the lower ureter usually occur about 2.5 cm. from the ureterovesical junction or occasionally at the pelvic brim. Those near the bladder, in benign disease, most frequently occur while the surgeon is trying to control hemorrhage. Surgery should never be desperate —if a vessel deep in the pelvis cannot be easily ligated, a primary ligation of the hypogastric artery will retard most of the bleeding. A hot laparotomy pad held firmly over the source of bleeding will control the loss of blood during the ligation. Difficult dissections in the presence of endometriosis, pelvic inflammatory disease, intraligamentary fibroids, and tuberculosis contribute their share of injuries. Adnexal disease in the presence of endometriosis or chronic salpingo-oophoritis may involve the ureter higher up, with injury to it during the clamping of the infundibulopelvic pedicle. In radical pelvic surgery for malignant disease, the stripping of the ureter or a difficult operation results in a certain percentage of fistulas in the experience of all pelvic surgeons. The ureter may be injured during radical surgery but could not conceivably be ligated, since it is mobilized and visible throughout its pelvic course. Radiation, especially interstitial radium with insertion of needles in the parametrium, causes some injuries. The lateral displacement of the ureters in pregnancy spares them during delivery, so that a fistula after vaginal delivery is extremely rare. Injuries to the ureters have occurred during cesarean section especially with a ruptured uterus, requiring an emergency hysterectomy.

Cauterization, conization, and other procedures on the cervix can cause sufficient edema about the ureteral orifices that partial occlusion and an ascending infection may result. Postoperative bleeding from the vaginal flaps after hysterectomy, especially if it is retroperitoneal, will cause considerable edema of the bladder base and frequently makes catheterization of the ureters technically impossible.

Injuries may be unilateral or bilateral. The latter are extremely rare. The ureters may be ligated, severed completely or incompletely, kinked, or otherwise compromised.

Symptoms, Diagnosis, and Psychosomatic Aspects of Disease

Injuries to the ureters discovered at the operating table present a much different problem than those that become evident during the postoperative period. The diagnosis of an injured ureter in the course of a difficult dissection is not simple. Catheters may be passed retrograde from the pelvic brim—a procedure with considerable merit but seldom employed. The continuity of the ureter is unequivocally determined. The patient may be cystoscoped while the abdomen is still open and catheters passed up from the bladder. If necessary, a cystotomy is performed and the ureters are catheterized retrograde by direct visualization. Any of these procedures with immediate correction of ureteral damage is preferable to the disaster a compromised ureter presents when discovered a week after operation.

The signs and symptoms of late ureteral injury are divided into those associated with unilateral injury and those associated with bilateral injury. A completely ligated ureter on one side may be symptomatic and cease to function, and its demise may never be suspected by the surgeon. More often there is flank pain and sepsis due to the obstruction. A ureter that is ligated and sloughs causes a ureterovaginal fistula. An acute pyelonephritis and ureteritis develop, with flank pain, sepsis, and subsequent leakage of urine from the vagina. The acute symptoms may subside with the establishment of drainage. Extravasation of urine into the peritoneum results in the signs and symptoms of acute peritonitis. The many courses a fistula may take will modify the signs and symptoms accordingly (see Chapter 11, page 225). Complete bilateral ligation results in anuria and, within forty-eight hours, the beginning symptoms of nitrogen retention. Both ureters may slough and drain into the vagina or create all kinds of bizarre pathways for drainage.

The diagnosis of late ureteral injuries requires complete urologic studies. These studies are emergencies for the most part if permanent damage to the urinary tract or the death of the patient from uremia is to be prevented. It would be difficult to name the exception when a patient with ureteral injury is too sick for an intravenous pyelogram. This is the first urologic procedure employed. The pyelogram may show the site of obstruction, bilateral or unilateral, or the course or pathways that extravasated urine is following, or it may present the surgeon with a picture of bilateral shutdown of the kidneys. Retrograde studies are then undertaken to further clarify the renal damage that, by this time, is usually more ominous and recalls the admonition to confirm the continuity of the urinary tract before closing the abdomen or vaginal vault during the primary operation. Rarely can a catheter be passed beyond the site of obstruction. A filiform catheter or one of the other variations may be employed to pass the point of stricture or angulation. Such a study is interesting but adds little to the solution of the problem, since it is time consuming and only confirms the disquieting evidence that one or both ureters have been damaged. The bladder is filled with methylene blue solution, a tampon is placed in the vaginal vault, and clear urine leaks from the vagina since there is no connection with the bladder. With bilateral ligation, the patient is anuric and catheters cannot be passed up either ureter. The presence and course of some fistulas may be elusive. Dyes of different colors may be introduced into the ureters and bladder to trace the source of the urinary drainage.

The psychosomatic aspects of this complication are charged with depressive features. The patient may develop considerable resentment toward the surgeon if the facts and circumstances surrounding the complication are concealed. Patients readily recognize the concern of all about them and the fact that their postoperative course is abnormal. Within the limits of the individual patient's comprehension, the details of the diagnostic tests and the possible cause of the ureteral damage are explained. Reassurance is given and consultation sought to plan the patient's management.

Surgical Anatomy of the Pelvic Ureter

The pelvic ureter begins at the pelvic brim where it crosses the common iliac vessels. On the right it lies just lateral to the inferior vena cava before entering the pelvis and is covered anteriorly by the ileum and its mesentery. On the left, just above the pelvic brim it is about 1.5 cm. lateral to the aorta and is covered anteriorly by the sigmoid colon and its mesocolon. After entering the pelvis, the ureter inclines laterally and posteriorly to conform to the curvature of the lateral pelvic wall.

In the presence of endometriosis or pelvic inflammatory disease, the technique of scooping the tubo-ovarian mass up out of the cul-de-sac to "free things up" before the beginning of the hysterectomy will scoop up the ureters.

They are then laid in the operative field for possible ligation or injury. Preoperative ureteral catheterization—in fact, a more useful procedure here than catheters in a radical operation where the ureters are going to be mobilized and extensively visualized—is a better procedure. The selection of patients in whom the presence of ureteral catheters will aid the surgeon should be a compliment to the operator and not offend his vanity regarding his knowledge of pelvic anatomy. In practice, the more one studies the complexities of the anatomy of the pelvis, the more one desires any additional guides available in the operating room.

At the level of the ischial spines the ureter bends gently medially and anteriorly toward the cervix. Here it lies upon the obturator internus and obturator fascia and crosses the obliterated hypogastric artery, the obturator vessels, and the obturator nerve. It now passes behind the uterine, superior, and middle vesical arteries and is about 8 to 12 mm. lateral to the supravaginal portion of the cervix. Drawing the uterus to the opposite side of a ureter will slightly increase the distance from the ureter to the cervix. Inflammation, extension of tumor, or fibrosis from radiation will make the ureter more adherent, and it thus more closely follows the line of traction. This maneuver will be used to help ascertain operability in the early part of an extended radical hysterectomy. The ureters are mobile, retroperitoneal, small, and elastic. Their normal course and variations, and the probable direction of displacement by pregnancy, inflammation, tumors, endometriosis, and other pelvic lesions, should be constantly reviewed and studied by the gynecologist.

The ureters then pass obliquely forward along the upper sides of the vagina until they are about 5 cm. apart and about 3 to 4 cm. below the vesicouterine reflection. The intramural portion of the ureter curves further medially so that the ureteral orifices are about 2.5 cm. apart in the collapsed bladder. These distances are all subject to some variation, depending on the length of the anterior wall of the vagina, its contraction from previous surgery, x-ray, or radium, or its distortion by the tumor.

The ureteral canal is an artifact created by dissecting the ureter from the connective tissue extensions of the branches of the hypogastric artery, vein, and nerves. When the uterine artery and, later, the middle and sometimes the superior vesical arteries are resected with the connective tissue, it would appear that the roof of a canal has been opened. The floor of the canal then consists of the pudendal, middle hemorrhoidal, and vaginal (inferior vesical) vessels and their connective tissue extensions. It is evident that in order to denude the ureter completely, the vessels comprising the so-called roof and, depending on how vigorously the surgeon attacks the remaining tissue, some of the vessels of the so-called floor must be ligated.

The abdominal ureter receives its blood supply from the renal and ovarian vessels. Because of the rich anastomosis of vessels in the periureteral sheath, this source of blood is important after the ureter is deprived of most of its blood supply in the pelvis. It receives branches from the common iliac, hypogastric, uterine, and middle vesical arteries and anastomoses with vessels from the bladder. Despite this, radical surgery deprives the terminal segment of the ureter of much of its blood supply when it is resected from its normal bed.

Indications and Surgical Principles

The various operations or combination of operations that may be employed are as follows: deligation of the ureter, deligation with an indwelling ureteral catheter, ureterostomy or pyelostomy, ureteroureteral anastomosis, ureterovesical implantation, reconstruction of the ureter with a vesical flap, ureterosigmoidoscopy, and nephrectomy. After accidental ureteral injury, the aim is to re-establish the continuity of the urinary tract as near as possible to its normal setting. Injured ureters, recognized at the primary operation, can be managed by one of the methods to be described. The point of ligation or damage to the ureter will determine whether a ureteroureteral anastomosis or a ureterovesical im-

plantation, with or without a bladder flap is feasible.

The injuries diagnosed during the postoperative period present a much more difficult problem. They can be divided into the early postoperative attempts for restoration of the urinary tract and later surgery, with temporary diversion of the urine by nephrostomy or nephrostomies. If the patient is critically ill and the full extent of the lower urinary tract damage is not entirely clear, it is best to delay the reconstructive surgery for several months. The early attempts at correction are always technically difficult and require the utmost care in the management of the patient's general nutrition and electrolytes to ensure healing. Deligation of a ureter at this time is difficult and hazardous. It may result in a more complicated urinary problem. In general, the continuity of the tract is best established by reimplantation of the ureter into the bladder as near to the original orifice as possible. A simple tube flap may be developed from the bladder wall if the ureter is shortened and cannot be transplanted without tension. Under some circumstances, and frequently as a palliative procedure, the ureter is placed in the bowel. With a normal functioning kidney and excretory tract on the other side, a nephrectomy may be resorted to if several attempts at reconstruction on the involved side fail or if it appears from the beginning that the kidney may be lost.

Preoperative Care and Anesthesia

The patient is given urinary antiseptics in addition to a wide-spectrum antibiotic. Fluids and electrolytes are regulated as indicated by appropriate laboratory studies, measurement of intake and output, and record of daily weight. The general nutrition of the patient is maintained by blood and replacement of proteins as indicated. The optimum time for surgery, which may be a prolonged procedure, is determined for each patient unless the extent of the complication is such that renal failure makes it an emergency operation. Lesions recognized during the primary operation and corrected then are not complicated by the above factors. General anesthesia is preferred.

ACCIDENTAL LIGATION OF THE URETER
Steps of the Operation

1. Plate 75, *A,* shows the approach to an accidentally ligated ureter. The left ureter had been ligated during a total hysterectomy and the blood supply of its terminal part is compromised. The abdomen is open, with the vaginal vault retracted to the right with Allis clamps.

2. The ureter is identified at the pelvic brim and a piece of rubber dam passed under it for traction (Plate 75, *A*). A small longitudinal incision is made in the ureter until the mucosa bulges through and a small (No. 4 or No. 5 Fr.) catheter passed down to the point of obstruction (Plate 75, *A* and *B*). The opposite end is passed up to the kidney pelvis later. The incision in the ureter is closed transversely at the conclusion of the procedure by several interrupted sutures of 0000 chromic catgut on atraumatic needles. A small flap of adjacent peritoneum is tagged over the closure (Plate 75, *C* and *D*).

3. The peritoneum is incised just lateral to the ureter, which is retracted medially. The peritoneum over the course of the hypogastric vessels is dissected laterally to expose the vessels and the uterine branches. The uterine artery and veins are ligated lateral to the ureter to decrease the bleeding in the field (Plate 75, *A*).

4. The point or points of ligation and the condition of this segment of the ureter is determined. The ureter shown in Plate 75, *A,* was damaged close to the bladder. A ureteroneocystostomy is the operation of choice. Damage more proximally may be treated by ureteroureterostomy if there are unmistakably viable segments above and below the injury and the ureter can be anastomosed without tension (Plate 75, *E* and *F*). The ends are brought together with interrupted sutures of 0000 chromic catgut on atraumatic needles. The sutures should not pass into the lumen and should accurately approximate mucosa to mucosa. The anastomosis may also be done side to side or end to side. An end-to-end anastomosis restores the normal course of the ureter—a surgical principle that is observed whenever possible. A small splinting catheter is left in place.

URETERONEOCYSTOSTOMY
Steps of the Operation

1. A cystotomy is performed to help identify the landmarks about the bladder base. The operation can be done without this if the operative field is not obscured. The ureter is resected and the distal stump ligated with a transfixion suture of 00 chromic catgut. An oblique incision, passing downward and medially, is made through the bladder wall. The intravesical opening of this incision emerges just above and lateral to the original orifice (Plate 75, *G*). The bladder wall should be normal; if not, another area is selected.

2. A fish-mouth incision is made in the terminal ureter, and traction sutures of 00 chromic catgut are placed in the edge of each flap (Plate 75, *H*). Instrumental handling of the ureter is avoided as with any plastic flap.

3. A hemostat is inserted from within the bladder out through the implantation site. The traction sutures are grasped in the clamp, and the ureter is drawn into the bladder (Plate 75, *G* and *I*).

4. The traction sutures are threaded on fine needles and passed back through the adjacent bladder wall to anchor the flaps. These are tied on the outside to just approximate the tissues without strangulation (Plate 75, *J* and *K*). A few sutures are used to anchor the ureter at the point of entrance into the bladder wall (Plate 75, *J*). They should be placed in the adventitia of the ureter and into the bladder wall without constricting the anastomosis.

5. If the operation is done without a cystotomy, the bladder opening is enlarged so the needles anchoring the flaps of the end of the ureter can be passed into the bladder and back through its wall through the site of anastomosis. The bladder wall is subsequently closed about the ureter with interrupted sutures.

6. A No. 4 or No. 5 Fr. ureteral catheter is used to splint the anastomosis. It may be placed up to the kidney pelvis and down to the bladder from the pelvic brim, if this method of exploration was used, or passed retrograde from the site of anastomosis. If a cystotomy was performed, it can be passed retrograde from the interior of the bladder.

7. A peritoneal flap is developed and sutured over the site of anastomosis, and the peritoneum from the pelvic brim to the bladder is closed to place the ureter in its retroperitoneal bed. During this closure a soft rubber drain is placed retroperitoneally along the lateral pelvic wall down to the site of anastomosis. It is brought out of the lower part of the wound. An alternate method is to provide drainage by opening a portion of the vaginal vault, from which the drain can emerge.

PLATE 75

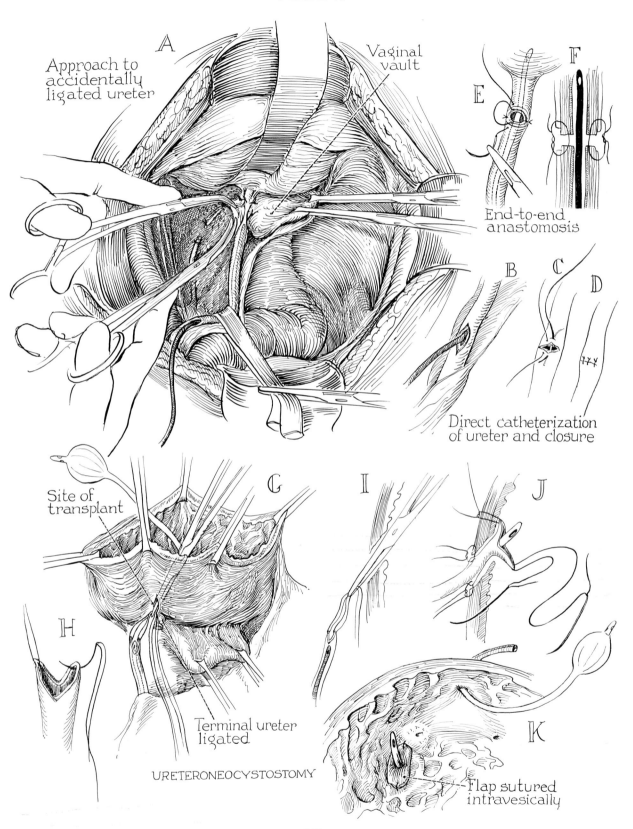

A — Approach to accidentally ligated ureter

Vaginal vault

E

F — End-to-end anastomosis

B   C   D — Direct catheterization of ureter and closure

G — Site of transplant

H

Terminal ureter ligated

URETERONEOCYSTOSTOMY

I   J

K — Flap sutured intravesically

542

8. The bladder is closed around a _suprapubic cystostomy tube._ If the operation was done without a cystotomy, an indwelling catheter is left in the bladder.

Postoperative Care

The patient's intake and output are carefully measured and the usual blood and urine chemistry studies made (see following discussion on Management of Electrolyte Abnormalities in Gynecologic Surgery). The drain is withdrawn a few centimeters each day and, with a successful transplant, may be removed completely on the fourth or fifth day. The indwelling catheter or suprapubic drainage catheter is left in place for ten days. With a successful anastomosis the patient is free of fever and drainage by this time. Urinary antiseptics or combinations of drugs, depending on the sensitivity tests, are continued for fourteen days. Other supportive measures are instituted as required.

MANAGEMENT OF ELECTROLYTE ABNORMALITIES IN GYNECO- LOGIC SURGERY
General Considerations

Patients with uncomplicated gynecologic operations, as well as comparable procedures in other organ systems, seldom present difficult electrolyte problems in their postoperative care. Patients with radical cancer surgery or operations requiring bowel resection or urinary tract diversion are not as readily managed. Meticulous attention must be given to fluid and electrolyte balance. Gynecologic patients with cardio-vascular-renal or respiratory complications require a systematic evaluation of their daily fluid requirement as they would with any other type of surgery.

Parenteral Fluids After Uncomplicated Gynecologic Surgery

An infusion of 5 per cent glucose in water is started prior to any major gynecologic procedure. Whole blood is replaced volume for volume if there is a loss of about 500 ml. as estimated from the drapes and sponges. A more accurate estimate can be obtained by weighing the sponges and measuring the blood loss in the suction bottle. Additional 5 per cent glucose in water is given to bring the total volume of blood and fluid to 2,500 ml. The first day after the operation the average patient will require 500 ml. of 5 per cent glucose in saline solution and 1,000 ml. of 5 per cent glucose in water. She will usually retain enough additional fluids by mouth to stay in fluid balance. With early mobilization and an adequate intake and output, parenteral fluids after the first postoperative day are necessary in less than 25 per cent of patients. A progressive diet allows the patient to proceed from clear liquids to a general diet within a few days. Since no laboratory tests or calculations can compare with the gastrointestinal tract and kidneys in deciding what the body needs, the gynecologist is spared any mental effort once the patient is retaining fluids and the bowel sounds are active.

Fluid and Electrolyte Management After Radical Surgery or Postoperative Complications in Pelvic Surgery
The Basic Plan

A basic plan for management of fluids and electrolytes includes the measurement of intake and output, a record of the body weight, an estimate of the insensible or unmeasured loss of fluids and electrolytes, attention to the patient's nutritional requirements and proteins, studies of the plasma electrolyte concentrations, and a plan for the patient's intake. Special situations will require attention to other details. In practice it is best to make the calculations in the morning, using data accumulated up to 6 A.M. The intake and output up to this time may not represent a complete twenty-four-hour period, but if urine excretion appears to be normal, an arbitrary amount of fluid for urine formation is prescribed, and this can be changed during the day if urinary output is less than anticipated.

On the electrolyte and fluid work sheet (Chart VIII), 500 ml. of 5 per cent glucose in D/W is marked in the Intake section under Water for Urine, and 500 ml. glucose in

CHART VIII

ELECTROLYTE AND FLUID WORK SHEET

—— LEAVE IN CHART

—— PLEASE, WHEN FINISHED SEND TO ——

THE NEW YORK HOSPITAL

Patient (Last name) (First name)

(History No.)

		M S W D Sep.
(Sex)	(Age)	(Marital Status)

(Location) (Service) (Date)

DATE								
WEIGHT								
CHANGE IN WEIGHT								
OUTPUT	URINE							
	EMESIS							
	SUCTION							
	TOTAL OUTPUT							
LOSS	INTAKE—OUTPUT							
INTAKE — SALINE SOLUTION FOR	URINE							
	SUCTION							
	TOTAL							
	5% SALINE SOLUTION							
INTAKE — WATER FOR	URINE							
	SUCTION							
	INSENSIBLE LOSS							
	TOTAL							
	TOTAL FLUID							
POTASSIUM CHLORIDE (mEq.)								
ALBUMIN (Gm.)								
BLOOD	SODIUM							
	POTASSIUM							
	CHLORIDE							
	CO_2 CAPACITY							
	PROTEIN A/G							
	N.P.N.							

AVERAGE PLASMA ELECTROLYTE CONCENTRATION

DEPARTMENT OF OBSTETRICS AND GYNECOLOGY, THE NEW YORK HOSPITAL-CORNELL MEDICAL CENTER*

Nonpregnant

SODIUM	139	± 2	mEq./L.
POTASSIUM	4.5	± 0.3	mEq./L.
CHLORIDE	105	± 3	mEq./L.
CO_2 CAPACITY	27	± 2	mM. /L.
PROTEIN A/G	6.5	$^{4.25}/_{2.25}$	Gm.%
N.P.N.	27	± 2	mg.%

*Laboratories under the direction of Dr. Roy W. Bonsnes, Chemist, Associate Professor of Biochemistry in Obstetrics and Gynecology, Cornell University Medical College.

N/S is marked under Saline Solution for Urine. This is a total of 1,000 ml. for urine formation. An additional 1,000 ml. of 5 per cent glucose in D/W is prescribed in the section Water for Insensible Loss. The 2,000 ml. of fluids prescribed starts the basic plan in operation the morning after surgery. It can be modified during the day for any unusual loss of fluids or, conversely, for any marked retention.

The output for urine, emesis, and suction from the end of the operation to 6 A.M. of the first postoperative day is recorded even though there may not be a full twenty-four-hour period at this time. If there is a large emesis or considerable suction, this loss is replaced—one half by glucose in saline solution and one half by glucose in water. If the suction tube has been passed into the bowel, glucose in saline solution is used to replace the loss. The 2,000 ml. of fluid in the basic plan plus any unusual losses are now added up and given so the infusion can be completed by the end of the day. As prophylaxis against a potassium deficiency, 60 mEq. of potassium chloride is added and diluted throughout the total volume of fluids to be given (Chart VIII). The patient is weighed on a stand-up or stretcher scale if available. Weight is corrected for clothing, or the patient is weighed with the same clothing, dressings, tubes, etc., each day.

The following day a full twenty-four-hour calculation can be made. In the second column of Chart VIII the intake and output are recorded for the various factors. A blood sample is drawn for electrolyte studies and such other factors as indicated. The output of urine, emesis, and suction is added. The intake during the period is added from all the sources. Unless the patient has a severe diarrhea, is losing excessive amounts of fluids and serum from large open wounds, or some unusual situation is complicating the calculations, the intake less the measured output is around 700 to 800 ml. This represents the insensible loss of fluid and is placed on the work sheet as Intake minus Output. Now the total measured output can be added to the insensible loss and the fluids calculated for the day. Potassium is

replaced prophylactically, and when the blood plasma electrolyte values are returned from the laboratory, the intake of sodium and chloride can be changed if there are marked variations from the normal.

Common Electrolyte Abnormalities Encountered in Pelvic Surgery
Hypochloremic Alkalosis

Prolonged vomiting or the necessity for gastric suction for bowel decompression produces a selective loss of chloride from the extracellular fluids. Chemically the patients show an alkaline urine, an increased blood pH, and an elevated plasma bicarbonate that has displaced plasma chloride lost by gastric drainage. The potassium and sodium become depressed from renal excretion. With an increasing alkalosis the normal reabsorption of bicarbonate of 22 to 28 mEq. per liter of filtrate permits the excretion of bicarbonate that coincidentally initiates an increased renal excretion of sodium and potassium. Without correction, this can go on to a potassium deficit, with a hypokalemia added to the hypochloremic alkalosis. Therapy consists of replacement of the excess sodium loss. If the chlorides cannot be brought to normal levels by the increase of saline solution infused, ammonium chloride can be added for chloride replacement.

Hypokalemic Alkalosis

A less frequent mechanism of potassium deprivation is found in the syndrome of hypokalemic alkalosis. In this syndrome the urine is acid, potassium and chlorides are decreased in the plasma, and bicarbonate and pH are elevated, while sodium remains normal. The mechanism is complex, but the essential feature is the failure of the kidneys to excrete bicarbonate. The subsequent cellular shifts of electrolytes, particularly intracellular loss of potassium, result in an intracellular acidosis and an extracellular alkalosis. Clinically, loss of potassium from the gastrointestinal tract, diuresis of potassium during therapy with the adrenal steroids or ACTH, debilitation, long-continued administration of parenteral fluids free of potassium, cardiac failure and mercurial diuretics, and starvation have all been accompanied with a negative body potassium balance. A positive diagnosis of this syndrome is essential since it does not respond to treatment with sodium or ammonium chloride. Replacement of the potassium deficit by meat extracts or intravenous therapy is required.

Hyperchloremic Acidosis

The syndrome of hyperchloremic acidosis after ureterointestinal transplants in gynecologic surgery has the following characteristics: There is an elevated chloride (110 to 125 mEq. per liter) and a decreased carbon dioxide combining power. Depending on the severity of the intoxication and renal function, there may be a moderate elevation of the nonprotein nitrogen and blood urea nitrogen. It is not uncommon for a potassium deficiency to exist with the hyperchloremic acidosis. The syndrome arises from a summation of renal defects and an ammonium chloride intoxication from colonic absorption. The renal lesion can be compared to a lower nephron nephrosis resulting from ascending infection, hydronephrosis because of stricture, and increased intracolonic pressure. We have seen a patient in whom only one kidney had been transplanted succumb suddenly with many of the features of a hyperchloremic acidosis. She did not, however, have a normal kidney on the opposite side. The increased ammonia formation in the bowel results in an increased absorption of ammonia.

The management and prevention of this syndrome necessitates a low salt diet. Deficiencies of sodium are made up without chloride in the acute cases. The colon is evacuated frequently to reduce pressure and minimize the length of contact of the urine with the mucosa. Potassium is given if there is reasonably good renal function and the plasma levels are depressed. When the pH and CO_2 are low, sodium bicarbonate or lactate is given intravenously. Studies of the acid-base balance indicate that about one-half of the bicarbonate administered will go to the intracellular compartment. If about 20 per cent of the body weight is extracellular fluid, then for a woman weighing 60 kilograms the bicarbonate replacement to raise the CO_2 10 mEq. would be as follows:

$$20\% \text{ of } 60 = 12; \quad 12 \times 10 \times 2 = 240 \text{ mEq.}$$

It is unwise to raise the CO_2 precipitously while studying the patient so, depending on the original level, a fraction of this amount is given to cause a gradual shift to a normal acid-base balance in the plasma.

References

Adams, R. H., and Pritchard, J. A.: Bacterial Shock in Obstetrics and Gynecology, Obst. & Gynec. 16: 387, 1960.

Baer, S., and others: Clinical Experiences With Warfarin (Coumadin) as an Anticoagulant, J. A. M. A. 167: 704, 1958.

Benson, R., and Hinman, F.: Urinary Tract Injuries in Obstetrics and Gynecology, Am. J. Obst. & Gynec. 70: 467, 1955.

Berry, R. E.: "Third Kidney" Phenomenon of the Gastrointestinal Tract, A. M. A. Arch Surg. 81: 193, 1960.

Best, C., and Taylor, N.: The Physiological Basis of Medical Practice: A Textbook in Applied Physiology, ed. 6, Baltimore, 1955, Williams & Williams Co., pp. 31-32.

Bettman, R. B., and Kobak, M. W.: Relative Frequency of Evisceration After Laparotomy in Recent Years, J. A. M. A. 172: 1764, 1960.

Binder, A. S., and Mitchell, G. A.: The Control of Pelvic Hemorrhage by Ligation of the Hypogastric Artery, South. M. J. 53: 837, 1960.

Blalock, J. B., Meyer, K., and Dukes, W. F.: Ligation of Inferior Vena Cava for Thromboembolic Disease, Rhode Island M. J. 42: 441, 1959.

Bonsnes, R.: Personal communication.

Browne, A. F., and others: Staphylococcic Wound Infections: Study of Wound Infections in Several Thousand Hernia Cases, J. A. M. A. 170: 1274, 1959.

Brunschwig, A., and Brockunier, A.: Postoperative Rupture of Major Vessels After Radical Pelvic Operation, Am. J. Obst. & Gynec. 80: 485, 1960.

Cantarow, A., and Trumper, M.: Clinical Biochemistry, ed. 5, Philadelphia, 1955, W. B. Saunders Co., pp. 297-298.

Caswell, H. T., and others: A Three-year Study of Staphylococcal Disease With Observations on Control, Surg., Gynec. & Obst. 110: 527, 1960.

Clifton, E.: Fibrinolysin as an Agent for Treatment of Thromboembolic Accidents, J. A. M. A. 175: 302, 1961.

Coon, W. W., MacKenzie, J. W., and Hodgson, P. E.: A Critical Evaluation of Anticoagulant Therapy in Peripheral Venous Thrombosis and Pulmonary Embolism, Surg., Gynec. & Obst. 106: 129, 1958.

Dalai, S. J., Plentl, A. A., and Bachman, A. L.: The Application of Pelvic Venography to Diagnostic Problems Associated With Cancer of the Female Genital Tract, Surg., Gynec. & Obst. 98: 735, 1954.

Dale, W. A.: Wound Complications, Surg., Gynec. & Obst. 108: 492, 1959.

Deaton, H. L., and Anlyan, W. G.: Treatment of Thrombophlebitis With Streptokinase-Streptodornase, J. A. M. A. 172. 1891, 1960.

Dineen, P., and Pearce, C.: A Ten Year Study on Wound Infections, Surg., Gynec. & Obst. 106: 453, 1958.

Duffy, L. T.: Intraperitoneal Hemorrhage From a Ruptured Coronary Vein of a Uterine Myoma, Obst. & Gynec. 15: 746, 1960.

Everett, H., and Mattingly, R.: Urinary Tract Injuries Resulting From Pelvic Surgery, Am. J. Obst. & Gynec. 71: 502, 1956.

Farabeuf, L. H.: Les vaisseaux sanguins des organes génitourinaires, du périnée, et de pelvis, Paris, 1905, Masson et Cie.

Forbes, G., and Perley, A.: Estimation of Total Body Sodium by Isotopic Dilution. Studies on Young Adults, J. Clin. Invest. 30: 558, 1951.

Gansau, H.: Significance of Cavography for the Demonstration of Thromboses of the Pelvic Veins and of Recurrent Tumors of High Localization From Genital Cancers, Geburtsh. u. Frauenh. 18: 566, 1958.

German, G. B., Schellenger, E. A. Y., and Haines, R. A.: Massive Retroperitoneal Hemorrhage Due to Rupture of Ovarian Vein Following Normal Delivery, Am. J. Obst. & Gynec. 74: 658, 1957.

Hancock, J. C., Jr., Dulaney, A. D., and Caldwell, M. G.: The Incidence and Character of Staphylococcus Aureus From Nose and Rectum of Obstetric Patients, South. M. J. 52: 1525, 1959.

Harkins, H.: Fluids and Metabolism; Shock, Burns, Wound Healing, and Infection, Surg., Gynec. & Obst. 112: 231, 1961.

Hayward, R. H., and others: An Experimental Study of the Role of the Colonic Mucosa in Hyperchloremic Acidosis, Surg., Gynec. & Obst. 112: 357, 1961.

Hoover, N. W., and Ivins, J. C.: Wound Debridement, A. M. A. Arch. Surg. 79: 701, 1959.

Howard, J. M.: Fluid Replacement in Shock and Hemorrhage, J. A. M. A. 173: 122, 1960.

Howland, W., and others: Treatment of Adrenal Cortical Insufficiency During Surgical Procedures, J. A. M. A. 160: 1271, 1956.

Ingelman-Sundberg, A.: Repair of Vesicovaginal and Rectovaginal Fistula Following Fulguration of Recurrent Cancer of the Cervix After Radiation. In Meigs, J.: Surgical Treatment of Cancer of the Cervix, New York, 1954, Grune & Stratton, Inc., p. 419.

Kinch, R. A. H.: Hypofibrinogenemia in Pregnancy and the Puerperium, Am. J. Obst. & Gynec. 71: 746, 1956.

Kobak, A. J., and Wishnick, S.: Potassium Permanganate Burn of the Vagina Followed by Bowel Obstruction, Am. J. Obst. & Gynec. 70: 409, 1955.

Kownatski: Die Venen des weiblichen Beckens und ihre praktische operative Bedeutung, Wiesbaden, 1907, J. F. Bergmann.

Kresky, B., and Elias, H. L.: Epidemiology of Staphylococcic Infection in Nursery of Small Community Hospital, J. A. M. A. 171: 1080, 1959.

Leemann, R. A.: The Chronic Obstruction of the Pelvic Veins and Its Surgical Treatment, Schweiz. med. Wchnschr. 88: 397, 1958.

McClellan, J. T., and Hyden, W. H.: Glove Powder Granuloma in Peritoneal Cavity, J. A. M. A. 170: 1048, 1959.

McNickle, H. F.: The Prevention of Primary Postoperative Thrombosis, A. M. A. Arch. Surg. 79: 775, 1959.

Marin, H. M., and others: Coagulation Changes in Experimental Phlebothrombosis, Surg., Gynec. & Obst. 110: 541, 1960.

Miller, J. N.: Hyponatremia: A Complication of the Treatment of the Edema of Pregnancy, Obst. & Gynec. 16: 587, 1960.

Muller, R. F., and Figley, M. M.: The Arteries of the Abdomen, Pelvis, and Thigh. I. Normal Roentgenographic Anatomy. II. Collateral Circulation in Obstructive Arterial Disease, Am. J. Roentgenol. 77: 296, 1957.

Ochsner, A.: Surgery: Indications for and Results of Inferior Vena Caval Ligation for Thromboembolic Disease, Postgrad. Med. 69: 321, 1960.

Olnick, H. M., Weens, H. S., and Rogers, J. V.: Radiological Diagnosis of Retained Surgical Sponges, J. A. M. A. 159: 1525, 1955.

Pommerenke, W. T.: The Neglected Pessary, Obst. & Gynec. 1: 226, 1953.

Randall, H., and Roberts, K.: The Significance and Treatment of Acidosis and Alkalosis in Surgical Patients, S. Clin. North America 36: 315, 1956.

Riva, H. L., and others: Intra-aortic Transfusion: Discussion of Technic and Report of 5 Cases, Obst. & Gynec. 11: 537, 1958.

Roberts, K., Parker, V., Randall, H., and Walker, J.: Common Electrolyte Abnormalities Encountered in Bowel Surgery, S. Clin. North America 35: 1189, 1955.

Roberts, K., DeCosse, J., and Randall, H.: Fluid and Electrolyte Problems in the Surgery of the Aged, Bull. New York Acad. Med. 56: 180, 1956.

Rosenthal, A. H.: Rupture of the Corpus Luteum, Including Four Cases of Massive Intraperitoneal Hemorrhage, Am. J. Obst. & Gynec. 79: 1008, 1960.

Sheller, H.: Gunshot Wounds of the Urinary Bladder, Am. J. Surg. 16: 301, 1932.

Singleton, A. O., Davis, D., and Julian, J.: The Prevention of Wound Infection Following Contamination With Colon Organisms, Surg., Gynec. & Obst. 108: 389, 1959.

Smith, G. K., and others: Exposure and Suction Drainage in the Management of Major Dissective Wounds, Surg., Gynec. & Obst. 107: 532, 1958.

Smith, R., Rodman, T., and Pastor, B. H.: A Comparative Study of Prothrombinopenic Anticoagulant Drugs; Bishydroxycoumarin, Diphenadione, Anisindione, and Acenocoumarol, J. A. M. A. 174: 1917, 1960.

Stein, A. A., and Wiersum, J.: The Role of Renal Dysfunction in Abdominal Wound Dehiscence, J. Urol. 82: 271, 1960.

Sweeney, W. J.: A Case of Hypofibrinogenemia Following Vaginal Surgery, Am. J. Obst. & Gynec. 72: 446, 1956.

Trumble, E. A.: Clinical Experience With Intramuscular Warfarin Sodium (Coumadin Sodium), Surg., Gynec. & Obst. 107: 303, 1958.

Tuller, M. A.: Amniotic Fluid Embolism, Afibrogenemia, and Disseminated Fibrin Thrombosis, Am. J. Obst. & Gynec. 73: 273, 1957.

Valenti, C.: Limb Edema of Pelvic Etiology in Women; Its Evaluation by Means of Pelvic Venography and a Lymphatic Function Test, Am. J. Obst. & Gynec. 73: 380, 1957.

Verney, E. B.: Some Aspects of Water and Electrolyte Excretion, Surg., Gynec. & Obst. 106: 441, 1958.

Wanke, R., Eufinger, H., and Diethelm, L.: Anatomy and Surgery of the Left Common Iliac Vein. A Contribution to the So-Called Congenital Status Varicosus, Deutsche med. Wchnschr. 85: 640, 1960.

Wegryn, S. P., and Harron, R. A.: Pelvic Phlebography, Obst. & Gynec. 15: 73, 1960.

Weseley, A. C., Neustadter, M. I., and Levine, W.: Massive Intraperitoneal Hemorrhage of Ovarian Origin During Anticoagulant Therapy, Am. J. Obst. & Gynec. 73: 683, 1957.

Wesley, R. H.: Internal Hemorrhage Following Gynecological Operations, Am. J. Obst. & Gynec. 80: 6, 1960.

Winkelman, N. W.: Femoral Nerve Complications After Pelvic Surgery; a Report of Six Cases, Am. J. Obst. & Gynec. 75: 1063, 1958.

31 · Perforation of the Uterus

Etiology and Pathogenic Anatomy

Perforations of the uterus occur (1) during the course of gynecologic and obstetric surgery, (2) during the course of misguided efforts at abortion, and (3) rarely as a result of flying missiles. Many of the perforations that occur in the first group are the work of skilled gynecologic surgeons called upon to make a diagnosis or perform a curettage in difficult cases. Some are the result of the work of less skilled surgeons who do not appreciate some of the simple precautions in performing a dilatation and curettage. The cases of perforation of the uterus that are included in the literature are usually due to something bizarre, such as the case reported of a hard, rubber pessary being lost in the pelvic cavity and found in the jugular vein. *The cases that should be called to everyone's attention are those where the operator fails to perform a careful examination under anesthesia to ascertain the exact position of the uterus before he introduces some instrument through the cervix.* After a careful examination under anesthesia, the surgeon forms a mental picture of the depth of the uterine cavity and the direction it takes. The procedure of measuring the uterine cavity prior to curettage should not be followed in pregnancy, malignancy, atrophic uteri, or other lesions that make the uterine wall more friable. If a perforation is suspected, the surgeon avoids the use of grasping or crushing instruments, since they are the prime offenders in necrosing bowel or omentum. If the curette or sound passes without resistance beyond the estimated depth of the uterine cavity, the surgeon presumes that the uterus has been perforated and abandons the procedure. The patient is ob-served to evaluate any injury to bowel, omentum, or a major vessel in the pelvis. Unusual structures can be found in the pelvis, and I have perforated the fundus of a uterus that had been radiated for benign disease, several decades before, and managed to introduce the exploring instrument into a Meckel's diverticulum adherent to the atrophic fundus. Most accidental perforations of the uterus occur during routine diagnostic curettage. The next most common cause occurs during dilatation and evacuation of the uterus for incomplete abortion. The instruments responsible for the perforation are usually small sharp curettes, uterine sounds, small cervical dilators, or ovum forceps. Any surgeon supervising a large service will soon become acutely aware of the simple precautions that are neglected when these accidents occur. The operator has usually followed the routine of attempting to sound a uterus when the organ is senile, probably the site of malignancy or a degenerated myoma, or recently pregnant and retroverted. Dilatation and curettage have been regarded as the first operation for the novice. However, he should learn how to open and close the abdomen, perform appendectomies, do varicose vein surgery, and repair simple hernias before he embarks on a surgical specialty.

Traumatic perforation of the uterus after misguided efforts at abortion is a different problem since the patient comes to the hospital subsequent to the injury rather than sustaining an accidental perforation during the course of surgery. Attempts at abortion by the patient, by some semiskilled ancillary medical personnel, or by an inept abortionist still occur. If the patient introduced some object herself, such as a hatpin, knitting needle, crochet hook, metal syringe, metal catheter, or other such object, it is unlikely that the perforation will be deep, since the pain and mechanical difficulties preclude perforation into the deeper tissues. It is the work of the unskilled or inept abortionist with instruments such as curettes, sounds, or ovum forceps that are incorrectly used that results in the tragic and fatal accidents. Particularly with grasping instruments are the omentum, intestine, mesentery, or large vessels within the pelvis torn and manipulated, with serious injury. The nonopaque urethral catheter is used in a considerable number of cases because of its ready availability and apparent usefulness for the intended purpose without the danger of a sharp object.

Symptoms and Diagnosis

The symptoms vary with the nature of the injury. If a large vessel has been perforated and the patient rapidly goes into deep shock, little confirmation is needed. Should the uterus have been perforated by some means several days prior to seeing the patient and a pelvic cellulitis or peritonitis has developed, the signs and symptoms will be those of intraperitoneal inflammation. The diagnosis can usually be based on the history, on the physical findings of a perforation or site of perforation in the vault of the vagina, and occasionally by the demonstration on x-ray examination of a radiopaque object. When the history is unreliable, the progression of the signs and symptoms of either bleeding or pelvic infection leads to the diagnosis. Clever abortionists have methods of avoiding external wounds on the cervix. The closest scrutiny of the cervix and vaginal vault reveals no evidence of manipulation. In the obscure cases the possibility of acute appendicitis, acute pyelitis, and other urologic or gastrointestinal causes of an acute abdomen are excluded.

Treatment and Surgical Principles

1. If a perforation is suspected in the course of a routine dilatation and curettage, the operator stops any further manipulation immediately. If blood is not already on call, a sample is sent for typing and crossmatching so that blood is immediately available. Anesthesia is stopped and the patient observed for signs of shock. In many cases, especially in the elderly patients with a small atrophic uterus, there is a minimal amount of bleeding and the patient need only be observed for several days for any signs of other injury. Antibiotic therapy is started and is continued until the danger of any intrapelvis infection has passed. The patient can be readmitted in several weeks and the diagnostic procedure repeated.

2. A major hemorrhage may result from the exploring instrument passing through the uterus and perforating a major vessel. In Plate 76, A, is illustrated the perforation of a uterus through the site of an endometrial carcinoma with myometrial invasion. The probe meets little resistance passing through the wall at the site of the malignancy but goes on to perforate the hypogastric vein before meeting the resistance of the sacrum. This represents a major catastrophe, and the patient soon shows signs of a massive intra-abdominal hemorrhage and shock. Immediate laparotomy and control of the bleeding are necessary if the patient is to survive (see Hemorrhage From Hypogastric Vessels, page 527).

3. Injury to the bowel is the result of perforation with a grasping instrument that inadvertently crushes omentum or bowel (Plate 76, B). This situation may arise in a patient with a retroverted uterus in whom the operation is performed for the removal of the retained products of conception. The ovum forceps passes through the anterior wall of the uterus, and bowel or omentum is grasped by the instrument. The surgeon thinks that fetal parts or placental products are held by the instrument and he attempts to extract the tissue. The traction, plus the crushing effect of the forceps, readily lacerates the bowel or omentum. Immediate laparotomy is necessary when this accident is diagnosed or is suspected, since the extent of the damage to the bowel must be ascertained.

4. A foreign body may be retained after an attempted abortion, and the location of the object will determine whether it can be removed vaginally or whether a laparotomy is necessary. If the object is radiopaque, x-ray and fluoroscopy may help in determining the position of the object and the route by which it can be removed. Proctoscopy and cystoscopy can be done to determine whether or not the object has perforated either the rectosigmoid or bladder. If the object was passed through the uterus and is thought to be lying free in the pelvis, an exploratory colpotomy could be done and the object removed through

PLATE 76

PERFORATION OF THE UTERUS
WITH LACERATION OF A MAJOR VESSEL

A

Sound meets little
resistance before
impinging on
pelvic wall

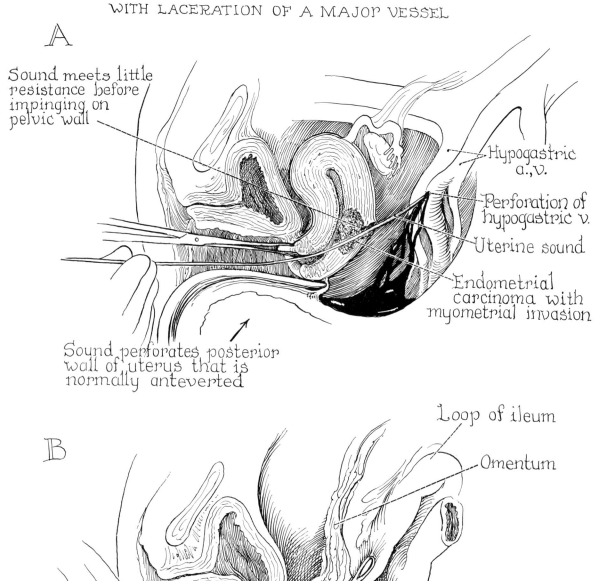

Hypogastric
a., v.

Perforation of
hypogastric v.

Uterine sound

Endometrial
carcinoma with
myometrial invasion

Sound perforates posterior
wall of uterus that is
normally anteverted

Loop of ileum

Omentum

B

Perforation of the ant.
wall of the uterus

PERFORATION OF A RETROVERTED UTERUS
BY OVUM FORCEPS WITH CRUSHING INJURY
TO BOWEL AND OMENTUM

this approach. The surgeon should satisfy himself that no further injury to the bowel or other structures has been done through the limited exploration that can be done through the posterior fornix.

5. Perforation of the uterus by a tandem containing radium or other radioactive substance, with subsequent irradiation of the bowel or bladder, is infrequent. Surgeons using these substances for the treatment of pelvic malignancies are more likely to be skilled in pelvis surgery, and the position of the uterus and the shape of the tandem and colpostat to be used will have been carefully studied and planned in advance of the surgery. X-rays taken after the insertion of radium to ascertain the position of the sources and to calculate the tumor dose will usually confirm the position of the radiation sources.

6. Drainage may be necessary after a perforation of the uterus, particularly if it has been neglected and there is a pelvic abscess. Drainage through the vaginal vault into the posterior fornix is the ideal method of draining such pelvic infection.

As a final word of caution, the introduction of some instrument or instruments to ascertain the damage that has been done when a perforation is suspected is rarely productive of any additional information and may compound the injury.

References

Adcock, L. L., and Hakanson, E. Y.: Vascular Collapse Complicating Septic Abortion, Am. J. Obst. & Gynec. 79: 516, 1959.

Deane, K. P., and Russell, K. P.: Enterobacillary Septicemia and Bacterial Shock in Septic Abortion, Am. J. Obst. & Gynec. 79: 528, 1960.

Decker, W., and Zaneski, B.: Accidental Perforation of the Uterus, Am. J. Obst. & Gynec. 66: 349, 1953.

Dodds, R.: Misguided Efforts at Abortion, Brit. M. J. 1: 921, 1935.

Kobak, A.: Potassium Permanganate Burn of the Vagina Followed by Bowel Obstruction, Am. J. Obst. & Gynec. 70: 409, 1955.

Veprovsky, E., and Ostreich, L.: Traumatic Perforation of the Uterus Following Attempted Self-Induced Abortion With a Rubber Catheter, Am. J. Obst. & Gynec. 68: 1615, 1954.

Zakin, D., Godsick, W., and Segal, B.: Foreign Bodies Lost in the Pelvis During Attempted Abortion With Special Reference to Urethral Catheters, Am. J. Obst. & Gynec. 70: 233, 1955.

32 · Cardiac Arrest and Fibrillation; Tracheotomy and Tracheostomy

Introduction

The instances of cardiac arrest extend well beyond the induction room for anesthesia, the operating room, and the recovery room or hospital bed. Myocardial infarction, drug reactions, drownings, electric shock, and a multitude of conduction diseases of the heart result in a sudden cessation of the circulation when some patients may be saved by temporary oxygenation of the brain by cardiac massage. Although we are concerned in this text with those arrests that occur during gynecologic surgery where instruments and facilities for intubation are immediately available, nevertheless external cardiac massage may restore artificial ventilation and circulation more promptly than open cardiac massage. Every operating suite should be equipped with cardiotonic drugs, an apparatus for ventricular defibrillation, and other drugs and apparatus for pulmonary and cardiovascular support.

Pathophysiologic Mechanisms of Cardiac Arrest

Three types of cardiac arrest occur. The most common is a ventricular asystole or standstill. Second is ventricular fibrillation which may ensue as a result of cardiac massage or during the recovery period. And third, an ineffective systole is occasionally seen. Seldom can one attribute an individual instance of cardiac arrest to a single cause. There are multiple causal elements. Hypoxia or anoxie almost always exists when the diagnosis is made. Altered vagal stimulation, the depth of anesthesia and preoperative medication, acidosis and hypercapnia, electrolyte shifts, and the existence of known heart disease or previous myocardial infarction, all may play a part in this catastrophe. Patients who have been given cortisone and antihypertensive medications may go into shock more readily, providing the state of hypoxia leading to a cardiac arrest.

The basic cardiac physiology is altered in three ways. There may be decreased conductivity, decreased contractility, or enhanced excitability. Some elements of all three derangements may be present. Cardiac arrest is caused by decreased conductivity. An ineffective systole represents decreased contractility plus other factors. If the myocardium is abnormally excitable and the conduction system fails, fibrillation results.

The open chest treatment of this emergency places the physician and surgeon in the position of making a difficult decision under the best circumstances. Beyond the operating room it is even more difficult and has not been clarified in many states and other countries insofar as the medicolegal aspects are concerned. External massage provides a method of treatment that can be employed not only during the time that a diagnosis is being established, but also should a true cardiac arrest exist. Thus, in the operating room when the anesthetist or surgeon might encounter this emergency, external massage would be instituted and internal massage resorted to, depending on the stage of the operation and whether the surgeon was already in the abdomen where cardiac massage could be done through the diaphragm.

Oxygenation to the brain must be established before irreversible damage occurs. Hypoxia of the brain for three to five minutes may result in serious impairment. Since it is difficult to know in these acute emergencies the state of oxygenation of the brain, at the least suspicion of cardiac arrest, cardiac resuscitation by external massage can be instituted. This provides a proved method of establishing some circulation which, when combined with some method of oxygenation, might avert permanent sequelae.

Diagnosis of Cardiac Arrest

Electroencephalographic and electrocardiographic tracings are taken during the course of thoracic and cardiac surgery to determine the degree of hypoxia or impending fibrillation. Except during extensive gynecologic procedures and in a poor-risk patient, these tracings are not made even where such facilities are available. As soon as the pulse and blood pressure are not obtainable, the surgeon is notified. If the abdomen is open, the aorta is palpated. If there is no pulse, the chest is immediately opened and massage begun.

Surgical Principles and Treatment

It is better to open the chest and find a heart that is still active than to procrastinate and restore life to a decerebrate patient who will constitute a difficult nursing problem or have to be institutionalized. Anesthesia is stopped and artificial respiration with 100 per cent oxygen in a closed circuit is begun. The patient is intubated only if necessary for obstruction so as not to interrupt the aeration of the right lung field. Drugs are injected directly into the left ventricle for their effect on the coronary circulation. The anesthetist is consulted on the selection of agents so a specific, desirable effect is obtained. Procaine is used to decrease myocardial irritability. It is contraindicated if the heart is dilated and sluggish. Five milliliters of 1 per cent procaine hydrochloride is injected into the left ventricle. A topical application of the same solution has been used on the exposed myocardium. Stimulation of the myocardium with epinephrine is used if the heart is sluggish and flaccid. One milliliter of a 1:1,000 solution is diluted to 10 ml. with normal saline

solution and injected into the ventricle. At any time that the heart contracts, the massage is interrupted for a moment and the situation reappraised. By this time it may have been possible to obtain an electrocardiographic tracing to support the diagnosis of ventricular fibrillation if such is observed by direct observation of the myocardium. This is quite rare, but a defibrillator, when available, can convert the fibrillation into a normal rhythm in many instances. The technique of cardiac massage and the anatomic landmarks are shown in Plate 77, *A* to *F*.

CLOSED CHEST CARDIAC MASSAGE

Closed chest cardiac massage for cardiac arrest has been demonstrated to be an effective method of maintaining cerebral perfusion while defibrillation is effected if this is possible. Rhythmic sternal compression is made while mouth-to-mouth breathing or other means of oxygenation of the patient is carried out. Depending on the facilities available, closed chest or direct fibrillation is attempted.

The procedure is not without complications. Fractured ribs, hemothorax, rupture of the internal mammary vein, hemopericardium, bone marrow emboli, liver injuries, and fracture of the sternum have been reported. Nevertheless, the procedure should be instituted immediately upon making the diagnosis of cardiac arrest since it may save a few individuals who would otherwise expire.

TRACHEOTOMY AND TRACHEOSTOMY

Together with cardiac massage, tracheotomy and tracheostomy are emergency procedures that every physician should master whether necessitated in or out of a hospital and without concern as to whether the doctor has had surgical training. Medicolegal considerations notwithstanding, many lives are saved by this operation. For a person to breath freely, a complex of nervous processes plus free air passages are needed. Thus, the causes of this emergency vary greatly, but all may be encountered in the course of a gynecologic practice.

PLATE 77

A

B

C

D

E

F

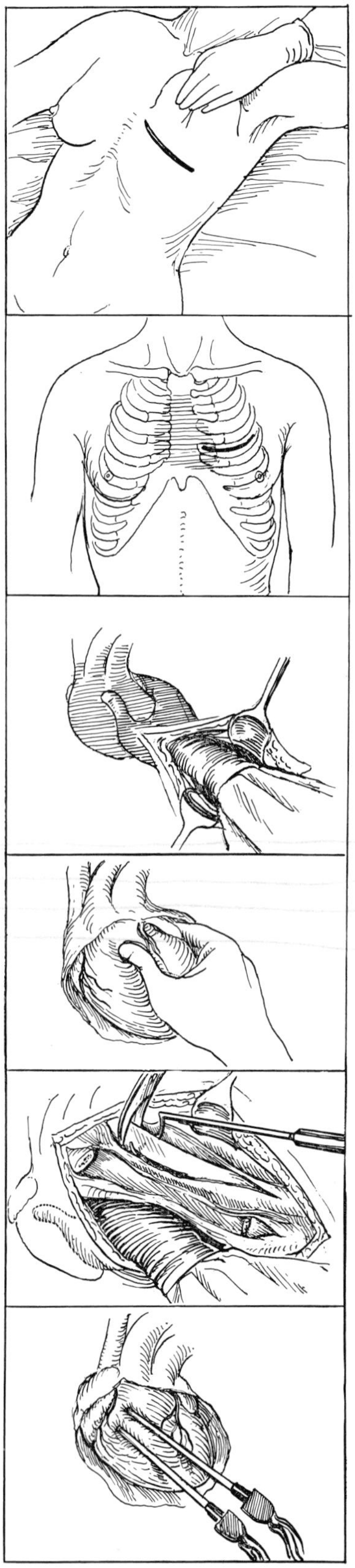

STEPS OF THE OPERATION

1 The breast is elevated and the 4th interspace is quickly entered. The transthoracic approach is the most effective method.

2 The incision extends from the sternum to the mid-axillary line. The pericardium is opened if ventricular fibrillation is suspected or to improve the efficiency of the massage.

3 The heart is grasped so that compression effectively empties the ventricles by as even a distribution of pressure as the hand permits.

4 A rate of massage of 60-80 per minute allows for re-filling of the ventricles. The surgeons alternate massaging the heart without interruption.

5 Ribs are resected for better exposure. Two-hand massage and compression of the thoracic aorta is now possible.

6 If ventricular fibrillation is recognized, rather than arrest, a defibrillator is employed when available.

PLATE 78

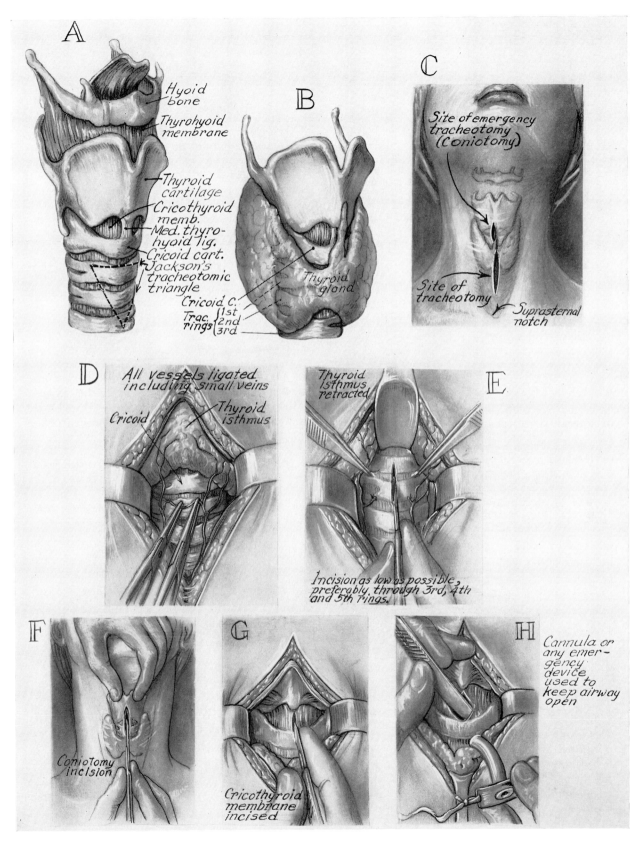

A
Hyoid bone
Thyrohyoid membrane
Thyroid cartilage
Cricothyroid memb.
Med. thyro-hyoid lig.
Cricoid cart.
Jackson's tracheotomic triangle
Cricoid C.
Trac. rings { 1st 2nd 3rd

B
Thyroid gland

C
Site of emergency tracheotomy (Coniotomy)
Site of tracheotomy
Suprasternal notch

D
All vessels ligated including small veins
Cricoid
Thyroid isthmus

E
Thyroid isthmus retracted
Incision as low as possible, preferably through 3rd, 4th and 5th rings.

F
Coniotomy incision

G
Cricothyroid membrane incised

H
Cannula or any emergency device used to keep airway open

555

Etiology and Pathologic Anatomy

More people have probably died from obstructive laryngeal dyspnea after the impaction of food than from any causes following routine elective surgery. The most common cause is an acute infective laryngotracheitis with edema in children. However, like cardiac arrest, the unexpected may happen, and the air passage should be opened by tracheotomy before the patient drowns in her own secretions or aspirations. Delay usually results in a hasty operation performed high in the trachea that may be followed by stenosis, perichondritis, and difficult decannulation.

Surgical Anatomy

Some of the details of the surgical anatomy of the larynx and trachea are shown in Plate 78, *A*. The important landmarks for the high operation (coniotomy) are the thyroid cartilage, the cricothyroid membrane, and the cricoid cartilage. Jackson's tracheotomic triangle has its base just below the cricoid cartilage and its apex at the suprasternal notch. This is the site of the standard operation. Plate 78, *B*, shows an enlargement of the area with the isthmus of the thyroid indicated. The isthmus is transected during the low operation.

High Versus Low Operation

The high operation should almost never be done unless the surgeon has only makeshift tools and no warning whatsoever. If it has to be done and the tracheotomy must remain even for a few days, the standard operation should be performed and the high operative site closed. Bleeding from the thyroid isthmus during the standard operation can be controlled without difficulty with a minimum of instruments.

Steps of the Operation
High Tracheotomy or Coniotomy

Should the rare occasion occur where the surgeon is without even a few instruments and the patient is in a state of acute asphyxia, an incision is made just below the thyroid cartilage and through the cricothyroid membrane or median thyrohyoid ligament (Plate 78, *C*). Obviously there are no steps to this procedure since the operator is simply making a stab wound into the trachea or just above in a desperate effort to prevent a death from asphyxia. Plate 78, *F, G,* and *H*, shows the high operation and the possibility that, in a hospital, some tracheotomic cannula or other device would be used to keep the airway open.

Standard Tracheotomy

1. If the respiratory difficulty is gradual, the operation would probably be performed by an otolaryngologist with the usual surgical setup for the operation. However, presuming that a tracheotomy set is not everywhere available for the acute emergencies, instrument sets of some kind are available with sufficient instruments to perform the low operation quickly and without difficulty.

2. An incision is made through skin and fascia from the thyroid notch to the suprasternal notch. The cricoid cartilage is palpated, and the ribbon muscles separated below this point and retracted laterally (Plate 78, *C* and *D*).

3. It may be possible to retract the thyroid isthmus upward, but, if it should appear that it was so broad that it would slip down toward the tracheotomy site, it is best to divide the isthmus. All bleeding points are meticulously ligated after the patient's airway has been re-established (Plate 78, *D*).

4. An incision through the tracheal cartilages as low as possible is made preferably through the third, fourth, and fifth tracheal rings (Plate 78, *E*). A tracheotomic cannula or some emergency hollow device is inserted into the trachea.

Postoperative Care

While arranging for the otolaryngologist to take over the care of the tracheotomy, an aspirating apparatus and oxygen tank are kept beside the patient. Any secretions coughed into the new airway must be quickly removed to prevent aspiration, therefore constant nursing attendance is essential.

References

Adelson, L.: A Clinicopathologic Study of the Anatomic Changes in the Heart Resulting From Cardiac Massage, Surg., Gynec. & Obst. 104: 513, 1957.

Adriani, J.: Some Causes of Cardiac Arrest, J. Louisiana State M. Soc. 107: 219, 1955.

Baden, E., and Wadem, W.: Cardiac Arrest During Cesarean Section, Am. J. Obst. & Gynec. 66: 202, 1953.

Bellville, J., and Artusio, J.: The Electroencephalogram in Cardiac Arrest, J. A. M. A. 157: 508, 1955.

Davis, P. H., Compere, E. L., and Bergan, J. J.: The Management of Cardiac Arrest, J. A. M. A. **170**: 1050, 1959.

Greene, D. G., and others: Cinefluorographic Study of Hyperextension of the Neck and Upper Airway Patency, J. A. M. A. **176**: 570, 1961.

Hosler, R.: A Manual on Cardiac Resuscitation, Springfield, Ill., 1954, Charles C Thomas, Publisher.

Jackson, C., and Jackson, C. L.: Surgery of larynx and trachea and endoscopic surgery of bronchi. In Waltman, W., editor: Lewis practice of surgery, Hagerstown, Maryland, 1955, W. F. Prior Co., vol. 4, chap. 7, p. 1.

Kouwenhoven, W. B., Jude, J. R., and Knickerbocker, G. G.: Closed-Chest Cardiac Massage, J. A. M. A. **173**: 94, 1960.

Mandel, M. M., and Berry, R. G.: Human Brain Changes in Cardiac Arrest, Surg., Gynec. & Obst. **108**: 692, 1959.

Reid, L. C., Del Missier, P. A., and Hinton, J. W.: Cardiac Arrest: A Review, New York J. Med. **58**: 4035, 1958.

Safar, P., and others: Ventilation and Circulation With Closed-Chest Cardiac Massage in Man, J. A. M. A. **176**: 574, 1961.

Sealy, W., Young, W., and Harris, J.: Studies on Cardiac Arrest. The Relationship of Hypercapnia to Ventricular Fibrillation, J. Thoracic Surg. **28**: 447, 1954.

Section X · REGIONAL ABDOMINAL SURGERY INCIDENT TO GYNECOLOGY

33 · Abdominal Incisions

Surgical Anatomy of the Abdominal Wall

The surgical anatomy of the abdominal wall cannot be reviewed too frequently by the regional surgeon. Especially below the umbilicus is the gynecologic surgeon confronted with the details of the anatomy—particularly if he does radical surgery. We should all form the habit of being perpetual anatomists.

Beneath the skin—in the lower abdomen—the superficial fascia divides into two layers: the subcutaneous, thin, and fatty layer (Camper's fascia) and a deep, membranous, and more elastic layer (Scarpa's fascia). The deep layer of the superficial fascia blends over the inguinal ligament into the fascia lata of the thigh. The continuations of the superficial and deep layers of the superficial fascia into the perineum and urogenital diaphragm are described in the anatomy of the vulva (page 298). The deep fascia of the abdomen is very thin in the inguinal region and intimately invests the external oblique muscle. It is scarcely recognizable but takes a definite part in the make-up of the fascial structures of the vulva.

The cutaneous nerves arise from the fifth to the twelfth thoracic nerves, the anterior cutaneous branch of the iliohypogastric nerve, and the ilioinguinal nerve (Plate 79, A). These nerves curve forward and downward between the internal oblique and transversalis muscles. The thoracic nerves terminate as anterior cutaneous branches after piercing the rectus sheath. The anterior cutaneous branch of the iliohypogastric nerve terminates after piercing the aponeurosis of the external oblique muscle just above the subcutaneous inguinal ring. The ilioinguinal nerve passes through the subcutaneous ring to innervate the skin of the labia majora and medial aspect of the thigh. The anterior branches supply the internal oblique and transverse abdominal muscles as they pass forward between them, and the terminal anterior cutaneous branches supply the rectus muscles. The anterior branch of the last thoracic nerve innervates the pyramidalis muscle (Plate 79, A).

The lateral cutaneous branches of the thoracic nerves pass between the digitations of the external oblique and supply this muscle. Posterior divisions of these lateral cutaneous branches are directed backward to the latissimus dorsi. The lateral cutaneous branch of the twelfth thoracic does not divide into an anterior and posterior division but descends over the crest of the ileum, behind the anterior superior iliac spine, to innervate the gluteal skin. Knowledge of the facts that the skin of the abdomen is innervated by the lower seven intercostal nerves and the iliohypogastric and ilioinguinal branches of the anterior division of the first lumbar nerve and that these same nerves contain the motor branches to the abdominal muscles is used by the surgeon in physical diagnosis. The abdominal viscera and the peritoneum are innervated by branches from the celiac plexus, which arises from the same cord segments and ganglia as the motor and sensory somatic nerves. This fact explains the referred pain and muscle spasm characteristic of peritoneal irritation from pelvic and abdominal disease.

The cutaneous arteries, derived from the aortic intercostal arteries, accompany the cutaneous nerves. Those accompanying the anterior cutaneous nerves, piercing the rectus sheath, come from the superior and inferior epigastric vessels. Other superficial arteries arise from the femoral artery in the fossa ovalis. The superficial external pudendal artery supplies the skin of the labia and clitoris; the superficial epigastric artery, the skin over the lower abdomen anteriorly; and the superficial circumflex iliac artery, the skin of the lower abdomen more laterally along the line of the inguinal ligament. The veins accompany these arteries and drain into the greater saphenous vein near its junction with the femoral vein (Plate 79, B and E).

Five pairs of muscles with their aponeuroses form the abdominal wall (Plate 79, A to D). The external oblique muscle arises, by eight digitate processes, from the outer surfaces and lower borders of the lower eight ribs. The fibers pass obliquely downward, ending in a strong aponeurosis. The aponeurosis (tendon) of the external oblique muscle is thinner superiorly where it inserts into the xiphoid process and thickest inferiorly where its insertions into the anterior superior iliac spine and pubic tubercle form the inguinal ligament. Between the xiphoid process and pubic tubercle it fuses with the aponeurosis of the internal oblique muscle, forming the anterior sheath of the rectus, and then inserts into the linea alba (Plate 79, C and D).

The aponeuroses of the external and internal oblique muscles do not fuse exactly parallel with the lateral border of the rectus muscle.

It is an oblique or semilunar line, often called by that name (Plate 79, A). Compared with the internal oblique muscle, the aponeurosis of the external oblique muscle contributes very little in the lower abdomen to the formation of the rectus sheath (Plate 79, C and D).

The internal oblique muscle arises from the lateral half of the grooved abdominal surface of the inguinal ligament, from the anterior two thirds of the iliac crest, and from the posterior lamella of the lumbodorsal fascia. The general direction of the muscle fibers is upward and medialward. The posterior fibers are inserted into the cartilages of the lower four ribs. The middle portion forms a strong aponeurosis which splits into two lamellae, a superficial and a deep. The superficial lamella fuses with the aponeurosis of the external oblique muscle to form the anterior sheath of the rectus muscle. The posterior lamella fuses with the aponeurosis of the transverse abdominal muscle to form the posterior rectus sheath. Below the semilunar fold of Douglas the aponeurosis of the internal oblique muscle passes entirely in front of the rectus, and here the posterior sheath of the rectus is less well developed, the muscle resting on the transversalis fascia (Plate 79, B and D). The lowest fibers, from their origin on the inguinal ligament, arch downward and medialward and join the lowermost fibers of the transverse abdominal muscle. These fibers pass in front of the rectus to insert on the pubic crest and iliopectineal line, behind the lacunar ligament and reflex inguinal ligament. They have been called the conjoined tendon by some anatomists—this exaggerates their strength and importance in a hernia repair.

The transverse abdominal muscle originates from the lateral third of the inguinal ligament and the anterior two thirds of the internal lip of the crest of the ilium, from the inner surfaces of the costal cartilages of the lower six ribs, and, through the medium of the lumbodorsal fascia, from the spinous and transverse processes of the lumbar vertebrae. Anteriorly the fibers of the transverse abdominal muscle end in a strong aponeurosis that is inserted into the linea alba, the pubic crest, and the iliopectineal line. Some lower fibers join with the internal oblique fibers to form the inguinal falx that inserts into the pubic crest and iliopectineal line. This inguinal falx is poorly defined in many females, particularly if the round ligament is very attenuated. The three flat abdominal muscles—external oblique, internal oblique, and transversalis—originate and insert with a different direction to their fibers. This arrangement greatly increases the total strength of the combined muscles and, except for special operations necessitating the transverse incision of the group, entrance to the abdomen should be obtained by splitting the muscles in the direction of their fibers. In pelvic infections the abdominal wound may be grossly contaminated, and if not controlled by proper drainage and antibiotics, pus can dissect between the mucles and work its way to the points of origin and insertion of these large flat structures. An abscess may extend from the attachments of the muscles and fasciae to the inguinal ligament up to the costal margin. It could extend laterally to the lumbar fascia and medially to the aponeuroses forming the sheaths of the recti. A seroma or hematoma of the abdominal wall would form with the same limitations.

The pyramidalis is a small, triangular-shaped muscle which originates from the front of the pubis and the ligaments of the symphysis and inserts into the linea alba. It is supplied by the twelfth thoracic nerve (Plate 79, *A* and *B*).

The rectus abdominis muscle is straplike in outline and originates from the pubic crest and ligaments in front of the symphysis (Plate 79, *B*). It inserts by three large slips into the anterior aspect of the costal cartilages of the fifth, sixth, and seventh ribs and by a small slip into the xiphoid process. Three irregular tendinous inscriptions break the muscle into segments. The anterior sheath of the rectus is formed by the fusion of the aponeurosis of the external oblique muscle with the anterior layer of the aponeurosis of the internal oblique muscle. The posterior sheath of the rectus is formed from the fusion of the posterior layer of the aponeurosis of the internal oblique muscle with the aponeurosis of the transverse abdominal muscle. The posterior sheath is absent superiorly where the rectus inserts over the costal cage. It is absent inferiorly below the semilunar fold of Douglas, where all three aponeuroses unite and pass anteriorly to form the anterior rectus sheath (Plate 79, *B* to *D*).

The deeper arteries and veins of any magnitude supplying the abdominal muscle mass are the inferior deep epigastric vessels, some branches of the deep circumflex iliac vessels, the last two intercostal vessels, the superior epigastric (branches of the internal mammary) artery and vein, and the abdominal divisions of the lumbar arteries. The superficial vessels are small by comparison. The superficial veins are very distinct when varicose or when taking part as an alternative blood channel in cases of obstruction of the vena cava. In general the blood drains from the umbilicus and above to the axilla. The veins in the subumbilical region drain into the femoral vein. The lymphatic drainage is essentially the same as the venous (Plate 79, *E*). The nerve supply to the abdominal muscles has been described.

Indications and Surgical Principles in the Selection of an Abdominal Incision

1. The abdominal incision selected for pelvic surgery must provide adequate exposure regardless of other considerations. After this consideration, other less important factors such as postoperative pain, possibility of postoperative hernia, and cosmetic result are considered. In any incision, tissue planes in which seromas, hematomas, and abscesses may form are not opened unnecessarily.

2. Fat is cleaned a short distance adjacent to the incision of the rectus sheaths and the aponeurosis of the oblique muscles so it does not intervene between the edges of strong tissue.

3. A postoperative hernia or dehiscence of a wound in a debilitated patient is frequently a greater surgical problem than the primary indication for operation.

4. The drainage of abdominal wounds in gynecologic surgery is frequently best done through the cul-de-sac of Douglas. This results in fewer ad-

PLATE 79

LOWER ABDOMINAL INCISIONS
(SUPERFICIAL LAYERS)

A

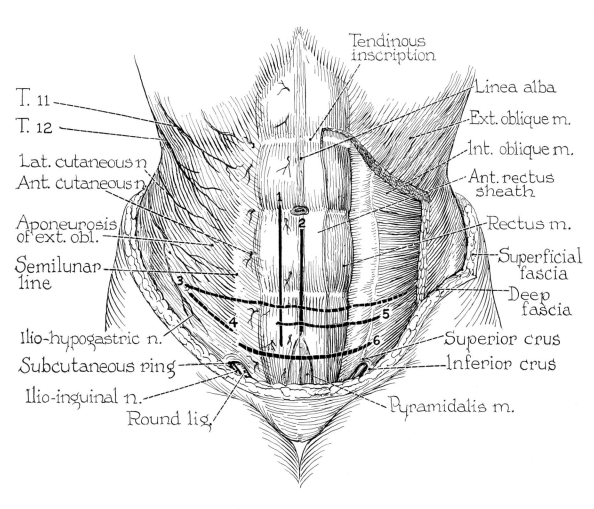

T. 11

T. 12

Lat. cutaneous n.

Ant. cutaneous n.

Aponeurosis of ext. obl.

Semilunar line

Ilio-hypogastric n.

Subcutaneous ring

Ilio-inguinal n.

Round lig.

Tendinous inscription

Linea alba

Ext. oblique m.

Int. oblique m.

Ant. rectus sheath

Rectus m.

Superficial fascia

Deep fascia

Superior crus

Inferior crus

Pyramidalis m.

1. Rectus and paramedian
2. Midline
3. Interiliac
4. McBurney and Gridiron
5. Half interiliac
6. Pfannenstiel

PLATE 79 (Continued)

B LOWER ABDOMINAL INCISIONS
(DEEP LAYERS)

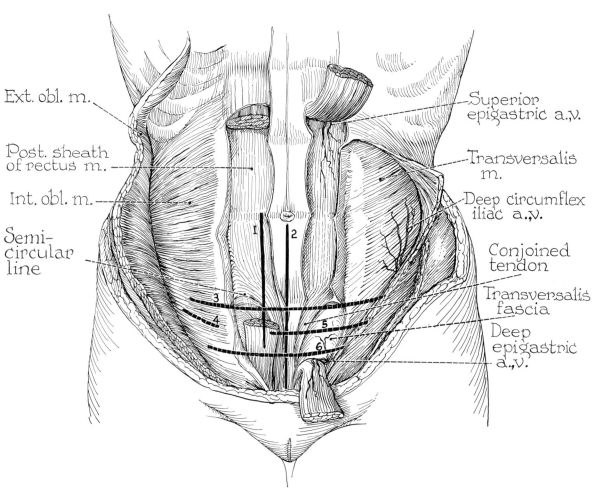

Ext. obl. m.

Post. sheath
of rectus m.

Int. obl. m.

Semi-
circular
line

Superior
epigastric a.,v.

Transversalis
m.

Deep circumflex
iliac a.,v.

Conjoined
tendon

Transversalis
fascia

Deep
epigastric
a.,v.

1. Rectus and paramedian
2. Midline
3. Interiliac
4. McBurney and Gridiron
5. Half interiliac
6. Pfannenstiel

PLATE 79 (Concluded)

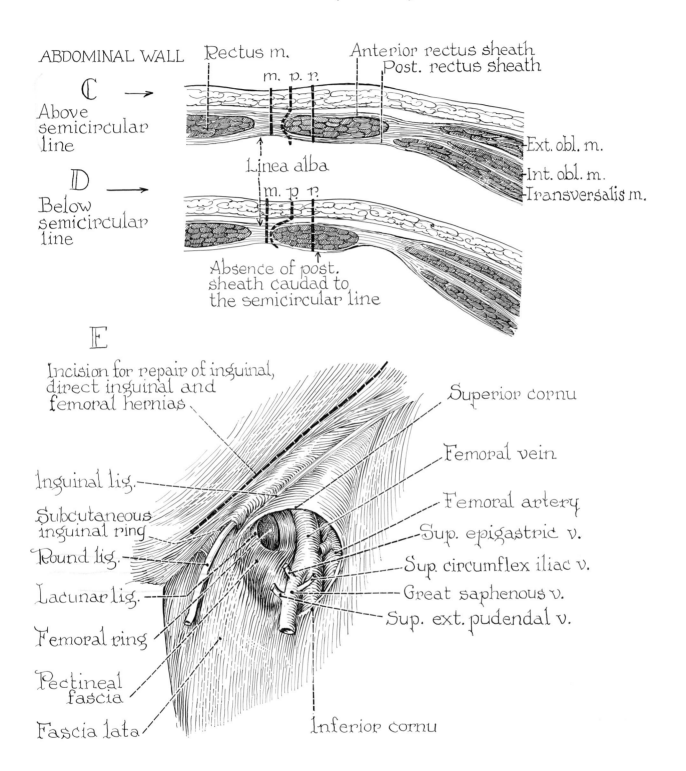

ABDOMINAL WALL   Rectus m.   Anterior rectus sheath

Post. rectus sheath

C →

Above
semicircular
line

m. p. r.

Linea alba

D →

Below
semicircular
line

m. p. r.

Ext. obl. m.

Int. obl. m.

Transversalis m.

Absence of post.
sheath caudad to
the semicircular line

E

Incision for repair of inguinal,
direct inguinal and
femoral hernias

Superior cornu

Femoral vein

Femoral artery

Inguinal lig.

Sup. epigastric v.

Subcutaneous
inguinal ring

Sup. circumflex iliac v.

Round lig.

Great saphenous v.

Lacunar lig.

Sup. ext. pudendal v.

Femoral ring

Pectineal
fascia

Fascia lata

Inferior cornu

SURGICAL ANATOMY OF THE FOSSA OVALIS

hesions and less morbidity than drains presenting from the abdomen.

5. The peritoneum and transversalis fascia are closed by a continuous or interrupted mattress type of suture so that wide serosal surfaces (peritoneum) are approximated without intervention of any of the peritoneal fat.

6. A lower midline incision, if extended, should either remove the umbilicus or cut the umbilical stalk free from the posterior rectus sheath. This permits better closure, with the peritoneum and transversalis fascia in the midline. The upper portion of the incision is closed with its layers in a different sagittal plane than the peritoneum and helps to prevent a postoperative hernia.

7. There are advantages to both transverse and longitudinal incisions in the abdomen. Transverse abdominal incisions, when mastered by the surgeon, are technically just as simple as the classical longitudinal incisions held in so much favor in the past. Transverse incisions, in general, result in less postoperative pain, and the patient therefore requires less sedation, is able to breathe deeper and to turn more frequently in bed, and responds to early ambulation with more enthusiasm. Transverse incisions produce less tension on the wound edges, and they less often dehisce or herniate. Transverse wounds are generally stronger than longitudinal wounds and in most instances give a more pleasing cosmetic result. Particularly is this true of the Pfannenstiel incision just above the mons pubis and extending along the natural folds of the abdominal skin. Longitudinal incisions are preferred to transverse lower abdominal incisions for exposure in short, obese women with a large panniculus. Such patients have a short distance between the ala of the ischium and the costal margin. Longitudinal incisions are preferred when a transverse incision would cause distortion of the lower inguinal regions that may be desired as a site for a cutaneous ureterostomy or a colostomy.

8. An interiliac incision (Maylard-Bardenheuer) cuts through all layers in a transverse plane. A modification of the interiliac incision (Cherney), with detachment of the recti from the pubis rather than transection, gives exceptionally wide exposure. In the latter incision the recti are reattached to the anterior rectus sheath on its underside just above their previous origin from the pubis. This is anatomically sound and prevents the development of a fascial defect above the symphysis. In this incision a large abdominal panniculus can be lifted up and out of the opera-

tor's field. This cannot be done with the classical Pfannenstiel type of incision. An interiliac incision permits of all gynecologic and urologic operations in the pelvis and is particularly suitable for radical dissections. When the muscles are not transected, their nerve supply is not interrupted, which is an added advantage. The aponeuroses of the oblique abdominal muscles, the transversalis fascia, and the peritoneum are divided at slightly different levels and subsequently are in different planes during the closure. As in all transverse incisions, the powerful oblique abdominal muscles do not pull at right angles to the line of closure. This is not true of the recti, which run longitudinally in the midline. However, the recti are segmented by their tendinous inscriptions and do not exert their entire force at the line of reattachment. In addition, the recti, being reattached to the underside of the anterior rectus sheath caudad to the incisions in the skin and anterior rectus sheath, splint, in a sense, the transverse incision between the iliac crests.

Technique of the Common Incisions Used in Gynecology
Rectus Incisions

Plate 79, A, shows the superficial layers of tissue that are incised in a left or right rectus incision. In the lower abdomen the superficial and deep layers of the superficial fascia and the deep fascia would be included. Upon reaching the anterior rectus sheath, this sheath is incised longitudinally, exposing the belly of the rectus muscle. In the lower edge of the incision is seen the pyramidalis muscle on that side (Plate 79, A). The rectus muscle is split in the direction of its fibers to expose the posterior rectus sheath above the semicircular line. The transversalis fascia is seen below the semicircular line where the posterior sheath is absent (Plate 79, B to D). The posterior sheath is incised together with the transversalis fascia. The peritoneum is picked up and incised in a longitudinal direction. This incision serves admirably for extension in the event that exploration or surgery of the upper abdomen becomes necessary. For purposes of description of the author's technique of the opening and closing of an abdominal wound, this incision is described in detail later. However, this is not to be construed as being the most ideal incision for benign gynecologic surgery where transverse incisions are commonly used.

Paramedian Incision

A paramedian incision is done the same as a rectus incision with the exception that the belly of the muscle is not split in the direction of its fibers. In this incision the medial edge of the rectus is retracted to the same side as the skin incision in order to expose the posterior sheath, transversalis fascia, and peritoneum (Plate 79, *C* and *D*). In the closure of this incision the muscle is allowed to fall back into its former bed rather than requiring suture, as does the rectus incision. A paramedian incision is not used if it is anticipated that a colostomy may be placed in the wound.

Midline Incision

A midline incision is made from above the symphysis pubis to below the umbilicus (Plate 79, *A* to *D*). After being carried down through skin and subcutaneous tela and through the anterior sheath of the rectus along the linea alba, the incision is continued through the linea alba, exposing the transversalis fascia. The dome of the bladder and the insertions of the pyramidalis muscles are identified. The operator frequently sees the urachus in the midline, and his incision through the peritoneum should be high enough to avoid the dome of the bladder. A lower midline incision can be extended into the upper abdomen by excision of the umbilicus or by passing to the right or the left of this structure with an oblique extension. If the incision is extended by an oblique cut, the urachus is detached from the umbilicus. The peritoneum and transversalis fascia in the immediate periumbilic area are closed by this maneuver in a slightly different sagittal plane than the remainder of the wound. This helps prevent an incisional hernia that frequently originates about the umbilicus after this incision.

Interiliac Incision

An interiliac incision passes between the iliac crests in a gentle caudad curve (Plate 79, *A* and *B*). After being carried down through the superficial and deep layers of the superficial fascia and the deep fascia, the anterior sheath of the rectus, plus the aponeurosis of the internal and external oblique muscles, is incised. The fibers near the origin of the transversalis may be incised or retracted for exposure. The bellies of the recti are incised transversely and the deep epigastric vessels ligated. The transversalis fascia and peritoneum are incised transversely, which allows for very adequate exposure in the pelvis.

The Cherney modification of this incision was referred to under Indications and Surgical Principles in the Selection of an Abdominal Incision. Here, the recti are resected from their insertion on the pubic tubercles rather than cut directly across. In the closure of the modified interiliac incision the detached recti are resutured to the undersurface of the anterior rectus sheath just above the symphysis. When the muscles are cut directly across, as in the classic interiliac incision, no attempt is made to resuture the bodies of the muscles together. The closure of these incisions utilizes the interrupted silk technique subsequently described for a left rectus incision.

McBurney and Gridiron Muscle-Splitting Incisions

The McBurney and Gridiron muscle-splitting incisions are used primarily in performing appendectomies. They are utilized, when enlarged, for exposure of the pelvic structures on the lateral pelvic wall—the ureter and the common iliac, external iliac, and hypogastric arteries and veins (Plate 79, *A* and *B*). The McBurney incision is in an oblique direction above the inguinal ligament and is modified in length and position, depending on the size of the patient and, in an acute appendicitis, on the point of maximum tenderness. The gridiron incision, while utilizing the same muscle-splitting technique in the deeper layers, is more transverse in its location. After incision of the skin and subcutaneous tela, the aponeurosis of the external oblique muscle is split in the direction of its fibers. The fibers of the internal oblique muscle are split by insertion of a Kelly clamp, and the fibers of the transversalis are separated by the knife handle. The peritoneum is picked up and incised in the general direction of the skin incision. If the incision is utilized as a retroperitoneal approach to the pelvic structures on the lateral pelvic wall, the peritoneum is not incised but is dissected medially to expose the vessels and ureter.

Half Interiliac Incision

The half interiliac incision is employed on the left side to expose the sigmoid colon. It is performed as one half of an interiliac incision with the middle portion passing over the midline (Plate 79, A and B). The level of this incision above the pubis or below the umbilicus is varied, depending on the position of the lesion.

Pfannenstiel Incision

The Pfannenstiel incision is a low transverse incision through skin, subcutaneous tela, and anterior rectus sheath, together with the aponeurosis of the external and internal oblique muscles and the fibers of the transversalis (Plate 79, A and B). The rectus and pyramidalis are not disturbed. They are separated in the midline by sharp dissection to expose the posterior rectus sheath, transversalis fascia, and peritoneum. The peritoneum and transversalis fascia are incised in a longitudinal direction, with care exercised not to injure the bladder at the lower edge of the incision. It is an anatomically sound incision and gives adequate exposure for most minor, benign pelvic surgery. It does not allow adequate exploration or visualization of structures in the upper abdomen.

DETAILS OF OPENING AND CLOSING THE ABDOMEN (ILLUSTRATED BY LOWER LEFT RECTUS INCISION)
Steps of the Operation

1. The incision is made through the skin and subcutaneous tela 2 to 3 cm. from the midline and extends from just above the pubic ramus to just below the umbilicus (Plate 80, A).

2. The area of the incision is draped with skin towels held in place by skin clips and a few interrupted sutures (Plate 80, B). It is particularly important to protect the incision from the region of the umbilicus.

3. The incision is carried down through the skin and subcutaneous tela until the anterior sheath of the rectus muscle is reached (Plate 80, C). This is cleaned of fat and areolar tissue for a few centimeters on each side of the point at which it will be incised.

4. Laparotomy pads are sutured to the subcutaneous tela and are inverted over the skin edges to protect the deeper layers of the wound (Plate 80, D).

5. The anterior rectus sheath is incised longitudinally for the full length of the incision (Plate 80, E).

6. The left rectus muscle is split in the direction of its fibers (Plate 80, F), and active bleeding points are clamped and tied. In performing this incision, the inferior epigastric artery and vein are cut and these are ligated. The generous anastomosis with the superior epigastric artery and vein permits this without compromising the blood supply to the muscle.

7. The peritoneum is incised by picking it up with smooth forceps (Plate 80, G), exercising care not to injure any bowel or omentum that may be adherent just underneath the peritoneum. After the incision into the peritoneal cavity, the index and middle fingers can be inserted while the peritoneal incision is extended the full length of the other layers (Plate 80, H).

8. In the closing of this incision a continuous running mattress suture is used so that the two edges of the peritoneum and transversalis fascia are broadly approximated (Plate 80, I). Interrupted sutures of fine silk that accomplish the same purpose may be used in this closure. If a running suture is used, the perforations in the peritoneum can be minimized by the use of 00 chromic catgut on an atraumatic needle.

9. The muscles are approximated by interrupted sutures of fine silk that just approximate the tissue without strangulation, and the fascia is closed with interrupted sutures of medium silk (Plate 80, J).

10. The deep fascia and the deep and superficial layers of the superficial fascia are closed with

PLATE 80

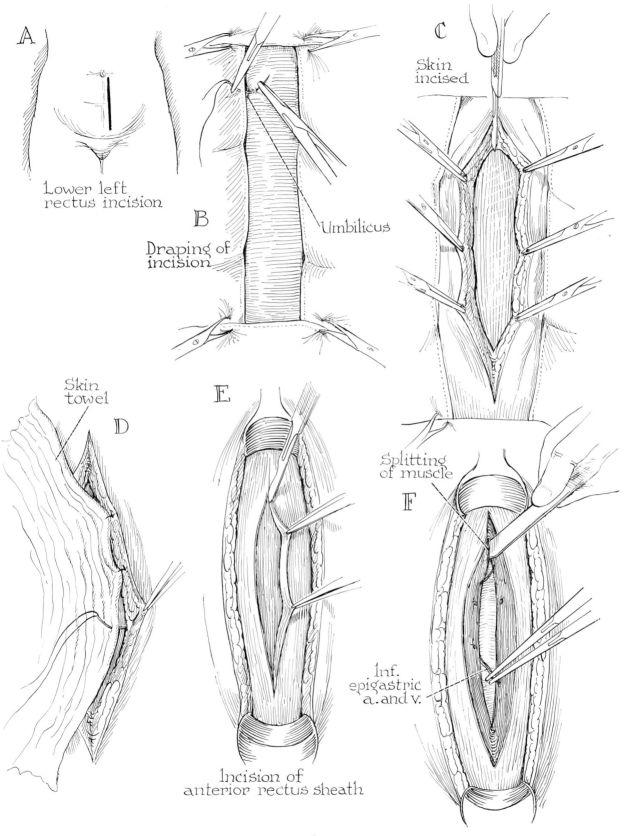

A

Lower left
rectus incision

B

Draping of
incision

Umbilicus

C

Skin
incised

Skin
towel

D

E

Incision of
anterior rectus sheath

Splitting
of muscle

F

Inf.
epigastric
a. and v.

567

PLATE 80 (Concluded)

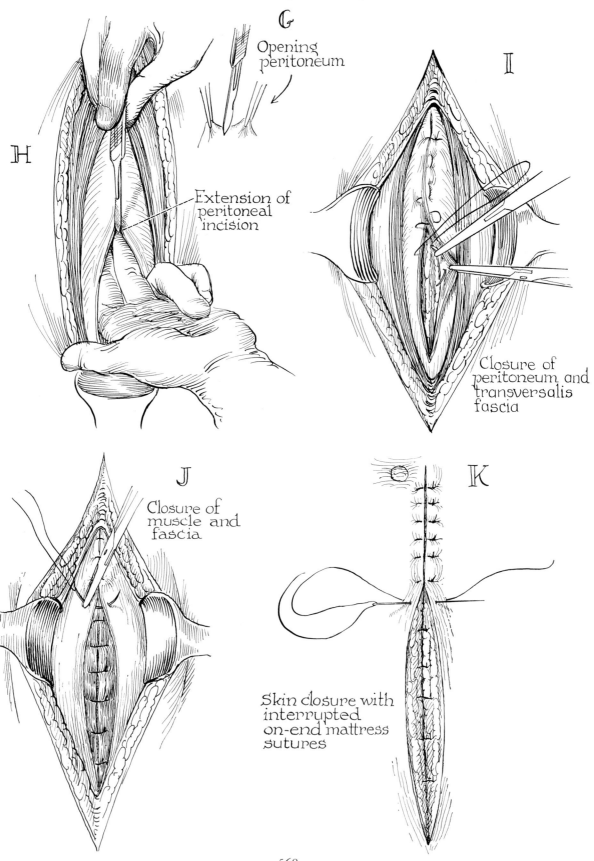

G
Opening
peritoneum

H

Extension of
peritoneal
incision

I

Closure of
peritoneum and
transversalis
fascia

J
Closure of
muscle and
fascia

K

Skin closure with
interrupted
on-end mattress
sutures

several interrupted sutures of fine black silk to obliterate dead space. The skin is closed with interrupted on-end mattress sutures of fine silk (Plate 80, *K*).

11. A sterile towel is placed over the incision and anchored by a few small pieces of adhesive tape until the patient is transported to her room and has reacted from the anesthetic. The towel is then removed and the wound left uncovered unless a large abscess has been drained or drainage tubes have been inserted in the wound for other reasons.

References

Baudelocque, C. A.: Nouveau procede pour pratiquer l'operation Cesarienne, Thesis, Paris, No. 132, 1823.

Cantrell, J. R., and Haller, J. A.: Peritoneal Reconstruction After Extensive Abdominal Wall Resection, Surg., Gynec. & Obst. 110: 363, 1960.

Colvin, E. M., and Wallace, F. T.: Transverse Abdominal Incisions, J. South Carolina M. A. 46: 277, 1959.

Daversa, B., and Landers, D.: Physiological Advantages of the Transverse Incision in Gynecology, Obst. & Gynec. 17: 305, 1961.

Doyle, L.: Abdominal Exposure, Australian & New Zealand J. Surg. 21: 20, 1951.

Maylard, A. E.: Direction of Abdominal Incisions, Brit. M. J. 2: 895, 1907.

Middleton, E. E.: Transverse Abdominal Incisions, Texas J. Med. 46: 154, 1950.

Milloy, F. J., Anson, B. J., and McAfee, D. K.: The Rectus Abdominis Muscle and the Epigastric Arteries, Surg., Gynec. & Obst. 110: 293, 1960.

Palumbo, L. T., Smith, A. N., and Lulu, D. J.: Nonsuture Closure of Clean Muscle-Splitting Abdominal Wounds, Preliminary Report of 117 Wounds, Surgery 41: 986, 1957.

Pfannenstiel, J.: Samml. klin. Vortr. Leipzig. No. 268 (Gynäk. No. 97): 1735, 1900.

Parker, W. S., and Christiansen, K. H.: Rupture of the Rectus Abdominis Muscle With Hematoma, A. M. A. Arch. Surg. 81: 655, 1960.

Silvis, R. S.: Abdominal Incisions for Operations on the Colon and Rectum, California Med. 82: 326, 1955.

Tenenblatt, W., and Cook, T. A.: Transverse Approach to Lower Abdomen, Obst. & Gynec. 3: 627, 1954.

Tollefson, D. G., and Russel, K. P.: Transverse Incision in Pelvic Surgery, Am. J. Obst. & Gynec. 68: 410, 1954.

Tollefson, D. G.: Transverse Abdominal Incisions in Obstetrics and Gynecology, West. J. Surg. 58: 308, 1950.

Williams, G. S.: The Low Transverse Muscle-Cutting Incision in Gynecological Surgery, Am. J. Obst. & Gynec. 67: 398, 1954.

Whitaker, W. G., Jr.: Transverse Abdominal Incisions, South. Surgeon 14: 143, 1948.

34 · Common Abdominal Hernias Corrected in the Course of Gynecologic Surgery

INGUINAL AND FEMORAL HERNIAS
General Considerations

The career of a gynecologist is one continuous study of the anatomy of the female pelvic floor and the forces that disrupt it. Gynecologic surgery for relaxations and reconstructions requires an intimate knowledge of the strength, pliability, and distensibility of structures supporting the pelvic and abdominal viscera. Hernias of the inguinal, femoral, and obturator regions are so simple in their mechanics compared with a vaginal or rectal procidentia, it is small wonder that gynecologic anatomists have ignored them. Perhaps, since we do not have to repair these simple hernias and still preserve such a vital structure as the spermatic cord, we tend to minimize the importance of a careful study of each hernia and individualization of each repair, just as we do in vaginal plastic surgery. Certainly a gynecologic surgeon who at one moment is guiding a patient through a driving labor and a forceful second stage and then retires to another room to reconstruct the pelvic floor is better equipped than any other surgeon to correct the force, direction of force, and other factors causing one of the minor hernias.

In an inguinolabial hernia the hernial fossa of the peritoneum can be seen at laparotomy hanging as an inverted sac in front of the round ligament. With the abdomen open and the patient in the Trendelenberg position, so common in pelvic surgery, the hernia reduces itself, and the sac is seen turned inside out, so to speak. This does not happen if omentum or bowel is adherent within the sac. It is difficult to comprehend how surgeons could have neglected, for so many years, the intra-abdominal approach for the repair of hernias, whether complicated or uncomplicated. The cure of the common inguinal and femoral hernias during the course of other gynecologic surgery adds little to the operating time. If the pelvic surgery can be done through a Pfannenstiel incision, the abdominal ring and fossa ovalis can be exposed with ease by extending the incision slightly and undermining the skin. The factors causing the hernia will be corrected from within the abdomen, where they should be. Additional support superficially is given by one or the other of the methods of hernia repair. It is amusing to speculate on how many hernias or potential indirect inguinal hernias must have been cured by surgeons suspending a uterus by imbricating, shortening, and drawing the round ligaments through the inguinal canal for anchorage to the external oblique aponeurosis. How many have been curing hernias for years by the logical route without knowing it? By coincidence, but reluctantly, a uterine suspension can be said to have some usefulness.

Etiology and Pathologic Anatomy

Anatomic factors and developmental defects are the basic causes of inguinal and femoral hernias in the female. While there is nothing comparable to the descent of the testis into the scrotum, a peritoneal process, the canal of Nuck, occurs to varying degrees along the round ligament. The damage and pressures sustained by women during pregnancy and parturition, together with the altered dynamics of the pelvic floor and intra-abdominal contents after repeated pregnancies, aggravate many potential hernias that become grossly recognizable and symptomatic. In the repair of an inguinal hernia, either direct or indirect, the extra-abdominal tissues are closed as if both existed. It should be assumed that if the patient has imperfect tissues that result in one type of hernia, she probably has a potential hernia of the other type. Study of such women will probably reveal varicose veins, cystorectocele, hemorrhoids with mucosal prolapse, and the other signs of poor fascial and connective tissue support.

Symptoms and Diagnosis

Most hernias are asymptomatic, with the patient becoming aware of the defect because of the protrusion. Pain or a dull ache, especially on lifting, may call the patient's attention to the area. The alterations of the body mechanics and changes in the position of the viscera during pregnancy undoubtedly contribute to herniation, but it is surprising how few hernias are recognized or become symptomatic during the actual pregnancy. Perhaps the looseness of the tissues, the hypertrophy of the round ligament, and the displacement of omentum and bowel into the upper abdomen change the signs and symptoms of this condition as it does many others. Strangulation is catastrophic when bowel is involved. Pain, nausea, vomiting, and other signs of intestinal obstruction ensue. Female patients are examined in the lithotomy and standing positions. The protrusion is palpated, particularly to determine whether it is above or below the inguinal ligament. In some obese patients, accumulations of fat in the lower abdomen or deposits in the areolar tissue of the femoral canal defy the most skillful palpation. The symptomatology and signs of recurrent, umbilical, incisional, obturator, and other special hernias are so varied that a characteristic description is not possible.

Surgical Anatomy of the Inguinal and Femoral Canals

The lower edge of the external oblique aponeurosis between the anterior superior iliac spine and the pubic tubercle folds back on itself to form the inguinal ligament (Plate 81, *A*). A rounded surface presents toward the thigh, while the abdominal aspect forms a shelf. The ligament describes a gentle curve in its course, the concavity of which is directed upward. Several extensions and landmarks are used in hernia repair. The lacunar ligament (Gimbernat) is a triangular process with its apex inserted into the pubic tubercle (Plate 81, *B* and *D*). Its upper side is an extension of the inguinal ligament, while its lower side is inserted for about 2.5 cm. into the iliopectineal line on the superior ramus of the pubis. The reflected inguinal ligament (triangular fascia, ligament of Cooper) is a triangular sheet of fibers woven into the aponeurosis of the external oblique muscle (Plate 81, *A* and *C*). The fibers originate from the medial end of the iliopectineal line together with the one side of the lacunar ligament. They pass upward and medialward under cover of the superior crus of the subcutaneous inguinal ring to insert into the linea alba. Some fibers pass across the midline to mingle with the fibers of the aponeurosis of the opposite external oblique muscle (Plate 81, *C*).

The internal or deep abdominal ring is situated in the transversalis fascia midway between the anterior superior spine of the ilium and the symphysis pubis (Plate 81, *B*). It lies about one half inch above the inguinal ligament. The internal ring is bounded above externally by the arched fibers of the transversalis muscle and below and internally by the deep epigastric vessels. The inguinal canal begins at the internal ring and passes downward and inward for 3 to 4 cm. to the external abdominal ring. The inguinal canal is bounded in front (anteriorly) by the aponeurosis of the external oblique for its entire length and by the internal oblique for its outer one third. Behind (posteriorly) its wall is formed by the transversalis fascia, conjoined tendon, and the

PLATE 81

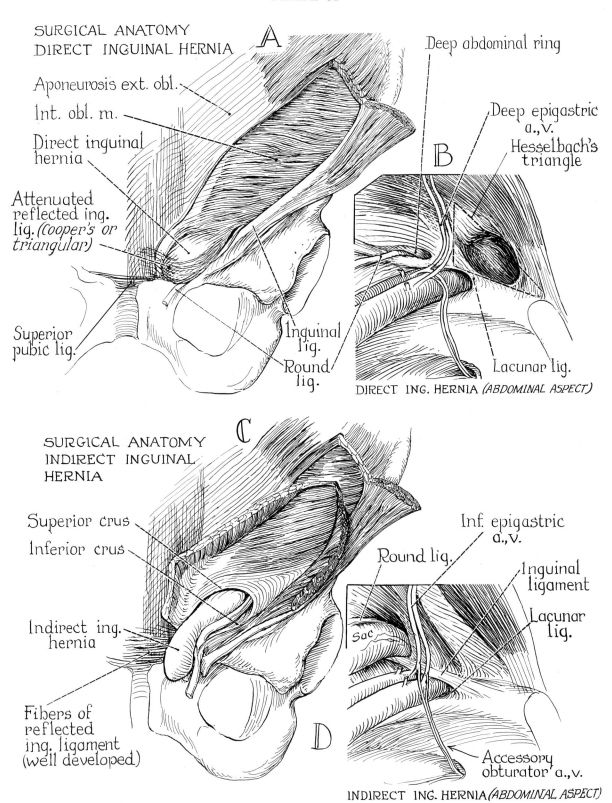

SURGICAL ANATOMY
DIRECT INGUINAL HERNIA

A

Aponeurosis ext. obl.

Int. obl. m.

Direct inguinal
hernia

Attenuated
reflected ing.
lig. *(Cooper's or
triangular)*

Superior
pubic lig.

Inguinal
lig.

Round
lig.

Deep abdominal ring

B

Deep epigastric
a., v.

Hesselbach's
triangle

Lacunar lig.

DIRECT ING. HERNIA *(ABDOMINAL ASPECT)*

SURGICAL ANATOMY
INDIRECT INGUINAL
HERNIA

C

Superior crus

Inferior crus

Indirect ing.
hernia

Fibers of
reflected
ing. ligament
(well developed)

Inf. epigastric
a., v.

Round lig.

Inguinal
ligament

Lacunar
lig.

Sac

D

Accessory
obturator a., v.

INDIRECT ING. HERNIA *(ABDOMINAL ASPECT)*

PLATE 81 (Concluded)

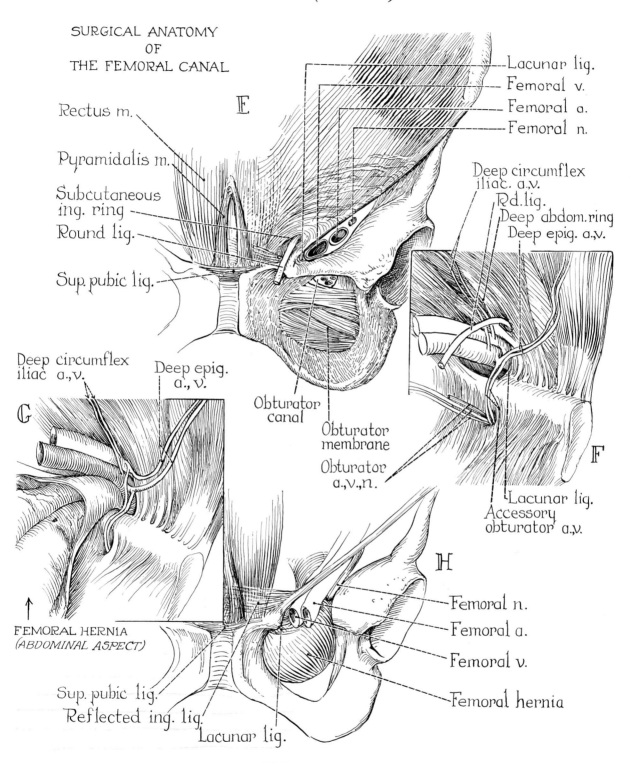

SURGICAL ANATOMY
OF
THE FEMORAL CANAL

Rectus m.

Pyramidalis m.

Subcutaneous
ing. ring
Round lig.

Sup. pubic lig.

E

Lacunar lig.
Femoral v.
Femoral a.
Femoral n.

Deep circumflex
iliac. a.,v.
Rd.lig.
Deep abdom.ring
Deep epig. a.,v.

Deep circumflex
iliac a.,v.

Deep epig.
a., v.

G

Obturator
canal

Obturator
membrane

Obturator
a.,v.,n.

F

Lacunar lig.
Accessory
obturator a.,v.

FEMORAL HERNIA
(ABDOMINAL ASPECT)

H

Femoral n.

Femoral a.

Femoral v.

Femoral hernia

Sup. pubic lig.
Reflected ing. lig.
Lacunar lig.

SURGICAL ANATOMY OF FEMORAL HERNIA

573

reflected inguinal ligament when the latter is prominently developed. Superiorly the wall or roof is formed by the approximated anterior and posterior walls. Inferiorly the floor is formed by the upper grooved surface of the inguinal ligament. The inguinal canal contains the round ligament (to whose circumference the internal ring closely corresponds), and small arteries derived from the deep epigastric and ovarian arteries. The deep epigastric artery passes upward and inward near the inner side of the internal abdominal ring. The interval between this artery and the outer edge of the rectus muscle is named Hesselbach's triangle (Plate 81, *B*). The base of this triangle —featured in the description of direct and indirect hernias—is formed by the inguinal ligament. The external (abdominal) ring is an interval in the aponeurosis of the external oblique muscle just above and to the outer side of the crest of the pubic bone (Plate 81, *C*). It is somewhat triangular in form: about 2.5 cm. from base to apex and about 1 cm. wide. It is bounded below by the crest of pubic bone, and its sides are formed by the margins of the aponeurosis that become somewhat thicker to gain the title of columns or pillars of the ring (superior and inferior crura —Plate 81, *C*). Fibers arching across the upper angle of the ring that strengthen it considerably are termed the intercolumnar fibers.

The femoral ring is the upper or abdominal opening of the femoral canal (Plate 81, *F* and *G*). It is not a true canal since it is closed by extraperitoneal fat, lymphatics, and lymph nodes. Medially it is bounded by the lacunar ligament and laterally by the femoral vein (Plate 81, *E* and *F*). Anteriorly it is bounded by the inguinal ligament and posteriorly by the pectineus muscle. The femoral canal occupies the medial division of the femoral sheath. It is about 2 cm. long from the femoral ring to the fossa ovalis (Plate 81, *G* and *H*). It is bounded laterally by the femoral vein, medially by the union of the iliac and transversalis fascia, behind by the iliac fascia, and in front by the transversalis fascia (Plate 81, *H*). Be-

cause of its rich contents of lymphatics, it has been called "the lymphatic canal." The fossa ovalis (saphenous opening) is an oval depression where the fascia lata diverges at different levels. There is actually no defect left by the fascia lata, since the deep layer of the superficial fascia fills up the opening. The upper extremity of the fossa ovalis blends with the lacunar ligament; the lower is at the point where the two parts of the fascia lata meet. The medial border is formed by the fascia lata (pubic or pectineal part) and the lateral border (falciform) by the iliac portion of the fascia lata. The greater saphenous vein gains entrance to the femoral vein by the fossa ovalis.

The femoral canal contains nerves, arteries, veins, and fatty connective tissue which resist the intra-abdominal pressure. When the capacity of the canal to resist is less than the pressure exerted, a hernia is extruded (Plate 81, *G* and *H*). Thus, the cure must divert the pressure by ligation of the sac and occlusion of the aperture.

Indications

Symptomatic hernias should be repaired surgically if there is no contraindication to surgery and anesthesia. Unequivocal hernias that may contain bowel or omentum provide the factors that lead to strangulation. Strangulation or irreducibility of a hernia requires immediate operation if the patient is ready for surgery and her electrolytes and fluids are such that she can tolerate the anesthetic and operation. The optimum time for such an operation is decided for each patient. Nonstrangulated or easily reducible hernias in infants and children may be observed for several years before electing surgery. Massive irreducible hernias in elderly, obese, poor-risk patients who have had no signs of subacute or chronic obstruction are better left alone. This is true as long as the contents function adequately in their ectopic location. Supports used in the nonoperative management of hernias are secured only after study and recommendation by the gynecologist.

Surgical Principles and Refinements in Technique

1. Muscle cannot be sutured to ligament and form a strong closure of a hernial defect. The approximation of the conjoined tendon (not conjoined, not a tendon, and usually not well developed in the female) to the shelving edge of the inguinal ligament is not surgically sound. Modifications of the original Bassini technique (Halsted, Tanner) that employ relieving incisions in the rectus sheath cannot compensate for a basic surgical and anatomic error.

2. The tissues used to repair an inguinal or femoral hernia should take the form of a graft or interposition of inert or vital tissues to obliterate the route of the sac.

3. Fatty deposits in the region of the external abdominal ring or fossa ovalis are justifiable causes of diagnostic errors. The gynecologist should be alert to the possibility that they coexist with a hernia containing bowel or omentum.

4. Nonabsorbable suture material (silk, wire, cotton) is preferred in hernia surgery. Complicated hernias may require fascial sutures or wire mesh of stainless steel or tantalum.

5. The round ligament serves no useful purpose in the adult female. Since it need not be carefully preserved, as the spermatic cord, the gynecologic surgeon may close the internal ring completely, and his herniorrhaphies should be stronger and recurrence rate lower.

6. As with the pelvic floor, the force and weight a hernia repair must carry in the erect position are compared to the force and weigh in the lithotomy position. The obese, short woman will direct her intra-abdominal pressure in a vertical direction in the erect position, while her large panniculus hangs forward, changing her center of gravity toward the hernial sites.

7. One should consider the surgical wisdom of repairing hernias in such patients by a combined extra-abdominal and intra-abdominal approach. If what little fibrous tissue that can be mobilized for the repair is infiltrated with fat and has lost its elasticity, one can hardly hope to create a firm union. Consideration is given to the use of tantalum mesh in the primary operation and not waiting until the recurrence to acknowledge the inadequacy of the patient's tissues.

8. In the intra-abdominal approach to hernia repair, remember to remove all the fat from the edges of the internal abdominal ring before it is obliterated. Explore for accessory sacs, and test the effectiveness of the closure by pushing with the finger to find weak areas near the obliterated ring.

Postoperative Care

The general nutritional requirements of the convalescent patient are maintained to promote wound healing. The wounds are best left open so sweat and skin secretions do not macerate the edges of the incision. Patients are mobilized early and reassured concerning this procedure. Abdominal binders, immobilization, and strapping of wounds invite thrombophlebitis and embolism that is potentially fatal, whereas the hernia may only have been mildly symptomatic.

INTRA-ABDOMINAL INDIRECT INGUINAL HERNIORRHAPHY
Steps of the Operation

1. Omentum or bowel is spontaneously reduced from the hernial sac with the patient in a high Trendelenburg position and the abdomen open. If the contents are adherent within the sac, they are reduced by sharp and blunt dissection. The femoral artery and vein, the deep epigastric artery and vein, and the abdominal aspect of the inguinal ligament are identified (Plate 82, A).

2. The sac is inverted into the abdomen, and the round ligament and the edges of the dilated internal abdominal ring are noted (Plate 82, B). An incision is made through the peritoneum at the base of the sac (Plate 82, B). Remnants of the transversalis fascia that will strengthen the closure are preserved.

3. Mattress sutures are placed through the anterior edge of the internal ring and the inguinal ligament. Fine and medium silk are used throughout the hernia repairs. Linen, steel wire, and tantalum are excellent materials and preferred by some surgeons. In a large hernia or one of long standing, it is not possible to identify the exact layers. The sutures will pass through the transversalis fascia and the edge of the internal oblique or conjoined tendon if the latter structure is well developed (Plate 82, C). The round ligament is deliberately cut and left to retract toward the uterus. If a hysterectomy has been performed, the portion of the round ligament between the internal ring and point at which it was resected during the hysterectomy can be left in its anatomic position to do no more harm nor no more good than it did before.

PLATE 82

INTRA-ABDOMINAL INGUINAL HERNIORRHAPHY

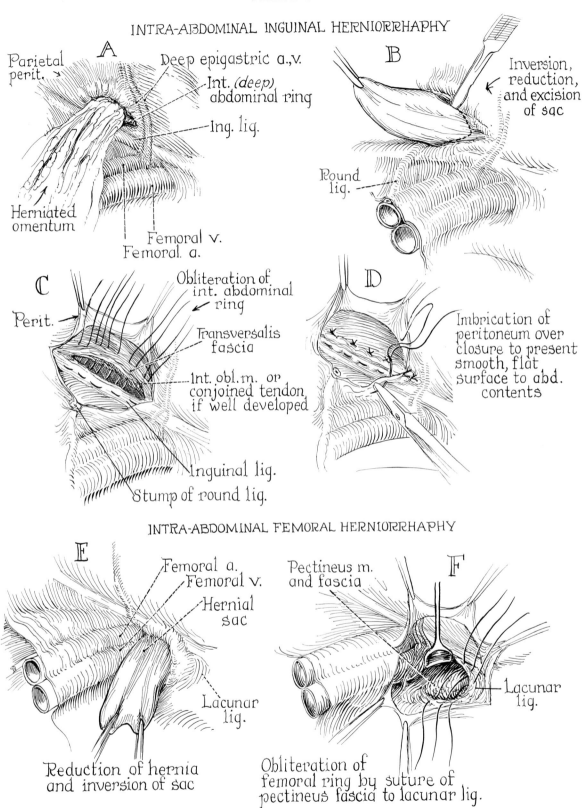

A

Parietal perit.

Deep epigastric a.,v.

Int. (deep) abdominal ring

Ing. lig.

Herniated omentum

Femoral v.
Femoral. a.

B

Inversion, reduction, and excision of sac

Round lig.

C

Obliteration of int. abdominal ring

Perit.

Transversalis fascia

Int. obl. m. or conjoined tendon if well developed

Inguinal lig.

Stump of round lig.

D

Imbrication of peritoneum over closure to present smooth, flat surface to abd. contents

INTRA-ABDOMINAL FEMORAL HERNIORRHAPHY

E

Femoral a.
Femoral v.

Hernial sac

Lacunar lig.

Reduction of hernia and inversion of sac

F

Pectineus m. and fascia

Lacunar lig.

Obliteration of femoral ring by suture of pectineus fascia to lacunar lig.

4. An anterior flap of peritoneum is imbricated over the inguinal ligament to present a smooth, flat surface to the abdominal contents (Plate 82, D).

5. The obliteration of the external abdominal ring is done during the closure of the abdominal incision if the herniorrhaphy is incidental to other pelvic surgery. If the hernia repair is the primary operation, additional support is gained by following the technique described later for an extra-abdominal inguinal herniorrhaphy.

INTRA-ABDOMINAL DIRECT INGUINAL HERNIORRHAPHY
Steps of the Operation

A direct hernia is reduced and the sac inverted in the same manner as the indirect hernia. The internal orifice of an intra-abdominal direct inguinal hernia is a congenital defect or weakness at the medial edge of the line of origin of the transversalis and internal oblique muscles. For the intra-abdominal closure of the neck of a direct hernial sac, the transversalis fascia and the edges of the transversalis and internal oblique muscles are sutured to the inguinal ligament or its extension toward the symphysis, the superior pubic ligament. Individual hernias may be dealt with by the use of fascial grafts or tantalum mesh in the primary repair.

INTRA-ABDOMINAL FEMORAL HERNIORRHAPHY
Steps of the Operation

1. The hernia is reduced and the sac inverted into the abdomen (Plate 82, E). An accessory obturator artery and vein may be encountered, and these can be ligated. The femoral artery and vein are usually displaced somewhat laterally by the hernia. They are retracted during the closure of the femoral ring and, at intervals, are allowed to fall back in their normal course and are observed for stricture or compression by the closure.

2. The lacunar ligament is sutured to the pectineus fascia to obliterate the femoral canal (Plate 82, F). The sutures are started medially and continue toward the femoral vein until the femoral ring is obliterated except for an adequate exit for the femoral vessels and nerve. Some of the deep inguinal lymphatics, nodes, and areolar tissue may have to be removed to avoid including these tissues in the line of closure.

3. The flaps of peritoneum are trimmed and imbricated to present a smooth surface to the abdominal contents. The exit sites for other hernias

—direct and indirect inguinal, obturator, lumbar, umbilical—are palpated so that defects in these locations can be corrected.

EXTRA-ABDOMINAL INDIRECT INGUINAL HERNIORRHAPHY
Steps of the Operation

1. The skin incision is made about 2 cm. above and parallel to the inguinal ligament. This is carried down through the superficial and deep fascia. The aponeurosis of the external oblique is cleaned of fat and areolar tissue over the external ring and for 6 to 8 cm. above.

2. The aponeurosis of the external oblique muscle is incised in the direction of its fibers from the external ring to a point 6 to 8 cm. above. The hernia is reduced by sharp and blunt dissection (Plate 83, A). No attention need be given to the round ligament, which may or may not be identified on the lateral side of the sac.

3. The sac is incised (Plate 83, A) and its contents are reduced and replaced within the abdomen. Adherent bowel or omentum that is dissected free is observed to ensure that it has an adequate blood supply and has not been damaged. The neck of the sac is dissected free through the inguinal canal to the internal ring.

4. The neck of the sac is ligated flush with the parietal peritoneum (Plate 83, B). The round ligament may be included in this suture since its preservation is unnecessary.

5. The ends of the suture from the ligation of the sac are passed under the internal oblique muscle and through the internal and external oblique muscles and tied (Plate 83, C).

6. Several interrupted sutures are used to obliterate the inguinal canal (Plate 83, C). A flap is now developed from the external oblique aponeurosis that will cover the area of the dilated external ring and extend further medially to be sutured to the fibers of the reflected tendon as they pass toward the midline.

7. Plate 83, D, shows the flap developed from the aponeurosis of the external oblique sutured to the reflected inguinal ligament. This gives a strong closure over the former site of the abdominal ring.

8. The aponeurosis of the external oblique is imbricated by mattress sutures (Plate 83, D). The upper flap is sutured to the inguinal ligament in the area from which the flap was cut to cover the region of the external ring. The final appearance

PLATE 83

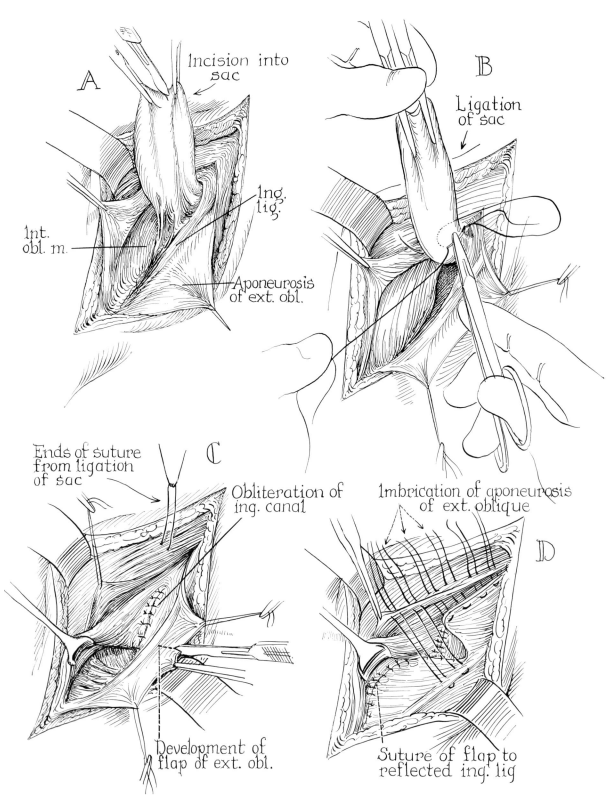

A

Incision into sac

Int. obl. m.

Ing. lig.

Aponeurosis of ext. obl.

B

Ligation of sac

C

Ends of suture from ligation of sac

Obliteration of ing. canal

Development of flap of ext. obl.

D

Imbrication of aponeurosis of ext. oblique

Suture of flap to reflected ing. lig

is that of a gentle S-curve when the imbrication is completed.

EXTRA-ABDOMINAL DIRECT INGUINAL HERNIA
Steps of the Operation

A direct inguinal hernia can be repaired by the technique illustrated in Plate 83, *D*. The sac which is medial to the deep epigastric vessels is tied off flush with the parietal peritoneum. A similar flap is developed from the aponeurosis of the external oblique muscle. It is sutured to the reflected inguinal ligament as near to the linea alba as possible. The imbrication is done in the same way except that the lower part of the upper flap should be mobilized so it can be brought down to the insertion of the inguinal ligament into the pubic tubercle or even more medially along the superior pubic ligament.

EXTRA-ABDOMINAL FEMORAL HERNIORRHAPHY
Steps of the Operation

1. An incision is made just above and paralleling the inguinal ligament. The incision is carried down through the superficial and deep layers of the superficial fascia and the deep fascia. The aponeurosis of the external oblique muscle is cleaned of fat and areolar tissue about 2 cm. above the inguinal ligament. It is cut in the direction of its fibers.

2. The internal oblique and transversalis muscles are split and retracted medially to expose the neck of the sac. If the sac reduces easily, this can be done at this time, converting it into an inguinal hernia. Plate 84, *A*, shows the position of the sac and its reduction.

3. The sac is ligated flush with the parietal peritoneum, and the dilated femoral ring is explored (Plate 84, *B*).

4. The reduction of the sac, particularly if it is adherent, can wait until the exposure of the fossa ovalis. This is done by dissection of the skin and superficial fascia from the fascia lata a sufficient distance below the inguinal ligament to expose the femoral vessels and the femoral canal emerging in the fossa ovalis. The skin and subcutaneous tela are readily retracted.

5. The reduction in size of the femoral canal below the inguinal ligament is accomplished by suturing the medial end of the inguinal and base of the lacunar ligament to the fascia of the pectineus muscle (Plate 84, *C*). Mattress sutures of medium silk are placed beginning at the medial side of the ring (Plate 84, *C*). The dilated fem-

oral canal is reduced so the femoral vessels and nerves pass through it without constriction. Enlarged deep inguinal lymphatics and fat that might intervene in the suture line are removed. This is especially important if they are enlarged and infected from the drainage of chronic skin infections of the feet and lower extremities.

6. A flap is fashioned from the lower side of the aponeurosis of the external oblique (Plate 84, *D*). This is cut so it can be folded over the inguinal ligament and sutured to the pectineus fascia to partially obliterate the femoral ring. Medially this flap is sutured to the transversalis fascia and fibers of the reflected inguinal ligament (Plate 84, *D*).

7. The internal oblique muscle is approximated with a few interrupted sutures, and the aponeurosis of the external oblique muscle is imbricated as previously shown for an inguinal herniorrhaphy.

OTHER COMMON HERNIAS
UMBILICAL HERNIA

Umbilical hernia is an all-inclusive term to cover several types of hernias about the umbilicus that can range from a massive defect in the abdominal wall with protrusion of the abdominal viscera to a small herniation about the umbilicus in an adult that requires no treatment. Clinically, umbilical hernias are divided into three groups: congenital hernia into the umbilical cord, umbilical hernias in the newborn infants, and umbilical hernias in adults. Cases of herniation into the cord may be so severe as to be incompatible with life and offer no hope for replacement of the ectopic viscera into an abdominal cavity. The obstetrician should exercise care in tying the cord in the less severe types of this hernia. A knuckle of bowel is readily included in the cord tie. These hernias are also known as funicular hernias, omphaloceles, and amniotic hernias. Several plastic repairs may be necessary to enclose the viscera completely, and the stages of the operation should be spaced along with the growth of the child. A small umbilical hernia, covered with skin and with no defect in the muscle development of the abdominal wall, is observed for spontaneous closure. A small dressing of sponge rubber is held in place with a binder to keep such a hernia reduced as the infant

PLATE 84

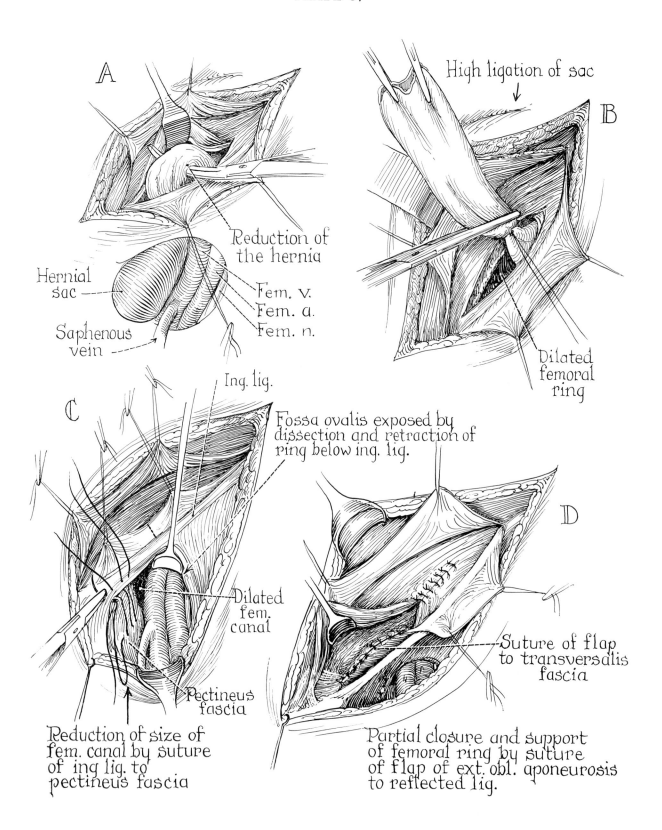

A

Reduction of the hernia

Hernial sac

Fem. v.
Fem. a.
Fem. n.

Saphenous vein

High ligation of sac

B

Dilated femoral ring

C

Ing. lig.

Fossa ovalis exposed by dissection and retraction of ring below ing. lig.

Dilated fem. canal

Pectineus fascia

Reduction of size of fem. canal by suture of ing. lig. to pectineus fascia

D

Suture of flap to transversalis fascia

Partial closure and support of femoral ring by suture of flap of ext. obl. aponeurosis to reflected lig.

grows older. If there is evidence of obstruction or if it fails to reduce in size after six to eight months' observation, a herniorrhaphy is done. Through a small, curved subumbilical incision, the sac is reduced and tied off flush with the adjacent parietal peritoneum. The fascia is closed transversely and may be imbricated if the defect is large. The adult variety of this hernia is usually repaired during some other abdominal surgery. The defect may be closed intra-abdominally, extra-abdominally, or by a combination of both approaches. The umbilicus can be excised should this facilitate the closure of the defect. The rectus sheaths may be imbricated across the midline as indicated.

INCISIONAL HERNIA

Incisional hernias present a varying picture, depending on their location in the abdominal wall and the type of incision employed at the primary operation. Frequently the wound was infected or had developed a seroma or hematoma. The sac is seldom well defined, and the hernia presents as a large bulge composed of skin, subcutaneous tela, and peritoneum. Bowel and omentum are almost invariably adherent within the sac and are meticulously dissected free during the operation. The method of closure depends on the ability of the operator to define and dissect the original layers of the abdominal wall. Usually two layers other than the skin and subcutaneous tela are developed for the closure. The peritoneum, transversalis fascia, and remnants of the abdominal muscles are imbricated as a deep layer. The rectus sheath is imbricated in the opposite direction and slightly different sagittal plane. If the hernia is lateral to the recti, the full thickness of the abdominal wall and peritoneum may have to be imbricated as one layer in the closure. Tantalum mesh has proved itself superior to other materials presently available for the closure of large defects where sufficient strong fascia and muscle cannot be mobilized for the closure. The mesh is fitted to the defect, the edges turned under, and sutures of tantalum wire used to anchor the mesh to the adjacent abdominal wall. Mattress sutures of tantalum wire are placed a centimeter back from the turned-under edge, down through the mesh into strong tissue at the edge of the defect, and back up through the mesh to be tied.

RARE HERNIAS

Posterior vaginal hernias, lumbar hernias, sciatic hernias, and obturator hernias are uncommon and may only be discovered accidentally if their points of exit from the abdominal cavity are routinely palpated during a laparotomy. The repair of these hernias follows the general principle of obliteration of the defect and presenting the abdominal contents with a smooth, solid surface at the site of the original hernia.

References

Anson, B. J., and Ashley, F. L.: Anatomy of Region of Inguinal Hernia; Parietal Coverings of Round Ligament of Uterus, Quart. Bull. Northwestern Univ. M. School 15: 32, 1941.

Anson, B. J., Morgan, E. H., and McVay, C. B.: Surgical Anatomy of the Inguinal Region Based Upon a Study of 500 Body-Halves, Surg., Gynec. & Obst. 111: 707, 1960.

Brown, R. K.: Umbilical Hernia Repair by Layer Closure of Posterior and Anterior Rectus Sheaths, Surg., Gynec. & Obst. 110: 363, 1960.

Burton, C. C.: A Description of the Boundaries of the Inguinal Rings and Scrotal Pouches, Surg., Gynec. & Obst. 107: 142, 1957.

Burton, C. C.: Fascia Lata, Cutis, and Tantalum Grafts in Repair of Massive Abdominal Incisional Hernias, Surg., Gynec. & Obst. 109: 621, 1959.

Gibson, L. D., and Gaspar, M. R.: A Review of 606 Cases of Umbilical Hernia, Internat. Abstr. Surg. 109: 313, 1959.

Handelsman, J. C.: A Technique for Increasing Abdominal Capacity in the Repair of Massive Ventral Hernia, Surg., Gynec. & Obst. 109: 751, 1959.

Harrison, J. H.: A Teflon Weave for Replacing Tissue Defects, Surg., Gynec. & Obst. 104: 584, 1957.

Hertzler, A. E.: The Peritoneum, vol. 1, St. Louis, 1919, The C. V. Mosby Co.

Jacobson, P.: Inguinal Herniorrhaphy From the Intra-abdominal Perspective, Am. J. Surg. 71: 797, 1946.

Jacobson, P.: Intraabdominal Approach to Inguinal Herniorraphy, Am. J. Surg. 79, 557, 1950.

Janelli, E., and Stevenson, A.: The Henry Approach to Femoral Hernia, New York J. Med. 55: 2191, 1955.

Keasling, J. E.: Incarcerated Femoral Hernia Containing an Ovary, J. A. M. A. 170: 2184, 1959.

LaRoque, P. G.: An Improved Method of Removing Hernia From Within, Ann. Surg. 79: 375, 1924.

LaRoque, P. G.: The Intraabdominal Method of Removing Inguinal and Femoral Hernia, Arch. Surg. 24: 189, 1932.

LaRoque, P. G.: The Intrabdominal Operation for Femoral Herniorrhaphy, Ann. Surg. 75: 110, 1922.

McDougal, W.: Purse-string Suture Repair of Indirect Inguinal Hernia, Am. J. Surg. 91: 227, 1956.

McVay, C. B., and Chapp, J. D.: Inguinal and Femoral Hernioplasty, Ann. Surg. **148:** 499, 1958.

Mason, M. S., and Raaf, J.: Use of Homologous Dura Mater in the Repair of Hernias, A. M. A. Arch. Surg. **82:** 856, 1961.

Nyhus, L. M., Condon, R. E., and Harkins, H. N.: Clinical Experiences With Preperitoneal Hernial Repair for All Types of Hernia of the Groin, Am. J. Surg. **100:** 234, 1960.

Ogilvie, H.: Hernia, Baltimore, 1959, Williams & Wilkins Co.

Poth, E.: A Basic Concept in the Use of the Rectus-Pyramidalis Sheath and Transplants in the Repair of Hernias, Surg., Gynec. & Obst. **111:** 515, 1960.

Pualwan, F.: Operative Aspects of Richter's Hernia, Surg., Gynec. & Obst. **106:** 358, 1958.

Rack, F. J., and Webb, E. A.: Sliding Hernia. Experiences With Thirty-Three Cases With a Report of Two Cases in Infants, Ohio M. J. **50:** 441, 1954.

Roesel, R. W.: Richter's Hernia, Nebraska M. J. **45:** 460, 1960.

Schwarts, W.: Lumbar Hernias, J. Kentucky M. A. **52:** 673, 1954.

Usher, F. C.: Knitted Marlex Mesh; an Improved Marlex Prosthesis for Repairing Hernias and Other Tissue Defects, A. M. A. Arch. Surg. **82:** 771, 1961.

Usher, F. C., and others: Marlex Mesh, a New Plastic Mesh for Replacing Tissue Defects, A. M. A. Arch. Surg. **78:** 138, 1959.

Usher, F. C., Cogan, J. E., and Lowry, T. I.: A New Technique for the Repair of Inguinal and Incisional Hernias, A. M. A. Arch. Surg. **81:** 847, 1960.

Usher, F. C.: A New Technique for Repairing Large Abdominal Wall Defects, A. M. A. Arch. Surg. **82:** 870, 1961.

Zimmerman, L. M., and Anson, B. J.: Anatomy and Surgery of Hernia, Baltimore, 1953, Williams & Wilkins Co.

35 · Intestinal Surgery Incident to Gynecologic Procedures

SURGERY OF THE SMALL BOWEL IN GYNECOLOGY
General Considerations

The third part of the ileum frequently occupies the upper part of the true pelvis and becomes involved in pelvic disease. Resection of damaged or obstructed segments secondary to pelvic operations is required in gynecology. Cancer surgeons are constantly developing new techniques for the use of isolated segments of the small bowel for repair of organs and diversion of the urinary stream.

Surgical Anatomy and Principles

The mesenteric small intestine is divided into the jejunum and the ileum. It is approximately 4 meters in length in the living body and decreases from a diameter of about 4 cm. at the duodenum to about 2.5 cm. at the lower end. The jejunum begins at the duodenojejunal flexure opposite the second lumbar vertebra, where it is in contact with the inferior surface of the pancreas and the root of the transverse mesocolon. The suspensory ligament of Treitz, an important landmark, descends from the left crus of the diaphragm to the terminal duodenum, passing to the left of the celiac artery and behind the pancreas. The coils of the jejunum tend to occupy the upper left quadrant of the abdomen.

The mesentery is a double layer of peritoneum that encloses and supports the jejunum and ileum and their vessels, nerves, and lymphatics. It is about 15 cm. long and extends from the duodenojejunal flexure obliquely downward and to the right and then across the transverse duodenum, the great vessels, and the vertebral column to the ileocecal junction. The attachment of the mesentery to the small bowel is much longer than its root—corresponding to the combined lengths of the jejunum and ileum. The length of the mesentery, from parietal to visceral attachments, ranges from 15 to 25 cm. The length of its proximal and distal portions is less than the center.

The lower portion of the small bowel, the ileum, occupies the lower right side of the abdominal cavity, with its lower portion in the true pelvis. It then passes upward over the brim of the pelvis to terminate at the ileocecal junction.

The small intestine has four layers: mucosa, submucosa, muscularis, and serosa. The mucosa is lined with a simple cylindrical epithelium, underneath which is a fibrous lamina propria limited externally by a muscularis mucosa. The inner surface of the mucosa presents many numerous transverse folds (circular plica) which are made up of the mucosa and submucosa and extend from one half to two thirds around the lumen. They are better developed in the jejunum and absent in the terminal ileum. This may aid in intestinal localization.

The mesenteric small intestine receives its arterial supply from the superior mesenteric artery. This artery runs between the layers of the mesentery and gives off six or seven large branches and several small branches. The first two or three of the larger branches divide into ascending and descending branches (intestinal arteries) that join together to form a single row of arches. At the beginning of the second quarter of the jejunoileum two tiers of arches are formed. From the middle half of the small bowel to the ileocecal junction two or more tiers may be present, and the complexity of the arches increases and the caliber of the vessels decreases. From the arches, vasa recta pass to the mesenteric border of the bowel. These straight vessels are longer in the proximal small bowel and become progressively shorter distally as the complexity of the arches increases. Study of the arterial supply helps indicate the part of the intestine that a given coil belongs to. Veins accompany the arteries, and the superior mesenteric vein joins the splenic to form the portal vein. Lymphatics of the mucosa and muscular coats of the small intestine join to form a rich plexus throughout the thickness of the bowel wall. The efferent lymphatic vessels (lacteals) pass through the nodes of the mesentery to reach the cisterna (receptaculum) chyli. The nerve supply to the small bowel is from the superior mesenteric plexus, which is continuous with the lower part of the celiac plexus. The nerve fibers are chiefly sympathetic, but part of them takes origin from the vagus nerve. A Meckel's diverticulum is found in a small percentage of patients. This is a blind tube, averaging about 5 cm. in length; it is located, on the average, about 80 cm.—with wide variations—above the ileocecal junction.

RESECTION OF THE SMALL BOWEL
Indications and Surgical Principles

Minor injuries to the small bowel are frequent occurrences in gynecologic surgery, particularly in the presence of pelvic inflammatory disease or endometriosis. Small areas of damage to the bowel or perforations are repaired by closure in a transverse direction with one or more layers of seromuscular sutures of fine silk. In general, if the normal mesenteric blood supply can be preserved to a section of the bowel and the damaged portion closed without constriction, this is preferable to a resection and anastomosis. The blood supply to an area of anastomosis can never approximate the normal. Intestinal obstruction due to ad-

hesions or volvulus after pelvic surgery or due to some pelvic disease is a surgical emergency. It may require only the release of the constricting band or volvulus or may require resection of extensive segments of the small bowel. In the following operation a segment of small bowel was nonviable after being dissected free of an extensive endometrial implant.

Steps of the Operation

1. A wedge of mesentery is outlined well beyond the vascular bed of the necrotic segment of bowel (Plate 85, A). The peritoneum is incised with a No. 15 blade, and the vessels coursing through the mesentery are clamped, cut, and tied up to the mesenteric border of the small bowel. The mesenteric border is cleared of fat and areolar tissue for several centimeters at each point where the bowel is to be divided.

2. Long Kocher clamps are placed across the bowel, which is divided between clamps (Plate 85, A). The everted edges of the bowel mucosa are wiped with alcohol before proceeding with the end-to-end anastomosis.

3. Angle or corner sutures of fine black silk are placed at the mesenteric and antimesenteric ends of the bowel (Plate 85, B). As the divided ends of the bowel are held together by the clamps, interrupted Lembert seromuscular sutures are placed in the bowel 0.5 cm. or less apart (Plate 85, B).

4. The clamps are rotated 180 degrees to expose the opposite surface of the bowel, and sutures are placed in the same manner (Plate 85, C).

5. When all of the sutures are placed, the clamps are opened and gently withdrawn as the sutures are pulled tight. The angle or corner sutures are tied first, and then each of the intervening sutures is tied first on one side and then on the other. The line of anastomosis is observed. Any part of the suture line requiring additional sutures for complete closure is approximated. If there has been an obstruction or if distention of the bowel is anticipated during the postoperative period, a second series of sutures can be used to reinforce the first suture line.

6. The mesentery is closed with several interrupted sutures of fine silk. Care is exercised to prevent the perforation of any vessels within the mesentery. The adequacy of the lumen of the bowel at the point of anastomosis is tested by the thumb and index finger. The bowel is allowed to fall back in the abdomen in its natural position.

PLATE 85

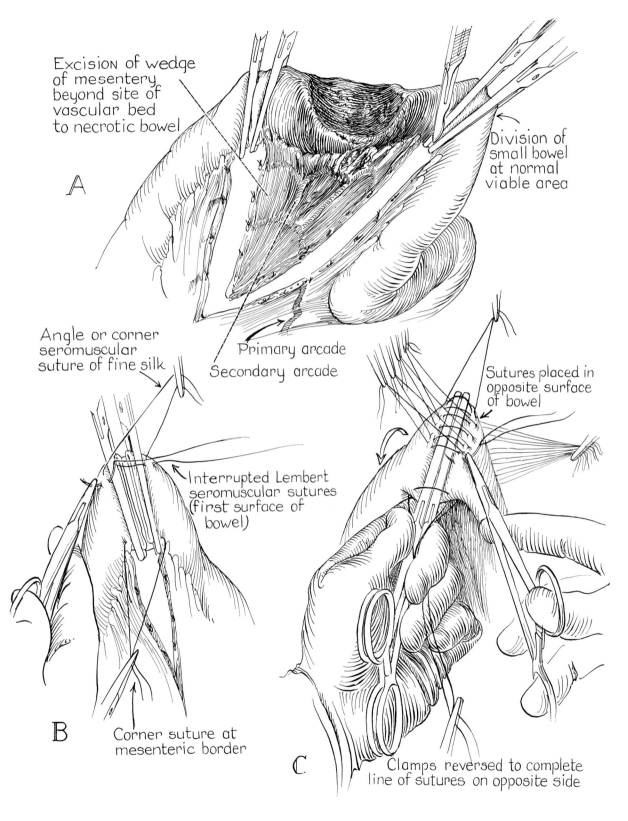

Excision of wedge of mesentery beyond site of vascular bed to necrotic bowel

Division of small bowel at normal viable area

A

Angle or corner seromuscular suture of fine silk

Primary arcade

Secondary arcade

Interrupted Lembert seromuscular sutures (first surface of bowel)

Sutures placed in opposite surface of bowel

B

Corner suture at mesenteric border

C

Clamps reversed to complete line of sutures on opposite side

Postoperative Care

A nasal suction tube is placed and passed beyond the pylorus. A fluid balance sheet is started and the intake and output of fluids recorded. Electrolytes are regulated to replace each milliequivalent of loss. (See Management of Electrolyte Abnormalities in Gynecologic Surgery, page 543.) The nasal tube can be clamped on the third postoperative day or sooner, depending on the degree of abdominal distention and the bowel sounds. Clear liquids are started in the absence of severe distention or other unfavorable signs. A progressive diet is given, depending on the patient's progress, and solid foods are instituted in the regimen as soon as tolerated. Penicillin and a wide-spectrum antibiotic are given in the usual dosage.

APPENDICITIS AND PROPHYLACTIC APPENDECTOMY
General Considerations

The gynecologist performs an appendectomy in most instances as a prophylactic procedure. Its removal is rarely contraindicated in pelvic surgery and is most commonly performed during a hysterectomy or myomectomy. There is no contraindication to the performance of a prophylactic appendectomy with an uncomplicated cesarean section. When radical pelvic surgery is undertaken, removal of the appendix becomes essential so that any confusing symptoms in the postoperative period are not ascribed to the appendix. This is equally true if the patient is subjected to radiation following pelvic surgery, and particularly if intraperitoneal radioactive gold is contemplated.

Etiology and Pathologic Anatomy

No specific etiologic agent is concerned with appendicitis, but several predisposing causes are of interest to the gynecologist. The incidence of disease is higher during periods of acute respiratory infections. Infrequently there is a history of indiscretion in the diet and overeating immediately preceding an acute attack. While the enlargement of the uterus during pregnancy, which displaces the cecum upward, probably adds to the possibility of appendicitis and the kinking and obstruction that may precede the development of an acute attack, it is more probable that the constipation accompanying pregnancy is a more important predisposing cause. Any factor, however, that tends to angulate the appendix causes impaction of its contents and a resultant stasis in its blood supply that may initiate an attack of acute appendicitis.

The specimens seen in acute appendicitis show two types of lesions. The milder form may emerge imperceptively into the more severe type of appendicitis as the disease progresses. In the acute catarrhal type the appendix is more turgid than normal, there is minimal reddening, and the vessels are slightly distended. On histologic examination such an appendix would show only an inflammatory reaction involving the mucosa. In the acute, diffuse form there is an inflammation of all of the muscular, submucous, and peritoneal coats of the appendix, and one segment of the appendix may be more involved than another due to the presence of a concretion within the lumen of the organ. The appendix is swollen and may be moderately red or an intense scarlet in color. As the disease progresses, yellowish-green, dark areas indicate necrosis and impending perforation. In the more intense type of this infection, where there has been a thrombosis of the arterial blood supply, the appendix, within a relatively short time, becomes a dirty, gray-green color and necrotic throughout. With an infection as acute as this, the appendix perforates, with the formation of a local appendiceal abscess or a local peritonitis. Some cases progress to general peritonitis despite efforts of the omentum and small bowel to wall off the area of rupture. While most surgeons do not feel that there is a type of chronic appendicitis in which a series of mild attacks damage the appendix, it is probable that some acute attacks do subside spontaneously, and the appendix subsequently shows scar tissue and adhesions to other viscera. Culture of the peritoneal fluid about the wall of an inflamed appendix reveals the enteric group of bacteria that are normal inhabitants of the cecum.

Symptoms and Diagnosis

In more than half of the patients an attack of acute appendicitis begins with acute abdominal pain. This pain is frequently epigastric in location and later becomes centered in the right lower quadrant. Frequently the patient raises the knees and jackknifes the thighs on the abdomen for relief. In some patients the onset is not so acute. They simply feel out of sorts for a day or two preceding the onset of epigastric pain. Following the onset of pain, nausea and vomiting may occur. As the disease progresses, a low-grade fever may develop, but a high fever is not the rule.

In dealing with a pregnant patient in whom appendicitis is suspected, the position of the appendix during the various weeks of pregnancy must be appreciated. The pain will tend to be higher as the uterus enlarges, but this is not characteristic of a retrocecal or retrocolic appendix, in which the pain may localize in the flank.

On physical examination the abdomen should be gently palpated, beginning with the left lower quadrant, proceeding to the left upper quadrant, and then to the right lower quadrant. Presence or absence of muscle spasm should be noted and the expression of the patient observed on deep pressure over the area. The intensity of rebound tenderness may suggest the extent of peritoneal inflammation, but the test should be done gently, particularly in the presence of a pregnant uterus.

The laboratory findings are helpful in the diagnosis. At first the urine may tend to be concentrated because of the lack of fluid and due to the vomiting and fever. If the appendix has ruptured and involved the bladder in a pelvic peritonitis, albumen and pus cells may be found in the urine. At other times the presence of a clear urine helps to differentiate acute appendicitis from acute right-sided pyelonephritis. Especially is this true in the pregnant patient. The white blood count in appendicitis may run anywhere from 12,000 to 20,000 cells. Counts above 20,000 should put the surgeon on the lookout for some other site of infection, since counts of this magnitude are more characteristic of pelvic inflammatory disease or acute pyelonephritis.

A differential diagnosis of acute appendicitis from other pelvic conditions is a recurrent problem to the gynecologist. The presence of pelvic inflammatory disease with a periappendicitis may simulate a primary inflammation of the appendix. A hemoperitoneum from a ruptured ovarian follicle may also simulate the signs and symptoms of an early appendicitis. A ruptured tubal pregnancy may, in its early stages, simulate appendicitis, but the development of shock and a mass in the pelvis will clarify the diagnosis in due time. Acute pyelonephritis, which occurs oftenest in pregnant women, and more on the right side than on the left, frequently presents a difficult differential diagnostic problem. A catheterized urine may clarify this situation, although it may be necessary to pass a ureteral catheter and obtain a specimen from the kidney pelvis itself.

Surgical Principles

Most surgeons agree that there is only a very rare indication for the expectant treatment of acute appendicitis. This is particularly true in the pregnant female. The rupture of the appendix, with subsequent pelvic peritonitis or generalized peritonitis, causes serious complications in the presence of the enlarged and pregnant uterus. The surgical anatomy of the appendix is discussed with the anatomy of the colon and cecum (see page 591).

Steps of the Operation

1. Where little doubt exists as to the diagnosis, a McBurney or gridiron excision is satisfactory for removal of the appendix. Should doubt exist as to the presence of other pelvic pathology, a right lower rectus incision affords greater exposure of the contents of the pelvis and is easily extended to perform other surgery.

2. On entering the abdomen, the anterior longitudinal band is identified, and Babcock clamps are applied along this band. As these clamps are successively applied toward the terminal portion

PLATE 86

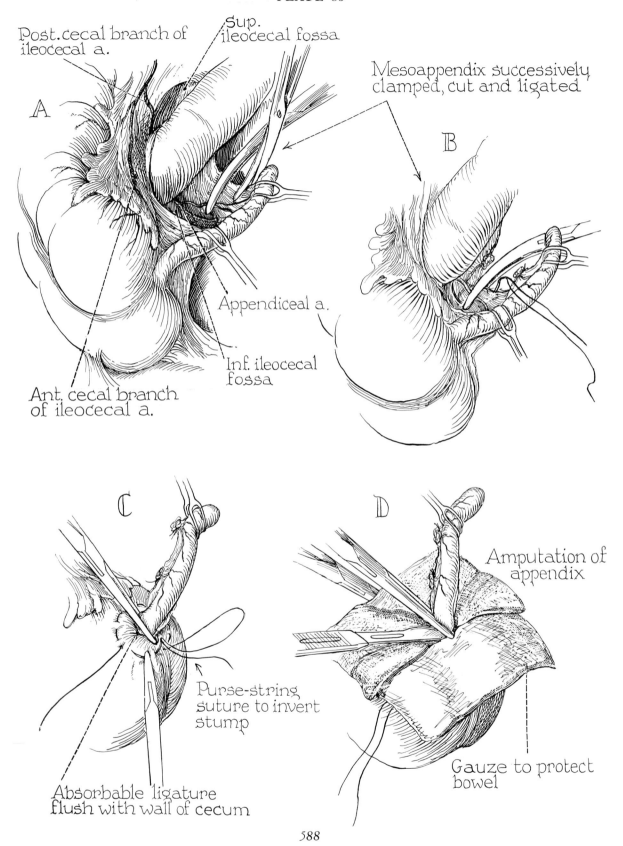

A

Post. cecal branch of
ileocecal a.

Sup.
ileocecal fossa

Mesoappendix successively
clamped, cut and ligated

B

Appendiceal a.

Inf. ileocecal
fossa

Ant. cecal branch
of ileocecal a.

C

Purse-string
suture to invert
stump

Absorbable ligature
flush with wall of cecum

D

Amputation of
appendix

Gauze to protect
bowel

PLATE 86 (*Concluded*)

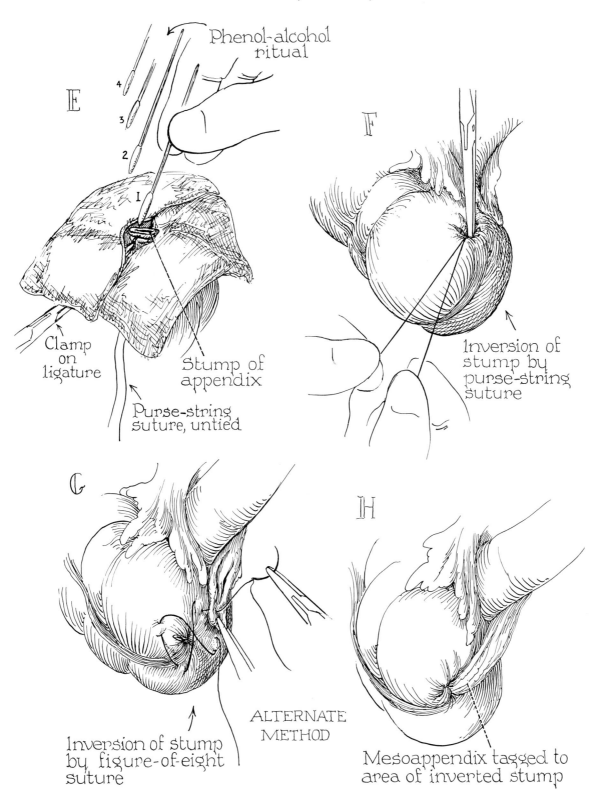

Phenol-alcohol
ritual

E

4
3
2
1

Clamp
on
ligature

Stump of
appendix

Purse-string
suture, untied

F

Inversion of
stump by
purse-string
suture

G

Inversion of stump
by figure-of-eight
suture

ALTERNATE
METHOD

H

Mesoappendix tagged to
area of inverted stump

of the cecum, the appendix will come into view unless it is retrocecal in position. General traction is made on the cecum by means of a wet gauze sponge, and the cecum is drawn into the incision to expose the entire length of the appendix. In Plate 86, *A,* are shown some of the anatomy of the appendix and cecum and the first step in the excision of an appendix that lies at or near the pelvic brim. Kelly clamps are successively placed along the mesoappendix, and the mesoappendix is cut. With each successive bite of the Kelly clamps, the mesoappendix is ligated with fine silk sutures. The appendiceal artery, which arises from the posterior cecal branch of the ileocecal artery, is usually located at or near the junction of the terminal ileum with the cecum.

3. In Plate 86, *B,* is shown the technique of ligating the appendiceal artery. While some operators prefer to ligate the appendiceal artery at the beginning of the appendectomy, with ligation of the mesoappendix by one large tie, the method of successively clamping, cutting, and ligating the mesoappendix allows for every variation in the length of the appendix and position of the mesoappendix.

4. A purse-string suture is placed around the base of the appendix with the ends left long. A straight hemostat is used to crush the appendix at its junction with the cecum, the clamp is moved a few millimeters toward the distal end of the appendix, and an absorbable ligature is placed flush with the wall of the cecum (Plate 86, *C*).

5. A straight clamp is used to grasp the ligature placed at the base of the appendix, and the other straight Halsted clamp is moved further distally on the appendix preparatory to amputation. Several gauze sponges are placed around the base of the appendix in order to protect adjacent bowel from the caustic phenol solution used later. The appendix is amputated (Plate 86, *D*), and all the instruments that have touched the organ are placed in a separate basin from the rest of the operative field.

6. The stump of the appendix is successively treated with phenol applicators and two alcohol applicators, followed by a dry applicator. This procedure is shown graphically in Plate 86, *E*.

7. The stump of the appendix is grasped with a straight hemostat and is inverted as the purse-string suture is tied (Plate 86, *F*).

8. An alternate method of inverting the appendiceal stump is shown in Plate 86, *G.* This consists of passing a double figure-of-eight mattress suture about the stump of the appendix and also into the adjacent segment of the mesoappendix. This is a faster method and effectively inverts the stump and sutures the mesoappendix over the area of operation.

9. The final appearance of the inverted stump by the alternate method is shown in Plate 86, *H.* The area about the inverted stump and all of the ligated points on the mesoappendix are then inspected for any bleeding before the abdomen is closed.

Postoperative Care

Patients who have had a routine prophylactic appendectomy in conjunction with other pelvic surgery require no special postoperative care. If the operation has been performed for an acute appendicitis, particularly if there is free fluid in the abdomen or if the appendix has ruptured, antibiotics effective against the enteric group of organisms are given. After removal of a simple unruptured appendix fluids are started as soon as tolerated by the patient and are supplemented by intravenous fluids. In the presence of a generalized peritonitis, no fluids are given by mouth, and gastric suction is instituted to combat postoperative distention. The presence of a pregnant uterus requires that the patient be kept in bed for forty-eight to seventy-two hours and sedated heavily in an effort to prevent a premature labor. Hormones, such as Releasin, under study for their effectiveness in preventing premature labor, may be administered when the uterus is irritable or premature labor is threatened. A prophylactic appendectomy performed at the time of cesarean section does not require any modification in the routine of management of patients after this operation.

SURGERY OF THE COLON IN GYNECOLOGY
General Considerations

The gynecologist is more commonly concerned with the cecum and sigmoid colon than with the other divisions of the large bowel. Especially in radical pelvic surgery should the pelvic surgeon be prepared to resect or divert the bowel.

Surgical Anatomy and Principles

The large intestine is made up of the cecum, ascending, transverse, descending, and sigmoid colons, and the rectum. The cecum lies in the right iliac fossa, continues as the ascending colon upward to the hepatic flexure, then crosses the abdomen (transverse colon) below the stomach to the spleen, makes a sharp bend (splenic flexure), and passes downward as the descending colon. At the left iliac fossa it forms the loop of the sigmoid colon and passes into the pelvis to continue as the rectum to the anal orifice. It varies in width from 3 to 8 cm. and is about 130 cm. long. Three longitudinal muscular bands (taenia coli), 12 mm. wide and 1 mm. thick, extend the length of the colon from the appendix to the rectosigmoid junction. These bands are shorter than the bowel itself and cause sacculations (haustra) as the bowel adjusts itself. Between the sacculations are folds (semilunar plicae) which involve the full thickness of the large bowel and project into its lumen. All three bands start at the base of the appendix but divide into distinct structures. One band is anterior on the ascending and descending colons and inferior on the transverse colon. A second is posteromedial on the ascending and descending colons and posterior on the transverse colon. The third is posterolateral on the ascending and descending colons and anterosuperior on the transverse colon. Along the free surface of the colon, especially near the taeniae, are pouches of peritoneum containing fat (epiploic appendages).

The cecum is that part of the colon below the iliocecal junction. It is quite variable in shape but is generally about 7.5 cm. broad and about 6 cm. long. It lies in the right iliac fossa, with its apex or lowest point projecting just beyond the medial border of the iliopsoas. Four common variations in the shape of the cecum are found. In the most common type of cecum the part to the right of the anterior longitudinal band is better developed than the part to the left. This creates a false apex, since the apex is anatomically and developmentally at the base of the appendix. In the second type there are two bulging sacculi of about equal size, with the appendix arising between them. In the third type, the cecum is fetal in appearance, with a conical shape (the appendix forms the true apex) and the three bands meeting at the base of the appendix, approaching it almost equidistantly. In the fourth type, a retrocecal appendix results. In this type the development of the cecum to the right of the anterior longitudinal band is excessive and the segment to the left of the band is atrophic, causing rotation of the base of the appendix posteriorly under the iliocecal junction. The form of the cecum and its redundancy are factors in several pelvic operations. The long conical types hang over the pelvic brim to become involved in lesions of the right adnexa. The cecum is mobilized during radical dissections and surgery involving the right ureter. Diversion of the urinary stream to an isolated loop of the terminal ileum involves the anatomy of the cecum. The right ureter may be transplanted in the cecum or brought retroperitoneally beneath it for a ureterocutaneous transplant.

The ileocecal junction is situated at the posteromedial aspect of the upper border of the cecum. The ileum passes into the cecum obliquely from below, upward and to the right. Two lips, a superior and inferior, project into the lumen of the large bowel and form a slit about 1.2 cm. long. This acts as a valve, but its efficiency is more dependent on the oblique course the ileum takes as it joins the cecum. Two fossa are fairly constant about the cecum. The superior ileocecal fossa is created by a fold of peritoneum enclosing the anterior cecal branch of the ileocolic artery. The pouch opens downward. A second pouch, the inferior ileocecal fossa, is created by a fold of peritoneum passing from the ileum to the mesentery of the appendix. This fold does not contain blood vessels.

The appendix arises from the cecum at a variable distance from the ileocecal junction (usually about 2.5 cm.). The average length of the appendix is between 8 and 10 cm. The mesoappendix is not a true mesentery but a fold continuous with the lower layer of the mesentery of the ileum. The appendiceal artery arises from the ileocolic artery and runs in the free edge of the mesoappendix. The appendicular artery passes behind the terminal ileum to reach the appendix. Thus, distention of the cecum or pressure from a large ovarian neoplasm can compress the circulation to the appendix. This is most frequently seen in volvulus of the terminal ileum. Gynecologists must wage an unending battle to prevent unnecessary surgery performed for the right lower quadrant pain syndrome and called a "chronic appendicitis." Surgeons who do not appreciate the many causes of right lower quadrant pain are not skilled in the diagnosis of abdominal and pelvic disease in women. They fail to realize the ever-changing picture of all the pelvic organs—bladder, uterus, tubes, ovaries, rectum—that occurs with the menstrual cycle. The gynecologist must master the diagnosis of all the common abdominal conditions for he is confronted daily with a complexity of abdominal pains.

The ascending colon is 20 cm. or less in length, extending from the cecum to the inferior surface of the liver, where it forms the right colic or hepatic flexure, which continues as the transverse colon. The ascending colon is covered in front and on the sides by peritoneum but may have a short mesocolon. The colon ascends between the quadratus lumborum and psoas and passes in front of the right kidney, and its hepatic flexure is at the level of the second lumbar vertebra.

The transverse colon is smaller in diameter than the ascending colon but is 40 to 50 cm. in length. It describes an arch, with its convexity downward and forward. It begins at the hepatic flexure and ends at the splenic flexure. Above it are the stomach, liver, and gall bladder, and at the left, the spleen. It has a short mesocolon, often lacking to the right of the midline, the root of which is connected to the posterior abdominal wall and anterior border of the pancreas.

The descending colon is 25 to 30 cm. in length and extends from the spleen to the pelvic brim. A fold of peritoneum, the phreno-colic ligament, suspends the region of the splenic flexure to the diaphragm on a level with the tenth and eleventh ribs. Posteriorly the descending colon is in contact with the lower pole of the left kidney and passes downward between the quadratus lumborum and psoas. It frequently develops a mesentery which merges into the sigmoid mesocolon in the left iliac fossa.

The sigmoid colon extends from the descending colon to the rectum and averages about 40 cm. in length. It does not matter where you say the descending colon ends and the sigmoid colon begins so long as the make-up of the mesocolon and its contained vessels is understood in the operation. The sigmoid colon descends first along the left pelvic wall, crosses transversely and downward to the right, and once more turns toward the left to the midline and forms a junction with the rectum opposite the second or third sacral vertebra. The sigmoid mesocolon has a line of attachment to the parieties beginning over the psoas and at the point of bifurcation of the left common iliac vessels. It proceeds downward, curving slightly to the right, to terminate about the second or third sacral vertebra. It may measure from 3 to 8 cm. from parieties to bowel at some points, and this predisposes to rotation and volvulus at this location.

The large intestine has four coats: mucosa, submucosa, muscularis, and serosa. The mucosa lacks villi and plicae but contains many solitary lymph follicles. The submucosa resembles that of the small intestine. The muscularis has a continuous circular layer, while the outer longitudinal layer is represented by the three taenia coli. The serosa differs from the small intestine only in the possession of the epiploic appendage. The wall of the appendix is frequently thicker than the rest of the colon and in young persons has closely packed or confluent lymph nodules so as to be an "abdominal tonsil."

The blood supply of the large intestine is from the superior mesenteric artery, the inferior mesenteric artery, and the middle hemorrhoidal branch of the hypogastric artery. The ileocolic artery is the first branch to be given to the colon from the superior mesenteric artery. The ileocolic artery divides into two divisions. The inferior division anastomoses with the terminal intestinal artery (also from the superior mesenteric artery) to form an arch, from the convexity of which branches proceed to the terminal ileum, cecum, and appendix. The superior division anastomoses with the right colic artery. The right colic artery arises from about the middle of the concavity of the superior mesenteric artery and passes to the right behind the peritoneum to the middle of the ascending colon. It divides into two branches: a descending, which anastomoses with the ascending (superior) branch of the ileocolic artery, and an ascending, which anastomoses and forms an arch with the middle colic artery. The middle colic artery arises from the upper part of the concavity of the superior mesenteric artery, and, passing downward and forward between the layers of the transverse mesocolon, divides into two branches. The right branch anastomoses and forms an arch with the ascending branch of the right colic artery. The left branch anastomoses with the left colic branch of the inferior mesenteric artery. The inferior mesenteric artery supplies the descending colon, the sigmoid colon, and the greater part of the rectum. It arises from the aorta—toward its left side—about two inches above the division of the aorta into the common iliac arteries. It passes downward in the sigmoid mesocolon and gives off the left colic artery, which passes in front of the lower pole of the kidney and divides into ascending and descending branches. The ascending branch anastomoses with and forms an arch with the descending branch of the middle colic artery. The descending branch anastomoses with and forms an arch with the uppermost sigmoidal artery. The sigmoid arteries run obliquely downward and outward behind the peritoneum and across the psoas to the sigmoid colon. The lowermost sigmoidal artery anastomoses and forms an arch with the superior hemorrhoidal artery. The superior hemorrhoidal artery is the terminal branch of the inferior mesenteric artery and descends in-to the pelvis between the folds of the mesocolon and mesorectum and crossing, in its course, the left ureter and left common iliac vessels. Opposite the middle of the sacrum it divides into two branches which descend one on either side of the rectum. These main branches break up into smaller straight vessels which pierce the muscular coat of the rectum and eventually anastomose with similar branches from the middle hemorrhoidal artery. The branches of the superior hemorrhoidal artery do not form arches and frequent anastomoses as do the arteries of the colon. The main trunk of the superior hemorrhoidal artery usually receives a large anastomotic branch from the last of the sigmoidal arteries. This branch should be looked for in surgery of the upper rectum and ligation of the hemorrhoidal artery done above this junction, which is usually well above the promontory of the sacrum. The form of the sigmoidal and superior hemorrhoidal vessels must be studied before ligation. Some arrangements preclude ligation of the superior hemorrhoidal artery at the pelvic brim without necrosis of the bowel.

The efferent lymphatic vessels of the large bowel follow the blood vessels and pass through corresponding lymph nodes in the various regions. The superior mesenteric plexus is formed chiefly from the lower part of the celiac plexus but receives fibers from the right vagus nerve and celiac (semilunar) ganglia. Its filaments follow the distribution of the arteries and innervate identical regions of the large bowel. The inferior mesenteric plexus is derived chiefly from the left side of the aortic plexus. Its filaments follow the course of the inferior mesenteric artery and anastomose with other nerves as arteries anastomose with arteries.

RESECTION OF LARGE BOWEL
Indications and Surgical Principles

Resection and end-to-end anastomosis of the large bowel by a gynecologist is usually the result of the involvement of the sigmoid or rectosigmoid in gynecologic disease. Extension of female genital cancer to involve the large bowel may require resection as a palliative procedure. In some instances the bowel is damaged by radiation or radium therapy, and particularly if the sigmoid is adherent to a cervical stump carcinoma that is managed with the use of radium. Endometriosis may implant on the sigmoid colon and cause a constricting lesion that simulates a malignancy. The sigmoid and rectosigmoid may be damaged during the course of surgery for extensive pelvic inflammatory disease. When the sigmoid is being resected for malignancy, the major vessels in the root of the mesentery are clamped, cut, and ligated before the remainder of the bowel to be resected is mobilized. In doing so, some of the lymphatic channels are interrupted. Theoretically, at least, this might prevent some spread of the carcinoma. A heavy, braided silk tie can be put around the bowel above and below the actual lesion in the colon on the presumption that cancer cells in the bowel lumen are not spread during the manipulation necessary to perform the resection and anastomosis. This might prevent implants in the suture line. A simple closed anastomosis and resection of the sigmoid with an end-to-end anastomosis is shown in detail.

Steps of the Operation

1. A wedge-shaped incision is made on both sides of the peritoneum of the sigmoid mesentery, which, when extended to the antimesenteric border of the bowel, will result in the resection of a segment that adequately clears the lesion and permits the anastomosis of healthy bowel (Plate 87, A).

2. The sigmoidal vessels are identified, and the areolar and lymphatic tissue in the root of the mesentery are carefully dissected free as these vessels are ligated. The excision of the lymphatic bed is not necessary if the resection is done for benign disease. The superior hemorrhoidal artery is preserved, provided the extent of the lesion does not require a lower resection and anastomosis in the rectosigmoid (Plate 87, A and B).

3. The peritoneum in the lateral gutter is incised, and the lower portion of the descending colon and the sigmoid are mobilized to resect the involved segment of bowel and allow for anastomosis without tension.

4. Long Kocher clamps are placed across the bowel after a few centimeters of the mesenteric side of the bowel have been cleared of fat and areolar tissue. The clamps are obliquely placed so the antimesenteric border of the bowel is slightly shorter than the mesenteric side. The bowel is resected with a knife, and the edges are touched with phenol and alcohol, followed by dry applicators (Plate 87, B).

5. By a similar technique the bowel beyond the lesion is resected and the segment removed with its sigmoid mesocolon attached.

6. The ends of the bowel are brought together with clamps, and angle or corner sutures are placed on the mesenteric and antimesenteric angles of the bowel (Plate 87, C). Interrupted sutures of fine silk are placed at intervals of 0.5 cm. or less, first on the anterior and then on the posterior surface of the bowel (Plate 87, C).

7. All of the sutures are left untied until sutures have been placed around the entire circumference of the bowel (Plate 87, D). By rotating the clamps back and forth through 180 degrees, the site of anastomosis can be inspected and additional sutures placed as needed.

8. The clamps are removed as the sutures are drawn together (Plate 87, E). The sutures are individually tied and cut.

9. The suture line is inspected for any portions that may require additional sutures, and if necessary a complete second row of sutures is placed. The bowel is tested for patency and the mesentery brought together by interrupted sutures of fine silk.

Postoperative Care

Blood is replaced as necessary during the course of the operation. Postoperatively, appropriate records are maintained of the intake and output of fluids. Electrolyte requirements are met for each twenty-four-hour period. If decompression of the bowel by short suction tube is indicated, the loss of chloride from this source is calculated on the fluid balance sheet. The patient is mobilized early and is encouraged to move about in bed to prevent phlebitis. If the patient has considerable distention and a long suction tube is used, nothing is given by mouth for the first twenty-four to forty-eight hours after the operation. Clear liquids are then started, and a progressive diet is

PLATE 87

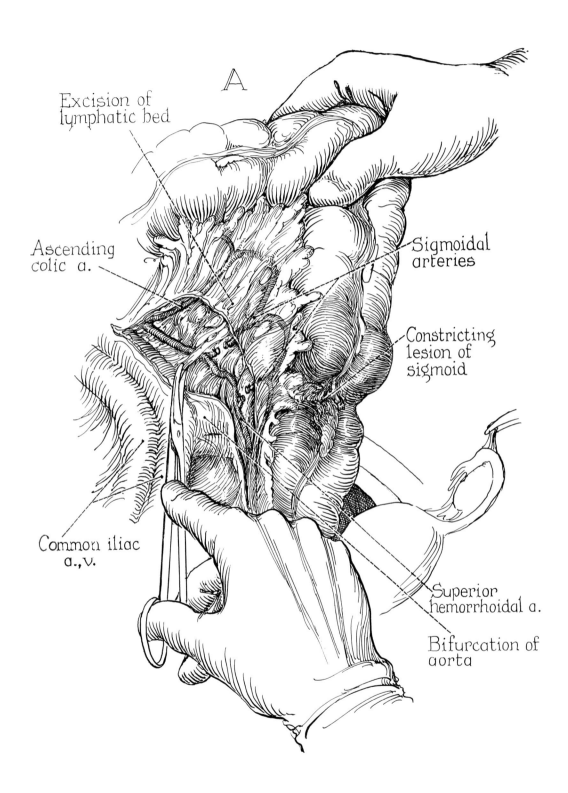

A

Excision of
lymphatic bed

Ascending
colic a.

Sigmoidal
arteries

Constricting
lesion of
sigmoid

Common iliac
a., v.

Superior
hemorrhoidal a.

Bifurcation of
aorta

PLATE 87 (Concluded)

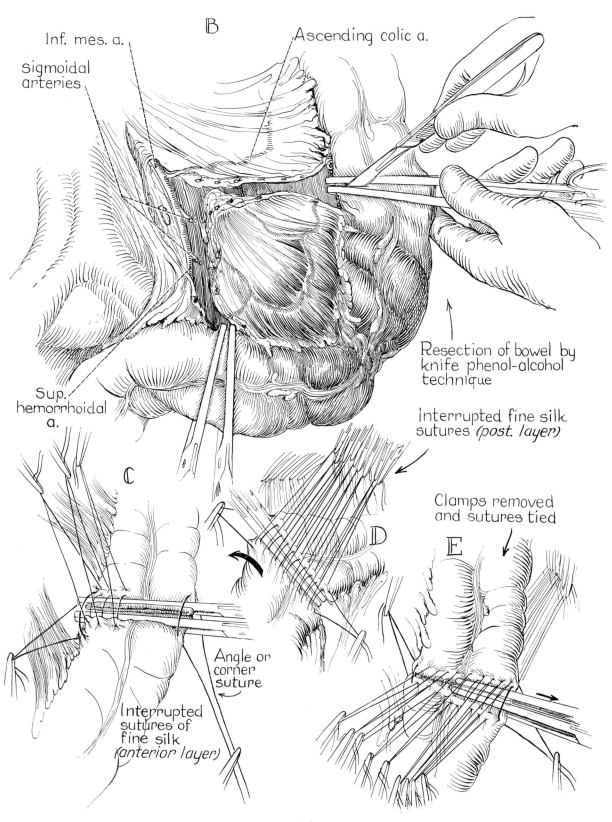

B

Inf. mes. a.

Sigmoidal arteries

Ascending colic a.

Sup. hemorrhoidal a.

Resection of bowel by knife phenol-alcohol technique

Interrupted fine silk sutures *(post. layer)*

C

Clamps removed and sutures tied

D

E

Angle or corner suture

Interrupted sutures of fine silk *(anterior layer)*

introduced as soon as possible. A wide-spectrum antibiotic to which the enteric group of organisms is sensitive is given. Routine orders for sedation and catheterization are left. The patient may have a spontaneous bowel movement due to the mild laxative effect of the antibiotics and the preoperative preparation of the bowel. Any leak at the line of anastomosis or infection at the site of operation will have manifested itself by the sixth or seventh day. At this time the anastomosis is usually well healed, and a low enema that is siphoned back may be given to stimulate peristalsis.

Transverse Colostomy
Indications and Surgical Principles

A transverse colostomy is frequently indicated in gynecology for large bowel obstruction due to recurrent pelvic cancer. Since the prognosis is poor, the colostomy is often a permanent one. A preliminary transverse colostomy may be done before exploring the pelvis to ascertain whether or not a lesion is operable. For some reason most transverse colostomies are performed as an emergency procedure during the night. Patients with terminal cancer can be spared an additional anesthetic and operation if the imminence of obstruction in the pelvis is appreciated at time of exploration and the colostomy performed during the primary procedure.

Steps of the Operation

1. A small transverse incision or an upper right rectus incision is made.

2. A loop of the transverse colon is mobilized and brought into the incision together with the adjacent omentum.

3. The omentum is incised to expose the transverse mesentery (Plate 88, *A*).

4. An avascular area just adjacent to the bowel is selected and opened to admit a glass rod (Plate 88, *A*).

5. While the bowel is retracted by a piece of rubber dam, a glass rod is inserted to prevent retraction of the loop during the early postoperative period (Plate 88, *B*).

6. The peritoneum is sutured to the anterior rectus sheath, and the ends of these sutures are left long so they can be anchored to the serosa of the bowel at several places (Plate 88, *B*).

7. If the surgeon anticipates that he may later wish to apply clamps to the spur between the distal and proximal loops of the colostomy, the mesenteric sides of the loop of bowel are approximated by a few interrupted sutures to facilitate this procedure.

8. The skin incision is closed around the bowel (Plate 88, *C*), allowing one finger on each side between the fascia and the bowel wall.

9. In forty-eight to seventy-two hours the bowel is opened by the actual cautery or knife (Plate 88, *C*). If an acute obstruction is present, a purse-string suture is placed in the bowel toward the distal loop and a soft rectal tube tied in place for decompression at the time of operation.

Postoperative Care

In addition to the management of intestinal obstruction by intubation and electrolyte control, the care of the skin and other measures for the function of a colostomy are instituted. The glass rod is removed on or about the eighth day or sooner if the wound is healing well and the danger of retraction of the loop of bowel is passed. The skin is covered with tincture of benzoin or other protective ointments. The distal and proximal loops of the colostomy are irrigated with warm saline solution beginning on the fourth or fifth day, and a well-lubricated finger is passed into the stomas to determine the adequacy of the openings. The patient is given instruction on the management of her colostomy as early in the postoperative period as possible. The institution of daily enemas, regular eating habits, and the use of productive devices are explained and taught in detail.

Permanent Left Inguinal Colostomy
Indications and Surgical Principles

The gynecologist most commonly performs a permanent left inguinal colostomy after a pelvic exenteration for cancer of the cervix. If, during this procedure, the ureters have been transplanted into the bowel and a wet colostomy is the result, such a colostomy must be

PLATE 88

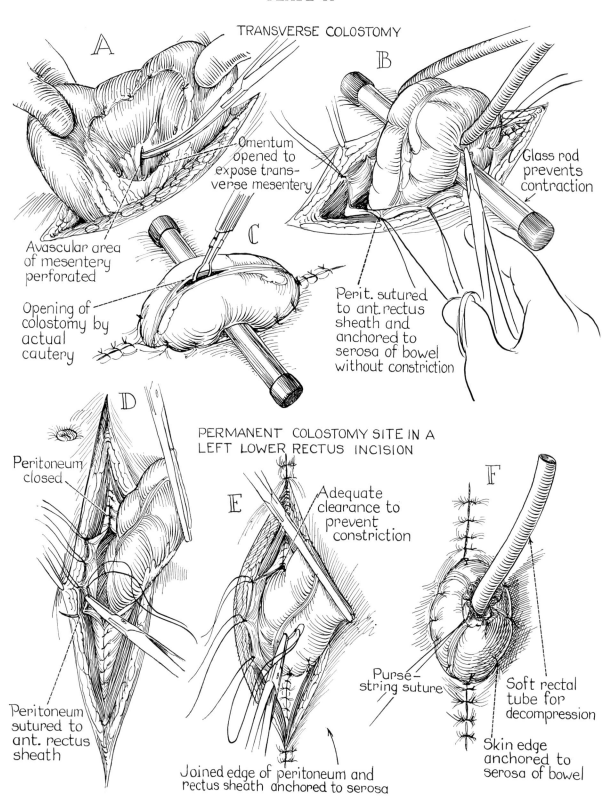

TRANSVERSE COLOSTOMY

A

Omentum opened to expose transverse mesentery

Avascular area of mesentery perforated

Opening of colostomy by actual cautery

B

Glass rod prevents contraction

C

Perit. sutured to ant. rectus sheath and anchored to serosa of bowel without constriction

PERMANENT COLOSTOMY SITE IN A LEFT LOWER RECTUS INCISION

D

Peritoneum closed

Peritoneum sutured to ant. rectus sheath

E

Adequate clearance to prevent constriction

Joined edge of peritoneum and rectus sheath anchored to serosa

F

Purse-string suture

Soft rectal tube for decompression

Skin edge anchored to serosa of bowel

left open at the operating table in order that the urine discharged into the bowel is left in contact with the bowel mucosa for as short a period of time as possible.

Steps of the Operation

1. The end of the bowel is brought out through some part of the original incision. In Plate 88, D, it is brought out approximately at the middle of a left lower rectus incision.

2. The peritoneum is sutured to the anterior rectus sheath, and the ends of these sutures are left long (Plate 88, D).

3. The peritoneal edge is sutured to the serosa of the bowel in several places to anchor the bowel so that approximately 4 to 5 cm. of bowel are above the skin surface (Plate 88, E).

4. The bowel is anchored in several places to the skin surface (Plate 88, F). A purse-string suture is placed around the opening of the bowel and a soft rectal tube inserted for a short distance (Plate 88, F).

Postoperative Care

The general instructions for the care as outlined for the transverse colostomy apply here.

INTESTINAL OBSTRUCTION
General Considerations

Mechanical obstruction in gynecologic surgery is most frequently a sequel to pelvic cancer, although it is seen after or due to endometriosis, pelvic inflammatory disease, myomectomies, and cesarean sections. The terminal ileum and left colon are most frequently involved.

Etiology and Pathologic Anatomy

The obstruction develops from extrinsic pressure from masses of pelvic cancer or kinking due to adhesions to the pelvic organs or the postoperative site. Rarely an endometrioma of the sigmoid causes an annular constriction that cannot be differentiated from cancer by x-ray or until a frozen section is done.

Symptoms and Diagnosis

Obstructions seen by the gynecologist are not usually acute such as those resulting from an intussusception, volvulus, or incarcerated hernia. These types of acute obstruction can occur with an underlying gynecologic cause. The onset is marked by abdominal distention, pain, and borborygmi. As the distention increases, there are nausea and vomiting. Strangulation of the bowel is evidenced by a worsening of the patient's general condition and signs of shock if a large segment of bowel is gangrenous. X-rays are taken in the prone and upright positions for evidence of a fluid level.

Preoperative Preparation and Anesthesia

Multiple fluid levels usually indicate that surgery will be necessary. They also indicate that the patient is in a negative fluid and electrolyte balance or soon will be. Since this must be corrected before surgery, an opportunity for conservative treatment of a nonstrangulated obstruction is provided. Many varieties of tubes have been developed for decompression of the bowel. They may be divided into the "long-tube deflations" and the "short-tube deflations." All have their exponents, but the simple rule that the tube should ensure drainage and deflation not far above the obstruction will govern the selection in most patients. A stomach tube will deflate the stomach plus the upper ileum due to regurgitation of the contents of the upper bowel into the stomach. Lower down, decompression of the bowel becomes more difficult, and the tube may have to be passed almost to the ileocecal junction.

A tube can be dangerous if a feeling of complacency develops in the surgeon while bowel becomes gangrenous and electrolytes are disturbed. The pouring of fluid into the obstructed bowel adds a third body compartment to the repository for electrolytes. This "third-space" syndrome can be deceptive even to the most fluid-conscious surgeon, and he should use all the clinical and laboratory facilities available to have the patient in electrolyte and fluid balance before operating.

With intestinal obstruction and well-defined fluid levels, the induction of a general anesthetic results in the relaxation of the pylorus and duodenum. An active reverse peristalsis occurs—not just a simple regurgitation. The amount of vomitus, often with a fecal odor, is frequently several liters or more, depending on the length of time the obstruction has existed. There is no tube of any diameter, or method of suction of any efficiency, that can handle the volume of vomitus forcefully propelled backward through the esophagus into the larynx. Any tube that exists only acts as an efficient splint along which the vomitus is carried. Therefore, spinal anesthesia or pre-induction intubation of the patient under local anesthesia is mandatory unless the patient be condemned to death or to an inevitable stormy postoperative course.

Treatment

A subacute obstruction may be managed by decompression, attention to fluids and electrolytes, and repeated films to observe the bowel. Surgical intervention may be relatively simple, with the release of a constricting band, or extensive bowel resection may be necessary. When dealing with recurrent pelvic malignancy, it is unwise to temporarily relieve an obstruction of the left colorectum, only to be faced with an emergency transverse colostomy shortly thereafter. It is better to anticipate the future obstruction and save the patient an additional surgical procedure.

PARALYTIC ILEUS

Paralytic ileus follows gynecologic surgery where there has been an extensive dissection or infection. The patient shows a distended abdomen with absent or only occasional bowel sounds. An x-ray reveals general bowel distention without a gas pattern that is organized.

The treatment consists of decompression, attention to fluid and electrolyte balances, gentle irrigation of the lower colon, and repeated x-rays and clinical observations in the event the adynamic ileus is masking a mechanical obstruction. When bowel sounds reappear, Prostigmin or other bowel muscle stimulants may be given.

References

Baker, J., Margetts, L., and Schutt, R.: The Distal and Proximal Margin of Resection in Carcinoma of the Pelvic Colon and Rectum, Ann. Surg. 141: 693, 1955.

Boynton, P. S., and Bonsnes, R. W.: Intestinal Obstruction After Pelvic Surgery, Am. J. Obst. & Gynec. 73: 149, 1957.

Crandon, J.: Nutrition in Surgical Patients, Mod. Med. 23: 95, 1955.

Dennis, C.: Current Procedure in Management of Obstruction of Small Intestine, J. A. M. A. 154: 463, 1954.

Eiseman, B., and others: A Long Sump for Operative Decompression of Obstructed Bowel, Surg., Gynec. & Obst. 110: 631, 1960.

Fine, J.: The Cause of Death in Acute Intestinal Obstruction, Surg., Gynec. & Obst. 110: 628, 1960.

Garry, J.: Abdominal Surgery During Pregnancy, Obst. & Gynec. 10: 660, 1957.

Glenn, F., and Dineen, P.: Recent Advances in Surgery of the Small Intestine, New York J. Med. 57: 2397, 1957.

Gregg, R.: Emergency Resections of the Colon, Mod. Med. 23: 101, 1955.

Hampton, C.: Fundamentals of Surgery in Contaminated and Infected Wounds, J. A. M. A. 154: 1326, 1954.

Hoyer, A. J., and Solheim, K.: The Therapy of Acute Small Bowel Obstruction, Surg., Gynec. & Obst. 109: 555, 1959.

Maynard, A., and Turell, R.: Therapy of Acute Left Colon Obstruction, Mod. Med. 23: 126, 1955.

McGrew, E., Laws, J., and Cole, W.: Free Malignant Cells in Relation to Recurrence of Carcinoma of the Colon, J. A. M. A. 154: 1251, 1954.

Morton, J. H., and Hibbard, L. T.: Unexpected Intestinal Rupture in Association With Pregnancy, Obst. & Gynec. 14: 214, 1959.

Myers, H. C.: The Management of Abdominal Injuries, Surg., Gynec. & Obst. 109: 629, 1959.

Sargent, C. W., Adams, F. M., and Westfall, C. H. P.: Postpartum Intestinal Obstruction, Obst. & Gynec. 9: 735, 1957.

Tyson, E. R., and Spaulding, E. H.: Should Antibiotics Be Used in Large Bowel Preparation? Surg., Gynec. & Obst. 109: 623, 1959.

36 · Retroperitoneal Pelvic Tumors

General Considerations

Extraperitoneal tumors are usually found by the gynecologist during a pelvic exploration for a mass the origin of which was not clear. The possibility of a retroperitoneal tumor is frequently anticipated, even though such tumors are statistically uncommon. The obstetrician may accidentally come upon such tumors, near the pelvic brim and out of the reach of the examining finger, when a cesarean section is done for failure of the presenting part to engage.

Etiology and Pathologic Anatomy

The classification of Lovelady and Dockerty divides the tumors into four groups: congenital anomalies, neurogenic tumors, bone tumors, and a miscellaneous group. This is useful since it not only catalogues the tumor, but also suggests the method of management. In the congenital group are included ectopic kidneys that certainly should not be removed or disturbed if there is functional renal tissue and no impairment of the excretory system. Teratomas and meningoceles are also included in the congenital group. Neurofibromas are the most common neurogenic tumors reported in Lovelady's series, while other tumors of the spinal cord and meninges are encountered. Bone tumors, benign and malignant, are seen on x-ray or diagnosed if they cause dystocia during labor. In the miscellaneous group are found tumors of muscle, fibrous tissue, metastatic cancer, and some that defy histologic classification.

Symptoms and Diagnosis

The symptoms of retroperitoneal pelvic tumors are variable and result from the involvement of nerve trunks, pressure on major vessels, and distortion and displacement of the bladder or rectum. Low back and sacral pain, leg pain or sciatica, and rectal pain and tenesmus are common. I have seen two patients with the presenting symptom of swelling and edema of one extremity. Difficulties with urination may arise. The symptoms are not characteristic, and diagnosis is usually made by bimanual examination or exploration of the pelvis. X-rays, cystoscopy, and proctoscopy may clarify the location of the mass.

Indications and Surgical Principles

The treatment is surgical removal or a combination of surgery and radiotherapy for the malignant lesions. Tumors low on the sacrum may be approached vaginally if they are not fixed to major structures that would cause injury to vessels and nerves not easily exposed from the vagina. Ureteral catheters are inserted prior to exploration, and the hypogastric vessels are ligated at the pelvic brim if the tumor involves lower branches that must be excised with the mass. Lateral and oblique films during retrograde urography may prepare the surgeon for the position and distortion of the ureter. Radiosensitive tumors may respond to deep x-ray therapy. This is particularly true of the malignant lymphomas with a retroperitoneal pelvic mass. In other instances of incomplete resection palliative therapy is given or subsequent radium or radon is implanted in localized masses of tumor. Other masses may be suitable for radiation by iridium[192] in nylon ribbons or cobalt[60] made up in essentially the same way. These newer sources require appropriate training in their use, and their general availability is limited at this time.

References

Albers, D. D., Milla, A. B., and Vickers, P. M.: Presacral Tumor With a Large Dystrophic Calcification Confused With Urologic Disease, J. Urol. **82**: 384, 1959.

Blakey, M.: Multiple Retroperitoneal Smooth Muscle Tumours, J. Obst. & Gynaec. Brit. Emp. **67**: 1000, 1960.

Crowley, L. V.: Adenocarcinoma Arising in Presacral Enterogenous Cyst, A. M. A. Arch. Path. **69**: 64, 1960.

Disch, R., and Sawyer, D.: Sacrococcygeal Teratomas, New York J. Med. **56**: 1654, 1956.

Gruhn, J. G., Hughes, J. C., and Addibert, C. O.: Tumors of the Peripheral Nervous System of Gynecological Interest: Report of a Case of a Neurilemmoma Within the Right Broad Ligament Mimicking an Ovarian Cyst, Am. J. Obst. & Gynec. **78**: 1334, 1959.

LiCalzi, N., McElwain, J. W., and Alexander, R. M.: Sacrococcygeal Teratomas: A Preliminary Report of Two Cases in Adults, Dis. Colon & Rectum **3**: 449, 1960.

Lovelady, S., and Dockerty, M.: Extragenital Pelvic Tumors in Women, Am. J. Obst. & Gynec. **58**: 215, 1949.

Norfleet, C. M., and others: Ureteral Obstruction Due to Retroperitoneal Lymphatic Cyst (Cystic Lymphangioma), J. Urol. **81**: 737, 1959.

Scanlan, D. B.: Primary Retroperitoneal Tumors, J. Urol. **81**: 740, 1959.

Wanke, R.: Surgical Therapy of Chronic Obstruction of the Pelvic Veins, Chirurg. **26**: 161, 1955.

Section XI · PEDIATRIC GYNECOLOGIC SURGERY

37 · Surgical Principles in Pediatric Gynecologic Surgery

General Considerations

Pediatric surgery has emerged as a subspecialty because of the problems children present. Gynecologists are faced not only with the differences in size, blood and fluid calculations, and the unintentional lack of cooperation, but also with a female child who may have already attached great emotional significance to her sexual organs. Before the age of 4 years a female child usually regards an examination of the genitalia as she would an examination elsewhere. Shortly after the age of 4 years, with individual variations, the surgeon must evaluate the psychic trauma against the good that his examination makes possible. This applies to minor gynecologic complaints such as vulvovaginitis rather than to lesions with more serious consequences. In skilled hands, the risk of an anesthetic is inconsequential compared with the information the surgeon may obtain by a complete investigation with the child relaxed and asleep.

Surgical Anatomic Considerations in Operations on the Prepubertal Pelvic Organs

The genital organs of a female child are not small imitations of the adult organs. They are in a state of growth and change each year through childhood, puberty and adolescence.

Although the female child may be afflicted with diseases analogous to those in the adult, the reactions are decidedly different. In hospitals where the pediatric house staff has not had specific training in the examination of female children, it is a revelation to read the report of the physical examination in which the physician has attempted to record his findings in terms of what he recalls of the examination of the adult, middle-aged multipara. The vulva of a child, compared with the adult, protrudes and is fragile and delicate and must be handled with the most delicate touch. The length and redundancy of the foreskin varies, as does the size and development of the clitoris. The number of children requiring circumcision ranges from none in the opinion of some gynecologists to a rare instance in the experience of others. The indication for circumcision is recurrent infection. Surgeons who perform this operation for the cure of tactile stimulation and chronic masturbation should be oriented as to the location of the hypothalamus. It is well known among sexologists that neither the size, nor the shape, nor the form of the genital apparatus has any great influence on sexual drives or satisfactory coitus.

The hymen has many normal variations, one of which is a bifid opening. I have examined three children who had been subjected to a

603

multitude of studies, including a work-up for the adrenogenital syndrome, and found nothing more than a bifid hymen. In two of these, complete renal studies, including cystoscopy, were done to exclude concomitant urinary anomalies. The attention to the urinary tract in a patient with a possible genital tract anomaly is commendable. The anxiety caused the parents during these studies of normal children emphasizes the necessity of the training of pediatric specialists and others dealing with large numbers of children in the examination of the genitalia of female infants and adolescents.

The vagina of the female child could not be more striking in contrast to the adult parous woman. The parous lower genital tract has smooth walls and is highly distensible, and the reflection of the vaginal mucosa on the cervix may be distorted by scar tissue from birth injuries. The infant vagina, by contrast, lacks distensibility and the mucosa is thrown up into folds and crypts. The mucosa covering the portio vaginalis of the cervix contains the same crypts and folds as the remainder of the vagina, but the mucosa is reflected on the small conical cervix without distortion. In addition, the infant vaginal mucosa is thin and fragile due to the lack of estrogenic stimulation. The infant vagina is therefore less resistant to bacterial infections and the infections are more difficult to treat since the organisms are protected from local therapy by the many crypts and form foci for recurrent infections.

The endocervix of a female child is devoid of mature glands and has little functional activity. In length it may represent one half or more of the cervix and uterus combined. Infections do not localize in these immature glands, so that upper genital tract infections are a rarity in the prepubertal female. The uterus is a small midline structure that grows slightly larger as the child approaches puberty. Its relative increase in size is disturbing to the uninformed, since it may be smaller in the first few years of life than it was at birth. The influence of the mother's estrogenic hormone on the uterus ceases with delivery, and the

organ reverts to an inactive state until the ovaries awaken at puberty. A small, anteflexed uterus is not infantile but a variation of the adult type. Realization of this will avoid harmful treatment with its profound psychosexual effects. It could at least protect the adolescent girl from some grotesque procedure such as the insertion of a stem pessary to "straighten out the uterus."

The ovaries show more progressive development than the uterus. They vary in size among immature children but seem to have a more consistent growth than the uterus and lower genital tract. This is logical since they must soon assume the regulation of the menstrual function and their role in the development of the secondary sexual characteristics. The Fallopian tubes in an infant are long and convoluted. As the female child approaches puberty, they tend to straighten out and assume their adult position. The shape and depth of the pelvic cavity is so different from that of the adult that the examiner must learn to interpret his findings in terms of size and space. Female infants have a narrow and elongated pelvic cavity. This is occupied by the urethra, bladder, vagina, rectum, genital organs, and the connective tissue extensions from the parietal connective tissue containing the vessels, nerves, and lymphatics. In a child of 4 or 5 years, the uterus and cervix are in a straight line and are the size of a small lead pencil. The bladder is an abdominal organ, an anatomic fact that may spare the diagnostician the embarrassment of mistaking urinary retention for a large tumor. Because of the compactness of the pelvic organs and lack of mobility and pliability, culdoscopy and exploratory colpotomy are not feasible.

Examination of the Female Child

The pediatrician has accustomed the child to examination of the abdomen and rectal palpation. This fact is utilized in examining the genitalia by simulating abdominal palpation with one hand while exploring the genitalia with the other. Likewise, a finger in the rectum distracts the female infant from any manipulation of the genitalia in many instances. Since the rectal examination is the best method of palpating the uterus and adnexal regions in the rigid shelf the prepubertal pelvis presents, vaginal examination need not be done even under anesthesia. In the small child the surgeon feels the uterus as a ridge between the sheaths of the broad ligament. It is relatively fixed and immobile. One can exclude masses in the adnexal region, but a description of the size and shape of the ovaries and tubes is pure imagination. The combined examination with a finger in the rectum and a blunt probe in the vagina is useful in exploring for foreign bodies, vaginal septa, and other anomalies. A simple endoscope of any kind or a McCarthy panendoscope makes an excellent colposcope for viewing the upper reaches of the vagina. This can be done without anesthesia in a cooperative child. Various sizes of nasal specula should be available for vaginal examination. Culture tubes and materials for spreads are the same as those used for an adult, except that the introduction of a cotton applicator is more disturbing to the child than is a warm glass rod. Transabdominal pneumoperitoneum with multiple x-rays has been studied as a diagnostic aid in obscure cases. The x-ray films may reveal a suspected anomaly of the genital tract. While it is advantageous to avoid a laparotomy, this may be the only method of providing information concerning the inguinal canals, the presence of an inguinal testis, biopsy of the ovaries, or directly visualizing suspected anomalous structures.

Handling of the Tissues

The tissues of the female genitalia of a child are fragile, and only the most delicate touch and instruments are used. Retraction should be accomplished by fine sutures on the edges of a wound whenever possible. Sutures of 0000 and 00000 silk and 000 and 0000 catgut have sufficient strength to hold the child's tissues.

Preoperative Care and Anesthesia

The psychic preparation of the child for even a minor procedure will relieve much anxiety. In simple terms, depending on the age and insight the patient may have, she is told why something has to be done and that it will not hurt while it is being done and is given reassurance that the doctor will see that it will hurt as little as possible afterward. If the lesion is serious, the child may be dehydrated and in acidosis or alkalosis. This and any other deficiencies are corrected before surgery if time permits. The oxygen requirements of a child are almost twice those of an adult, and an inhalation anesthesia that permits maximum oxygenation is preferable. A major gynecologic operation should not be started until a polyethylene catheter or cannula has been introduced into a vein and is working. Surgeons accustomed to the blood loss in certain operations on adults are sometimes unaware that a much smaller loss in a child represents a percentage of the total blood volume sufficient to cause shock.

References

Allen, E.: Pelvic Examination of the Preadolescent and Adolescent Girl, Am. J. Obst. & Gynec. 68: 1311, 1954.

Ball, T. L.: Pediatric and Adolescent Gynecologic Surgery, S. Clin. North America 37: 501, 1957.

Chandler, L.: Symposium on Total Care of Surgical Patient: Preoperative and Postoperative Care in Infants and Children, S. Clin. North America 34: 1463, 1954.

Gross, R.: Surgery of Infancy and Childhood, Philadelphia, 1953, W. B. Saunders Co.

Jackson, K.: Psychologic Preparation as a Method of Reducing the Emotional Trauma of Anesthesia in Children, Anesthesiology 12: 293, 1951.

Kunstadter, R., and Tulsky, A.: Diagnostic Transabdominal Pneumoperitoneum in Children, Am. J. Obst. & Gynec. 68: 819, 1954.

Levy, D.: Psychic Trauma of Operations in Childhood, Am. J. Dis. Child. 69: 7, 1945.

Potts, W.: Pediatric Surgery, J. A. M. A. 157: 627, 1955.

Schauffler, G.: Pediatric Gynecology, Obst. & Gynec. 5: 391, 1955.

Wilson, D.: Further Observations on the Age of Menarche, Brit. M. J. 2: 4684, 1950.

38 · Tumors, Foreign Bodies, and Minor Gynecologic Surgery in Children

General Considerations

Tumors of the genital tract are relatively uncommon in children. Perhaps since the genital organs are relatively static until the menarche, this is reflected in the incidence of new growths. Tumors of bone, blood, and the nervous system are more common since these systems are undergoing rapid growth.

OVARIAN TUMORS

The most common ovarian tumors are ovarian cysts, carcinomas of the ovary, teratomas, and granulosa cell tumors. The small funnel of the child's pelvis permits limited expansion for any lesion, so abdominal enlargement is an early sign. Pain due to torsion, degeneration, or pressure on surrounding structures is present in more than half of the cases. There is frequently considerable delay in making the diagnosis. The tumors are removed surgically after careful study and examination under anesthesia. A rare tumor of the upper vagina or cervix is the botryoid sarcoma. This is of mesodermal origin, containing muscle, cartilage, and other mesodermal derivatives. It is highly malignant, and the only chance for survival has been radical surgery.

FOREIGN BODIES

Foreign bodies are most frequently found in children up to the age of 6 years. Whether inserted by the child herself or a playmate, there is no more dire psychosexual significance than if it were inserted into the ear, nose, or anus. Safety pins, crayons, pencils, coins, and a myriad of small toys have been found. A persistent vaginal discharge tinged with blood is the usual symptom. Diagnosis is established by x-ray and the combined probe-rectal finger technique to sound for the object. In most cases the foreign bodies are removed under anesthesia to avoid injury to the delicate tissues.

MINOR SURGERY OF THE VULVA IN CHILDREN

Several common operations about the vulva are described. The delicacy with which the tissues must be handled cannot be overemphasized. Despite the slight anesthetic hazard, these minor operations are best done as soon as recognized and before the child attaches much significance to the genitalia or the mother makes a major issue out of the lesion by recurrent attention to it.

DEHISCENCE OF AGGLUTINATED LABIA
Indications and Surgical Principles

The separation of agglutinated labia usually can be done as an office procedure. Obstinate cases are better done under anesthesia, for a more complete examination can be done without psychic trauma to the child. The medical management of a vulvovaginitis is carried out prior to the operation. Cultures, local and systemic estrogens, education of the mother, and specific antibiotic therapy are jointly undertaken by the pediatrician and the gynecologist.

Steps of the Operation

1. A nasal speculum is introduced and a small malleable spatula, frequently used by eye surgeons,

PLATE 89

DEHISCENCE OF AGGLUTINATED LABIA

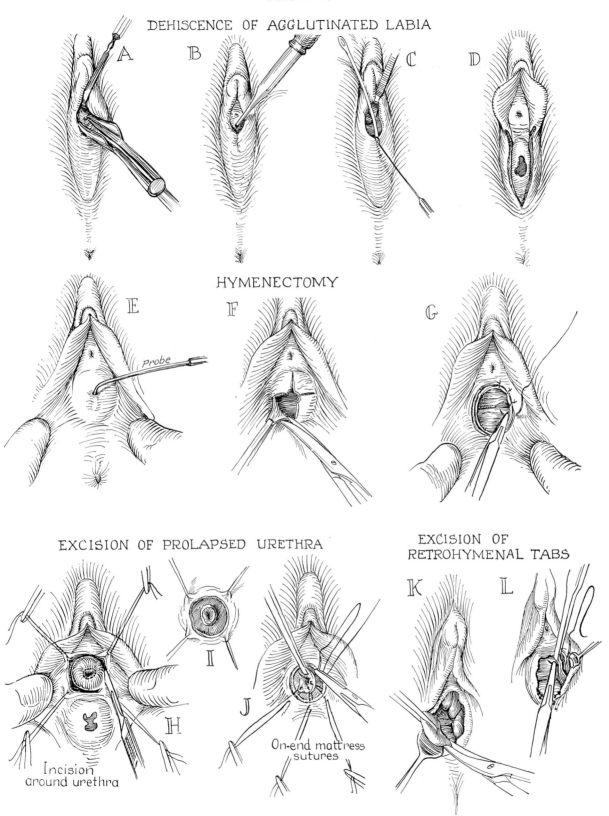

HYMENECTOMY

probe

EXCISION OF PROLAPSED URETHRA

Incision around urethra

On-end mattress sutures

EXCISION OF RETROHYMENAL TABS

is used to visualize the external urethral meatus (Plate 89, *A*).

2. When the procedure is done in the office, a few drops of 10 per cent cocaine or Xylocaine jelly, 5 per cent, are placed in or near the urethral meatus for its limited local anesthetic value (Plate 89, *B*).

3. The malleable spatula is used to protect the external urethral meatus while a grooved director is introduced behind the agglutinated labia. A membrane hook or similar instrument is used to dehisce the agglutinated labia. It may be necessary to sharply incise some long-standing cases (Plate 89, *C*).

4. Plate 89, *D,* shows the appearance after the labia minora have been separated and the hymenal orifice is evident. In addition to taking cultures of the upper vagina, a vaginoscopy is done. Congenital anomalies of the genital tract are excluded by this examination and cystoscopy and proctoscopy.

HYMENECTOMY
Indications and Surgical Principles

Hymenectomy is indicated for an annular, rigid hymen diagnosed during a premarital examination. The gynecologist feels that attempts at intercourse would either be impossible or be so traumatic as to seriously disturb the sexual life of the couple. In children it is indicated for a pinhole hymen that precludes adequate drainage. A persistent vulvovaginitis may exist. Other varieties of the normal hymen may cause the same situation. A hymenectomy is also done for imperforate hymen, which is usually diagnosed shortly after the menarche. This creates a different surgical problem and has been discussed in Chapter 3 (page 66). The surgical principles involved in a hymenectomy are (1) an adequate incision that allows ample room for coitus and (2) careful attention to the approximation of tissues so as not to cause scarring about the base of the hymen.

Steps of the Operation

1. In Plate 89, *E,* is shown a pinhole hymen. This is explored by a small probe to determine whether a septum or other congenital anomaly of the lower vagina exists.

2. A cruciate incision is made in the hymen, and the four quadrants are excised (Plate 89, *F*).

3. The edges are approximated by fine interrupted sutures of 000 chromic catgut on atraumatic needles (Plate 89, *G*).

EXCISION OF PROLAPSED URETHRA
Indications and Surgical Principles

Prolapse of the urethra is corrected as soon as recognized. It represents a surgical emergency if areas have become thrombosed, with subsequent swelling and edema that cause urinary retention. The condition occurs in young children, usually in the wake of whooping cough or some other infectious process causing violent coughing. It occurs at the other extreme of life, in the aged, where retraction of the mucous membrane of the vestibule causes a partial prolapse of the lining of the urethra. Severe coughing superimposed upon this may result in a complete extrusion. It is to be compared with a prolapse of the rectum and is a condition entirely different from urethral caruncle.

Steps of the Operation

1. Four traction sutures are placed about the prolapsed urethra (Plate 89, *H*). A circular incision is made about the external meatus and prolapsed mucosa (Plate 89, *H*).

2. The swollen and thrombotic urethral mucosa, together with a small portion of the muscularis of the external meatus, is excised (Plate 89, *I*).

3. On-end mattress sutures of 000 chromic catgut on atraumatic needles are used to approximate the mucous membrane of the vestibule to the mucosa of the urethra. The sutures include some of the muscular wall of the external meatus for hemostasis (Plate 89, *J*).

EXCISION OF RETROHYMENAL TABS
Indications and Surgical Principles

Embryologically the immediate retrohymenal area is thought to represent the lowermost portion of the vagina formed from the Müllerian ducts. Occasionally there is a complete retrohymenal membrane that is imperforate and causes hematocolpos and hematometra. Redundant tabs of a retrohymenal membrane may be disturbing to the patient and interfere with normal sexual intercourse. They are removed and any constriction of the vagina is corrected.

Steps of the Operation

1. The individual tabs of retrohymenal tissue are grasped and excised at the base (Plate 89, *K*).

2. These tabs are excised and the base closed with fine, interrupted sutures of 000 catgut on atraumatic needles (Plate 89, *L*). The operator assures himself that an adequate introitus exists and the subsequent contraction of the base of the excised retrohymenal tabs will not cause dyspareunia.

HYDROCELE OF THE CANAL OF NUCK
General Considerations

A hydrocele of the canal of Nuck is also known as a pudendal, labial, or Nuck's hydrocele. It has been described by the terms hydrocele feminae or hydrocele muliebris. It is a form of congenital indirect inguinal hernia.

Etiology and Pathologic Anatomy

Hydrocele of the canal of Nuck is congenital in origin, and not infrequently it is accompanied by a benign tumor of the labia majora. Such was the case in the patient upon whom the operation to be described was done.

Symptoms and Diagnosis

A typical picture of Nuck's hydrocele is an elongated swelling (sausage-like) that extends along the course of the round ligament and distends the labia majora. Such swellings, if observed for several months, will enlarge and distort the terminal urethra in some patients. Differentiation from a solid or cystic tumor in the area is not difficult, since transillumination is used as a routine diagnostic procedure. However, a hydrocele of the canal of Nuck may exist together with a tumor of the labia majora.

Indications and Surgical Principles

A hydrocele of the canal of Nuck is corrected surgically before the female child becomes psychologically conscious of her genital organs. The tumor may be observed to enlarge and distort the terminal urethra and other adjacent structures. Injection therapy has no place in the correction of this condition. The principles of surgery require that the sac be ligated and transfixed high along the course of the round ligament. The latter structure need not be preserved. A routine hernia repair is done, as is the proper procedure for any congenital hernia. A hydrocele of the canal of Nuck can provide a very difficult dissection. It frequently descends far down on the labia and lacks the rather simple identification of layers seen in the common adult varieties of hernias. Particularly when seen in conjunction with a benign tumor of the labia, it is frequently adherent to the structures surrounding it and is not distinct or reducible.

Preoperative Care and Anesthesia

No special preoperative care is necessary. The large varieties may cause a cystitis due to obstruction of the urethra, indicating appropriate urinary antiseptics. A general anesthesia, after induction by rectal Pentothal, is ideal in the hands of a competent anesthetist.

Steps of the Operation

1. Plate 90, *A*, shows a moderately large hydrocele of the canal of Nuck and a hemangioma of the labia majora. The tumor was intimately associated with the hernia. The vulva was distorted, and pressure upon the urethra caused the child to cry when she urinated. On one occasion she had urinary retention for thirty-six hours.

2. A small incision paralleling and just above the inguinal ligament is made and carried down through the skin and the superficial and deep layers of fascia. The aponeurosis of the external oblique muscle is identified and is incised in the direction of its fibers. The round ligament is identified with the hernial sac extruding from the external or abdominal ostium of the inguinal canal. A finger is inserted to avoid injury should an ovary or tube be drawn into the field by traction on the sac. The smallest instruments available are used for this type of surgery, and the dissection is carried out with a minimum of trauma (Plate 90, *B*).

3. The sac of the hernia is ligated as high as possible (Plate 90, *C*), and in doing so the round

PLATE 90

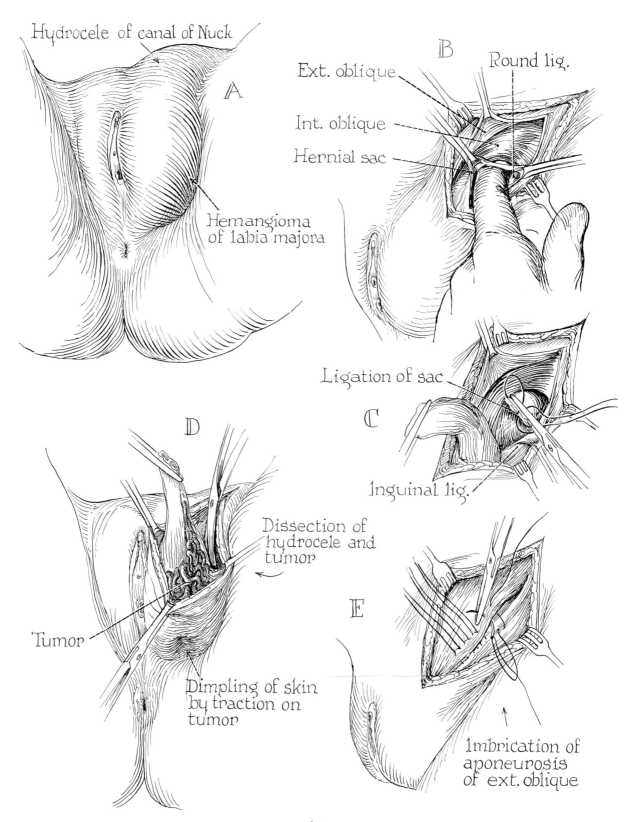

Hydrocele of canal of Nuck

A

Hemangioma of labia majora

B

Ext. oblique

Round lig.

Int. oblique

Hernial sac

Ligation of sac

C

Inguinal lig.

D

Dissection of hydrocele and tumor

Tumor

Dimpling of skin by traction on tumor

E

Imbrication of aponeurosis of ext. oblique

ligament is sectioned. The direction of the sac is changed by passing the ends of the suture used for ligation of the sac through the edges of the internal oblique muscle and the beginning of the conjoined tendon. The internal inguinal ring is obliterated.

4. The sac extends into the left labia majora, where it ends in a moderately large hemangioma intimately attached to the skin (Plate 89, *D*). The remnants of the round ligament plus the sac are used as traction in the subsequent dissection of the tumor (Plate 90, *D*). This could be completely removed by sharp and blunt dissection without extending the incision used for the hernia repair. The entire mass is removed by this means.

5. The aponeurosis of the external oblique muscle is imbricated as shown in Plate 90, *E*. As in a hernia repair in the adult female, the obliteration of the sac and the closure of the internal ring are the fundamental principles of the repair. The imbrication of the fascia is not so important but adds something to the strength of the closure.

Postoperative Care

The child can be up and around as soon as she has reacted from the anesthetic. No other special postoperative care is necessary, except to watch for urinary retention.

References

Ariel, I. M., and Pack, G. T.: Cancer of Infancy and Childhood, New York J. Med. **60**: 404, 1960.
Baber, M., Rosser, E., and Lavertine, J.: Carcinoma of the Cervix Uteri in an Infant, Brit. M. J. **1**: 392, 1951.
Bailey, W. C., and others: Rhabdomyosarcomas in Childhood; a Review of 14 Cases, A. M. A. Arch. Surg. **82**: 943, 1961.
Brack, C. B., and Guild, H. G.: Urethral Obstruction in the Female Child, Am. J. Obst. & Gynec. **76**: 1105, 1958.
Brayton, D., and Lewis, G. B.: The Use of Hypothermia in General Pediatric Surgery, Ann. Surg. **145**: 304, 1957.
Burns, E., Pratt, A., and Hendon, R.: Management of Bladder Neck Obstruction in Children, J. A. M. A. **157**: 570, 1955.
Butt, J.: Ovarian Tumors in Children, Am. J. Obst. & Gynec. **69**: 833, 1955.
Caldwell, J., Jr.: Foreign Body in the Vagina for Twenty Years, Am. J. Obst. & Gynec. **66**: 899, 1953.
Calgano, P. L.: Parenteral Fluid Therapy in the Pediatric Surgical Patient, New York J. Med. **60**: 1252, 1960.
Callel, F.: Sarcoma of the Vagina in the Case of a Girl of Fifteen Months, Riv. medicoquirurgica de Oriente **4**: 99, 1943.
Carache, H.: Tumors in Children, New York J. Med. **55**: 1953, 1955.
Chenoweth, C. V., and Clawater, E. W.: Interstitial Cystitis in Children, J. Urol. **83**: 150, 1960.
Creadick, R.: Sarcoma Botryoides, Am. J. Obst. & Gynec. **68**: 567, 1954.
Crissey, J., Osborne, E., and Jordon, J.: Lichen Sclerosus et Atrophicus in Children, New York J. Med. **55**: 1953, 1955.

Daniel, W. W., Koss, L. G., and Brunschwig, A.: Sarcoma Botryoides of the Vagina, Cancer **12**: 74, 1959.
Dargan, L.: Sarcoma Botryoides, Obst. & Gynec. **2**: 127, 1953.
Dargeon, H.: The Diagnosis and Management of Neoplastic Diseases in Childhood, M. Clin. North America **31**: 498, 1947.
Deakin, R.: Congenital Bladder Neck Obstruction in Children, J. Urol. **78**: 384, 1957.
Delascio, D., and Schor, H.: Foreign Bodies in the Vagina of Children, Rev. de ginec. e d'obst. **1**: 425, 1939.
De Queiroz, A. P., and Freitas, A. L.: Granulosa Cell Tumor of the Ovary With Precocious Puberty in a Patient of 6 Years (Tumor de celulas da granulosa do ovario, com puberdade precoce em paciente de 6 anos), An. brasil. ginec. **43**: 1, 1957.
Donovan, E. J., and Stanley-Brown, E. G.: Inguinal Hernia in Female Infants and Children, Surg., Gynec. & Obst. **107**: 663, 1958.
Duckett, H. C., Davis, C. D., and McCall, J. B.: Sarcoma Botryoides: A Clinical and Pathologic Review of 4 New Cases, Obst. & Gynec. **9**: 517, 1957.
Epstein, B. S.: Subcutaneous Urography in Infants, J. A. M. A. **164**: 39, 1957.
Goldstein, I. R., and Potts, W. J.: Inguinal Hernia in Female Infants and Children, Ann. Surg. **148**: 819, 1958.
Gross, R., Holcomb, G., and Swan, H.: Treatment of Neurogenic Urinary and Fecal Incontinence in Children, Arch. Surg. **66**: 143, 1953.
Hamm, F. C., and Waterhouse, K.: Changing Concepts in Lower Urinary-Tract Obstruction in Children, J. A. M. A. **175**: 854, 1961.
Hammond, D. O.: A New Pediatric Gynecologic Examining Instrument for Use in Diagnosis of Pediatric Vaginitis, Am. J. Obst. & Gynec. **80**: 85, 1960.
Hamperl, H., and Kaufmann, C.: The Cervix Uteri at Different Ages, Obst. & Gynec. **14**: 621, 1959.
Hanten, J. S., Galuszka, A. A., and Rotner, M.: Vesical Neck Contracture in Children, J. Urol. **82**: 218, 1959.
Harned, H. S., and Cooke, R. E.: Symptomatic Hyponatremia in Infants and Children Undergoing Surgery, Surg., Gynec. & Obst. **108**: 543, 1957.
Hastings, N., Pollock, W. F., and Snyder, W.: Retroperitoneal Tumors in Infants and Children, A. M. A. Arch. Surg. **82**: 950, 1961.
Hays, D. M.: Intussusception as a Postoperative Complication in Pediatric Surgery, Surg., Gynec. & Obst. **112**: 583, 1961.
Keeley, J. L., DeRosario, J. L., and Schairer, A. E.: Desmoid Tumors of the Abdominal and Thoracic Walls in a Child, A. M. A. Arch. Surg. **80**: 144, 1960.
Kook, H., Kamhi, B., and Hermann, H. B.: Trigonal Curtain Obstruction in a Female Child, J. Urol. **73**: 1026, 1955.
Knight, A.: Management of a Case of Uterine Sarcoma in a Nine Year Old Girl, Guthrie Clin. Bull. **9**: 94, 1939.
Leader, A. J.: A New Instrument for Contracted Bladder Necks in Children, J. Urol. **81**: 492, 1959.
Levene, M.: Congenital Retinoblastoma and Sarcoma Botryoides of the Vagina, Cancer **13**: 532, 1960.
McDonald, H. P., Upchurch, W. E., and Artime, M.: Bladder Dysfunction in Children Caused by Interstitial Cystitis, J. Urol. **80**: 354, 1958.
McGovern, J. H., Marshall, V. F., and Paquin, A. J., Jr.: Vesicoureteral Regurgitation in Children, J. Urol. **83**: 122, 1960.
McQuiston, W. O.: Anesthesia for Pediatric Surgery, S. Clin. North America **36**: 1441, 1956.
Maletta, T., and Horton, B.: Botryoidal Sarcoma of the Bladder in Children: A Case Report, J. Urol. **82**: 490, 1959.
Marcus, S. L.: Müllerian Mixed Sarcoma (Sarcoma Botryoides) of the Cervix, Obst. & Gynec. **15**: 47, 1960.
Mertz, J. L.: Peritonitis in Infants and Children, Hawaii M. J. **18**: 341, 1959.
Mestel, A. L., Farber, M. G., and Chabon, I.: Femoral

Hernia in Infancy and Childhood, A. M. A. Arch. Surg. **79**: 750, 1959.

Miller, T. R.: Sarcoma Botryoides, Am. J. Obst. & Gynec. **76**: 1172, 1958.

Miles, J. V., and Harris, L. E.: The Venostomy Procedure in Infants and Children, J. A. M. A. **161**: 619, 1956.

Nash, A., and Stout, A. P.: Malignant Mesenchymomas in Children, Cancer **14**: 524, 1961.

Ober, W. B., Smith, J. A., and Rouillard, F. C.: Congenital Sarcoma Botryoides of the Vagina: Report of Two Cases, Cancer **11**: 620, 1958.

Offergeld, H.: Foreign Bodies in the Vagina in Girls, Relation to Sexual Life, Monatschr. Kinderh. **46**: 29, 1930.

Parker, P., and Smith, P. L., and Rathmell, T. K.: Sarcoma Botryoides of the Bladder: Successful Therapy by Cystectomy, J. Urol. **82**: 494, 1959.

Politano, V. A.: Vesicoureteral Reflex in Children, J. A. M. A. **172**: 1252, 1960.

Radman, H. M., and Korman, W.: Ovarian Tumors in Children, Am. J. Obst. & Gynec. **79**: 989, 1960.

Rainer, E. H., and Bullough, J.: Respiratory and Cardiac Arrest During Anesthesia in Children, Brit. M. J. **2**: 1024, 1957.

Richardson, W. R.: Progress in Pediatric Cancer Surgery: Recent Advances in the Surgical Management of Neoplasms in Infants and Children, A. M. A. Arch. Surg. **82**: 641, 1961.

Sadove, M. S., and Frye, T. J.: Preoperative Sedation and Production of a Quiescent State in Children, J. A. M. A. **164**: 1729, 1957.

Schauffler, G.: Foreign Body in the Immature Vagina, California & West. Med. **50**: 411, 1939.

Schauffler, G. C.: Genital Bleeding in Infancy and Childhood, Clin. Obst. & Gynec. **1**: 784, 1958.

Scott, R. B.: Leukorrhea During Childhood, Am. J. Obst. & Gynec. **77**: 679, 1959.

Stickler, G. B., and Pinkel, D.: Serum Protein Fractions in Children With Malignant Tumors, Cancer **13**: 446, 1960.

Thompson, H.: Obstruction of the Vesical Neck in Children, New York J. Med. **56**: 361, 1956.

Thompson, H. T.: Obstruction of the Vesical Neck in Children, New York J. Med. **60**: 4377, 1960.

Thompson, I. M., and Coppridge, A. J.: The Management of Bladder Tumors in Children: A Study of Sarcoma Botryoides, J. Urol. **82**: 590, 1959.

Wilkins, L.: Masculinization of Female Fetus Due to Use of Orally Given Progestins, J. A. M. A. **172**: 1028, 1960.

Woodruff, J., and Everett, H.: Prognosis in Childhood Urinary Tract Infection in Girls, Am. J. Obst. & Gynec. **68**: 798, 1954.

Zapp, E.: Stenosis of the Vesical Neck in Early Childhood (Die Blasenhalsstenose des fuehen Kindesalters), Muenchn. med. Wchnschr. **99**: 11761, 1957.

39 · Adrenogenital Syndrome

General Considerations

The adrenogenital syndrome is due to a congenital hyperplasia of the adrenal glands. Before the role of cortisone in its management was understood, many patients went undiagnosed and were considered males with some form of hypospadias, and many plastic operations to make a penis out of the clitoris, and a male urethra out of a female urinary tract, were attempted. Varying degrees of the disease exist, and the role of the adrenal gland in the many variations is becoming clearer.

Etiology and Pathologic Anatomy

Histologically there is a hypertrophy of the reticularis layer with much lipid material in the cells. The fasciculata and glomerulosa layers are small in contrast. The width of the reticularis must be compared with a normal female infant in the same age period. However, when age groups are compared, there is a relative increase in the development of the reticularis in the older pseudohermaphrodites. The ovarian pathology varies with the severity of the disease. In the older pseudohermaphrodites there may be no primordial follicles and no developing or atretic follicles, and the ovarian cortex consists of ovarian stroma. In the less severe cases there may be abundant primordial follicles and a few antrum follicles but no evidence of ovulation at any time. Variations from this situation, to the finding of a normal ovary histologically, may be presumed if one accepts the fact that subclinical forms of the disease exist.

All the basic details of the steroid chemistry involved in the adrenogenital syndrome have not been clarified. With some logical presump-

tions to fill the gaps, a practical understanding of the medical treatment is possible. The basic defect is the failure of the fasciculata to produce cortisone. Cortisone suppresses ACTH (adrenocorticotrophic hormone) and its stimulating effect on the reticularis. Without this suppression, ACTH stimulates the reticularis to produce abnormal amounts of the virilizing compound that in turn suppresses pituitary gonadotrophins and that may be the precursor of the abnormal urinary 17-ketosteroids detected in severe cases. This suppression may be severe enough to inhibit FSH (follicle-stimulating hormone), with an absence of follicles in the ovary. The suppression may be less severe and allow the production of antrum follicles but cause a deficiency of ICSH (interstitial cell-stimulating hormone), with lack of estrogenic production and ovulation.

Classification

Jones and Jones have outlined a clinical classification that is useful for comparison among investigators and stimulates thought about the relationship of the adrenogenital syndrome to mild cases of hirsutism, amenorrhea, and even selected cases of infertility.

Group 1. *Female pseudohermaphrodites*—Marked virilization with severe anomalies of the urogenital sinus derivatives.

Group 2. *Postnatal virilization*—A milder form than Group 1; frequently not diagnosed until puberty.

Group 3. *Postpubertal hirsutism, oligomenorrhea, and infertility*—Menarche occurs but menstruation is scant. The secondary sex characteristics develop normally, and there are no abnormalities of the urogenital sinus derivatives except an enlarged clitoris in some patients. It is distinguishable from the Stein-Leventhal syndrome by elevated 17-ketosteroids with normal ovaries.

Group 4. *Postpubertal hirsutism, oligomenorrhea, and infertility with normal urinary 17-ketosteroids*—Differ slightly from Group 3 in that the 17-ketosteroids are normal. The onset of ovulatory menstruation under stimulation by cortisone suggests adrenal hyperplasia as the etiology.

Another clinical group may be added to the classification of Jones and Jones:

Group 5. *Potential group*—Further study of adrenal function may some time explain the large group of patients who have amenorrhea together with hirsutism, seborrhea, acne, increased libido, decrease in size of breasts and hips, and a variety of other unexplained symptoms.

Symptoms and Diagnosis

The signs and symptoms vary not only between each of the five groups of patients, but also in patients that may be intermediate between groups in the classification. The masculinization of the patient, the findings of some anomaly of the urogenital sinus derivatives, and the elevation of the 17-ketosteroids easily establish the diagnosis in the obvious cases. Since all gradations of the disease occur, one may expect to see a large group of patients in whom the condition may be suspected but is never proved.

Psychosomatic Aspects

The preparation of patients with the adrenogenital syndrome for acceptance of their anomaly is exceedingly difficult. Just how can you answer an adolescent who says, "What have I done to be like this?" How can the stigma of the condition be neutralized? It is obviously not a simple problem. The gynecologist, who may be the first to recognize the condition, must sense the symbolic meaning with which this disease is highly invested and not do anything that will hinder adaptation to the situation. Patients with this affliction are an interdisciplinary problem between the gynecologist and psychiatrist. Once the patient's instinctive desires to be a female are affirmed, both physicians can zero-in on the problem to prevent a sexual, social, and economic catastrophe.

Surgical Principles

The administration of cortisone or other derivatives under study and the extent of surgery to be performed are decided by the severity of the anomaly and the age of the patient. In children who may not experience the menarche for many years but who have an upper genital tract that shows possibilities of development and function later, the surgical correction of gross external genital anomalies should be done in childhood before the patient becomes sex conscious. Following complete healing of the wound, cortisone replacement therapy is given, with its effect and dosage governed by determination of urinary 17-ketosteroids. The creation of a functional vagina at the same time is dependent upon the surgeon's evaluation of the danger of contraction during the ensuing years. This, in turn, is governed by the severity of the anomalous development of the vagina and the probable functional capacity of the upper genital tract.

Patients with less severe defects who are near the expected menarche should have a complete operation, with a functional vagina connecting the upper genital tract to the vulva. The clitoris should be completely amputated if it is large and unsightly. Medical treatment can then be undertaken, with careful attention given to electrolyte disturbances. Finally, those patients with no congenital defects requiring plastic surgery are managed with medical treatment alone. Basal temperature charts, endometrial biopsies, and biochemical studies are done in the course of therapy. The treatment of each patient must be individualized, and the cortisone derivative used will most certainly be changing from time to time. The 17-ketosteroids will decrease on therapy with a dosage of cortisone varying from 75 to 150 mg. a day. Dr. Ephraim Shorr feels strongly that all grada-

PLATE 91

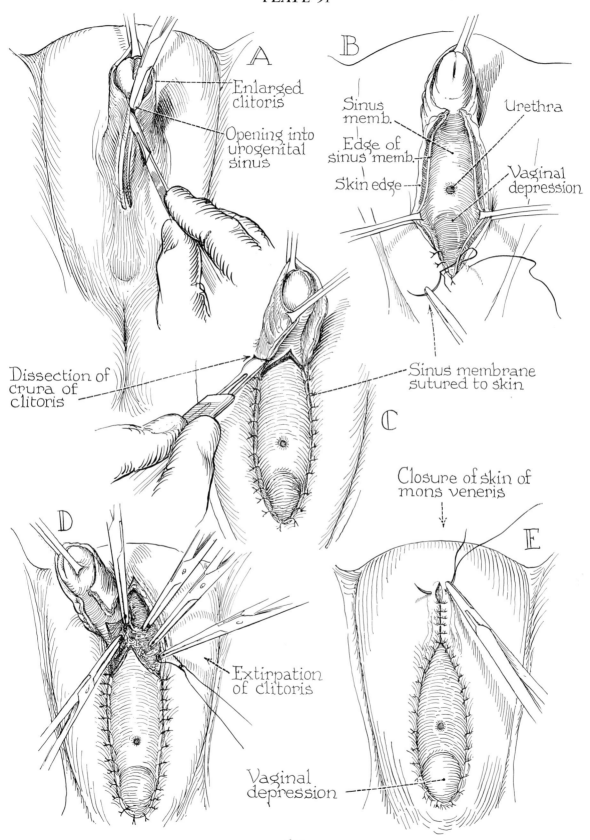

A — Enlarged clitoris — Opening into urogenital sinus

B — Sinus memb. — Edge of sinus memb. — Skin edge — Urethra — Vaginal depression

Dissection of crura of clitoris — Sinus membrane sutured to skin

C

Closure of skin of mons veneris

D — Extirpation of clitoris — Vaginal depression

E

tions of adrenal function exist, so that a fixed schedule can hardly be set for even a group of patients whose deficiency seems to be about the same clinically. He has noted an explosive effect in some patients with less severe disease, with a vaginal smear typical of ovulation. A flat glucose tolerance curve may be seen that is probably related to the metabolism of the glucocorticoids. The excretion of 17-ketosteroids, in patients in whom they are elevated, should be lowered to less than the usually accepted normal of 12 mg. in twenty-four hours. Creatinine determinations are run simultaneously to check on the accuracy of the urine collections.

Steps of the Operation

1. The clitoris is drawn sharply toward the mons veneris and a Kelly clamp inserted into the opening of the urogenital sinus (Plate 91, *A*). The clamp is opened slightly, and the skin forming the inferior aspect or floor of the urogenital sinus is incised.

2. This exposes the sinus membrane, urethra, and vaginal introitus. In the operation sketched the vagina was represented by a simple depression (Plate 91, *B*), and a vaginal reconstruction will be necessary at a later date. In some patients the vagina is found quite well developed and continuous with the other Müllerian duct derivatives. Such patients will have an infantile cervix and uterus also present, and in some cases structures approximating the normal development for the patient's age will be present. The edge of the sinus membrane is then sutured to the skin with interrupted sutures that roll over the skin edges in an attempt to simulate labia minora (Plate 91, *B*).

3. The entire clitoris and crura are excised (Plate 91, *C*), since any part of the organ left may react with hypertrophy to subsequent stimulation. The skin incisions about the clitoris should be planned for easy closure without attempts at using flaps or folds to simulate a clitoris. These simply atrophy or become a nubbin of distorted scar tissue that is unsightly and bears no resemblance to the normal clitoris. In patients already disturbed about their anomaly, such sensitive areas are better absent than bizarre in their appearance.

4. The clitoris has an abundant blood supply, and its amputation close to the periosteum of the symphysis will require the ligation of many bleeding points (Plate 91, *D*). This, of course, provides an adequate blood supply for the skin and sinus membrane that must be approximated in the anterior aspect of the field.

5. The skin of the mons veneris is undermined sufficiently to permit closure of the skin edges without tension (Plate 91, *E*). Interrupted sutures of 00 chromic catgut are used throughout.

Postoperative Care

The postoperative care after this simple procedure is no problem. If this operation in an older subject is combined with a vaginal reconstruction, the management of the vaginal graft or other technical problems must be dealt with. The wound is covered only with a sanitary napkin, and a heat lamp may be applied twice daily if for no other reason than to help the patient forget the irritation of the sutures. If no complications develop by the fourth or fifth day, the patient can be given sitz baths, and selected, irritating sutures can be removed. Those that do not fall out may be removed on subsequent days.

References

Allen, W. M., and Woolf, R. B.: Medullary Resection of the Ovaries in the Stein-Leventhal Syndrome, Am. J. Obst. & Gynec. 77: 826, 1959.

Behrman, H. T.: Diagnosis and Management of Hirsutism, J. A. M. A. 172: 1924, 1960.

Benson, R., Kolb, F., and Traut, H.: Hirsutism, Defemization, and Virilization, Obst. & Gynec. 5: 307, 1955.

Biggs, A. D., and Wied, D. M.: Management of Congenital Adrenogenital Syndrome, Am. J. Obst. & Gynec. 74: 200, 1957.

Bunim, J. J.: Clinical Uses and Hazards of Adrenal Steroids and Their Analogues in the Management of Rheumatic Diseases, Bull. New York Acad. Med. 33: 461, 1957.

Carpentier, P. J., and Potter, E. L.: Nuclear Sex and Genital Malformation in 48 Cases of Renal Agenesis, With Especial Reference to Nonspecific Female Pseudohermaphroditism, Am. J. Obst. & Gynec. 78: 235, 1959.

Chapple, C.: Possible Mechanisms of Some Congenital Defects, Am. J. Obst. & Gynec. 70: 711, 1955.

Coppedge, W. W., and Hasty, L. B.: Estrinism in a Girl 2½ Years of Age; With Minimal Ovarian Changes Suggestive of Thecosis, Am. J. Obst. & Gynec. 80: 637, 1960.

DeAlvarez, R. R., and Smith, E. K.: Congenital Adrenal Hyperplasia: Endocrine Patterns in Women and Effects of Cortisone Treatment, Obst. & Gynec. 9: 426, 1957.

Erez, N., and Yenen, E.: A Case of Adrenogenital Syndrome (Adrenal Pseudohermaphroditism), Am. J. Obst. & Gynec. 76: 877, 1958.

Evans, T., and Riley, G.: Pseudohermaphroditism, Obst. & Gynec. 2: 363, 1953.

Gold, J. J., and Frank, R.: The Borderline Adrenogenital

Syndrome: An Intermediate Entity, Am. J. Obst. &
Gynec. 75: 1034, 1958.

Greenblatt, R.: Cortisone in Treatment of the Hirsute
Woman, Am. J. Obst. & Gynec. 66: 700, 1953.

Heinbecker, P., O'Neal, L. W., and Ackerman, L. V.:
Functioning and Non-functioning Adrenal Cortical
Tumors, Surg., Gynec. & Obst. 104: 21, 1957.

Ingersoll, F. M., and McArthur, J. W.: Longitudinal
Studies of Gonadotropin Excretion in the Stein-
Leventhal Syndrome, Am. J. Obst. & Gynec. 77:
795, 1959.

Jailer, J. W., and others: Further Observations on Adrenal
Cortical Function During Pregnancy, Am. J. Obst. &
Gynec. 78: 200, 1957.

Jones, H., and Jones, G.: The Gynecological Aspects of
Adrenal Hyperplasia and Allied Disorders, Am. J.
Obst. & Gynec. 68: 1330, 1954.

Lash, S., and Lash, A.: Management of Anomalies of the
Genital Tract, Am. J. Obst. & Gynec. 70: 383, 1955.

LeVeen, H., and Pruit, A.: Role of Surgery in Therapy
of Adrenocortical Hypersecretion, J. A. M. A. 158:
1438, 1955.

Morris, J.: The Syndrome of Testicular Feminization in
Male Pseudohermaphrodites, Am. J. Obst. & Gynec.
65: 1192, 1953.

Peris, L. A.: Congenital Adrenal Hyperplasia Producing
Female Hermaphroditism With Phallic Urethra, Obst.
& Gynec. 16: 156, 1960.

Perloff, W. H., and others: Clinical Management of

Idiopathic Hirsutism (Adrenal Virilism), J. A. M. A.
167: 2041, 1958.

Philipp, E., and Stange, H. H.: Diagnosis of Intersexuality
Occurring With Rudimentary and Hypoplastic Gonads
(Zur Problematik der Zwitter mit rudimentaeren und
hochgradig hypoplastischem Gonaden), Geburtsh. u.
Frauenh. 18: 703, 1958.

Philpott, N., and Ross, J.: Congenital Uterine Anomalies
and Associated Complications of Pregnancy, Am. J.
Obst. & Gynec. 68: 285, 1954.

Quint, B. C., Parker, R. T., and Hamblen, E. C.: Uterine
Hypertrophy in the Presence of Androgen-Producing
Adrenal Tumor, Am. J. Obst. & Gynec. 73: 206, 1957.

Taylor, E., and Snow, R.: Adrenal Virilism in the Female
Child and Adult, Am. J. Obst. & Gynec. 67: 1307,
1954.

Ten Berge, B. S.: The Psychogenic Factor of the Adrenogenital Syndrome, Acta obst. et gynec. scandinav. 38:
379, 1959.

Vara, P., and Seiro, V.: A Case of Endocrinologically Active
Adrenal Adenoma With Hirsutism and Amenorrhea as
the Only Clinical Manifestation, Acta obst. et gynec.
scandinav. 38: 704, 1959.

Wharton, L.: Congenital Malformations Associated With
Developmental Defects of Female Reproductive Organs, Am. J. Obst. & Gynec. 53: 37, 1947.

Wilson, R. B., and Keating, F. R.: Pregnancy Following
Treatment of Congenital Adrenal Hyperplasia With
Cortisone, Am. J. Obst. & Gynec. 76: 388, 1958.

Section XII · GYNECOLOGIC SURGERY RELATED TO PREGNANCY

40 · Dilatation and Evacuation of the Uterus and the Surgical Management of the Incompetent Internal Cervical Os

DILATATION AND EVACUATION OF THE UTERUS
Indications and Surgical Principles

A dilatation and evacuation of the uterus are performed for the completion of an incomplete abortion, the evacuation of a missed abortion, the performance of a prophylactic abortion, the evacuation of the uterus for hydatidiform mole, and for the removal of the products of conception when the pregnancy has been terminated by radiotherapy for malignant pelvic disease.

The operation is not infrequently done for the removal of retained products of conception either in the immediate post-partum period or for persistent bleeding due to retention of fragments of the placenta several weeks after a full-term delivery. Until the twelfth week of gestation it is possible to terminate the pregnancy by dilatation and evacuation. After the twelfth week of pregnancy the size of the uterus and the bleeding encountered make it advisable to perform a laparotomy—abdominal hysterotomy. The pregnancy after the twelfth week can also be terminated by a vaginal hysterotomy. This is accompanied by marked bleeding and is more hazardous than the abdominal approach. The operation can be done after the twelfth week of gestation provided that you are dealing with an incomplete or missed abortion. The uterus had had time to involute, and the placenta is degenerating. Bleeding from the placental site is not profuse.

Many of the surgical principles already enumerated in the performance of a dilatation and curettage apply equally to a dilatation and evacuation of the uterus. Perforation of the uterus is not uncommon because of the softness of the uterine wall, particularly at the placental site. Only sharp curettes should be used, since smooth or serrated curettes simply slide over the surface of the retained products of conception. The larger the instruments used, the less the possibility of perforating the uterus. The cervix should be dilated to not less than a No. 15 Hegar dilator. This is not necessary in performing an ordinary diagnostic or therapeutic dilatation and curettage.

When the operation is performed for a hydatidiform mole, there is always a considerable loss of blood. The operator, if he deems it safe, should attempt to remove some of the superficial layers of the musculature to give the pathologist an opportunity to study the invasiveness of the mole. If the duration of the pregnancy has been misjudged chronologically, one may encounter a fetus of more than twelve weeks' gestation. The fetus must be crushed

618

to evacuate the uterus, and this requires considerable skill and experience. It is particularly difficult to remove the head of the fetus, which represents the largest diameter at this state of gestation. Should it become technically difficult or hazardous, the operator should stop at this time and proceed to evacuate the uterus abdominally. This operation can be exceedingly difficult in removing the products of conception from a large myomatous uterus in which the cavity is distorted either by a cervical myoma or myomas in the lower uterine segment. The fetus and placenta are behind these structures in the upper part of the cavity. Brisk bleeding is encountered under these circumstances, and it is difficult to be sure, in a distorted cavity, that all of the retained products have been removed. Should it become impossible to evacuate a myomatous uterus by the vaginal route, the operator resorts to an abdominal approach, particularly if uncontrolled bleeding ensues during the course of the procedure.

Carcinoma of the cervix in pregnancy presents some unusual problems that may necessitate a dilatation and evacuation of the uterus. In the early months of pregnancy the fetus may succumb as a result of the x-ray therapy, and in the majority of instances a spontaneous abortion will take place within a few weeks. However, should the products of conception not be passed or should bleeding ensue, the surgeon will have to decide whether the retained products can be removed vaginally without disturbing the malignancy. If not, and it is desired to retain the uterus for radium therapy, it should be evacuated from above. The surgeon may elect to do radical surgery in an early carcinoma of the cervix. The uterus and the pregnancy can be removed at the time of operation. Pregnancies beyond the twelfth week, in which a cervical carcinoma is diagnosed, will require an abdominal hysterotomy for evacuation of the uterus prior to the institution of therapy.

Steps of the Operation

1. A weighted retractor is placed in the posterior vagina and a Sims speculum used to retract the anterior vaginal wall and visualize the cervix. The cervix is grasped with a Jacobs tenaculum (Plate 92, *A*). Care is exercised not to tear the anterior lip. The uterus is not routinely sounded in a dilatation and evacuation (Plate 92, *A*), since the information to be gained is not worth the risk of perforation of the uterus by this instrument. The cervix is dilated up to a No. 15 Hegar dilator or larger, depending on the duration of the pregnancy and the contents to be evacuated. As in a nonpregnant uterus, the dilator should follow the curve of the uterine cavity (Plate 92, *A*), as determined by the preoperative bimanual examination. This examination is religiously done.

2. In Plate 92, *B,* is shown the direction the dilator takes in the event the uterus is retroverted and retroflexed. The curve of the cervical dilator is reversed to follow the direction of the uterine cavity and avoid perforation of the anterior wall of the uterus.

3. Except in very early miscarriages, a digital exploration of the uterine cavity with the index finger is possible after the cervix has been dilated. Plate 92, *C,* shows the technique of performing this digital exploration while the fundus of the uterus is manipulated by the abdominal hand. The tenaculum on the cervix is grasped by the middle, ring, and small fingers, and, as traction is made on the cervix, the index finger is introduced into the cavity and the position of the retained products determined.

4. The largest ovum forceps that can be admitted through the internal os is introduced into the uterine cavity, and the retained products of conception are grasped (Plate 92, *D*). If every gentle traction is made, it is possible to remove, intact, the entire retained placenta. More often, the retained placenta is removed piecemeal, first by the use of the ovum forceps and finally by the use of curettes.

5. In a retroverted uterus the retained products of conception are extracted by reversing the curve of the forceps and curettes (Plate 92, *E*). If the retroversion of the uterus is not recognized, the introduction of the curette along its normal curve may penetrate the anterior wall of the uterus. Once the retained products are grasped with the forceps, very gentle traction should be made in order to detach the tissue from the uterine wall and extract as much tissue as possible in one piece.

6. When the retained products have been brought to the external os, the tissue can be released and the open forceps introduced higher and higher

PLATE 92

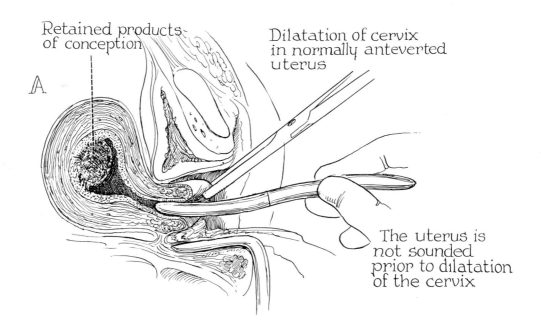

Retained products of conception

Dilatation of cervix in normally anteverted uterus

A

The uterus is not sounded prior to dilatation of the cervix

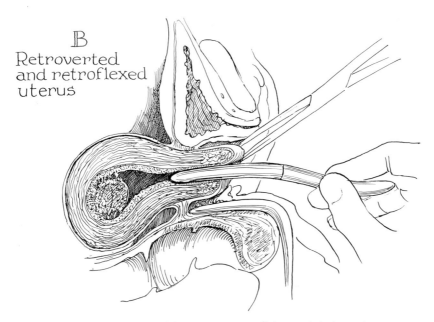

B
Retroverted and retroflexed uterus

The curve of the dilator is reversed to avoid perforation of the anterior wall of the uterus

PLATE 92 (Continued)

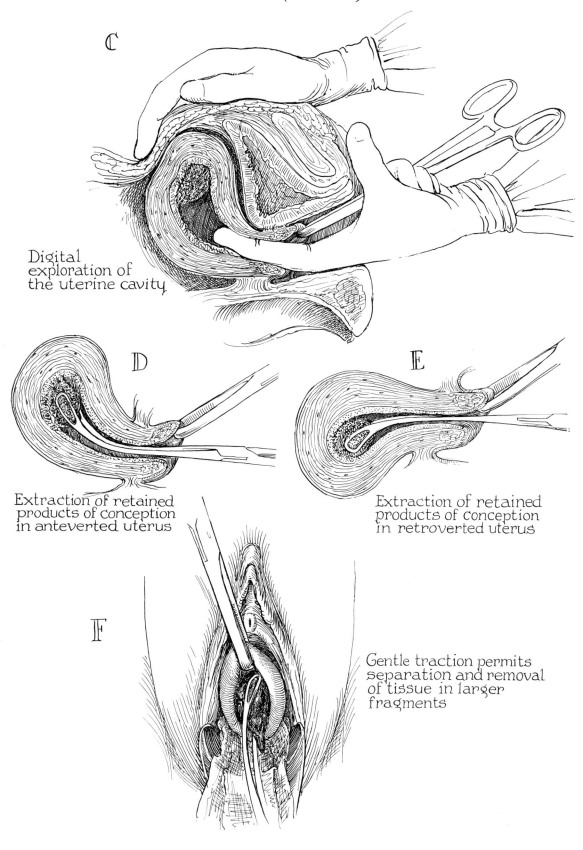

C

Digital
exploration of
the uterine cavity

D

Extraction of retained
products of conception
in anteverted uterus

E

Extraction of retained
products of conception
in retroverted uterus

F

Gentle traction permits
separation and removal
of tissue in larger
fragments

PLATE 92 (Concluded)

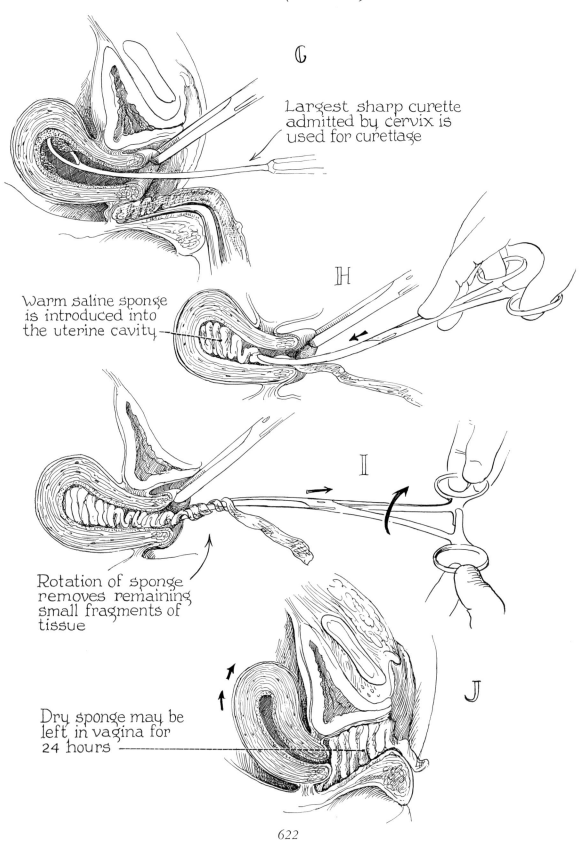

G

Largest sharp curette
admitted by cervix is
used for curettage

H

Warm saline sponge
is introduced into
the uterine cavity

Rotation of sponge
removes remaining
small fragments of
tissue

I

Dry sponge may be
left in vagina for
24 hours

J

in the canal in an attempt to gently extract all of the detached tissue (Plate 92, *F*).

7. After extraction of as much tissue as possible with the ovum forceps, the largest sharp curette available, or admitted by the cervix, is introduced into the uterus (Plate 92, *G*). A systematic curettage is done, curetting first the anterior wall; second, the posterior wall; third, the right uterine cornu; fourth, the fundus of the uterus, and finally the left cornu. This is repeated to permit removal of all of the tissue in the uterus.

8. A sponge saturated with warm saline solution is packed into the uterine cavity (Plate 92, *H*). The uterus will have contracted down considerably because of the stimulation of the curettage and the routine use of oxytocics.

9. The sponge introduced into the uterine cavity is rotated to impinge upon the wall of the uterus (Plate 92, *I*). Small fragments of tissue that may remain are removed in this way. This technique also stimulates the uterine musculature to contraction and reduces the amount of bleeding from the uterine sinuses that are opened up by the extraction of the retained products of conception.

10. If there is a small amount of oozing from the external os, a dry sponge or light pack may be left in the vagina for twenty-four hours (Plate 92, *J*). This does not increase the risk of infection but may necessitate catheterization of the patient.

Postoperative Care

Antimicrobial therapy is administered to patients with an incomplete abortion of several days' duration or if instrumentation is suspected.

OPERATION FOR AN INCOMPETENT INTERNAL CERVICAL OS
General Considerations

An incompetent internal cervical os is now recognized by many as a cause of premature labor, premature prolapse and subsequent rupture of the membranes, and spontaneous abortion. Much remains to be learned about this condition, but there is gradually accumulating in the literature sufficient experience to warrant a surgical approach when the history and physical findings suggest this cause of the patient's trouble.

Etiology and Pathologic Anatomy

Most cases are believed to follow a particularly traumatic delivery with disproportion due to a large infant, abnormal position, or injudicious interference before the patient was ready for delivery. I have seen the birth of a hydrocephalic infant apparently result in the incompetency of the internal os. The mother had three subsequent premature births, and on one occasion the prolapse of the membranes through the cervix in the sixth month of gestation was observed. None of her pregnancies resulted in a living child. Sketches of the operation performed on this patient for an incompetent internal os are shown in Plate 93. It is also conceivable that congenital variations in the fibromuscular make-up of the cervix might be a factor. Studies of the physiology of the uterine and cervical musculature may shed some light on the subject in the future.

Symptoms and Diagnosis

The case history reveals repeated abortions or pregnancies that terminate in the sixth or seventh month of gestation. Not infrequently there is a premature rupture of the membranes. One patient complained that as soon as her pregnancies had proceeded to the twentieth week or thereabouts, she started to feel as if "everything was coming out," although she had no prolapse of the pelvic floor. In some instances the obstetrician observes the membranes protruding from the cervix, which is prematurely effaced for the duration of pregnancy. In the nonpregnant patient it has been observed that the cervix is dilated without the usual resistance at the internal os. A No. 12 Hegar dilator is passed almost with the same ease as when dilating the cervix of a patient who has had a recent abortion. Hysterograms, by our present techniques, are not conclusive.

Surgical Anatomy and Principles

The cervical canal narrows at its junction with the endometrial cavity. In the immediate vicinity there is a transition from the normal myometrial layers to the fibromuscular pattern of the cervix. It is not possible to say with certainty that the thickness of the wall of the region of the internal os is less in this disease than it is normally, but one gets such an impression. In Plate 93, *B,* the incision at the internal os is diamond shaped. As this is closed, it tends to decrease the caliber of the internal os markedly when the two lateral points of the diamond are approximated. A small wedge is taken out of the anterior wall of the middle portion of the cervix, and at the distal end the incisions extend laterally. These lateral extensions are then continued as a conization of the distal part of the cervix. The disease is seldom seen in a patient with a perfectly normal, unlacerated external os. Were such a patient to be encountered, then the diamond-shaped incision at the internal os would not be continued to the external os, as was done in the operation sketched.

Preoperative Care and Anesthesia

Tubal patency and other infertility studies should obviously be normal before advising an operation for an incompetent internal cervical os, particularly if several years have elapsed since the last abortion or premature birth. Since a catheter or piece of rubber tubing will be left in the cervical canal for twenty-four hours postoperatively, a broad-spectrum antibiotic is started the day prior to surgery and continued postoperatively. Five hundred milliliters of whole blood are made available, since this operation, like a myomectomy, can result in considerable blood loss when the wall of the uterus is incised.

Steps of the Operation

1. Right-angle bullet tenacula are placed on the lateral aspects of the cervix to leave the anterior aspect free for the plastic procedure. The cervical canal is then slowly dilated up to a No. 12 Hegar dilator (Plate 93, *A*). This usually proceeds without difficulty and aids in confirming the diagnosis. Mechanical dilators that exert strong force are not necessary and may tear the cervix. A curettage is performed.

2. The full thickness of the vaginal wall is opened from the anterior fornix to a point a few centimeters above the region of the internal os (Plate

93, *B*). The bladder is advanced above the level of the internal os and retracted out of the field of operation. A diamond-shaped incision with a tail extending toward the external cervical os is then outlined (Plate 93, *B*).

3. The wedge of tissue outlined to lengthen the cervical canal and to decrease the caliber of the internal os is then excised by cutting down on a Hegar dilator (Plate 93, *C*). Specific bleeding points are ligated with fine chromic catgut, and the cervical canal is explored for evidence of any intrinsic pathology.

4. Usually the exocervix presents a cystic cervicitis, and a conization of the cervix is performed as part of the operation (Plate 93, *C*). This, in addition, lengthens the cervical canal to some extent.

5. The wall is then closed with interrupted sutures of 00 chromic catgut (Plate 93, *D*). Repeated soundings of the canal are done during the closure to note the effectiveness of the plication. Additional tissue can be removed as indicated.

6. The remainder of the closure is the same as that for a simple Sturmdorf amputation of the cervix. Hemostasis is effected about the external os, and anterior and posterior Sturmdorf sutures, are placed (Plate 93, *E*). The remainder of the anterior vaginal wall and lateral flaps of the cervix are closed with interrupted sutures (Plate 93, *E*).

Postoperative Care

A light vaginal pack is placed in the vagina. An indwelling catheter is left in place until the following morning, when the pack is removed. As with any vaginal procedure, a course of urinary antiseptic therapy is given prophylactically.

CIRCLAGE OF THE UTERINE CERVIX
Introduction

After the control of maternal deaths from hemorrhage, toxemia, and heart disease and the surgery of obstructive lesions of the female genital tract to correct infertility hopelessly stalled until such time as tissue transplantation is possible, American obstetrics in the past decade has placed its emphasis on improving perinatal mortality. One problem that has met with success and improvement in fetal salvage is the modern management of the incompetent cervical os. In this condition, either because of

PLATE 93

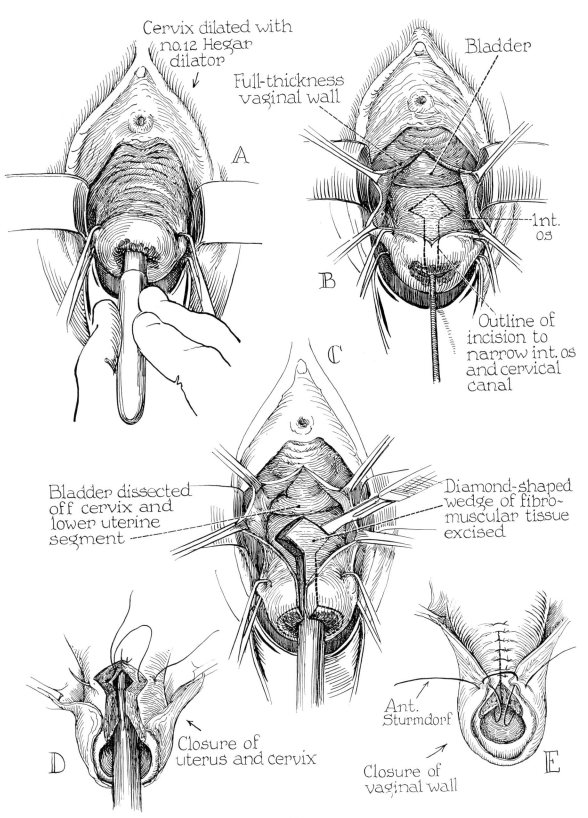

Cervix dilated with no. 12 Hegar dilator

Full-thickness vaginal wall

A

Bladder

Int. os

B

Outline of incision to narrow int. os and cervical canal

C

Bladder dissected off cervix and lower uterine segment

Diamond-shaped wedge of fibro-muscular tissue excised

D

Closure of uterus and cervix

Ant. Sturmdorf

Closure of vaginal wall

E

some unknown congenital defect, previous trauma of childbirth, or some as yet unknown hormonal influence, the internal portion of the neck of the uterus fails to stay closed as it should during the early part of pregnancy, finally relaxing in the weeks before delivery as seen in a normal uncomplicated pregnancy. Various operations have been devised to restore the competency of this region of the uterus both before conception takes place and in the event that it shows signs of weakening during the pregnancy, with surgery being performed during the pregnant state. These procedures are generally referred to as preconceptional circlage and postconceptional circlage of the uterine cervix. In effect, all of the operations devised entail the use of some material such as nylon, nylon threaded in polyethylene tubing, human or animal fascial strips, silk worm gut, and a variety of other substances used by various surgeons to encircle the incompetent area and narrow this portion of the neck of the uterus. Statistics vary from clinic to clinic and from operator to operator, but in general the precise diagnosis of the condition before pregnancy with appropriate surgery and prompt recognition of the condition or the impending dilatation during pregnancy with appropriate surgery has salvaged many infants who would have succumbed because of prematurity without the benefits of circlage. Should the surgeon be successful in carrying these patients at or near term, the question arises as to whether a cesarean section is a preferred form of delivery or some other method involving cutting of the material used to surgically make the internal os competent. After a successful circlage, the future childbearing capacity of the mother must be considered in the decision as to whether a cesarean section or vaginal delivery is effected.

Etiology and Pathologic Anatomy

Although extensive studies have been done on the fibromuscular structure of the cervix and a multitude of papers written concerning hormonal factors in its competency and subsequent dilatation just before and during labor, the region of the internal os of the cer-

vix is little understood. What we do know is that in some patients premature dilatation and effacement of the cervix occur repeatedly, causing the fetus to be lost. If diagnosed by intrauterine balloon studies as pioneered by Mann and associates before conception, a prophylactic circlage of the internal cervical os can be done. More frequently the diagnosis is made sometime after the twentieth week of pregnancy when the patient has leakage of amniotic fluid by transudation, actual bulging of the membranes through the external os, and dilatation and effacement of the cervix. In these patients a postconceptional circlage of the cervix has resulted in the salvage of many infants otherwise destined to add to our perinatal mortality.

Steps of the Operation
Postconceptional Circlage

1. Routine preparation of the external genitalia is done, but vigorous cleansing of the vagina and cervix is avoided to prevent rupture of the membranes.

2. The cervix is inspected anteriorly and posteriorly and gently palpated to determine the position of the cardinal and uterosacral thickenings. These are seldom evident in a pregnancy beyond the twentieth week, but their approximate level is determined since it is above this that the constricting suture should be placed.

3. The anterior lip of the cervix is grasped gently with an ovum forceps, carefully avoiding the amniotic membranes should they be visible or prolapsed (Plate 94, A).

4. While the anterior vaginal wall is gently pushed away from the cervix and gentle traction is made on the anterior lip of the cervix, an incision is made in the anterior vaginal wall at the approximate level of the internal os of the cervix.

5. It is seldom necessary to displace the bladder upward, but with a partially effaced cervix the normal landmarks are distorted and the proximity of the bladder appreciated.

6. The cervix is drawn anteriorly, and a posterior incision is made just above the level of the insertion of the uterosacral thickenings, as the operator can best determine, but short of an incision that would enter the cul-de-sac peritoneum (Plate 94, B).

PLATE 94

Postconceptional Circlage

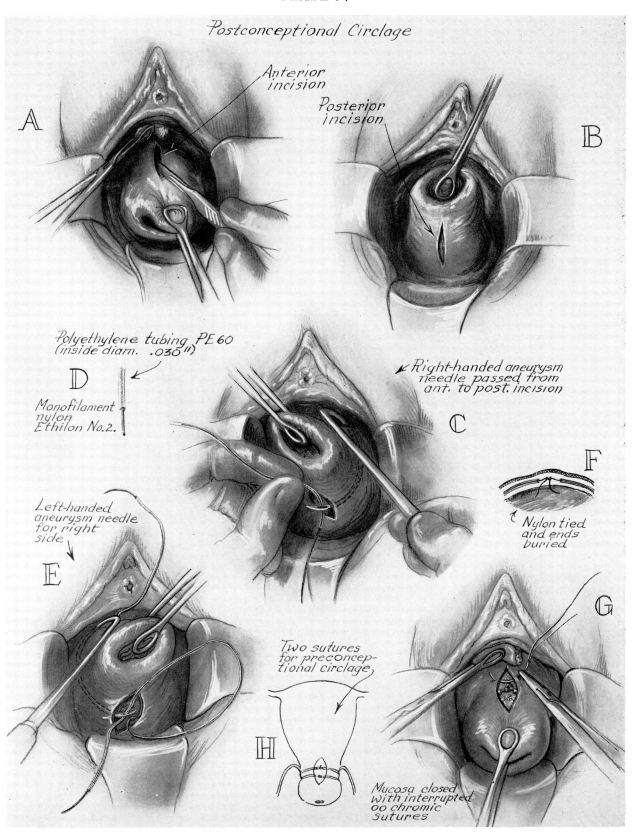

A — Anterior incision

B — Posterior incision

C — Right-handed aneurysm needle passed from ant. to post. incision

D — Polyethylene tubing PE 60 (inside diam. .030")

Monofilament nylon Ethilon No. 2.

E — Left-handed aneurysm needle for right side

F — Nylon tied and ends buried

G — Mucosa closed with interrupted oo chromic sutures

H — Two sutures for preconceptional circlage

627

7. A right-handed aneurysm needle is passed through or above the cardinal and uterosacral thickenings and deep to the full thickness of the vaginal wall (Plate 94, C). This area, normally vascular, is even more so during pregnancy. As the aneurysm needle is passed from the anterior to the posterior incisions in the vaginal mucosa, it should not be forced but gently guided through the tissues along the tissue planes of least resistance.

8. Monofilament nylon (Ethilon No. 2) that has been previously threaded through polyethylene tubing PE 60 (inside diameter 0.030) is introduced into the eye of the aneurysm needle (Plate 94, D). This end is then drawn out anteriorly and tagged with a clamp.

9. With a left-handed aneurysm needle for the right side, the procedure is repeated and the other end of the material used is drawn out anteriorly (Plate 94, E). Were the surgeon to prefer other sutures, linen, braided silk, or some other non-absorbable material, the procedure would be the same.

10. The ends of the sutures are now crossed and tightened until further constriction would cause them to cut into the tissue of the cervix. The operator notes this point by crushing the polyethylene tubing with a clamp where the sutures cross. The polyethylene cover of each end is then stripped off the nylon a few millimeters distal to this point. A square knot tied with the polyethylene will slip, whereas the nylon will not. On the other hand, the flexible polyethylene sleeve around the remainder of the cervix helps prevent a suture from cutting through cervical tissue (Plate 94, F).

11. Plate 94, F, shows the nylon suture tied. The ends are then threaded on a small round needle and countersunk into the immediate fibromuscular tissue of the cervix. Cut flush with the surface where the suture emerges, they will retract deep enough to prevent them from protruding into the vaginal wall where they could cause enough pressure to erode through. This may result in infection and necrosis and premature termination of the pregnancy.

12. The vaginal mucosa is then closed with interrupted sutures of 00 chromic catgut. The posterior incision is closed by the same technique (Plate 94, G).

Preconceptional Circlage

Preconceptional circlage of the cervix, with less bleeding and less of the aspects of the postcon-ceptional circlage insofar as being an emergency, permits the use of two sutures and much more time and deliberation as to their location. One suture should be placed just above the internal os of the cervix, and one below. The sutures should be tied down tight on a No. 4 Hegar dilator. When the dilator is removed, the fibromuscular tissue of the cervix should contract down to make the internal os competent or approximate its normal contour (Plate 94, H).

Postoperative Care

Patients having a postconceptional circlage are kept in bed for at least forty-eight hours and are heavily sedated. They are then gradually mobilized if there is no evidence of contractions or other complications. A wide-spectrum antibiotic is given since a wound infection would be disastrous. If viability of the infant is achieved and the patient goes into labor, a cesarean section is usually the most conservative method of delivery although some surgeons would elect to cut the band and allow vaginal delivery. Should the patient go into labor before viability of the infant, vaginal delivery is effected after releasing the polyethylene-nylon band. The postoperative care of patients having a preconceptional circlage is the same as for any vaginal plastic operation.

References

Adcock, L. L., and Hakanson, E. Y.: Vascular Collapse Complicating Septic Abortion, Am. J. Obst. & Gynec. 79: 516, 1960.

Anselmino, K. J.: The Operative Treatment of Cervical Incompetence (Zur operativen Behandlung der Insuffizienz des inneren Muttermundes und der oberen Zervix), Geburtsh. u. Frauenh. 18: 797, 1958.

Aren, P.: On Legal Abortion in Sweden; Tentative Evaluation of Justification of Frequency During Last Decade, Acta obst. et gynec. scandinav. (Suppl. I) 37: 1, 1958.

Asplund, J.: Uterine Cervix and Isthmus Under Normal and Pathological Conditions; Clinical and Roentgenological Study, Acta radiol. (supp. 91) p. 3, 1952.

Borglin, N. E., and Eliasson, G.: On the Effect of Methyloestrenolone on Histaminase Activity in the Plasma, on Excretion of Pregnandiol and Adreno-cortical Steroids in the Urine and on Vaginal Cytology in Threatened Abortion, Acta obst. et gynec. scandinav. (Suppl. I) 40: 14, 1961.

Borglin, N. E., and Willert, B.: Value of Histaminase and Pregnanediol Determinations in Suspected Illegal Abortion, Acta obst. et gynec. scandinav. 40: 59, 1961.

Brandy, J. R., and Peterson, J. H.: Review of 36 Shirodkar Operations, Am. J. Obst. & Gynec. 81: 1191, 1961.

Deane, R. M., and Russell, K. P.: Enterobacillary Septicemia and Bacterial Shock in Septic Abortion, Am. J. Obst. & Gynec. 79: 528, 1960.

Dunn, L. J., Robinson, J. C., and Steer, C. M.: Maternal Death Following Suture of Incompetent Cervix During Pregnancy, Am. J. Obst. & Gynec. 78: 335, 1959.

Durfee, R. B.: Surgical Treatment of the Incompetent Cervix During Pregnancy, Obst. & Gynec. 12: 91, 1958.

Fluhmann, C.: The Glandular Structures of the Cervix Uteri During Pregnancy, Am. J. Obst. & Gynec. 78: 990, 1959.

Friedman, S., and Hogans, C. W.: Removal From the Parametrium of a Nail Employed to Induce Abortion, Am. J. Obst. & Gynec. 76: 561, 1958.

Hunter, R. G., Henry, G. W., and Judd, C. S.: Physiologic or Dysfunctional Incompetence of the Cervix; Diagnosis and Surgical Treatment in the Nonpregnant Woman, Am. J. Obst. & Gynec. 81: 1183, 1961.

Ingelmann-Sundberg, A.: Intra-uterine Measurement of Pressure During Labor; Sources of Error, J. Obst. & Gynaec. Brit. Emp. 67: 629, 1955.

Javert, C. T.: Spontaneous and Habitual Abortion, New York, 1957, The Blakiston Division, McGraw-Hill Book Co., Inc.

Knapp, R. C., Platt, M. A., and Douglas, R. G.: Septic Abortion, Obst. & Gynec. 15: 344, 1960.

Lash, A. F.: The Incompetent Internal Os of the Cervix; Complications After Repair, Am. J. Obst. & Gynec. 81: 465, 1961.

Lash, A. F., and Lash, S. R.: Habitual Abortion: The Incompetent Internal Os of the Cervix, Am. J. Obst. & Gynec. 59: 68, 1950.

Lewis, G. C., and Reed, C. P.: Management of the Incompetent Cervix During Pregnancy, Obst. & Gynec. 13: 498, 1959.

Mann, E. C.: The Role of Emotional Determinants in Habitual Abortion. S. Clin. North America, p. 447, April, 1957.

Mann, E. C.: Habitual Abortion; a Report, in Two Parts, on 160 Patients, Am. J. Obst. & Gynec. 77: 706, 1959.

Mann, E. C., McLarn, W. D., and Hayt, D. B.: The Physiology and Clinical Significance of the Uterine Isthmus; Part I. The Two-Stage Intrauterine Balloon in the Diagnosis and Treatment of Cervical Incompetence, Am. J. Obst. & Gynec. 81: 209, 1961.

McCarthy, J. J., Erving, H. W., and Lauff, L. E.: Preliminary Report on the Use of Relaxin in the Management of Threatened Premature Labor, Am. J. Obst. & Gynec. 74: 134, 1957.

Mehta, C., and Mehta, A.: Puerperal Sterilization, J. Obst. & Gynec. India 8: 199, 1958.

Neumann, H. H., and Frick, H. C.: Occlusion of the Fallopian Tubes With Tantalum Clips, Am. J. Obst. & Gynec. 81: 803, 1961.

Page, E. W.: Incompetent Internal Os of the Cervix Causing Late Abortion and Premature Labor; Technique for Surgical Repair, Obst. & Gynec. 12: 509, 1958.

Palmer, R.: Physiology of the Isthmus Uteri and Its Part in Sterility and Habitual Abortion, Am. J. Obst. & Gynec. (supp.) 61A: 715, 1951.

Palmer, R., and Lacomme, M.: La Béance de l'orifice interne, cause d'avortements à répétition? Une observation de déchirure cervico-isthmique réparée chirurgicalement, avec gestation à terme consécutive, Gynéc. et obst. 47: 905, 1948.

Platt, M. A., Bonsnes, R. W., and Rubin, A. L.: Renal Failure Following Postabortal Clostridium Welchii Infection, Obst. & Gynec. 14: 482, 1959.

Rubovits, F. E., Cooperman, N. R., and Lash, A. F.: Habitual Abortion: A Radiographic Technique to Demonstrate the Incompetent Internal Os of the Cervix, Am. J. Obst. & Gynec. 66: 269, 1953.

Sheares, B. H.: Sterilization of Women by Intra-uterine Electro-cautery of the Uterine Cornu, J. Obst. & Gynaec. Brit. Emp. 65: 419, 1958.

Skajaa, T.: Central Spontaneous Rupture of the Cervix Uteri. A Complication of Induced Abortion, Acta obst. et gynec. scandinav. 40: 68, 1961.

Solomon, H. J.: Problems in the Treatment of the Incompetent Internal Os, J. Obst. & Gynaec. Brit. Emp. 67: 249, 1960.

Stromme, W. B., Wagner, R. M., and Reed, S. C.: Surgical Management of the Incompetent Cervix, Obst. & Gynec. 15: 635, 1960.

Taylor, E. S., and Hansen, R. R.: Incompetent Os of the Cervix as a Cause of Fetal Loss, J. A. M. A. 171: 1312, 1959.

Turell, R.: Repair of the Incompetent Internal Os of the Cervix, New York J. Med. 60: 524, 1960.

Turksoy, N.: The Management of Infected Abortion, Obst. & Gynec. 13: 399, 1959.

Youssef, A. F.: The Uterine Isthmus and Its Sphincter Mechanism: A Clinical and Radiographic Study, Am. J. Obst. & Gynec. 79: 1161, 1960.

Youssef, A. F.: The Uterine Isthmus and Its Sphincter Mechanism, a Radiographic Study; the Uterine Isthmus Under Normal Conditions, Am. J. Obst. & Gynec. 75: 1305, 1958.

41 · Ectopic Pregnancy

General Considerations

Antibiotic therapy should theoretically increase the incidence of ectopic pregnancies by converting severe infections of the tubes into milder cases with partial mechanical obstruction. To prove or disprove this contention would require a careful statistical study on a wide scope without the advantage of a control group, since specific therapy could hardly be denied patients with acute infections.

Etiology and Pathologic Anatomy

Infection of the upper genital tract, specific or nonspecific, postabortal or incidental to a ruptured appendix, produces a partially occluded tube with many recesses in which a fertilized ovum may lodge. Severe infections occlude the tube or tubes completely and do not create the conditions necessary for an ectopic implantation. The rare types of ectopic gestation, such as ovarian and intraligamentary pregnancies, are difficult to explain. An ovarian pregnancy is probably the result of a fertilized ovum being trapped in its follicle. Intraligamentary pregnancies are probably the result of erosion of the conception into the broad ligament through the mesovarium. Ectopic pregnancies occur in tubes that histologically have not been inflamed. Congenital diverticula may be responsible for these cases. The ovum finds an inhospitable resting place in the tube, with its thin walls and limited capacity for expansion. Implantations near the fimbriated end of the tube may terminate by expulsion of the conception into the peritoneal cavity and require no surgical intervention. In the middle and inner two thirds of the tube, unless the conception dies, distention of the tube and erosion of its walls can result in a severe hemorrhage. A cornual pregnancy, with the anastomosis of the ovarian artery and the ascending branch of the uterine artery in the field, can rupture, causing an alarming intraperitoneal hemorrhage. The rare death due to ectopic pregnancies includes many cornual implantations in which the patient died in shock. Death of an ectopic gestation without intraperitoneal hemorrhage is followed by vaginal bleeding since the decidual cast within the uterus is desquamated.

Symptoms and Diagnosis

The signs and symptoms of ectopic pregnancy vary from those associated with a massive intraperitoneal hemorrhage to the deception an unruptured ectopic pregnancy can create. Amenorrhea, followed by staining and vague pelvic discomfort, alerts the gynecologist to the possibility of a threatened abortion or an ectopic pregnancy. A tube distended by the conception is quite consistently tender on palpation and causes pain without manipulation. Examination reveals a uterus that is soft but not necessarily enlarged. A mass distinct from the ovary may be felt in the adnexal region. Rupture of the ectopic pregnancy is a more simple diagnosis. Blood spilled into the peritoneal cavity is irritating and gives rise to peritoneal symptoms. It may pool in the gutters or most dependent portions of the pelvis and refer signs and symptoms to these areas. Large clots in the cul-de-sac or within the broad ligament may give the patient the urge to urinate or defecate. The signs of shock appear if the blood loss is large or occurs within a short period of time. Pregnancy tests, if positive, contribute information in obscure cases, but the time involved in performing the tests limits their usefulness.

Treatment

Blood is made available and antibiotics or chemotherapy begun if there is evidence of infection. Preparations are made for a curettage, exploratory colpotomy, and a laparotomy. Examination under anesthesia may clarify the diagnosis and reveal a bulging cul-de-sac. Aspiration of the cul-de-sac under these circumstances is superfluous. The next step in the obscure cases is a dilatation and curettage. If no products of conception are found, but there is abundant tissue suggesting decidua, the next step is an exploratory colpotomy. This step is not done in the presence of a large, adherent, adnexal mass that would obviously present technical difficulties from this approach. The appendix cannot be removed from this approach under the usual circumstances and remains to complicate a differential diagnosis if the patient has subsequent pelvic disease. However, with the proper instruments, the vaginal approach to an ectopic pregnancy is not difficult and certainly is a minor procedure compared with the abdominal approach. Finally, a laparotomy may have to be performed to remove the products of conception or to control hemorrhage in the upper reaches of the pelvis. The appendix is removed, since the patients frequently present themselves later with pelvic disease and statistically have a greater chance for a second ectopic gestation.

Steps of the Operation
Vaginal Approach

1. An exploratory colpotomy is performed and the uterus retroverted and retrocessed by traction on the fundus (Plate 95, A).

2. An angle clamp is placed on the cornual end of the tube (Plate 95, A). If a few centimeters of the uterine end of the tube appear normal, the end can be left open as a snorkel-type of procedure, although the chances of conception are extremely remote.

3. In Plate 95, A, the tube cannot be spared, and a salpingectomy is performed by successively clamp-

ing, cutting, and tying the mesosalpinx. The ovary and its blood supply are preserved.

4. In Plate 95, B, the cornual end of the tube is inverted with several sutures. The opposite tube is inspected and the uterus replaced within the peritoneal cavity. The colpotomy incision is closed without drainage unless necessitated by a pelvic abscess.

Abdominal Approach

1. The abdomen is opened by an adequate lower abdominal incision with consideration for the necessity of further abdominal exploration or surgery of adjacent vital structures that may be involved.

2. The tube cannot be saved, so a salpingectomy is performed and the blood supply to the ovary carefully preserved (Plate 95, C).

3. The cornual end of the tube is either inverted or, if it appears normal, left open and the ovary sutured near the distal end (Plate 95, D).

4. Approximation of the round ligament and the ovarian ligament (Plate 95, E) prevents prolapse of the ovary into the cul-de-sac.

5. A few sutures are used to draw the round ligament over the cornua of the uterus and cover the operative site (Plate 95, F). An appendectomy is performed.

Postoperative Care

Antibiotic or chemotherapy is administered for several days after either the vaginal or abdominal operations as a prophylactic measure against any infection that might further compromise the remaining tube. Larger doses and prolonged administration are indicated in the presence of obvious pelvic inflammatory disease. The patient is mobilized early, and fluid and blood replacement is managed as indicated by oral intake or blood loss not replaced volume for volume in the operating room. If a tubal plastic procedure is done in conjunction with the primary operation and there is no gross inflammatory disease, some surgeons do a tubal insufflation with air or normal saline solution in the immediate postoperative period and repeat this as frequently as a week apart. I have been unable to achieve any more patent tubes and certainly no term pregnancies by the addition of this procedure.

PLATE 95

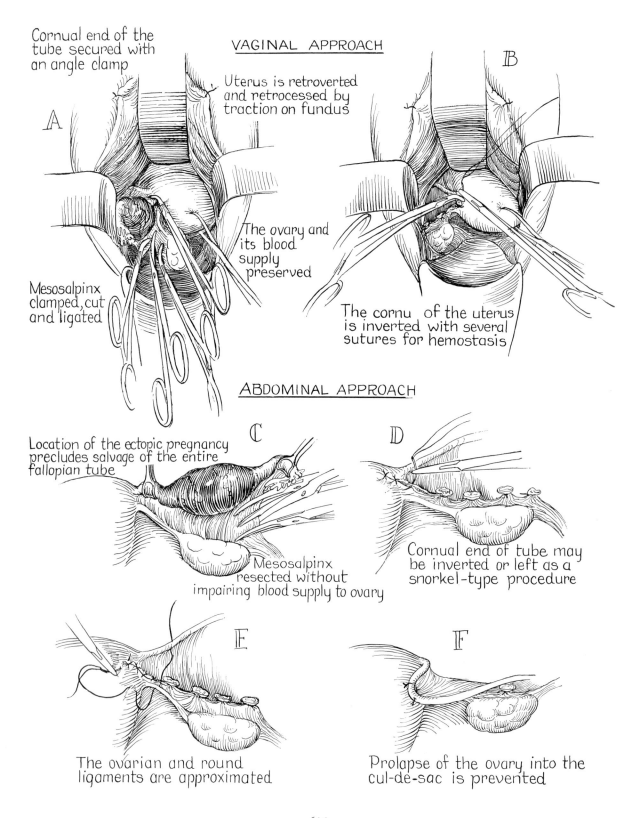

Cornual end of the
tube secured with
an angle clamp

VAGINAL APPROACH

Uterus is retroverted
and retrocessed by
traction on fundus

A

B

The ovary and
its blood
supply
preserved

Mesosalpinx
clamped, cut
and ligated

The cornu of the uterus
is inverted with several
sutures for hemostasis

ABDOMINAL APPROACH

Location of the ectopic pregnancy
precludes salvage of the entire
fallopian tube

C

D

Mesosalpinx
resected without
impairing blood supply to ovary

Cornual end of tube may
be inverted or left as a
snorkel-type procedure

E

F

The ovarian and round
ligaments are approximated

Prolapse of the ovary into the
cul-de-sac is prevented

References

Asherman, J.: Etiology of Ectopic Pregnancy: A New Concept, Obst. & Gynec. 6: 619, 1955.

Birch, H. W., and Collins, C. G.: Atypical Changes of Genital Epithelium Associated With Ectopic Pregnancy, Am. J. Obst. & Gynec. 81: 1198, 1961.

Bobrow, M., and Windelstein, L.: The Value of Centesis as a Diagnostic Procedure in Ruptured Ectopic Gestation, Am. J. Obst. & Gynec. 69: 101, 1955.

Crawford, E., and Hutchinson, H.: A Decade of Reports on Tubal Pregnancies Condensed From the Literature Plus Three Hundred Consecutive Cases Without a Death, Am. J. Obst. & Gynec. 67: 568, 1954.

DeAlvarez, R. R., and Nisco, F. S.: Ectopic Pregnancy: An 18-Year Analysis, Obst. & Gynec. 17: 536, 1961.

Grody, M., and Otis, R.: Ectopic Pregnancy After Total Hysterectomy, Obst. & Gynec. 17: 96, 1961.

Hall, R. E., and Todd, W. D.: The Suspected Ectopic Pregnancy; a Review of 500 Cases, Am. J. Obst. & Gynec. 81: 1220, 1961.

Page, H. G.: A Case of Ectopic Pregnancy Associated With Carcinoma of the Uterine Cervix, J. Obst. & Gynaec. Brit. Emp. 66: 976, 1959.

Wooten, E. L.: Use of Posterior Colpotomy in the Diagnosis and Treatment of Ectopic Pregnancy and Other Lesions of the Pelvis, Am. J. Obst. & Gynec. 80: 727, 1960.

42 · Ligation of the Fallopian Tubes

Indications and Surgical Principles

Ligation of the Fallopian tubes should become less and less frequent as certain chronic and disabling diseases are controlled. Like a therapeutic abortion, it is distasteful to many gynecologists regardless of religious considerations. Where there is little chance of fetal salvage, I seldom hesitate to perform a sterilization. The number of instances where one can say unequivocally that pregnancy is a threat to the mother's life are small indeed. The control of tuberculosis and the management of valvular heart disease by surgery have eliminated many of the former medical indications. Cesarean sections can be done by the low-flap technique and be repeated many times with a uterine scar that is scarcely recognizable. After quiet meditation I would rather ligate the tubes of a treatment-resistant psychoneurotic with an equally disturbed husband than for many of the accepted medical reasons. The operation then, although illegal and it cannot be done, would reduce the number of potential neurotics that plague our present society. Fortunately, most of these people are too immature to accept the responsibility of a child and use contraception or have an unwanted pregnancy terminated outside the profession. I have great respect for my colleagues in psychiatry, but they are likely to overevaluate pregnancy as a factor prompting suicide in a disturbed patient. The usual note recommending prophylactic abortion for psychiatric reasons contains a punch line suggesting that the patient will commit suicide should the pregnancy continue. New York is a large city, and each year some 800 persons take their own lives. Many other deaths cannot be positively proved to be suicides. In the year 1953, with many cases still under study and not yet classified, there were about 300 suicides of women in the childbearing age. *Only one had been found pregnant, and she may not have been aware of the fact.* The psychiatrists might argue that this proves many suicides were avoided by aborting disturbed patients. When one considers the number of emotionally disturbed women who are not aborted and do not commit suicide, pregnancy as a provocation to the act is of dubious importance.

Two of the many methods of tubal ligation are illustrated.

SIMPLE TUBAL LIGATION
Steps of the Operation

1. A segment of the tube is picked up with a Babcock clamp. The tube and mesosalpinx are crushed with a Kelly clamp (Plate 96, *A*).

2. The segment of tube is ligated with 00 chromic catgut (Plate 96, *B*).

3. The segment of tube is resected and sent to the laboratory for section (Plate 96, *C*). The same procedure is done on the opposite side.

CORNUAL RESECTION AND TUBAL IMPLANTATION IN THE BROAD LIGAMENT
Steps of the Operation

1. The tube is clamped, cut, and tied at the uterine cornu (Plate 96, *D*).

2. A wedge of the cornu of the uterus and a portion of the intramural tube are resected (Plate 96, *E*).

3. A channel is made in the broad ligament and the distal end of the tube buried (Plate 96, *F* and *G*).

PLATE 96

SIMPLE TUBAL LIGATION

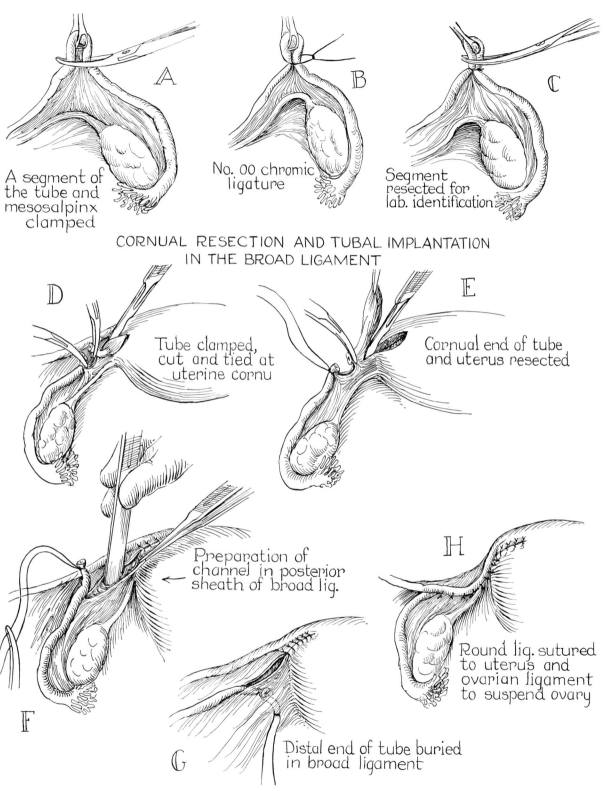

A
A segment of
the tube and
mesosalpinx
clamped

B
No. 00 chromic
ligature

C
Segment
resected for
lab. identification

CORNUAL RESECTION AND TUBAL IMPLANTATION
IN THE BROAD LIGAMENT

D
Tube clamped,
cut and tied at
uterine cornu

E
Cornual end of tube
and uterus resected

F
Preparation of
channel in posterior
sheath of broad lig.

G
Distal end of tube buried
in broad ligament

H
Round lig. sutured
to uterus and
ovarian ligament
to suspend ovary

4. The round ligament is sutured over the uterine cornu and to the ovarian ligament as shown in Plate 96, *H*.

Postoperative Care

No special postoperative care is indicated. Many patients react better to this operation if it is done by a cornual resection and they are told that successful reimplantation of the tubes is feasible. This situation might arise if the original indication for the ligation were later found amenable to treatment and no longer constituted a serious threat to the patient's life if she became pregnant.

References

Dieckmann, W. J., and Harrod, J. P.: Tubal Ligation (Sterilization) by a Modified Madlener Method, Am. J. Obst. & Gynec. **68:** 897, 1954.
Evans, T. N.: Simplified Method for Sterilization of the Female, Am. J. Obst. & Gynec. **66:** 393, 1953.
Hearin, W. C.: Tubal Ligation—Its Use and Abuse, Am. J. Obst. & Gynec. **72:** 1207, 1956.
Kohl, G. C.: Torsion of Uterine Tube Following Pomeroy Sterilization, Obst. & Gynec. **7:** 396, 1956.
McGraw, R. B.: Legal Aspects of Termination of Pregnancy on Psychiatric Grounds, New York J. Med. **56:** 1605, 1956.

INDEX

Numerals set in boldface type indicate pages on which charts or illustrations appear.

639

644